ESSENTIALS OF

Radiologic Science

SECOND EDITION

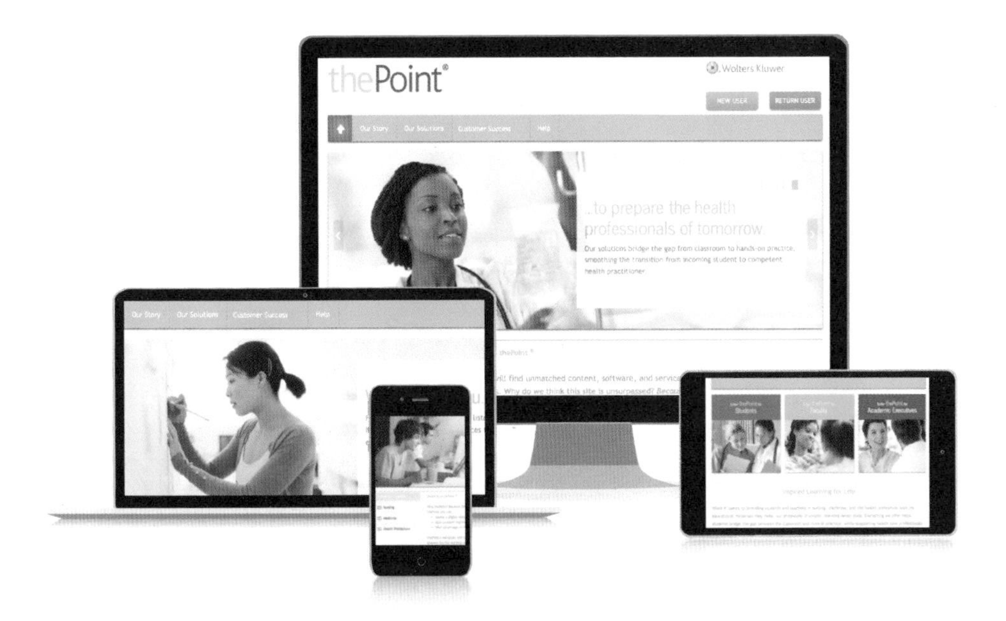

thePoint®

http://thePoint.lww.com

Provides flexible learning solutions and resources for students and faculty using ***Essentials of Radiologic Science, Second Edition***

Resources for students:

- Videos
- Animations
- Interactive Question Bank
- Exam Simulator

Resources for instructors*:

- Image Bank
- Test Generator
- PowerPoints
- Lesson Plans
- Answers to Text Review Questions
- LMS Cartridges

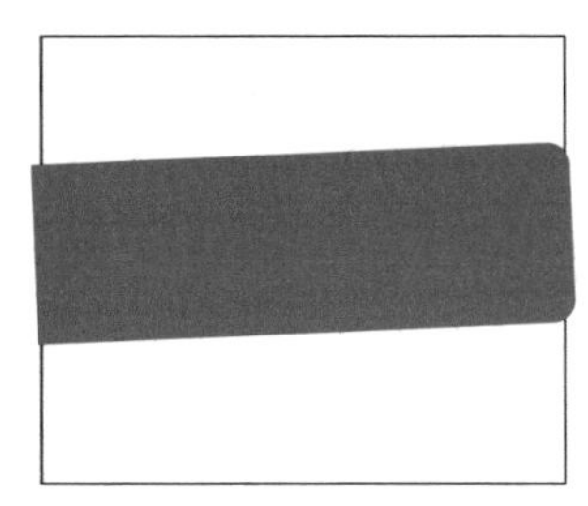

Note: Book cannot be returned once panel is scratched off.

Log on today!

Visit http://thePoint.lww.com to learn more about thePoint® and the resources available. Use the scratch off code to access the student resources.

*The faculty resources are restricted to adopters of the text. Adopters have to be approved before accessing the faculty resources.

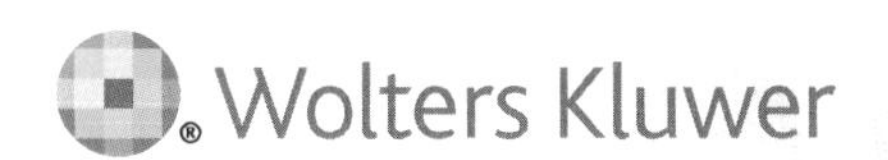

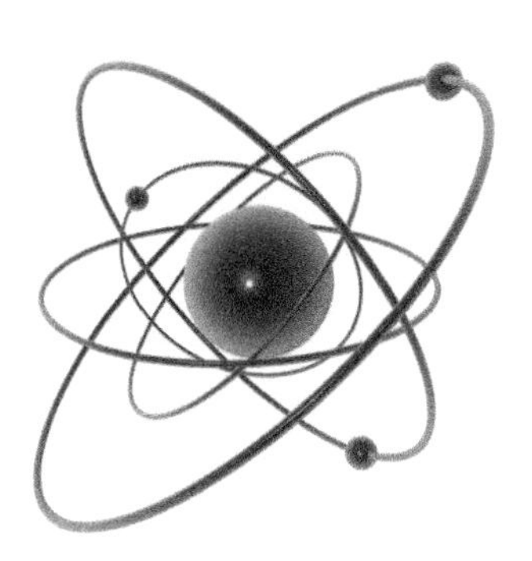

ESSENTIALS OF Radiologic Science

SECOND EDITION

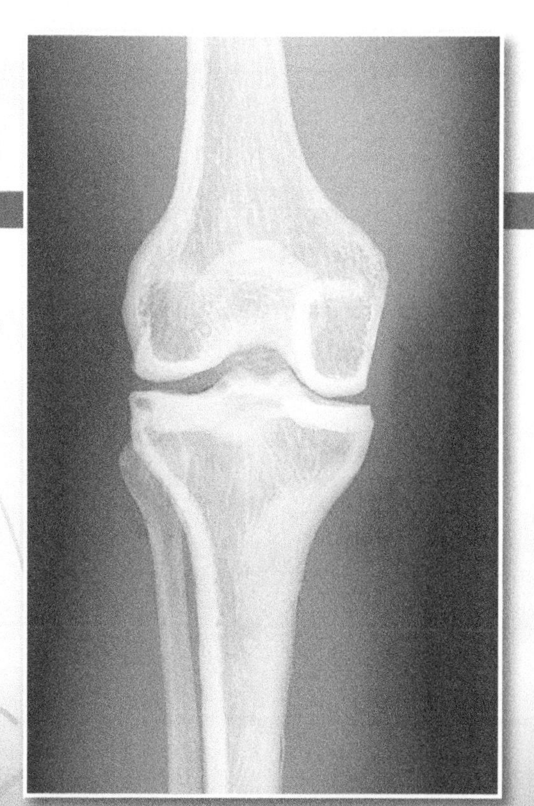

Denise Orth, MS, RT (R)(M)
Associate Professor and Clinical Coordinator
Allied Health Department
Fort Hays State University
Hays, Kansas

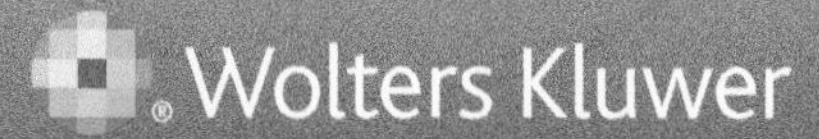

Wolters Kluwer
Philadelphia • Baltimore • New York • London
Buenos Aires • Hong Kong • Sydney • Tokyo

Acquisitions Editor: Jay Campbell
Senior Product Development Editor: Amy Millholen
Marketing Manager: Shauna Kelley
Production Product Manager: Kim Cox
Design Coordinator: Elaine Kasmer
Artist: Jonathan Dimes
Manufacturing Coordinator: Margie Orzech
Prepress Vendor: SPi Global

Second Edition

10 9

Printed in the USA

Library of Congress Cataloging-in-Publication Data
Names: Orth, Denise, author. | Preceded by (work): Fosbinder, Robert A. Essentials of radiologic science.
Title: Essentials of radiologic science / Denise Orth.
Description: Second edition. | Philadelphia : Wolters Kluwer, [2017] | Includes index. | Preceded by Essentials of radiologic science / Robert Fosbinder, Denise Orth. c2012.
Identifiers: LCCN 2016026301 | ISBN 9781496317278
Subjects: | MESH: Technology, Radiologic | Radiation Protection
Classification: LCC RC78.4 | NLM WN 160 | DDC 616.07/572—dc23 LC record available at https://lccn.loc.gov/2016026301

LWW.com

In Memorial

Robert A. Fosbinder, BA, RT(R), authored the original *Essentials of Radiologic Science*. The text book was instrumental in educating first- and second-year radiologic technology students about the wonders and dangers of producing radiation to image the human body. His work enlightened students to the many concepts and theories of the physics used in radiology. Robert was dedicated to the education of students in many facets of the radiologic sciences; his dedication was evident in his knowledgeable approach to delivering the material in a manner which engaged the student. His foundational work was an inspiration, and I trust the revisions in this second edition would meet his expectations. Robert's dedication to the radiologic sciences will forever be revered.

Reviewers

Yasmin Ali
Radiography Instructor
Dade Medical College
Miami, Florida

Brenda Cliff
Medical Radiation Technology Instructor
Cambrian College of Applied Arts and Sciences
Greater Sudbury, Ontario, Canada

Guillermina Colunga
Radiologic Technology Instructor
El Camino College
Hawthorne, California

Tammy Delker, MS, RT(R)
Radiologic Technology Program Director
Health Sciences Division
Indian Hills Community College
Ottumwa, Iowa

Anthony F. DeVito, MA, RT(R)
Radiologic Technology and Medical Imaging
School of Professional Studies
New York City College of Technology
Brooklyn, New York

Hernan Febres
General Radiologic Technologist
Dade Medical College
Miami, Florida

Pasquale Fiore
Medical Radiography Technology
Camosun College
Victoria, British Columbia, Canada

Cassandra Forbes
General Radiologic Technologist
Dade Medical College
Miami, Florida

Jennett Ingrassia, MSRS, RT(R)
Radiologic Technology and Medical Imaging
School of Professional Studies
New York City College of Technology
Brooklyn, New York

Catherine Kurimchak, RT(R), MS
Clinical Coordinator
Diagnostic Medical Imaging Program
Community College of Philadelphia
Philadelphia, Pennsylvania

Jennifer Little, MS, BSRT, ARRT(R), CRT
Radiologic Sciences Instructor
Department of Health Sciences
College of Health and Human Development
California State University, Northridge
Northridge, California

Galen Miller, RT(R)
Radiography Clinical Coordinator
Mid Michigan Community College
Harrison, Michigan

Selina M. Muccio, MEd, BA, RT(R)
Radiography Program Director
Pima Medical Institute, Denver Campus
Denver, Colorado

Catherine Nobles, RT(R), MED
Radiography Instructor
Houston Community College System
Houston, Texas

Rogelio Orta-Martin
General Radiologic Technologist
Dade Medical College
Miami, Florida

George Pales, PhD, RT (R) (MR) (T)
Radiography Program Director
Health Physics and Clinical Sciences
University of Nevada, Las Vegas
Las Vegas, Nevada

MaryJane S. Reynolds, MAIS, RT (R) (T)
Radiography Program Director
Pima Medical Institute
Houston, Texas

Deena Slockett, EdD
Assistant Professor
Department of Radiologic Sciences
Adventist University of Health Sciences
Orlando, Florida

Colleen Sutterley
Radiography Instructor
Bucks County Community College
Newtown, Pennsylvania

Beth L. Veale, PhD
Professor of Radiologic Sciences
Midwestern State University
Wichita Falls, Texas

Preface

Essentials of Radiologic Science has been designed with students and educators in mind. The textbook is designed to distill the information in each of the content-specific areas down to the essentials and to present them to the student in an easy-to-understand format. I have always believed that the difference between professional radiographers and "button pushers" is that the former understand the science and technology of radiographic imaging. To produce quality images, a student must develop an understanding of the theories and concepts related to the various aspects of using radiation. They should not rely on preprogrammed equipment and blindly set technical factors, as this is the practice of "button pushers." In this updated edition, I have made a special effort to design a text that will help the students achieve technical competence in using ionizing radiation safely.

First- and second-year students will be provided with the basic physics foundations from which to learn about the discovery of x-rays and use this knowledge to build upon the theories and concepts regarding the production of radiographic images. The inclusion of film-screen radiography transitioning into digital radiography will demonstrate the evolution of the field. Many essential concepts are valid in both film-screen and digital radiography; the student will learn these concepts as the foundation for their knowledge of the use of ionizing radiation to create a radiographic image.

The text book has been significantly updated with expanded content to include a brief history of radiography, basic mathematics review, formulating radiographic technique, and digital imaging. In all, 13 new chapters have been added! I have placed the chapters in an order to help the student and educator progress from one topic to another. The chapters can be used in consecutive order to build comprehension; however, each chapter can stand alone and can be used in the order that is appropriate for any program.

From the discovery of x-rays by Wilhelm Roentgen to modern day, there have been major changes in how radiography is performed and the responsibilities of the radiographer. The advancement of digital imaging and the elimination of film in a majority of imaging departments in the country have changed the required knowledge base for radiographers, which is different today than just a few years ago. This text addresses those changes and the way radiography students must be educated.

My goal is to make this text a valuable resource for radiography students during their program of study and in the future. The text covers the content areas of three of the content-specific areas contained in the registry examination: Physics, Radiographic Image Production, and Radiation Protection. The sections are independent and designed to be combined in whatever fits the instructor's current syllabus.

It is my hope that this text will exceed the expectations of students and educators in their use of this book. I hope that instructors find this book easy for their students to read and understand, and I know they will find it a useful addition to their courses.

Features

The text has many features that are beneficial to students as they learn about the fascinating world of radiography. Key terms are highlighted with **bold text** and are located at the beginning of each chapter as well as inside the chapter material. A glossary provides definitions for each key term. Other features include objectives, full-color design, in-text case studies with critical thinking questions, critical thinking boxes with clinical/practical application questions and examples, video and animation callouts, chapter summaries, and chapter review questions. One of the most exciting features of this text is the use of over 250 illustrations, radiographic images, photographs, and charts that provide graphic demonstration of the concepts of radiologic science while making the text visually appealing and interesting.

Ancillaries

The text has ancillary resources available to the students to further assist their comprehension of the material. Student ancillaries include a registry exam–style question bank, a chapter review question bank, videos, and animations. These animations complement the text with action-packed visual stimuli to explain complex physics concepts. For example, the topic of x-ray interactions contains an animation demonstrating the x-ray photon entering the patient and then undergoing photoelectric absorption, Compton scattering, or through transmission. Thus, the student can see how the exit radiation is made up of a combination of through transmitted and scattered photons. Videos provide the student with the "real world" example of different scenarios including venipuncture, taking vital signs, using correct body mechanics, hand hygiene, and patient rights.

Valuable resources for educators to use in the classroom are also included. Instructor resources include full-text online, PowerPoint slides, lesson plans, image bank, test generator, answer key for text review questions, and Workbook answer key. Their purpose is to provide instructors with detailed lecture notes that tie together the textbook and all the other resources offered with it.

Workbook

An *Essentials of Radiologic Science Workbook* is available separately to supplement the text and to help the students apply knowledge they are learning. The *Workbook* provides additional practice and preparation for the **ARRT** exam and includes registry-style review questions, as well as other exercises (crossword puzzles, image labeling) and a laboratory experiments section. All the questions in the *Workbook* are correlated directly with the text. Use of the *Workbook* will enhance learning and the enjoyment of radiologic science concepts.

Denise Orth

User's Guide

This User's Guide introduces you to the helpful features of *Essentials of Radiologic Science* that enable you to quickly master new concepts and put your new skills into practice.

Chapter features to increase understanding and enhance retention of the material include:

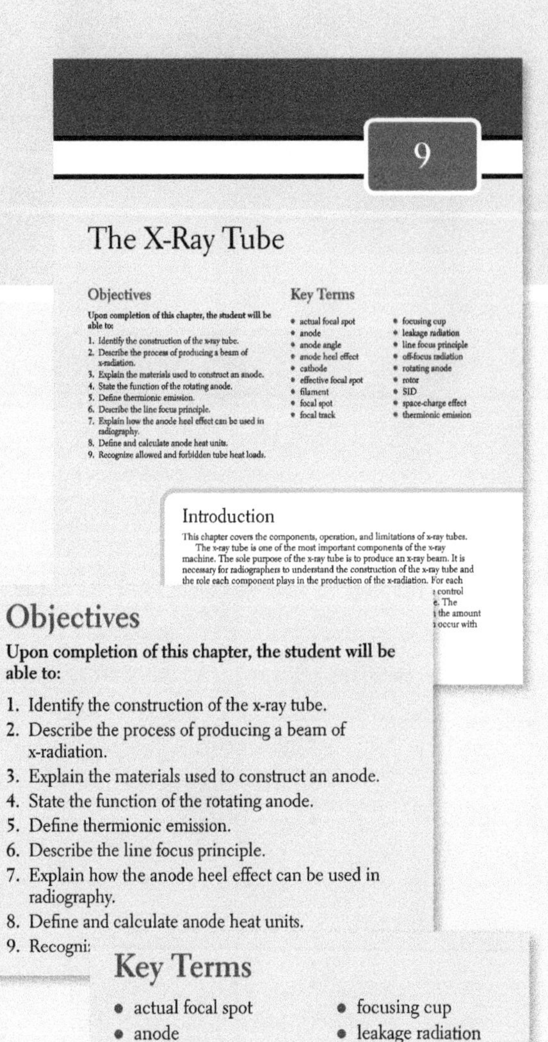
9

The X-Ray Tube

Objectives

Upon completion of this chapter, the student will be able to:

1. Identify the construction of the x-ray tube.
2. Describe the process of producing a beam of x-radiation.
3. Explain the materials used to construct an anode.
4. State the function of the rotating anode.
5. Define thermionic emission.
6. Describe the line focus principle.
7. Explain how the anode heel effect can be used in radiography.
8. Define and calculate anode heat units.
9. Recognize allowed and forbidden tube heat loads.

Key Terms

- actual focal spot
- anode
- anode angle
- anode heel effect
- cathode
- effective focal spot
- filament
- focal spot
- focal track
- focusing cup
- leakage radiation
- line focus principle
- off-focus radiation
- rotating anode
- rotor
- SID
- space-charge effect
- thermionic emission

Introduction

This chapter covers the components, operation, and limitations of x-ray tubes.

The x-ray tube is one of the most important components of the x-ray machine. The sole purpose of the x-ray tube is to produce an x-ray beam. It is necessary for radiographers to understand the construction of the x-ray tube and the role each component plays in the production of the x-radiation. For each

Objectives help you focus on the most important information to glean from the chapter.

Key Terms for the most important concepts are listed at the beginning of the chapters, bolded when mentioned first in the chapter and defined in the Glossary.

Critical Thinking boxes provide the opportunity to apply chapter material by answering practical application questions.

CRITICAL THINKING BOX 9.3

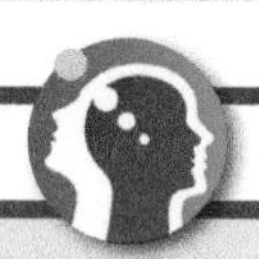

What are the HU produced if the exposure is made with a high-frequency circuit, 100 kVp, 200 mA, and 0.1 second?

CRITICAL THINKING BOX 9.4

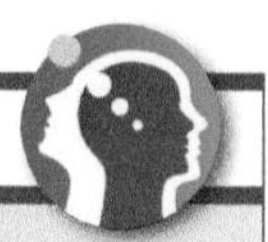

Five abdominal images are exposed with a phase circuit using 85 kVp and 135 mAs. What are the total HU generated?

Case Study

Mark is performing a barium study on a patient. During the exam, the high-frequency x-ray machine stopped producing the x-ray beam because the maximum amount of heat units, 350,000, was used during fluoroscopy. Mark needs to produce seven more images using 100 kVp and 250 mAs.

Critical Thinking Questions

1. What is the formula to determine heat units?
2. How many heat units will this set of exposures produce?
3. Using the anode cooling curve in Figure 9.16, how long must the anode cool before the additional exposures can be made?

Case Studies with Critical Thinking Questions use real-life scenarios to encourage learning and application of chapter concepts.

Video and Animation Callouts identify topics for which there are videos or animations available as part of the online ancillaries.

X-Ray Tube

thePoint® ***An animation for this topic can be viewed at http://thepoint.lww.com/Orth2e***

The major components of the x-ray tube are the cathode, anode, rotor/stator, glass or metal envelope, tube port, and tube housing. The tube components are sealed inside an evacuated (vacuum) glass or metal envelope. The vacuum allows the electrons to travel freely from the negative cathode to the positive anode. A thorough discussion of each component follows along with discussion for utilizing safe practices to extend the life of the x-ray tube.

Chapter Summary

1. The negative cathode of the x-ray tube contains the filament. Thermionic emission from the heated filament produces projectile electrons, which are accelerated to the positive anode.
2. The positive anode is a disk-shaped structure constructed of a high atomic number alloy with high thermal conductivity and a high melting point.

Chapter Summaries provide a synopsis of the chapter content and help to reinforce learning.

Review Questions

Multiple Choice

1. The anode heel effect is described by which of the following?

a. It causes greater radiation intensity on the cathode side.
b. It occurs because x-rays produced inside the cathode are attenuated.
c. It depends on mA and kVp.
d. It is reduced by dual focal spots.

2. Which best describes the line focus principle?

a. Makes the focal spot appear larger than it really is
b. Makes use of an angled cathode structure
c. Produces x-ray lines on the image
d. Spreads the heat over a larger part of the anode

Review Questions at the end of each chapter help you assess your knowledge.

Additional Learning Resources

Valuable ancillary resources for both students and instructors are available on thePoint companion Web site at http://thepoint.lww.com/Orth2e. See the inside front cover for details on how to access these resources.

Student Resources include a **registry exam-style question bank, a chapter review question bank, videos, and animations.**

Instructor Resources include **ebook, PowerPoint slides, lesson plans, image bank, test generator, answer key for text Review Questions, and answer key for Workbook questions.**

Acknowledgments

There are many individuals who have guided me in my career as a radiographer, educator, and professional. Over my professional career I have worked with radiographers who are dedicated to their field, students who are incredibly eager to learn and to ask questions to further their understanding of all subject matter, and the colleagues that I have had the pleasure to know. Each of you were instrumental in furthering my knowledge of the radiologic sciences.

I would like to thank Jay Campbell, Acquisitions Editor, for his encouragement to revise this second edition. He believed in my approach to the subject and expanding the text. His support has been unwavering.

To Amy Millholen, Senior Product Development Editor, a special thank you for your guidance in writing this edition. I can always count on you for advice on the project and for keeping me on track with deadlines. It was a pleasure working with Amy on both editions of this text.

A special thanks to the artists and production staff whose dedicated work and professionalism are evident in the quality of their work. Their expertise helped to provide a fresh, new look to the text and to bringing my vision to fruition.

To the reviewers of this text, you provided valuable feedback on content and art which was especially helpful in writing this text. I appreciate your efforts in challenging me to expand on the material to provide an in-depth explanation of the content.

Finally, I wish to express my deep gratitude to my husband Mark and our family for their unwavering support throughout this project. Your belief in me and this project has meant the world to me.

Denise Orth

Contents

PART IV: DIGITAL IMAGING AND PROCESSING

PART V: SPECIALIZED IMAGING TECHNIQUES

PART VI: RADIATION BIOLOGY AND PROTECTION

PART I

Physics for Radiologic Science

1

History of Radiologic Science

Objectives

Upon completion of this chapter, the student will be able to:

1. Define all the key terms in the chapter.
2. Describe the discovery of x-rays and natural radioactivity.
3. State the importance of each innovation in the process of producing an image.
4. Describe the importance of reducing radiation exposure.
5. List the basic principles of radiation protection.

Key Terms

- cathode ray tube
- fluorescence
- diaphragm
- thermionic emission

Introduction

The journey of the "invisible" ray began as an accidental discovery in Germany. The journey has been relatively short when compared to other areas of medical science. However, the journey has been filled with many fascinating advancements, which have greatly influenced physics and diagnostic medical imaging!

Discovering the "Invisible" Ray

The "invisible" ray has been studied by many scientists from the late 1800s through today. From the very beginning, scientists have been fascinated with the ray, and countless experiments have been performed to discover its many properties. The following discussion focuses on several scientists who were instrumental in researching the ray and in applying it to medical science for the betterment of patients.

Wilhelm Conrad Roentgen

Wilhelm Conrad Roentgen was an accomplished physicist and mathematician who was fascinated with energy (Fig. 1.1). Roentgen studied at the Polytechnic Institute in Zurich and was a professor of physics at the universities of Strasburg, Giessen, and Munich. While at the University of Würzburg, he served as a professor and director of the Physical Institute. He spent many hours in his lab where he conducted experiments with conduction of high-voltage electricity through a partially evacuated glass tube known as a Crookes tube. The Crookes tube was also called a **cathode ray tube**.

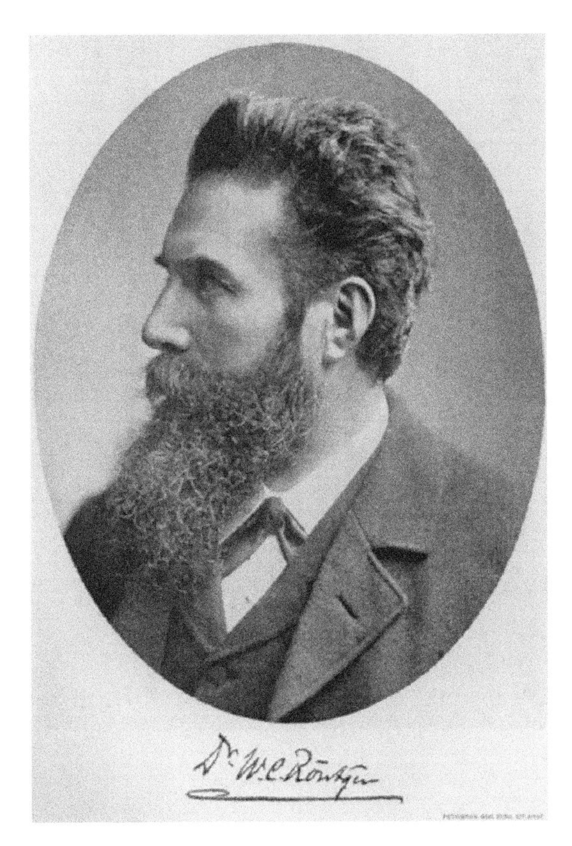

Figure 1.1. **Wilhelm Conrad Roentgen.**

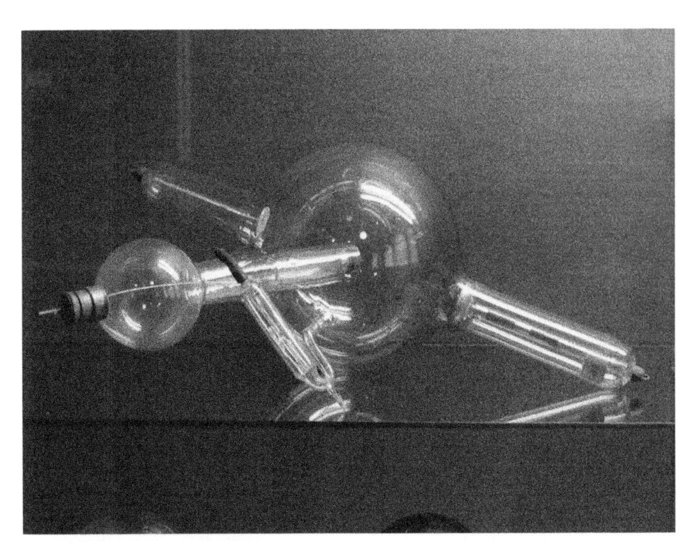

Figure 1.2. **Crookes tube used by Roentgen. (Photo by Daderot, CC-0-1.0.)**

Roentgen used a Crookes tube (Fig. 1.2), which contained a negatively charged cathode and a positively charged anode plate. On November 8, 1895, he surrounded the Crookes tube with black cardboard and darkened the lab. As the tube was energized, there was a glow, which was emitted from the tube. This indicated that the tube was properly energized and cathode rays were being emitted toward the anode.

While the room was darkened, Roentgen noticed a faint glow several feet away from the Crookes tube. The faint glow was coming from a piece of paper that was coated with barium platinocyanide. Roentgen theorized that when the cathode rays struck the glass wall of the tube, an unknown radiation was formed and traveled across the room, struck the coated paper, and caused it to fluoresce. To prove his theory, he conducted the experiment several more times. Each time he observed the glow of the barium platinocyanide–coated paper. The glow emanating during each experiment was fluorescence. **Fluorescence** is the ability of phosphors (barium platinocyanide) to emit visible light when stimulated by energy, which in this case was x-rays. Further experimentation revealed that paper, wood, and aluminum, among other materials, were also transparent to this new form of radiation. He discovered that it affected photographic plates, and because it did not noticeably exhibit any properties of light, he mistakenly thought the rays were unrelated to light. In view of the uncertain nature of the rays, he used his mathematician background and called the phenomenon x-radiation.

As a physicist, Roentgen was very excited about his discovery, but he knew he had to perform further experiments to more fully understand the potential of his discovery. While performing the experiments, he noticed that when he placed his hand between the Crookes tube and the barium platinocyanide–coated paper, he could see the bones in his hand. Imagine his wonder when he watched the bones in his hand move with this live fluoroscopic image! His curiosity about seeing his one hand led him to wonder if a static image could be produced. His wife, Anna Bertha, was the model for this experiment. He placed her hand on the coated paper and energized the Crookes tube. The exposure took several minutes to complete and became the first radiographic image of human anatomy (Fig. 1.3).

Roentgen deduced that the radiation traveled in straight lines in all directions and could penetrate less dense objects. Further investigation with objects of varying densities determined if these objects were transparent to the new form of radiation. Roentgen noticed partial shadows of the objects on the glowing screen; lead projected a solid shadow that blocked the mysterious rays. Over the next few weeks, Roentgen performed numerous experiments and meticulously chronicled the results of these experiments. Roentgen wanted to know as much as possible about this new form of radiation before he presented his research to colleagues. Figure 1.4 is a photograph of the room where Roentgen spent his time investigating the unknown rays.

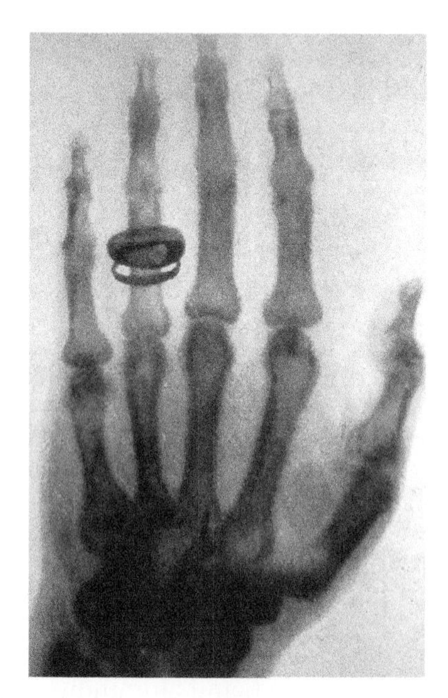

Figure 1.3. **Anna Bertha Roentgen's hand x-ray image showing the bones in her hand and her ring.**

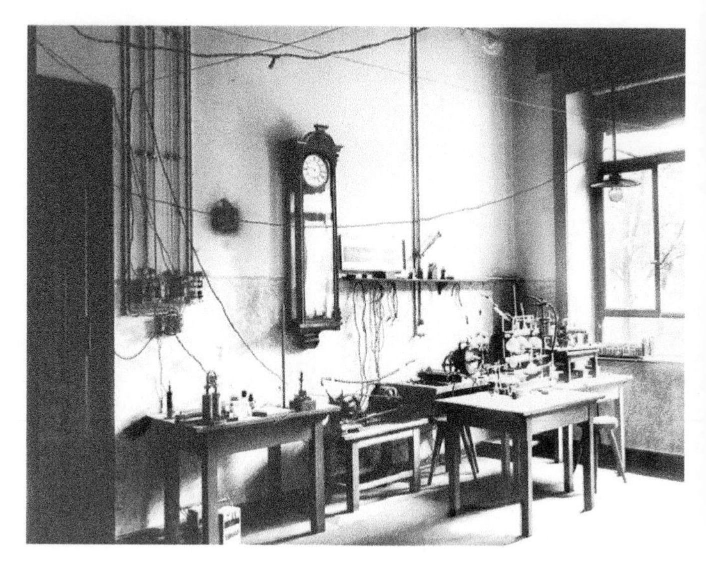

Figure 1.4. **Photograph of Roentgen's laboratory.**

On December 28, 1895, Roentgen presented a scholarly paper "On a New Kind of Rays" to the Würtzburg Physico-Medical Society. His new discovery caused quite a stir in the scientific and medical communities. The Roentgen rays caused skepticism and curiosity among researchers. Humans are naturally curious about all things "new." This curiosity is the driving force of discovery and invention. This natural curiosity leads many scientists to build their own devices, test and retest theories, and begin to perform experiments. To gain further knowledge about the x-rays, scientists used inanimate objects, animal and human tissue to determine the possible uses of x-radiation.

Roentgen realized the importance of his discovery and the potential impact it could have; however, he was very modest about his discovery. He chose not to patent his process but left it available for anyone to use. This was indeed an unselfish act, which allowed for many scientists to experiment with x-rays. These experiments would expand to become the field of radiology. Medical scientists researched the use of x-radiation to image living tissue to identify pathology. Through this research, scientists began to theorize that the x-ray could also be used to treat disease.

Medical researchers proved the tremendous value of Roentgen's discovery, and he was awarded the first Nobel Prize for Physics in 1901. A new branch of medicine, roentgenology, focused on the use of x-rays for medical purposes. The unit of radiation exposure was called the roentgen, which led to x-rays being called roentgen rays.

A Second Source of Radiation

The year following Roentgen's discovery of the invisible ray, another physicist was experimenting with crystals. Antoine Henri Becquerel was a French physicist who worked with crystals, which would phosphoresce after absorbing light. He theorized that these crystals were emitting x-rays. Becquerel experimented with photographic plates wrapped in black paper and phosphorescing crystals, which he had placed in the sun to absorb light. During one experiment, he was frustrated by a lack of sunshine and placed a crystal along with the wrapped photographic plate in a drawer. At some point, he processed the plate and was surprised to find it darkened! He realized that the crystal must be emitting rays continuously and not the light the crystal absorbed from the sun. Much like Roentgen, Becquerel's discovery was accidental and led to further experimentation with natural radioactivity.

Natural radiation was found to consist of three distinct forms of radiation, *alpha*, *beta*, and *gamma*. Physicists discovered that alpha rays consisted of heavy particles with a positive electrical charge, while beta rays were light particles with a negative electrical charge. It was determined that gamma rays were very high-energy rays, which Becquerel was "seeing" each time he developed a photographic plate. Becquerel received the Nobel Prize for Physics in 1903.

Thomas Edison

In 1896, Thomas Edison was an American researcher who performed many experiments in his own laboratories. He devised a fluoroscope composed of a fluorescent screen in a light-tight viewing cone made of metal. The device allowed real-time x-ray imaging. The tube was placed under the patient with the viewing cone above. The room was darkened, and very high-energy x-ray techniques were required to make the screen glow bright enough to see the anatomy with the viewing cone. Exposures took several minutes to adequately visualize the anatomy.

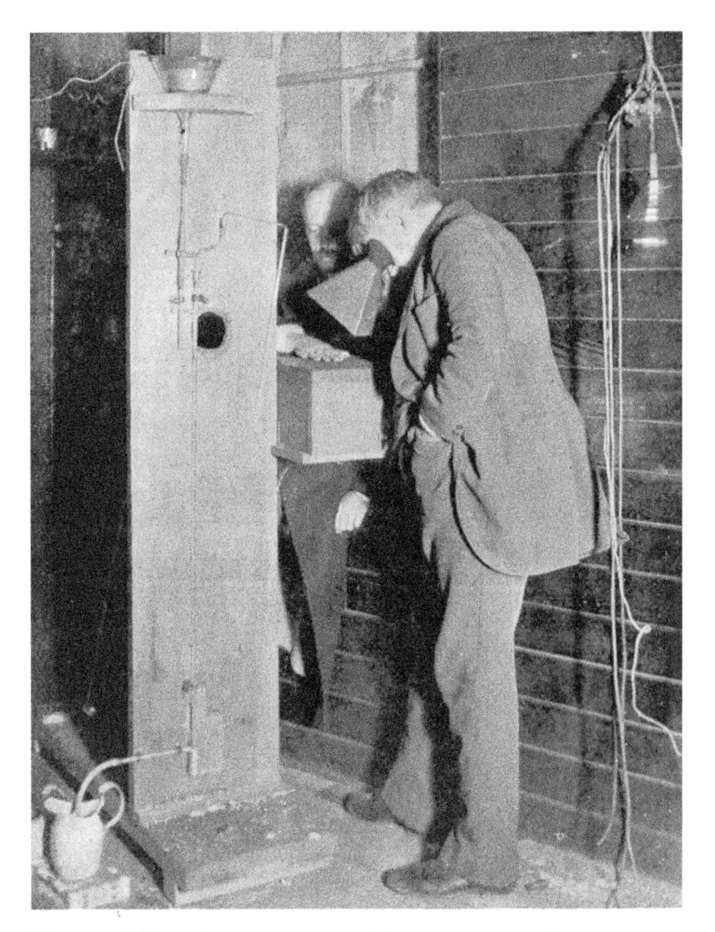

Figure 1.5. **Edison using a calcium tungstate fluoroscope to examine Clarence Dally's hand. Dally's hand is placed on the box that contains the x-ray tube. (This file comes from Wellcome Images, a website operated by Wellcome Trust, a global charitable foundation based in the United Kingdom. CC-BY-4.0.)**

Clarence Dally, Edison's assistant, participated in many experiments with the fluoroscope as seen in Figure 1.5. Dally was fascinated with x-rays and performed countless experiments while volunteering to be Edison's "patient." Because of the extensive exposure Dally received, he developed lesions on both upper extremities, which resulted in the amputation of both arms. Dally became the first human death from x-rays in 1904 just a few years after the exciting discovery by Roentgen. Edison stopped his research with x-rays after this tragic event. Edison recognized the potential value x-rays would have as an adjunct to surgery and locating objects within the body.

He also realized that in the hands of an inexperienced operator, x-rays were very dangerous. If Edison had continued his research, he would likely have had countless inventions involving x-rays.

As medical research progressed, individuals in the nonmedical community took a different view of the new ray. Entrepreneurs developed devices that were used for entertainment purposes or to block unscrupulous people from using "x-ray" vision to peer through clothing. Using x-rays became commercialized, and people were excited to "see" their skeletons. Fortunately, all of this did not distract the researchers who investigated the effect of x-ray on living tissue.

Notable Scientists

Within a year of Roentgen's discovery, Michael Pupin of Columbia University placed a film between two fluorescent screens. The screens were made of calcium tungstate, which was developed by Thomas Edison. Edison determined that certain chemicals would emit hundreds of light rays when stimulated by an x-ray. The overall effect of the exposure to the film was magnified because the film was mostly exposed to light. This great advancement meant lower techniques were required to produce a quality image. The new techniques were 1/50th those previously used for an exposure!

William Rollins, a Boston dentist, was fascinated by physics. Shortly after the news of Roentgen's discovery reached the Unites States, he began researching the properties of x-rays. Because of his primary field of dentistry, he directed his research of x-rays to visualize oral anatomy. By mid-1896, he had designed his own fluoroscope so that a dentist could observe portions of the oral cavity. Rollins reported in January 1898 the results of his initial research regarding the hazards of radiation. Tesla theorized that exposure to the x-rays created skin burns on the surface of the skin. Rollins tested this theory by applying a high potential across a highly evacuated tube. He suffered a severe burn and concluded that it was caused by a high-frequency electrical field surrounding the tube. It was 5 years later when he asserted that electrons from the cathode were most likely the cause of the burn. He firmly believed that it was necessary to be protected from x-rays. Rollins worked for many years to design x-ray tubes and related apparatus to improve the images, and through his work, he discovered that using filtration of the x-ray beam resulted in an improved image. He used aluminum plates to filter the beam and lead plates with a hole in the center, a **diaphragm**, to restrict the beam. The result of using these two principles was a significant reduction in radiation exposure to the patient and a higher-quality image that improved diagnosis.

In 1913, William Coolidge experimented with a new x-ray tube and improved on the Crookes tube significantly; the new tube was called the Coolidge tube (Fig. 1.6). He used a hot-cathode x-ray tube with a tungsten x-ray filament, which could withstand extreme temperatures created from using a high-voltage transformer. The tungsten filament allowed electrons to be boiled off the cathode in a process known as **thermionic emission**. Coolidge's

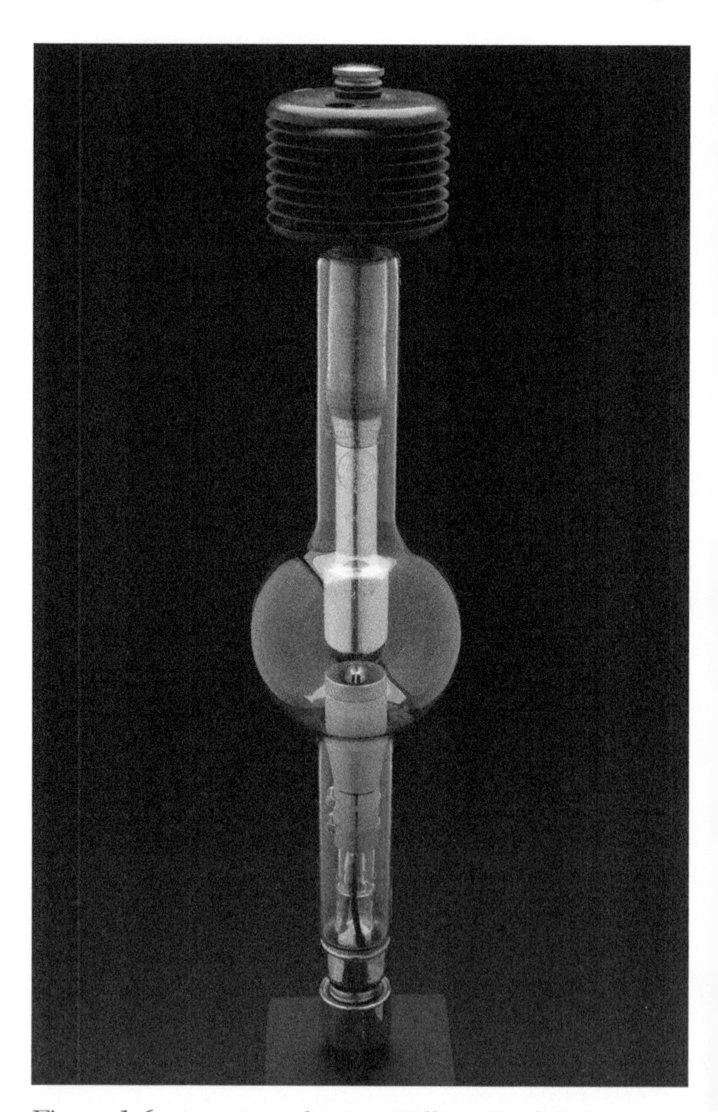

Figure 1.6. American physicist William Coolidge (1832–1919) patented his hot cathode tube in 1913. (This file comes from Wellcome Images, a website operated by Wellcome Trust, a global charitable foundation based in the United Kingdom. CC-BY-4.0.)

tube was a vacuum tube, which allowed the operator to select the x-ray intensity and energy separately for greater accuracy with each exposure. The Coolidge tube was recognized as being superior to the Crookes tube and was widely accepted by the medical community. The modern x-ray tubes are Coolidge tubes that have evolved over time.

In 1913, Dr. Gustav Bucky, a German radiologist, invented the stationary x-ray grid. His grid utilized lead strips that were thick enough to appear as lines on the x-ray image. To remove the lines, he developed a moving grid, which would move during the x-ray exposure. In 1915, Dr. Hollis Potter, an American radiologist, invented a moving grid to enhance the quality of diagnostic x-ray images. The grid consisted of lead strips, which prevented some of the scatter radiation from reaching the film. The lead strips caused white grid line artifacts, which degraded the image. To correct this effect, Potter developed an oscillating mechanism to move the grid back and forth during the exposure. The movement effectively blurred out the lines. Recognizing Bucky's earlier grid invention, Potter introduced the Potter-Bucky grid in 1921.

The first rotating anode was developed in 1929 by William D. Coolidge. The rotating anode allowed the tremendous heat generated during an exposure to be dispersed around the outer edge of the anode. This design allowed for higher techniques to be used for an exposure. A focused tube that used negatively charged bits to surround the filament was developed. This new configuration of the filament resulted in compressing the electron stream as it left the cathode and sped toward the anode. The electron stream converged on a small area on the anode. This was called the "small focal spot" and greatly improved image sharpness.

Essentially, the 50 years after Edison invented the fluoroscope, there were no advancements to this equipment. Fluoroscopic exposures required high x-ray techniques to make the screens glow bright enough to see anatomy. The exposures lasted several minutes, which resulted in excessive exposure to the doctors, radiographers, and patients. In 1948, the electronic image intensifier was developed. The image intensifier converted incident x-rays into an electron beam. Electrically charged plates focused the beam while speeding up the electrons. The fast-moving electrons then struck a small fluorescent screen at the top of the image intensifier tube. The fluorescent screen converted the electrons to light that was up to 5,000 times brighter than Edison's fluoroscope! This new development reduced the techniques necessary to produce the fluoroscopic image and allowed for the examinations to be completed in a shorter amount of time. The exposure to everyone involved in the examination was greatly reduced.

Since the discovery of x-rays in 1895, the field has constantly changed and evolved to improve on each subsequent invention. The stationary anode was replaced with a rotating anode, automatic exposure controls standardized exposures, and the automatic processor greatly reduced the time required to process film. No more dipping or dunking film in developer, fixer, and water! This process plus drying time could take up to 30 minutes or longer for each film! An eternity by today's standard. Currently, the new generation of radiography equipment is digital imaging. Roentgen would be very pleased to see how his "invisible" ray has lit the way for many other scientists to develop new equipment. Table 1.1 lists notable dates in the development of medical imaging.

Ushering in the Modern Era

The "newest" advancement in medical imaging occurred when digital imaging was developed. For nearly 80 years, there were improvements in equipment and designing screen cassettes, but none significantly improved the capturing of an image like digital imaging! The invention of computers brought about the computerization process of static x-ray images. This was called computed radiography or CR. In 1979, digital fluoroscopy was developed by connecting image intensifier technology to analog-to-digital converters, which were coupled with TV camera tubes to produce digital information. When computer technology advanced to the point where computers could handle huge amounts of the electronic signals, the digital image was born! CR became available in the early 1980s and employed a cassette with fluorescent screens. The new fluorescent screen materials were able to emit light after stimulation by a laser light. The emitted light has many different intensities, which contain the information about the patient's anatomy. The use of light-sensitive diodes converted the information into electrical signals, which were stored by a computer.

The advancement of computer technology with miniature electronic detectors brought about the next new advancement in obtaining a radiographic image. In 1996, direct digital radiography or DR was unveiled. DR allows the x-ray image to be captured directly by the electronic

TABLE 1.1 NOTABLE DATES IN THE PROGRESS OF MEDICAL IMAGING

Date	Event
1895	Roentgen discovers x-rays.
1896	First application of x-rays in diagnosis and therapy are made.
1901	Roentgen receives the first Nobel Prize in Physics.
1905	Einstein presents his theory of relativity and the famous equation $E = mc^2$.
1913	Bohr theorizes his model of the atom, which includes a nucleus and orbital electrons.
1913	Coolidge develops the hot-filament x-ray tube.
1920	Multiple inventors demonstrate the use of soluble iodine compounds as contrast media.
1921	The Potter-Bucky grid is announced.
1922	Compton describes the properties of scattering x-rays.
1923	Eastman Kodak introduces cellulose acetate "safety" x-ray film.
1925	The First International Congress of Radiology is convened in London.
1928	The roentgen (R) is defined as the unit of x-ray intensity.
1929	Forssman performs cardiac catheterization on himself!
1930	Multiple inventors present tomographic devices.
1932	DuPont adds blue tint to x-ray film.
1932	The U.S. Committee on X-ray and Radium Protection issues the first dose limits. Now the NCRP.
1942	An electronic photo-timing device is exhibited by Morgan.
1942	Pako introduces the first automatic film processor.
1948	Coltman develops the first fluoroscopic image intensifier.
1953	The rad is adopted as the unit of absorbed dose.
1956	Xeroradiography is demonstrated.
1956	Eastman Kodak presents the first automatic roller transport film processor.
1960	DuPont develops the polyester base film.
1963	Kuhl and Edwards demonstrate single-photon emission computed tomography (SPECT).
1965	Eastman Kodak presents the 90-second rapid film processor.
1966	Diagnostic ultrasonography enters routine use in medicine.
1972	DuPont develop single-emulsion film and one-screen mammography.
1973	Hounsfield completes development of the first computed tomography (CT) imaging system.
1973	The first magnetic resonance image is produced by Damadian and Lauterbur.
1974	Rare earth radiographic intensifying screen is first used.
1977	Mistretta demonstrates digital subtraction fluoroscopy.
1979	Allan Cormack and Godfrey Hounsfield win the Nobel Prize in Physiology or Medicine for CT.
1980	The first commercial superconducting MRI system is presented.
1981	The International System of Units (SI) is adopted by the International Commission on Radiation Units and Measurements (ICRU)
1982	Picture archiving and communications system (PACS) becomes available for use.
1983	Eastman Kodak develops the first tabular grain film emulsion.
1984	Fuji introduces laser-stimulable phosphors for CR.
1989	The SI is adopted by the NCRP and most scientific and medical societies.
1990	Toshiba presents the Helical CT.
1991	Elscint develops the two-slice CT.
1992	Mammography Quality Standards Act (MQSA) is passed.
1996	DR that uses thin-film transistors (TFTs) is developed.
1997	Swissray presents the charge-coupled device (CCD) digital radiography unit.
1998	General Electric introduces multislice CT.
1998	Amorphous silicon-cesium iodide image receptor is demonstrated for DR.
2000	General Electric produces the first direct digital mammographic imaging system.
2002	The 16-slice helical CT unit is presented.
2002	Positron emission tomography (PET) is available for routine clinical use.
2003	Paul Lauterbur and Sir Peter Mansfield receive the Nobel Prize for Physiology or Medicine for MRI.
2004	64-slice helical CT is presented.
2005	Siemens presents the dual-source CT.
2009	NCRP Report No. 160, *Ionizing radiation exposure of the population of the United States: 2006* is published.

detectors. The cassette with screens or plates that relied on the conversion of x-rays to light was no longer needed for the DR system to produce an x-ray image.

Whether using CR or DR, the electronic image provides the ability to postprocess the image. The image can be manipulated to affect contrast and brightness along with other manipulations without the need to repeat the exposure. Historically, any time the image needed to be improved for contrast, the radiographer would perform a repeat exposure because this was the only way to change the image. Computerization allows the manipulation to take place on either the radiographer's or radiologist's work station, which means that the patient isn't exposed to radiation for another image.

The traditional method of producing an image entailed a cassette, film, processor, and chemicals. The facility had to have a supply of film and chemicals available so that they did not run out of these essential items; this just added to the cost of the procedure. Technology has saved millions of dollars in chemical and film costs for imaging departments. More importantly, technology has dramatically reduced the overall radiation exposure to patients! The journey of x-ray imaging has progressed very rapidly in just over a century since Wilhelm Conrad Roentgen discovered the "invisible rays"!

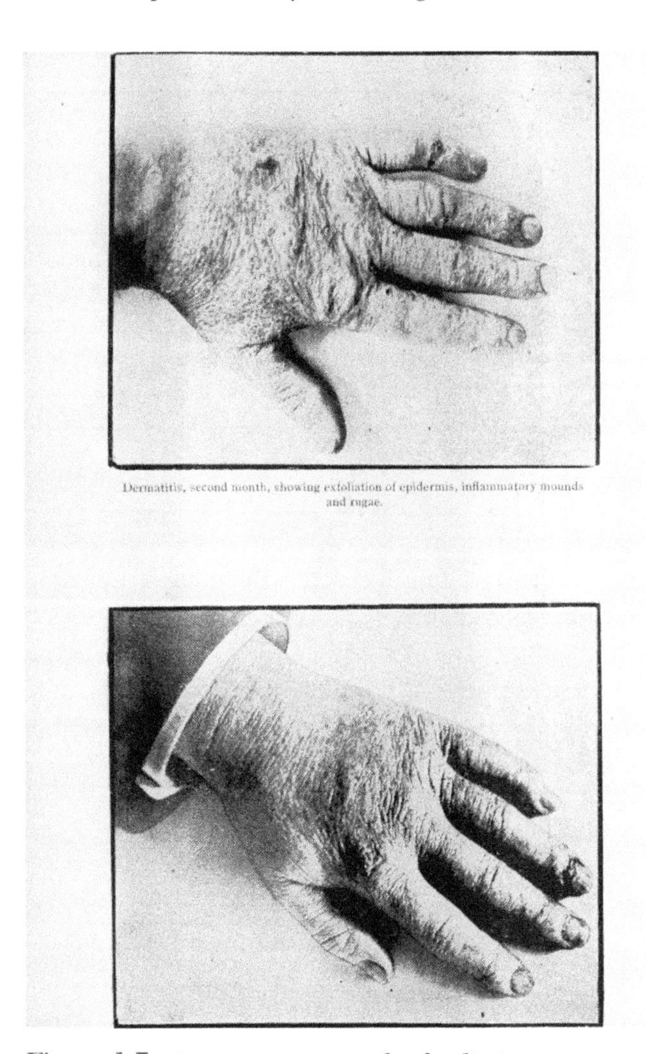

Figure 1.7. Dermatitis as a result of radiation exposure.

Dangers of Radiation

In the years since William Rollins researched the hazards of radiation, the medical industry has identified the causes of radiation injury, the processes used to assess the level of occupational radiation received by medical workers, and practices that must be used to protect the patient and medical worker from radiation.

Radiation Injury

In 1898, the effects of x-radiation were identified in researchers, physicians, and workers who were exposed to large doses. These people developed erythema, skin reddening and burning, from the large doses of radiation caused by the long exposures required to produce the images (Fig. 1.7). Physicians determined that this new method was to be used when there was a great enough reason. In the decades since Roentgen's discovery, other serious effects such as malignant tumors and chromosomal changes have been identified. The identification of the effects of radiation brought about the realization that individuals who work with radiation must follow safe practices to protect workers.

Radiation workers wear protective apparel such as lead gloves and aprons when in close proximity to a radiation exposure. Radiation dosimeters are a required device for all radiographers to wear in order to measure and document the amount of occupational exposure. All these efforts have been effective in reducing radiation exposure to radiographers.

Radiation Protection

Radiation protection principles are taught and emphasized during an educational program. As a radiographer progresses into a daily routine of performing

TABLE 1.2 **BASIC PRINCIPLES OF RADIATION PROTECTION**

Always apply the cardinal rules of radiation protection: time, distance, and shielding.
Never stand in the primary beam.
Always use collimation to restrict the field to the smallest size appropriate for the examination.
Always wear protective apparel when standing outside a protective barrier.
Wear an occupational radiation monitor outside the protective apron at the collar.
Never hold the patient during an exposure. Use mechanical devices to restrain a patient during an examination. If these are not available, have a family member or friend hold the patient.
Person holding a patient must always use or wear protective aprons, thyroid shields, and lead gloves.
Always use gonadal shielding for patients of childbearing age when the shield will not interfere with the image.

examinations, it becomes easy to be complacent or apathetic about practicing the core principles of radiation protection. This apathy is seen in poor practices, which results in an increase of radiation exposure to the worker. Unfortunately, these poor practices also increase the radiation exposure to patients! A lack of shielding and higher exposure factors used to produce an image has become more common in radiology departments. Radiation control practices have proven effective when they are followed.

The safe practices evolved into the three cardinal rules: time, distance, and shielding. When these rules are followed, the exposure to radiation can be significantly reduced to both the patient and radiographer while producing images to diagnose pathologies in all areas of the body. Table 1.2 introduces the Basic Principles of Radiation Protection. Following these practices and utilizing the information from this text make it easy to reduce radiation exposure. Chapter 31, Radiation Biology and Protection, and Chapter 33, Radiation Protection: Principle Concepts and Equipment, go into depth in discussing the dangers of radiation and protective methods, which must be used.

The implementation of safe practices has gone a long way in reducing radiation exposure to patients. X-radiation is a valuable tool in improving the lives of patients, but as with any type of radiation, its potential for harm is always present and must be respected. All students and radiographers must approach each exposure with the goal of producing a quality diagnostic image while minimizing the radiation exposure to the patient and health care workers.

Chapter Summary

1. Wilhelm Conrad Roentgen discovered x-rays on November 8, 1895. Antoine Henri Becquerel discovered natural radioactivity in 1896. Both physicists received the Nobel Prize for Physics.
2. Thomas Edison invented the fluoroscope in 1896. His assistant, Clarence Dally, was the first human death from x-rays in 1904.
3. Historically many scientists are acknowledged for improving upon Roentgen's processes.
4. The electronic image intensifier used electrically charged plates and a fluorescent screen to increase the brightness of the image.
5. Advancements in computerization and data storage brought about digital imaging in the early 1980s.
6. Safe practices must be followed to minimize radiation exposure to patients and health care workers.

Review Questions

Multiple Choice

1. X-rays were discovered in which year?
   a. 1890
   b. 1880
   c. 1901
   d. 1895

2. Electricity and __________ were used in experiments where x-rays were discovered.
   a. cathode ray tubes
   b. atomic structure
   c. magnetism
   d. ionization

3. X-rays were discovered when they caused a barium platinocyanide–coated plate to:
   a. vibrate
   b. burn
   c. fluoresce
   d. phosphoresce

4. Anna Bertha Roentgen's __________ was the first radiographic image of human anatomy.
   a. foot
   b. elbow
   c. hand
   d. knee

5. Roentgen discovered that __________ projected a solid shadow when exposed to x-rays.
   a. wood
   b. glass
   c. pottery
   d. lead

6. In which year did Roentgen receive the Nobel Prize for Physics?
   a. 1899
   b. 1901
   c. 1903
   d. 1896

7. Who was Thomas Edison's assistant who was documented as the first x-ray fatality?
   a. Becquerel
   b. Curie
   c. Dally
   d. Potter

8. William Rollins used __________ to filter the beam.
   a. lead
   b. aluminum
   c. tungsten
   d. molybdenum

9. Who was the first person to design a stationary x-ray grid?
   a. Potter
   b. Bucky
   c. Edison
   d. Curie

10. In which year were the effects of x-radiation first identified?
    a. 1898
    b. 1903
    c. 1950
    d. 1897

11. Image intensifiers create an image that is __________ times brighter than the original fluoroscopic images.
    a. 2,500
    b. 4,000
    c. 9,000
    d. 5,000

2

Basic Mathematics

Objectives

Upon completion of this chapter, the student will be able to:

1. Perform functions with fractions and decimals.
2. Perform calculations in scientific notation.
3. Apply basic math concepts to radiography formulas.
4. Identify the units of exposure, dose, and effective dose.

Introduction

In this chapter, the student will be exposed to radiographic formulas for the first time! The chapter includes select formulas that are the cornerstone for selecting the best technical factors for a given exposure. Radiography has many formulas to aid the student in making changes based on distances, types of grids, etc. There will be additional formulas to learn as the student progresses through the book.

Before we get into radiographic formulas, it will be helpful to review basic math principles. The student will review basic operations with fractions, decimals, rounding, and so on. Students will learn how to make conversions in a simple way and how to use scientific notation to simplify working with incredibly large or small numbers.

Basic Operations

Convert a Fraction into a Decimal

In radiography, we frequently work with ratios as fractions. Using a calculator, divide the denominator into the numerator.

EXAMPLE: Convert 6/8 into a decimal:

$$6 \text{ divided by } 8 = 0.75$$

Converting Percentages and Decimals

Percentages are used frequently to calculate new exposure factors. To convert a decimal to a percent, move the decimal point two places to the right.

EXAMPLE: Convert 0.483 into a percentage.

$$0.483 = 48.3\%$$

To convert a percent to a decimal, move the decimal point two places to the left.

EXAMPLE: Convert 78.3% to a decimal.

$$78.3\% = 0.783$$

Rounding a Number

The age old question is always "How many places to round after the decimal?" When comparing the numbers in the problem, determine the least number of decimal places to the right of the decimal point. A common practice is to use two digits to the right of the decimal point.

EXAMPLE: Solve and round 136.41 + 103.4613

136.41
103.4613
Answer: 239.8713
Round to: 239.87

Order of Operation

When solving complex problems, the established order of operation must be followed. If it is not precisely followed, the result will be an incorrect answer. The order of operation is as follows:

Step 1: Perform all operations inside the parentheses first.
Step 2: Next, apply all exponents.
Step 3: Multiplication and division are now applied.
Step 4: Last, perform all additions and subtractions.

Exercise 2.1

Use the steps to solve the equation

$$\frac{2(6+9)^2}{3^2} + 30$$

Step 1: Solve parentheses: Add $(6 + 9)^2$ = ______
Step 2: Apply exponents: Square the answer from Step 1 (15×15) = ______
Step 3: Square number underneath the equation (3×3) = ______
Step 4: Multiply Step 2 answer by 2, ______ Divide entire ratio, ______
Step 5: Add and subtract entire formula: 50 + 30, ______

Powers of 10

In science, either very large or very small numbers are often used. Two units, the millampere (mA) and kilovolt peak (kVp) are used when producing x-radiation. Table 2.1 includes the prefixes and symbols that provide a quick method of expressing numbers. To simplify equations and make it easier to use these types of numbers, the powers of 10 or exponents are very useful. Exponents are the number of times a number is multiplied by itself. There are three rules to follow when using exponents:

1. When multiplying an equation, **add** the exponents:

$$10^6 \times 10^8 = 10^{(6+8)} = 10^{14}$$

$$10^4 \times 10^{-9} = 10^{(4+(-9))} = 10^{(4-9)} = 10^{-5}$$

2. When dividing an equation, **subtract** the exponents:

$$10^4 \div 10^2 = 10^{(4-2)} = 10^2$$

TABLE 2.1 POWERS OF 10 AND SCIENTIFIC PREFIXES

Multiple	Prefix	Symbol
10^{18}	exa-	E
10^{15}	peta-	P
10^{12}	**tera-**	**T**
10^{9}	**giga-**	**G**
10^{6}	**mega-**	**M**
10^{3}	**kilo-**	**k**
10^{2}	hecto-	h
10	deka-	da
10^{-1}	deci-	d
10^{-2}	**centi-**	**c**
10^{-3}	**milli-**	**m**
10^{-6}	**micro-**	**µ**
10^{-9}	**nano-**	**n**
10^{-12}	pico-	p
10^{-15}	femto-	f
10^{-18}	atto-	a

Remember that subtracting a negative number creates a positive number.

$$10^7 \div 10^{-9} = 10^{(7-(-9))} = 10^{(7+9)} = 10^{16}$$

3. When exponents are multiplied the number is raised in power.

$$\left(10^5\right)^8 = 10^{(5\times 8)} = 10^{40}$$

Boldfaced prefixes and symbols are commonly used in imaging science.

Algebraic Expressions

Algebraic expressions are letters and/or numbers that are multiplied, divided, added, or subtracted. "x" is the unknown variable in algebraic equations, and there are four basic rules to follow when working with "x":

1. To add or subtract two numbers inside parentheses when the entire set is multiplied by another number, change the set to:

$$a(b+c) = a\times b + a\times c$$

$$a(b-c) = a\times b - a\times c$$

2. When a number is added to "x," the number must be subtracted from both sides of the equation to solve for "x."

$$x + a = c$$
$$x + a - a = c - a$$
$$x = c - a$$

3. To make an equation equivalent when the "x" is multiplied by a number, both sides of the equation must be divided by that number.

$$3x = 12$$
$$\frac{3x}{3} = \frac{12}{3}$$
$$x = \frac{12}{3}$$
$$x = 4$$

4. If both sides of the equation are ratios, then the equation must be cross multiplied to solve for "x."

$$\frac{x}{b} = \frac{c}{a}$$
$$\frac{x}{b} = \frac{c}{a}$$
$$xa = bc$$
$$x = \frac{bc}{a}$$

Scientific Notation

As stated previously, incredibly large and small numbers are used in science. Radiography has many formulas for setting techniques, physics, equipment, and radiation biology. Students who have an excellent grasp of using scientific notation will have an easier time of working the formulas.

We have already covered working with the powers of 10, the cornerstone for scientific notation. Determining the power of 10 is as easy as moving the decimal place to either the left or right. Of course, there are a few rules to follow, but once you have mastered them, scientific notation will make working problems much easier.

Converting Numbers to Scientific Notation

The first step to converting a number is to find the first *nonzero* or *significant* number. Move the decimal point to either the left or right to place the decimal point immediately after the first nonzero number. When the decimal point is moved to the left, the exponent is the number of places the decimal point was moved. When the decimal point is moved to the right, the exponent is expressed as a negative number.

Exercise 2.2

Express 34,100 in scientific notation.

Place decimal point two places to the left after first nonzero number: 3.4100

Answer: ______

Exercise 2.3

Express 0.086 in scientific notation.

Place decimal point after the first nonzero number or two places to the right: 8.6

Answer: ______

A caveat to the above rule is that it is acceptable to have two nonzero digits in front of the decimal point when working with large numbers.

Exercise 2.4

Express 56782.4 using scientific notation.

Move the decimal point three places to the left: 56.7824

Answer: ______

Calculations using Scientific Notation

To add or subtract numbers that are expressed in scientific numbers, convert the numbers using care to align the decimal points in the correct locations. The true magic of scientific notation is revealed when multiplying or dividing an equation. When multiplying two numbers follow these steps:

Exercise 2.5

$$\left(20 \times 10^{4}\right) \times \left(5 \times 10^{2}\right)$$

Step 1: Multiply the whole numbers: 20 × 5 = ______
Step 2: Add the exponents: 4 + 2 = ______
Step 3: Write answer with product from Step 1 multiplied by the exponent in Step 2: ______

Exercise 2.6

To divide an equation, perform the following steps:

$$\frac{6 \times 10^{12}}{3 \times 10^{4}}$$

Step 1: Divide the whole numbers: 6/3 = ______
Step 2: Subtract the exponents: 12 – 4 = ______
Step 3: Write the answer as the ratio from Step 1 multiplied by the exponent in Step 2: ______

Radiographic Formulas

This section provides an overview of some of the formulas used in radiography. This is not an extensive list of formulas found throughout the text. However, the student should strive to develop an understanding of these formulas and concepts to build a strong foundation for working with and solving radiography formulas.

Direct and Indirect Relationships

The basis for radiography formulas is direct and indirect relationships. It can be confusing when the phrases "directly related" and "directly proportional" are used. To shed light on these phrases, we must first define each.

Directly proportional means that an increase in one variable causes an exactly identical increase in another variable. When one variable doubles, the other variable must also double. The same is true when one variable is decreased.

EXAMPLE: mAs is directly proportional to image density. Double mAs, and the radiographic image turns out two times darker. Cut the mAs in half, and the resultant receptor exposure (density) on the image is one-half.

$$C = D$$

$$3C = 3D$$

This principle is also true if "*D*" is being multiplied by a factor. In the formula, C = ½ *D*, "*D*" is still directly proportional to "C." If "C" is doubled, then "*D*" must also double.

EXAMPLE: When C = 4, 4 = ½ *D*, *D* = 8.
When C = 8, 8 = ½ *D* = 16.

Notice that when "C" doubled from 4 to 8, "D" also doubled from 8 to 16. Therefore, "C" and "D" are directly proportional.

Exponentially proportional or related means that one variable is squared or cubed in the formula. When a small change is made in this variable, the other variable in the formula will experience a big change.

EXAMPLE: kVp is exponentially related to radiographic image density: kVp^2 = Density

Triple kVp and the resultant image is 3^2 or 9 times darker.

Setting up the formula: $C = \frac{1}{2} DB^2$, whereas "C" is directly proportional to "D" *and* exponentially proportional to "B."

Directly related means that a change in variable "C" causes a similar change in variable "D"; they go either up or down together. It does not specify if the relationship is proportional or exponential. It also does not specify the amount of change.

EXAMPLE: Setting up the formula: $C = \frac{1}{2} DB^2$. "C" is directly related to "D" and "B," because if one variable is changed, the other variables must also change.

Inversely proportional means that when two variables change, the change is in exactly the same proportion or magnitude. However, the change occurs in opposite directions. As one goes up by a factor, the other must go down by the same factor. If "C" is doubled, then "D" must be cut in half. When "C" is cut to 1/3, then "D" is tripled.

EXAMPLE: In the formula $C = DB$, "D" and "B" are inversely proportional. Let us set up this formula with numbers to see how it works.

When $C = 20$, $D = 10$, and $B = 2$,

$$20 = 10 \times 2$$
$$20 = 5 \times 4$$

As you can see when "D" was cut in half, "B" had to be doubled to keep the formula equal.

Calculating mAs

mAs is expressed as a formula, mAs = mA × seconds. mAs is used for every exposure, which makes it important for the student to be able to manipulate the formula when a mAs change is needed.

EXAMPLE: 100 mA × 0.25 s = **25 mAs**
300 mA × 0.4 s = **120**
500 mA × 100 ms (milliseconds or 0.1 second) = **50 mAs**

When an adjustment is needed in mAs, either milliamperage (mA) or exposure time (seconds) can be increased or decreased.

EXAMPLE: 100 mA × 0.1 s = **10 mAs**

To increase mAs to 30, either the mA or seconds will be changed:

100 mA × 0.3 s = **30 mAs**
300 mA × 0.1 s = **30 mAs**

When you want to maintain the mAs, either the mA or seconds will need to be changed.

EXAMPLE: 300 mA × 100 ms (0.1 s) = **30 mAs**

To maintain mAs at 30, you could use

150 mA × 200 ms (0.2 s) = **30 mAs**
75 mAs × 0.4 s = **30 mAs**

15% Rule

The 15% rule is used when an overall change in exposure is needed. The 15% rule uses changes in both kVp and mAs.

When kVp is increased 15% the exposure to the image receptor is increased. Multiply kVp by 1.15 (original kVp = 15%).

$$60 \text{ kVp} \times 1.15 = \mathbf{69\ kVp}$$

If a decrease in exposure is needed, multiply the kVp by 0.85 (original kVp – 15%).

$$60 \text{ kVp} \times 0.85 = \mathbf{51\ kVp}$$

When maintaining exposure, the kVp can be increased by 15% and the mAs must be divided in half.

$$60 \text{ kVp} \times 1.15 = \mathbf{69\ kVp\ and\ \tfrac{1}{2}\ mAs}$$

If kVp is decreased by 15%, the mAs must be doubled or multiplied by 2.

$$60 \text{ kVp} \times 0.85 = \mathbf{51\ kVp\ and\ mAs \times 2}$$

Inverse Square Law

This law is used to determine the intensity of radiation at a distance from the x-ray tube. This formula gives the student practice with inverse relationships.

$$\text{EXAMPLE}: \frac{I_1}{I_2} = \frac{(D_2)^2}{(D_1)^2}$$

The intensity of radiation at a 40-inch distance is 300 mR. What will be the intensity of the radiation if the distance is changed to 72 inches?

$$\frac{300\text{ mR}}{X} = \frac{(72)^2}{(40)^2} \longrightarrow \frac{300\text{ mR}}{X} = \frac{5184}{1600}$$

$$300\text{ mR} \times 1600 = 5184X \longrightarrow 480{,}000 = 5184X$$

$$\frac{480{,}000}{5184} = X \qquad \textbf{Answer: 92.59 mR}$$

mAs/Distance Compensation Formula

The standard SID in radiography is 40 inches; however, there are instances where the SID is increased to 72 inches. It is necessary to use this formula to determine the amount of change in mAs to produce a quality image.

$$\text{EXAMPLE: } \frac{mAs_1}{mAs_2} = \frac{(SID_1)^2}{(SID_2)^2}$$

An exposure was made using 15 mAs at a 40-inch SID. If the SID is increased to 72 inches, what is the adjustment that must be made to the mAs to maintain exposure to the imaging receptor?

$$\frac{15}{X} = \frac{(40)^2}{(72)^2} \longrightarrow \frac{15}{X} = \frac{1600}{5184}$$

$$15 \times 5184 = 1600X \longrightarrow 77{,}760 = 1600X$$

$$\frac{77{,}760}{1600} = X \qquad \textbf{Answer: 48.6 mAs}$$

Chapter Summary

1. Apply the order of operation working in progression from numbers in parenthesis; apply all exponents, multiply or divide, and finish with addition or subtraction.
2. Scientific notation makes calculations easier by using exponents for very large or small numbers.
3. When multiplying an equation with scientific notation, add the exponents. When dividing an equation, subtract the exponents.
4. Radiographic formulas use direct and indirect relationships to determine radiation intensity as well as making changes in exposure factors to maintain the mAs.
5. The inverse square law states that the intensity of the x-ray beam will either increase or decrease corresponding to the inverse square of the distance as it is changed from the source.

Case Study

JoAnn is experimenting on a radiographic phantom with a variety of mAs settings and SID changes. She wants to determine how the changes in distance will affect the mAs required for the subsequent exposures.

Critical Thinking Questions

1. Which radiographic formula will she use to determine the effect of distance on the x-ray beam intensity?
2. When the distanced is changed, how will the mAs be changed to maintain adequate exposure?

Review Questions

Short Answer

1. Solve for X.

$$X = \frac{3(7+2)^2 - 52}{40}$$

2. Convert 5/8 into a decimal.

3. Solve for X.

$$\frac{X}{9} = \frac{33}{8}$$

Convert each using scientific notation.

4. 0.25 =

5. 75,000 =

6. 0.000038 =

7. 287 =

8. 88,000,000 =

Solve using scientific notation.

9. $(3.2 \times 10^{6}) \times (7.2 \times 10^{-3})$

10. $\frac{9.6 \times 10^3}{4.1 \times 10^{-2}}$

Solve using radiographic formulas.

11. 100 ma × 0.25 s =

12. 60 kvp and 6 mAs were used to make an exposure. If the kVp is increased 15%, what is the new kVp? How will mAs change to maintain radiographic density?

13. Solve using the mAs/Distance Compensation Formula.

    Original mAs = 80
    Original SID = 40 inches
    New SID = 72 inches
    New mAs =

14. The intensity of radiation at a 40-inch SID is 300 mR. What is the intensity when distance is increased to 72 inches?

3

Basic Physics for Radiographic Science

Objectives

Upon completion of this chapter, the student will be able to:

1. Differentiate fundamental from derived units of measure.
2. Identify the principles of each of Newton's laws.
3. Discuss the characteristics of matter and energy.
4. Describe various forms of energy.

Key Terms

- inertia
- kinetic energy
- potential energy

Introduction

Understanding physics is essential for the radiographer to produce ionizing radiation in a safe and responsible manner. A guiding principle in radiography is to use the least amount of radiation necessary to produce an optimal diagnostic image. To accomplish this goal, radiographers must establish a foundation of general physics theories and concepts. A firm foundation will assist the student in understanding the production of x-radiation and how it is used in the imaging process.

Units of Measurement

Each day, we use units of measurement often without realizing it. We determine the weight of an object, how far it is to jump, and to determine the time of day. We use measurements to make sure other people understand us. In order for two people to come up with an answer to a given problem, it is necessary for them to use the same units of measurement that society has agreed to use. Having a standard of measurement makes it possible to remove uncertainty when performing experiments and to enhance reproducibility.

Physicists strive for certainty and simplicity when studying the interactions of mass and energy. To remove any uncertainty, they must eliminate the potential for errors to occur when different units of measurements are used. There are three basic quantities called fundamental units of measurement, which are *mass*, *length*, and *time*.

In science, it is necessary for individuals to be able to use measurements that are reproducible. The two systems of measurement are the British system and the *Systems Internationale d'Unites* (SI). The SI system uses kilogram to quantify mass, the meter for length, and the second to measure time. In relation to radiation, the SI system has specific units of radiation. For example, the SI unit for exposure is Coulomb/kilogram (C/kg) and the conventional unit is the Roentgen (R). Chapter 33 goes into depth in describing radiation dose limits for occupational exposure. Table 33-4 is a quick reference for units of radiation, and Table 33-5 lists the NCRP dose limit recommendations.

The three basic quantities of measure are the building blocks for the derived units. Derived units are combinations of one or more of the basic quantities. *Power, work, momentum, force, velocity*, and *acceleration* are the derived units, which are used in the production of x-radiation. In the radiologic sciences, there are special quantities of *exposure, dose, effective dose*, and *radioactivity*. Throughout this text, students will learn the theories and concepts that directly relate the special quantities to clinical practice.

Mass

Mass is the quantity of matter in a body and is not quantified by weight. Weight is the gravitational force placed on a body or object on earth. The weight of an object will change when the gravitational force is changed. Assume an astronaut has 94 kg of matter. On Earth, the astronaut would weigh 207 pounds, but when weighed on the moon, the astronaut's weight would be ~95 pounds. Yet, the astronaut's mass is still 94 kg! This occurs because the moon has a much weaker gravitational force than does the Earth. As you can see, the difference between mass and weight is the location of the body or object (Fig. 3.1).

On the moon:
Weight = 95 lbs
On earth:
Weight = 207 lbs

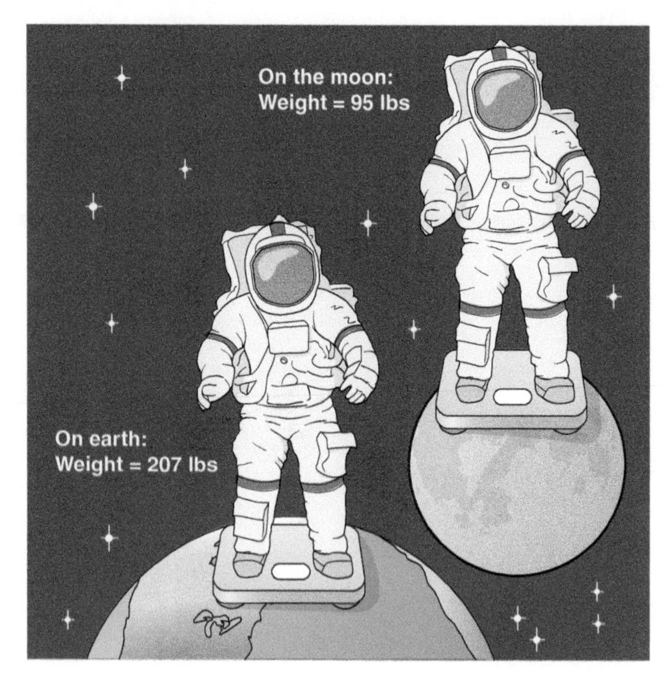

Figure 3.1. **Gravitational force affects the weight of an object on the Earth and the moon. The moon has a much weaker gravitational force than the Earth, which results in the astronaut weighing less on the moon, but the overall mass is unchanged.**

Although the weight of the astronaut changed, the overall mass did not change. The astronaut occupies space and has form regardless of location on earth or the moon; therefore, weight is the gravitational force on a body.

The British unit for weight is the pound, and the SI unit of mass is the kilogram. A kilogram is based on the mass of 1,000 cm^3 of water at 4°C. This is a constant measure that does not change.

Length

Originally, the standard unit of length (the meter) was defined as the distance between two scratches on a bar of platinum that is kept at the International Bureau of

Weights and Measures in Paris, France. The definition was updated in 1960 to reflect a more accurate measurement of the meter. The meter is now defined as the distance light travels in 1/299,792,458 second. The SI unit for length is the meter. The British system uses the foot as the measurement for length.

Time

The standard unit of time is the second (s). Previously, the second was defined in terms of the rotations of the Earth or the mean solar day. Time is now measured by an atomic clock that is based on the vibration of cesium atoms. The atomic clock is accurate to ~1 second in 5,000 years.

Velocity

Two terms are used to describe the motion of an object: velocity and acceleration. Velocity is also called speed and is the measurement of how fast the object is moving. When an object is moving, it changes its position over time, and the rate of the change is called speed. An example is a race car that is speeding around the track. When the driver wants to pass another car, the speed of the car must increase to overtake and pass the other car. In effect, the race car has changed its position on the track. How quickly the change is made will determine the speed of the race car or the distance the race car traveled over time.

Velocity is measured in kilometers per hour (miles per hour). The SI unit for velocity is meters per second (m/s). The equation for velocity is:

$$v = \frac{d}{t}$$

where v, velocity; d, distance traveled; and t, time. The derived quantity of velocity is determined by combining the fundamental quantities of length (d) and time (t).

CRITICAL THINKING BOX 3.1

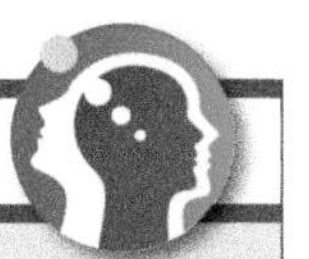

What is the velocity of a ball traveling 40 meters in 2 seconds?

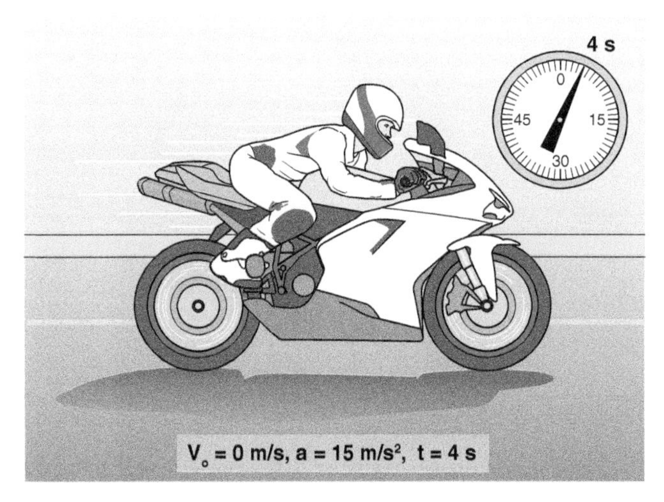

Figure 3.2. **A motorcycle is a common example of the relationships between original velocity, final velocity, and the amount of time required for acceleration to occur.**

Acceleration

Acceleration is the rate of change in velocity over time. When an object is traveling a constant speed, there is no acceleration. To reach the constant speed, the object had to start at zero and begin moving with increasing speed until it reached a final speed or velocity (Fig. 3.2). For example, a motor cycle driver wants to go 60 m/s, but in order to reach that speed, the driver must start at zero and continue accelerating until the final speed of 60 m/s is reached.

Acceleration is determined by subtracting the original velocity from the final velocity then dividing the resultant value by the amount of time used to reach final velocity. The unit of measure is m/s². The equation for acceleration is:

$$a = \frac{V_f - V_0}{t}$$

where V_f is final velocity, V_0 is original velocity, and t is time.

CRITICAL THINKING BOX 3.2

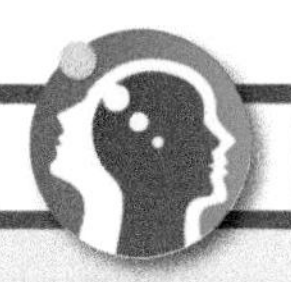

What is the acceleration of a motor cycle if the original velocity is zero, the final velocity is 60 m/s, and the travel time is 4 seconds?

Physical Concepts of Energy

Sir Isaac Newton, an English scientist, developed three principles to explain the laws of motion. Although he presented his work on the laws of motion in 1686, the laws are relevant today as the fundamental laws of motion.

Newton's First Law: Inertia

Newton's first law explains that if an object is not acted upon by an outside force, the object will not move. Objects at rest will remain at rest until the object is pushed, pulled, or acted on by an external force (Fig. 3.3). Objects in motion will stay in motion. The property of an object to resist a change in motion is called **inertia**. For example, a radiographer must use force to move a wheelchair. As long as force is applied, the wheelchair will continue to move until an opposing force or friction is used to slow down or stop the movement of the wheelchair.

Newton's Second Law: Force

To set a resting object in motion, we must push or pull the object. In order for the object to move, we must apply force. When we want to stop an object that is moving, we must apply an opposite force. The question becomes, how much force is needed to move an object? For us to move the object, we must use enough force to overcome the mass of the object. When this happens, the object will start to move and will build speed or it will accelerate (Fig. 3.4). Therefore, force is equal to the mass times acceleration. The SI unit of force is the newton (N).

$$F = ma$$

where F, force; m, mass; and a, acceleration.

CRITICAL THINKING BOX 3.3

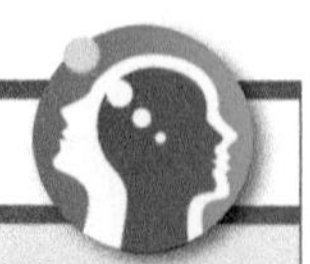

What is the force needed to move a 100-kg object at a rate of 20 m/s^2?

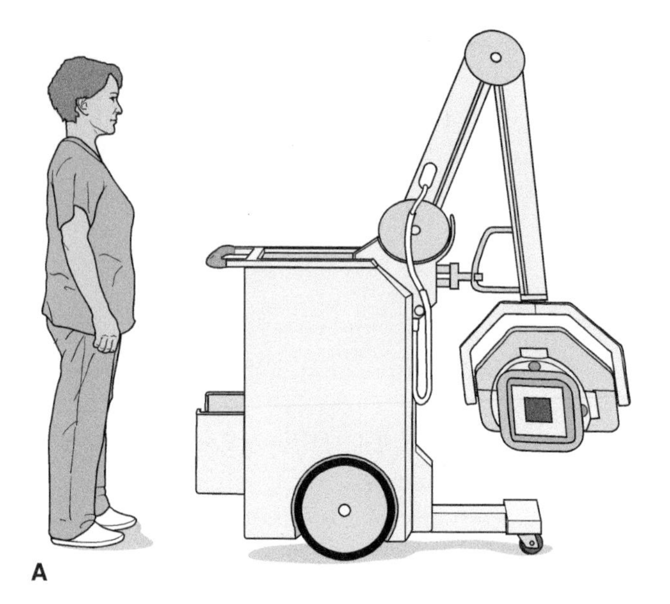

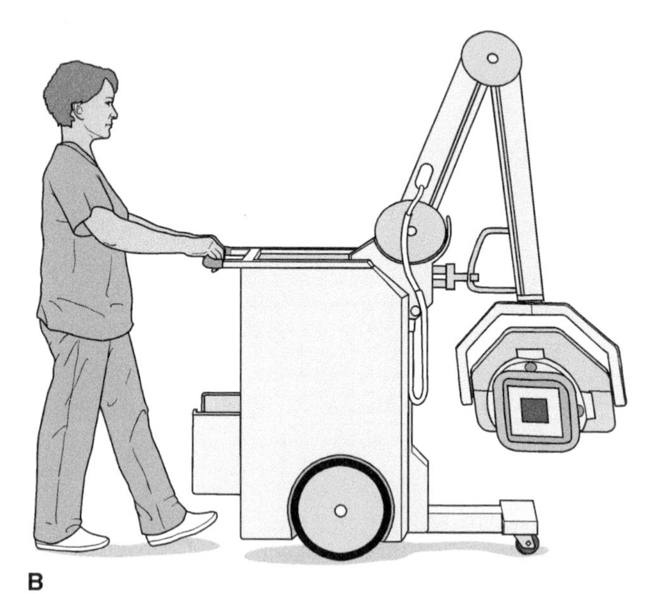

Figure 3.3. Newton's first law states that a body at rest will remain at rest (A), and a body in motion will remain in motion (B) until an outside force acts on the body to cause it to slow down or stop.

Newton's Third Law: Action Equals Reaction

Newton's third law states that for every action, there is an equal and opposite reaction. When force or action is applied to an object, the object pushes back with the same amount of force. A rocket sits on the launch pad; when the launch begins, the rocket pushes on the ground. The ground pushes back with equal but opposite force (Fig. 3.5).

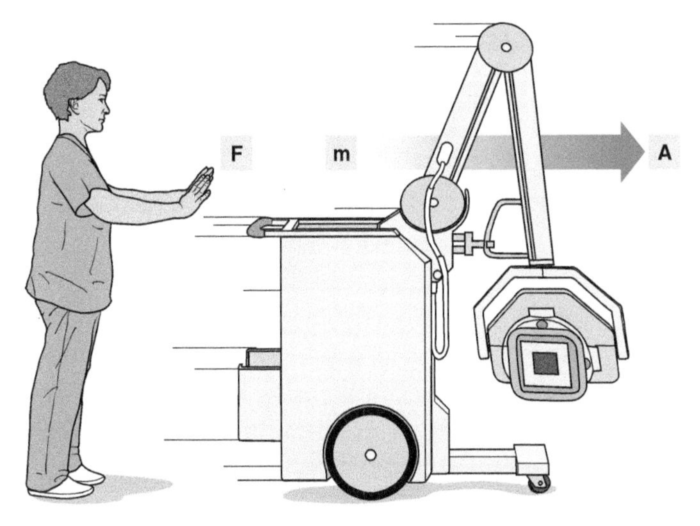

Figure 3.4. Newton's second law states that the force used to move an object must be equal to the mass of the object multiplied by acceleration.

Work

When a force acts on a body over distance, work is done. To lift an object, we must overcome the amount of gravity that is being applied to the object. For example, a cassette is lying on a counter. In order to pick up the cassette, we must use enough force to overcome gravity. The heavier the cassette, the more force we must use to pick up the cassette. As the cassette is lifted, work is being done. Work performed is force multiplied by the distance the object was lifted. If the object is lifted twice the distance, then twice the amount of work must be done. The SI unit for work is the joule (J).

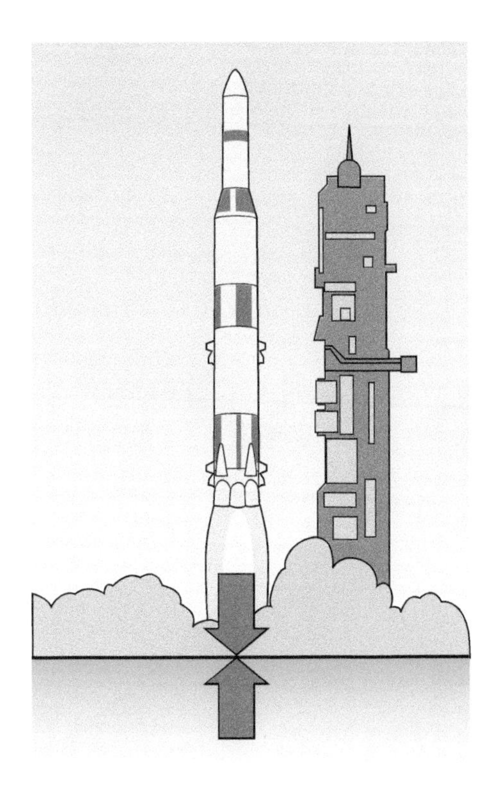

Figure 3.5. Newton's third law states that when an object pushes against an object, an equal reaction will occur. As the rocket takes off, it must push against the earth. The earth pushes back with equal reaction.

$$W = fd$$

where W, work done in joules; f, force in Newtons; and d, distance in meters.

CRITICAL THINKING BOX 3.4

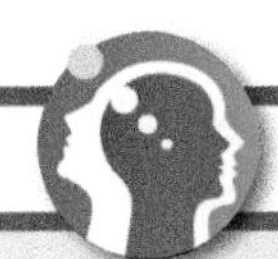

How much work is done when lifting a patient who weighs 222 N (50 lbs) a distance of 2 m? Change distance to 4 m and determine the new amount of work performed.

Energy

The expenditure of energy is the ability to do work. Energy is defined as the actual or potential ability to do work. Work and energy are measured in the same unit, joules, because the amount of work done must equal the amount of energy. There are two forms of mechanical energy: kinetic and potential. The energy is involved in the operation of machines and is relevant to the operation of an x-ray unit.

Every moving body can do work because of its motion. The energy of the moving body is called **kinetic energy**. Kinetic energy is expressed as:

$$KE = \frac{1}{2}mv^2$$

where m is the mass of the body in kg and v is the velocity in meters per second. Therefore, the amount of kinetic energy expended depends on the mass of the object and on the square of the velocity.

CRITICAL THINKING BOX 3.5

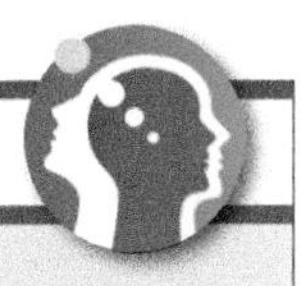

A 2,000-kg van starts to move and reaches a velocity of 15 m/s. Find the kinetic energy of the van.

You may be wondering how kinetic energy is used to produce x-ray photons! Let us look first at the formula. As you can see, velocity is much more important than mass; the energy changes proportionally to the mass, but it increases by the square of the velocity. The projectile electrons from the x-ray tube filament are incredibly tiny objects with very little mass, if the electrons are sped up to extreme velocities, they will be able to impart enough energy to the anode disc to produce x-ray photons.

Potential energy is stored energy. An object may have energy because of its position, which means it has the ability to do work. A parked mobile x-ray unit has stored energy by virtue of its state or position. When the brake is released, the unit will start to move. The movement of the mobile unit reflects that the potential energy in the unit is converted to kinetic energy with the motion of the mobile unit. Common examples of potential energy include a stretched rubber band and a coiled spring. These objects have stored or potential energy, which is waiting to be used. As the stretched rubber band flies through the air, the potential energy is converted to kinetic energy of motion (Fig. 3.6).

Law of Conservation of Energy

In the universe, the amount of energy is constant. It can be converted from one form to another, but it cannot be created or destroyed. Therefore, when energy is converted, it must be converted into an equivalent amount of energy. There are many types of energy in the universe, but we will concentrate of these forms of energy: mechanical, thermal, electrical, chemical, and electromagnetic. Electrical motors convert electrical energy to mechanical energy. Chemical energy converts into electrical energy in batteries, a steam engine converts heat into mechanical energy, and electrical energy is formed by the flow of electricity (Fig. 3.7). Electromagnetic energy is a form of energy that exists as an electric and magnetic disturbance. Each of these forms of energy is used to create the x-ray beam and resultant image.

Albert Einstein defined the universe as a continuum of space and time containing only mass and energy. Everything can be described as matter, energy, or both. Einstein developed this formula to express the relationship between matter and energy:

$$E = mc^2$$

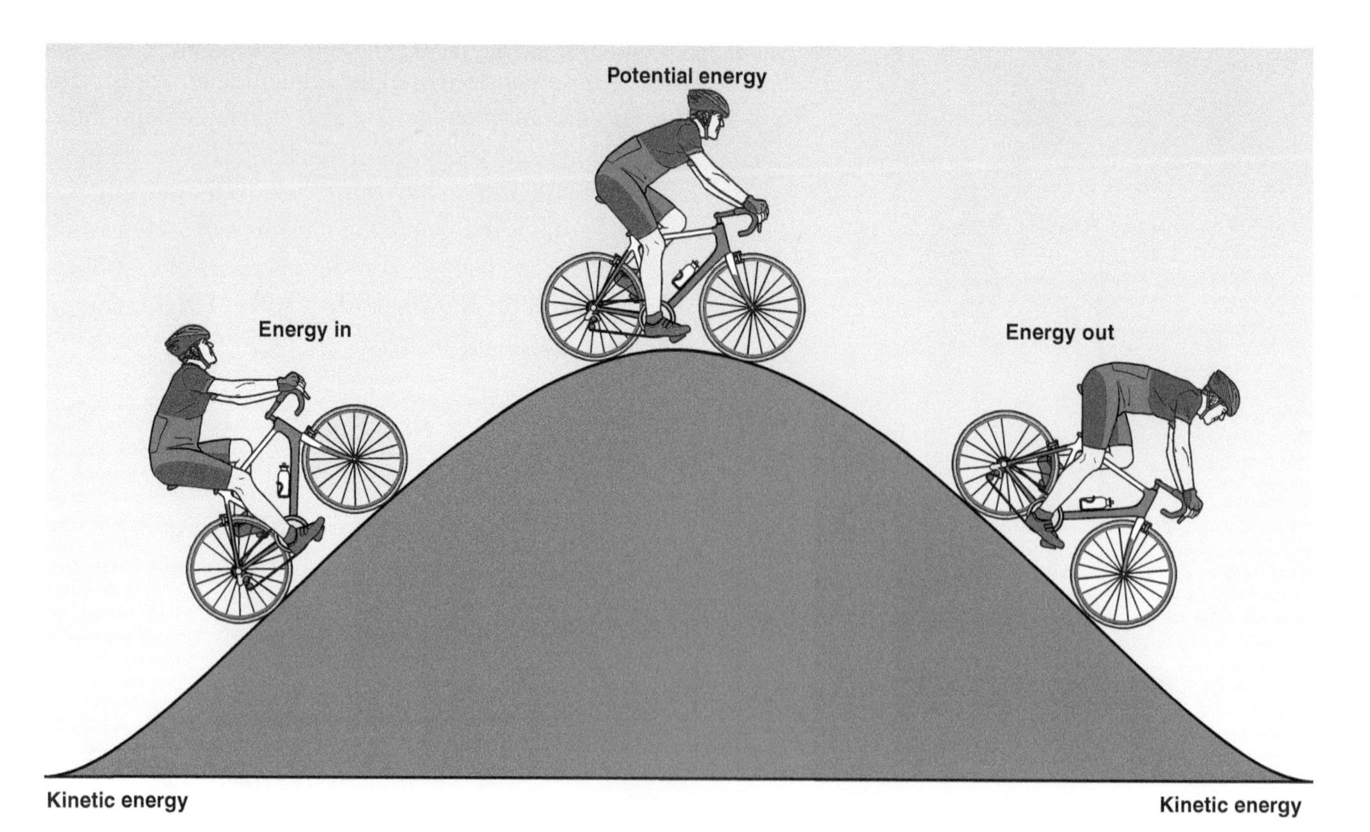

Figure 3.6. Demonstration of the relationship between kinetic and potential energy. Kinetic energy is seen when the bicycle is moving up and down the hill. When the bicycle stops at the top, it has potential energy because it is not moving but has the ability to move.

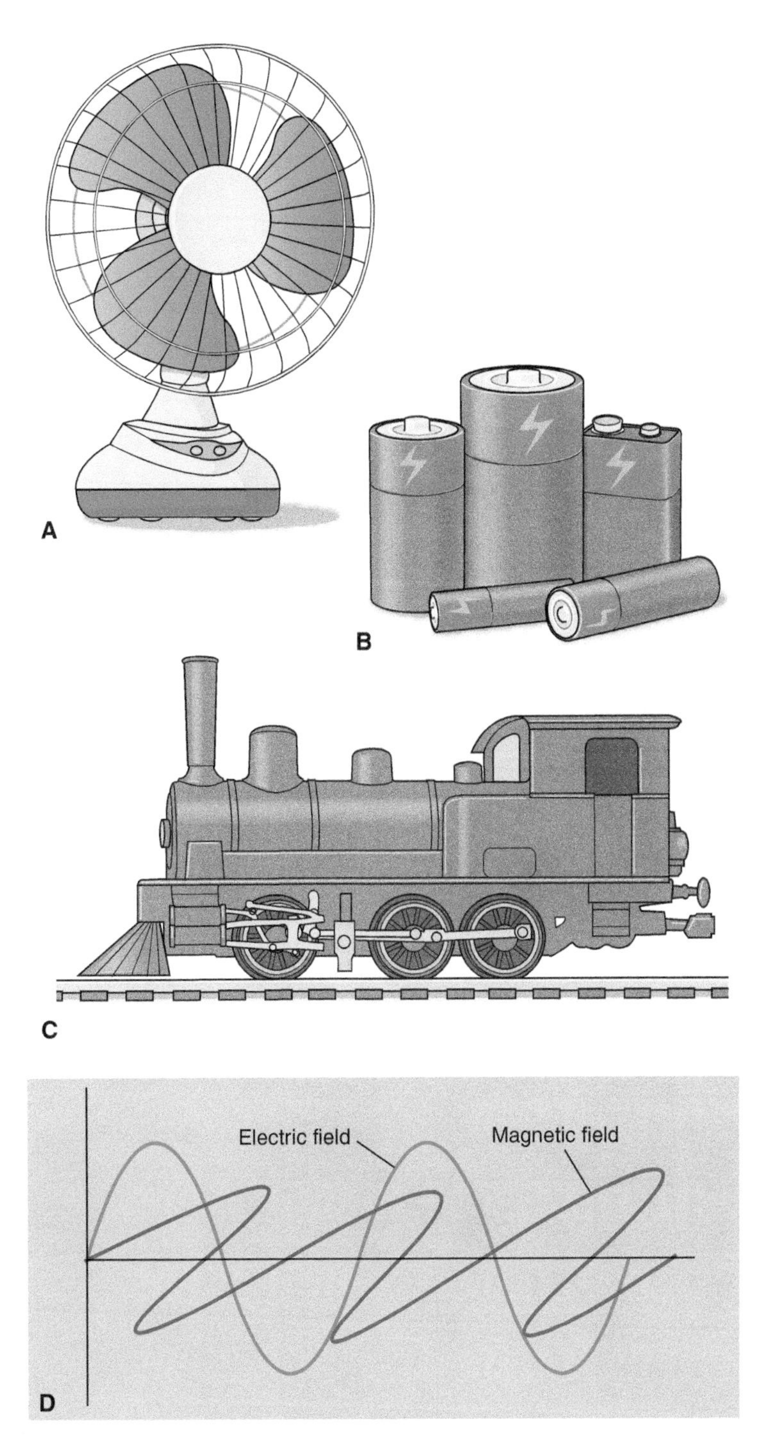

Figure 3.7. **Forms of energy. (A) Electrical to mechanical energy. (B) Chemical to electrical energy. (C) Thermal to mechanical energy. (D) Electromagnetic energy.**

where E, energy in joules; m, mass (the quantity of matter in an object); and c, the constant speed of light in a vacuum. The equation shows that matter can be transformed into energy, and energy can be transformed into matter. The total mass-energy of the universe is always conserved.

Chapter Summary

1. The units of measurement are established as a standard set of measurements that are used to produce consistent results.
2. Radiographers use the theories and concepts of matter and energy when a beam of x-radiation is produced.
3. Mass, length, and time are the fundamental units of measure, which combine to form the derived units of measure.
4. Sir Isaac Newton studied objects to determine how the objects' inertia would be affected by force. From his research, he developed the Laws of Motion.
5. All energy in the universe is constant; it may change forms from one type of energy to another, but it will only be changed and never destroyed.

Case Study

Brandi has the task of explaining kinetic and potential energy to her radiology class. She has researched these two kinds of energy to further her knowledge.

Critical Thinking Questions

1. How is kinetic energy different from potential energy?
2. What is the formula for kinetic energy?
3. When is potential energy converted into kinetic energy?

Review Questions

Multiple Choice

1. A car traveled at a rate of 95 m/s for 3 seconds. What is the acceleration of the car?

a. 3.16
b. 31.6
c. 285
d. 2.85

2. The unit for force is the:

a. joule
b. ohm
c. watt
d. newton

3. How much force is needed to move a 225-lb boulder 50 m/s^2?

a. 1,125
b. 4.5
c. 11,250
d. 45

4. What is the SI unit for mass?

a. Kilogram
b. Cubic meter
c. Pound
d. kg/m^3

5. **The fundamental units of measurement include:**

   a. mass
   b. power
   c. force
   d. momentum

6. **Acceleration occurs when the mass of an object is overcome by sufficient __________.**

   a. work
   b. force
   c. inertia
   d. weight

7. **A radiographer pushes a mobile x-ray unit weighing 1,050 pounds at a rate of 3 m/s^2. How much force was used to move the x-ray unit?**

   a. 315 N
   b. 30.5 N
   c. 3,150 N
   d. 350 N

8. **A radiography student lifts a 10-pound (44.4 N) sandbag 3.5 feet (1.06 m) onto an x-ray table. How much work is performed by the student?**

   a. 47 J
   b. 4.7 J
   c. 35 J
   d. 42 J

9. **Electric motors convert electrical energy converted into __________ energy.**

   a. electromagnetic
   b. chemical
   c. mechanical
   d. thermal

10. **Which law explains the concept that a moving object will continue to move until an outside force is applied in the opposite direction?**

   a. Law of conservation of energy
   b. Newton's first law
   c. Newton's second law
   d. Newton's third law

Short Answer

1. **Explain the relation between mass and weight. Define the unit of mass.**

2. **What is the fundamental unit of length?**

3. **What is the physical concept of work?**

4. **Discuss kinetic energy, and state the equation for kinetic energy. Give the unit for energy.**

4

Atomic Structure

Objectives

Upon completion of this chapter, the student will be able to:

1. Define atomic mass and atomic number.
2. Describe the Bohr model of the atom and its components.
3. Define electron binding energy.
4. Describe the process of ionization.
5. Identify the types of ionizing radiation.

Key Terms

- activity
- alpha particle
- atomic mass number
- atomic mass unit (AMU)
- atomic number
- beta particle
- covalent bonds
- electron binding energy
- half-life
- ion
- ion pair
- ionic bonds
- ionization
- isobars
- isomers
- isotones
- isotopes
- nucleons
- radioactive decay
- radioisotopes

Introduction

An understanding of nuclear and atomic structure together with how nuclei and atoms interact is fundamental to an understanding of how medical imaging uses radiation to produce diagnostic images. Students may be curious about why a thorough understanding of the atom is necessary for their programs of study. Key points to consider are

1. Interactions that occur in the x-ray tube occur at the atomic level. The resultant x-ray photons depend on how an electron interacts with an atom.
2. Interactions between an x-ray photon and human tissue also occur at the atomic level. This determines the dose delivered to the cells in the tissue.
3. When the x-ray photon exits the patient, it must interact with the image receptor at the atomic level. This interaction creates the x-ray image.

The basic principles of atomic structure are core concepts used throughout medical imaging. In this chapter, we discuss the fundamental units of radiation and how atomic structure and the ionization of atoms affect the formation of the radiographic image.

Atomic Models

thePoint® *An animation for this topic can be viewed at http://thepoint.lww.com/Orth2e*

Over several thousand years, scientists have studied the structure of matter. The Greeks studied the structure of matter several hundred years BC. They believed that there were four types of matter: air, earth, fire, and water and that all matter was a combination of these four types but in various proportions. The Greek term atom means "indivisible" and was used to describe the smallest part of matter that has the properties of an element. Over hundreds of years, many scientists discovered the electrical nature of the structure of the atom. In the early 1920s, scientists knew that atoms contained electrons and were electrically neutral. The Bohr model describes the atom as a central dense positive nucleus surrounded by electrons moving around the nucleus. The Bohr model more accurately describes the experimental observations and so is widely accepted today.

The major problem with the Bohr model was that the negative electrons would be strongly attracted into the positive nucleus resulting in the collapse of the atom. Bohr said that in an atom, electrons could only exist in shells or orbits around the nucleus and were forbidden to exist anywhere else. Although the Bohr model has been radically revised, his early model of the atom adequately describes the relationship of the nucleus of the atom to the orbital shells.

Figure 4.1 illustrates the essential features of the Bohr model of the atom. In the Bohr model, electrons move in orbits or shells around a dense central nucleus. The electrons are negative, and the nucleus is positive.

Matter

Matter has shape and form, occupies space, and has mass or inertia. In nature, matter is commonly found as a mixture of two or more substances. A mixture is in an impure form of indefinite composition. An example is rock salt; it is a mixture of certain minerals in a variety of combinations, which creates the various appearances of rock salt. A substance is defined as a material that has a definite, constant composition. Pure salt, sodium chloride, is an example of a substance. Substances may be either simple or complex. Simple substances, known as elements, cannot be broken down into by chemical means.

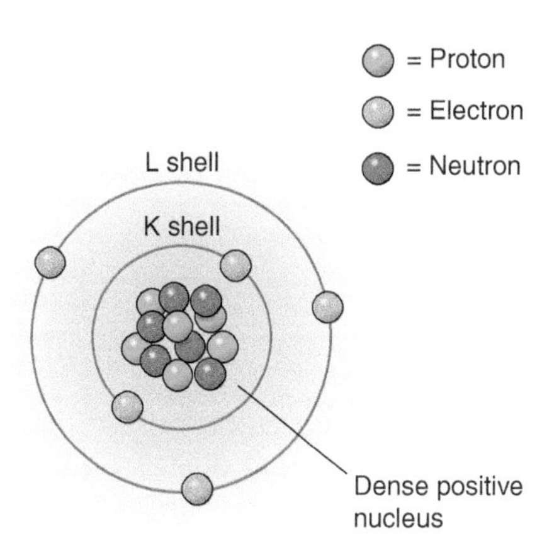

Figure 4.1. **Bohr model.**

The periodic table of elements lists 92 naturally occurring elements. When two or more elements are combined, a complex substance or compound is formed. A well-known example of a compound is salt. When an equal proportion of the element sodium (Na) is combined with the element chlorine (Cl), the two elements are held together by a strong electrochemical force called a bond. The bond forms a molecule of salt. If the salt molecule were to be broken into increasingly smaller particles, the salt molecule would still contain the same two elements. A molecule cannot be broken down by ordinary physical means like crushing because the salt molecule is made of two atoms. Even the smallest particle of salt has the same properties; therefore, each molecule of salt consists of an atom of sodium and an atom of chlorine. Atoms are the fundamental building blocks of nature, which can combine to form elements. Atoms are incredibly small but can be seen with electron microscopes. Although molecules cannot be broken down physically, they can be broken by electrical means into simple substances—elements.

Atomic Nucleus

At the center of the atom, the nucleus contains nuclear particles called nucleons. **Nucleons** are either protons or neutrons. Protons have a single positive charge and a mass of 1.673×10^{-27} kg. Neutrons are electrically neutral and have zero charge. The mass of a neutron is 1.675×10^{-2} kg. Essentially, the proton and neutron have almost the same mass, but the neutron is slightly larger. The nucleons make up the majority of the mass of an atom. Revolving around the nucleus of the atom are the orbital electrons. The electrons carry a negative charge and have a mass of 9.1×10^{-31} kg. The electrons revolve around the nucleus in fixed orbits like the solar system has planets that orbit the sun.

Atoms are considered neutral in charge when the number of protons equals the number of orbital electrons. The hydrogen atom has one proton and one electron, which make it electrically neutral. In this configuration, the atom is chemically stable.

Electron Shells

Electrons in an atom move around the nucleus in specific orbits or shells. The number of shells occupied in a particular atom depends on how many protons are there in the nucleus. There is a limit to the number of electrons that can occupy each shell. The shell closest to the nucleus is called the K shell and can hold no more than two electrons. If an atom has more than two protons within the nucleus, the additional electrons are located in shells further from the nucleus. Atoms with more protons in the nucleus have more electrons in the surrounding shells. The number of electrons in the shells must equal the number of protons in the nucleus of a neutral atom.

The shells are identified by shell number or letters of the alphabet: the closest shell to the nucleus is No. 1 and is called the K shell, the No. 2 shell is called the L shell, and so on to shell No. 7, the Q shell, in order of increasing distance from the nucleus. The order of the shell is important because the shell number designates the maximum number of electrons the shell can hold.

The maximum number of electrons that can be contained in a shell is given by the equation:

$$\text{Maximum number} = 2n^2$$

where n is the shell number. For shell number 3, called the M shell, the maximum number of electrons that can occupy the shell is 18 (Table 4.1).

TABLE 4.1 ATOMIC ELECTRON SHELLS

Shell Letter	Shell Number	Maximum Electron Number
K	1	2
L	2	8
M	3	18
N	4	32
O	5	50
P	6	72
Q	7	98

$$\begin{aligned}\text{Maximum number} &= 2[3]^2\\ &= 2\times 9\\ &= 18 \text{ electrons}\end{aligned}$$

Figure 4.2 illustrates the hell structure for hydrogen, carbon, and sodium. Hydrogen has a single electron in its shell. Carbon has six protons in the nucleus. It has two electrons in the K shell and four electrons in the L shell. Sodium has eleven electrons contained in three shells, two in the K shell, eight in the L shell, and one in the M shell.

Even though the maximum number of electrons that a shell can hold is $2n^2$, there is another rule that may override the maximum number. That overriding rule is the octet rule, which states that the outer shell of a chemically stable atom will only contain eight electrons or an octet of electrons.

Electron Binding Energy

Electron binding energy describes how tightly the electron is held in its shell. The negative electron is attracted to the positive nucleus by electrostatic forces. Electrons in shells closer to the nucleus have a stronger attraction. The electron binding energy is the energy required to remove the electron from its shell and is measured in a unit called an electron volt (eV). An eV is a very small unit of energy. Electron binding energies can be as small as a few electron volts or as large as thousands of electron volts.

The binding energy of electrons decreases as the orbital shells get farther away from the nucleus. The K shell always has the highest binding energy because its electrons are closest to the nucleus, and the Q shell has the lowest binding energy because it is farthest from the nucleus. Therefore, it takes less energy to remove a Q-shell orbital electron than a K-shell orbital electron. Atoms with fewer protons in the nucleus have lower binding energies, while atoms with more protons in the nucleus have higher binding energies. The difference in binding energies is because atoms with more protons have an increased positive charge. This means that electrons in atoms of high atomic number elements are bound more tightly than electrons in lower atomic number elements (Fig. 4.3). The binding energy of K-shell electrons in lead is much higher than the binding energy of K-shell electrons of hydrogen.

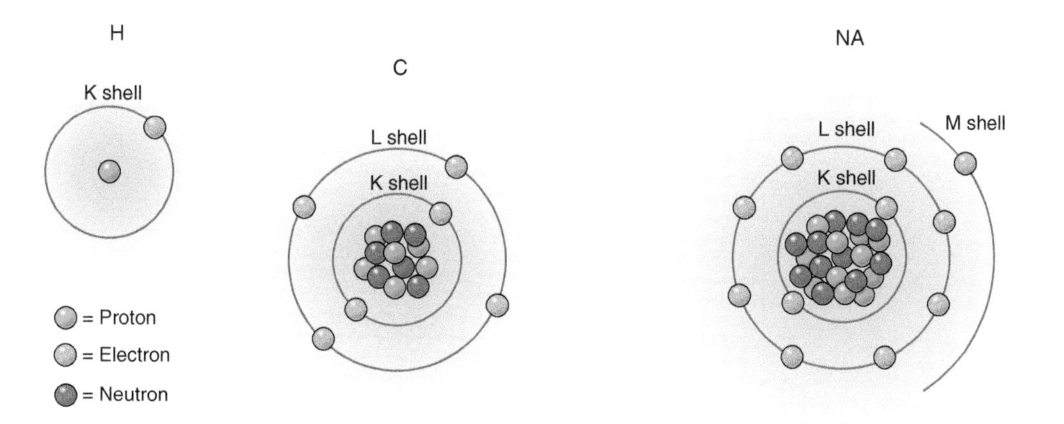

Figure 4.2. Electron shell structure of hydrogen, calcium, and sodium.(H) The electron shell structure of hydrogen (Z = 1). (C) Electron shell for carbon (Z = 6). (NA) Electron shell for sodium (Z = 11).

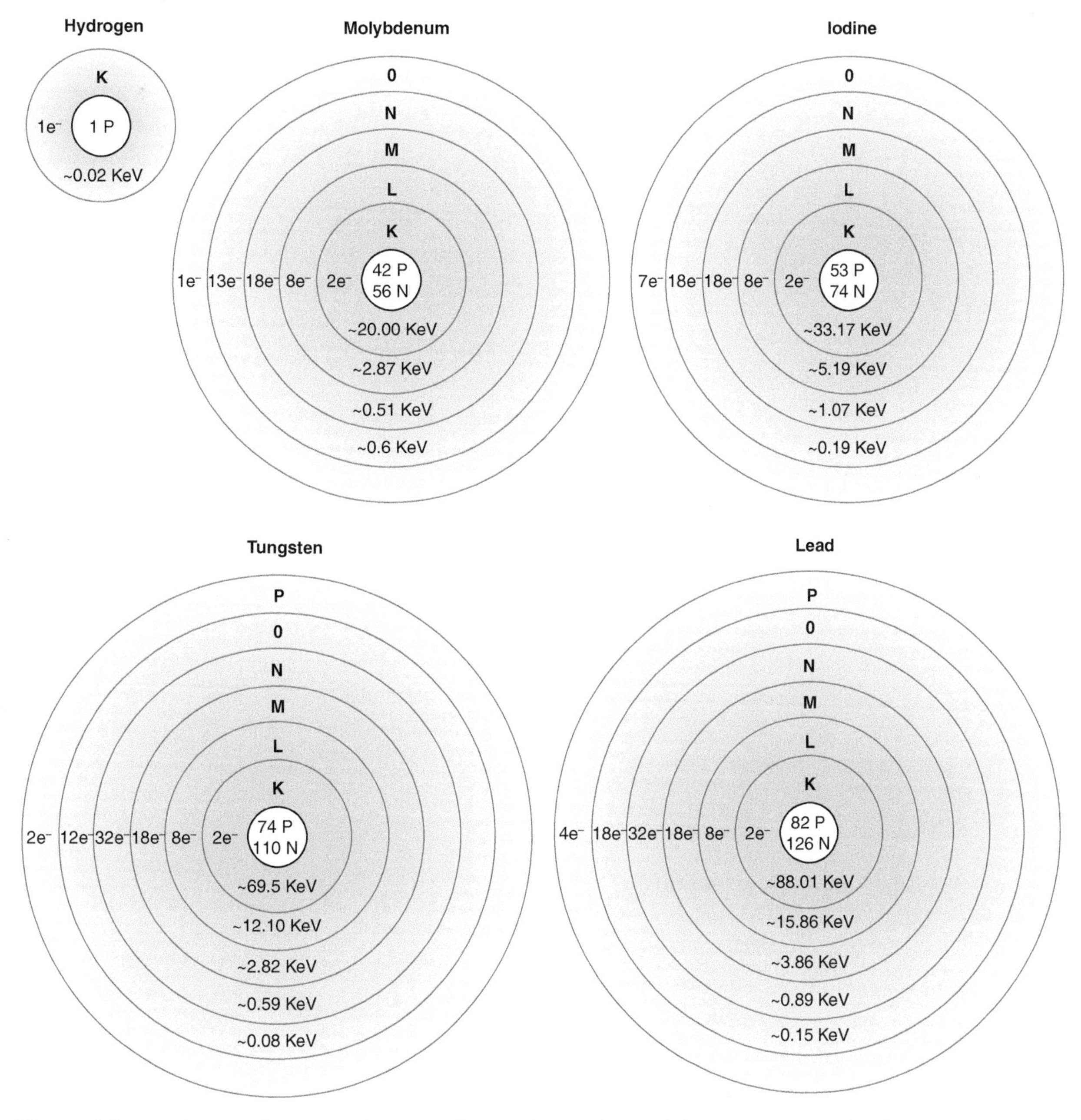

Figure 4.3. Binding shell energy. Electrons close to the nucleus will have the greatest binding energy.

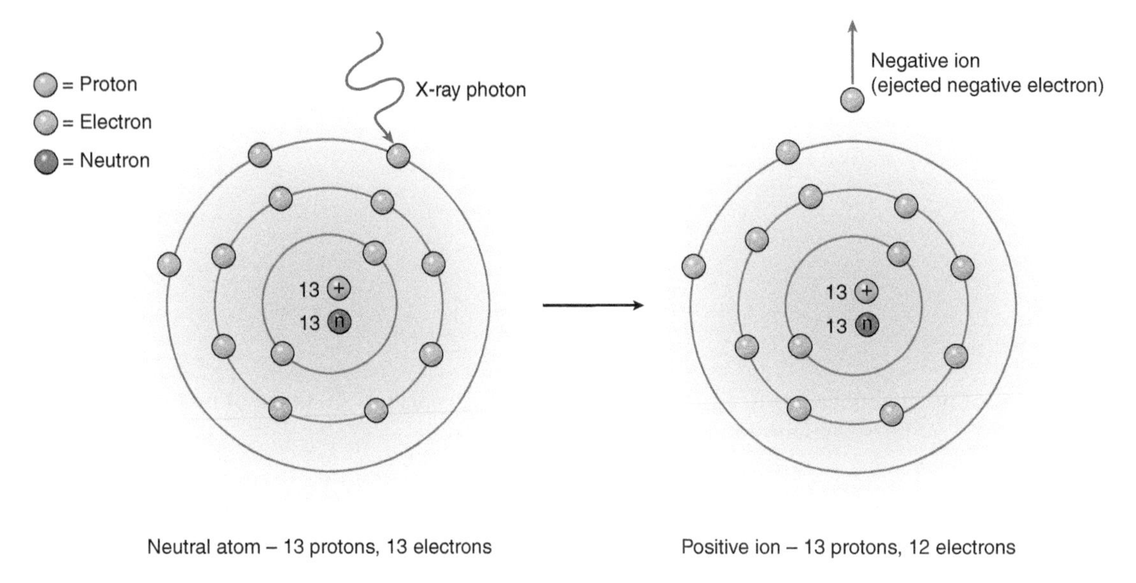

Figure 4.4. **Ion pair.**

Ionization

Ionization is the process of adding or removing an electron from its shell in the atom. When an electron is removed from an atom or when an electron is added to an atom, the atom becomes electrically charged and is called an **ion**. Therefore, if an electron is added, the atom is a negative ion because the atom has a higher negative charge, and if an electron is removed, the atom is a positive ion because it has a higher positive charge. Figure 4.4 shows the formation of a positive and a negative ion, also termed an **ion pair**. The energy available to form the positive and negative ions must be sufficient to overcome the binding energy of the orbital electron or ionization cannot occur. Ionization always results in the formation of a positive ion and a negative ion. Ions can expose film, activate radiation detectors, and produce biological effects.

Atoms

Now that you have an understanding of the components of an atom, we will discuss the characteristics that determine the placement of an element on the periodic table.

Atomic Mass

Because the proton and neutron masses are so small, the **atomic mass unit** (**AMU**) is used to describe the mass of an atom instead of the kilogram. The proton and neutron weigh almost exactly 1 AMU. The electron is about 2,000 times lighter than the nucleons. Table 4.2 gives the atomic mass in kilograms and in AMU along with the charge of the electron, the proton, and the neutron.

The **atomic mass number** is the mass of the atom in AMU. It is the sum of the protons and neutrons in the nucleus. The mass of the orbital electrons in an atom is so small that their contribution to the atomic mass is usually ignored. The atomic mass number is symbolized by "A." The atomic mass number is written above and to the left of the chemical symbol.

Atomic Number

The **atomic number** is equal to the number of protons in the nucleus. The atomic number is distinct for each element, and because of the arrangement of orbital electrons, the atom has distinct chemical properties that are different from those of other elements. The atomic number is symbolized by "Z." The symbol for carbon with six protons and six neutrons is ${}^{12}_{6}C$ (Fig. 4.5). The atomic number, Z, is always smaller than the atomic mass number A except for hydrogen

TABLE 4.2 ATOMIC MASS AND CHARGE

Particle	Mass in Kilograms	Mass in AMU	Charge
Proton	1.6726×10^{-27} kg	1	+1 (positive)
Neutron	1.6749×10^{-27} kg	1	0 (neutral)
Electron	9.109×10^{-31} kg	0	–1 (negative)

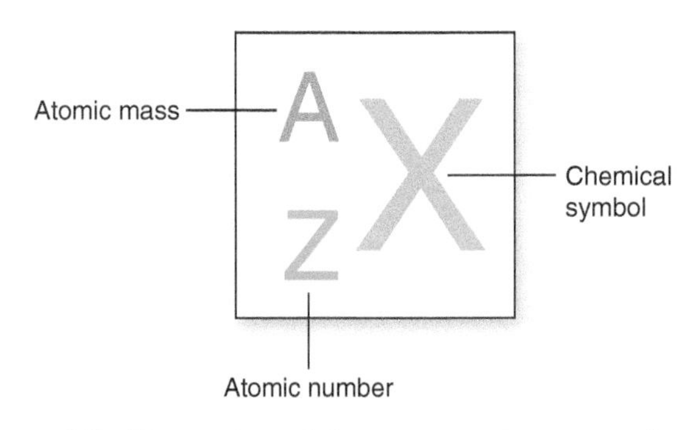

Figure 4.5. **Expression of element atomic mass and atomic number.**

where A and Z are equal. Table 4.3 gives the chemical symbol, atomic mass in AMU, atomic number, and K-shell binding energies of some elements of interest in radiology. Larger atoms with higher atomic numbers and larger atomic mass numbers have higher binding energies. The density and atomic numbers are important in radiographic imaging because elements with higher densities and higher atomic numbers are more effective in attenuating x-rays.

Periodic Table

The periodic table of elements lists the elements in ascending order of atomic number.

In the periodic table, the atomic number is located above the chemical symbol, and the atomic weight is listed below the symbol. The atomic weight shown on the periodic table is an average of the different isotope masses and is usually not a whole number. The chemical symbol for calcium is "Ca." Its atomic number is 20, and its atomic weight is 40.08 AMU.

Figure 4.6 presents the periodic table. The periodic table is arranged with elements where similar chemical characteristics lie underneath one another in a column, called a *group*, representing an increasing Z number as the table is read left-to-right. Fluorine, chlorine, bromine, and iodine all have similar chemical properties. That is, when combined with hydrogen, acids form, and when combined with sodium, salts form. Each row includes elements with the same number of orbital shells and is called a *period.*

The periodic table gets its name from the fact that the chemical properties of the elements are repeated periodically. The simplest element is hydrogen and has an atomic number of 1. The next heavier element is helium, a light inert gas with an atomic number of 2 and an atomic mass of 4. The first row or horizontal period of the periodic table is unusual because it contains only two elements. The first element in the second row is lithium. Lithium has an atomic number of 3 and has one electron in the L shell. This lone electron in the outer shell makes lithium chemically reactive. Each row in the periodic table ends with an inert nonreactive gas. They are inert because their outer electron shell is filled with eight electrons and thus has no need to combine with other atoms.

If the atomic number is increased by 1, the number of electrons in the outer shells also increases by 1 because atoms in nature are electrically neutral. Elements in

TABLE 4.3 **ELEMENTS OF INTEREST IN RADIOLOGY**

Element	Symbol	Atomic Mass (A)	Atomic Number (Z)	K-Shell Binding Energy (keV)
Hydrogen	$^{1}_{1}H$	1	1	0.014
Carbon	$^{12}_{6}C$	12	6	0.28
Nitrogen	$^{14}_{7}N$	14	7	0.40
Oxygen	$^{16}_{8}O$	16	8	0.5
Aluminum	$^{27}_{13}Al$	27	13	1.56
Calcium	$^{40}_{20}Ca$	40	20	4.04
Molybdenum	$^{98}_{42}Mo$	98	42	20.0
Iodine	$^{127}_{53}I$	127	53	33.2
Barium	$^{137}_{56}Ba$	13	56	37.4
Tungsten	$^{184}_{74}W$	184	74	69.065
Lead	$^{207}_{82}Pb$	207	82	88.0
Uranium	$^{238}_{92}U$	238	92	115.6

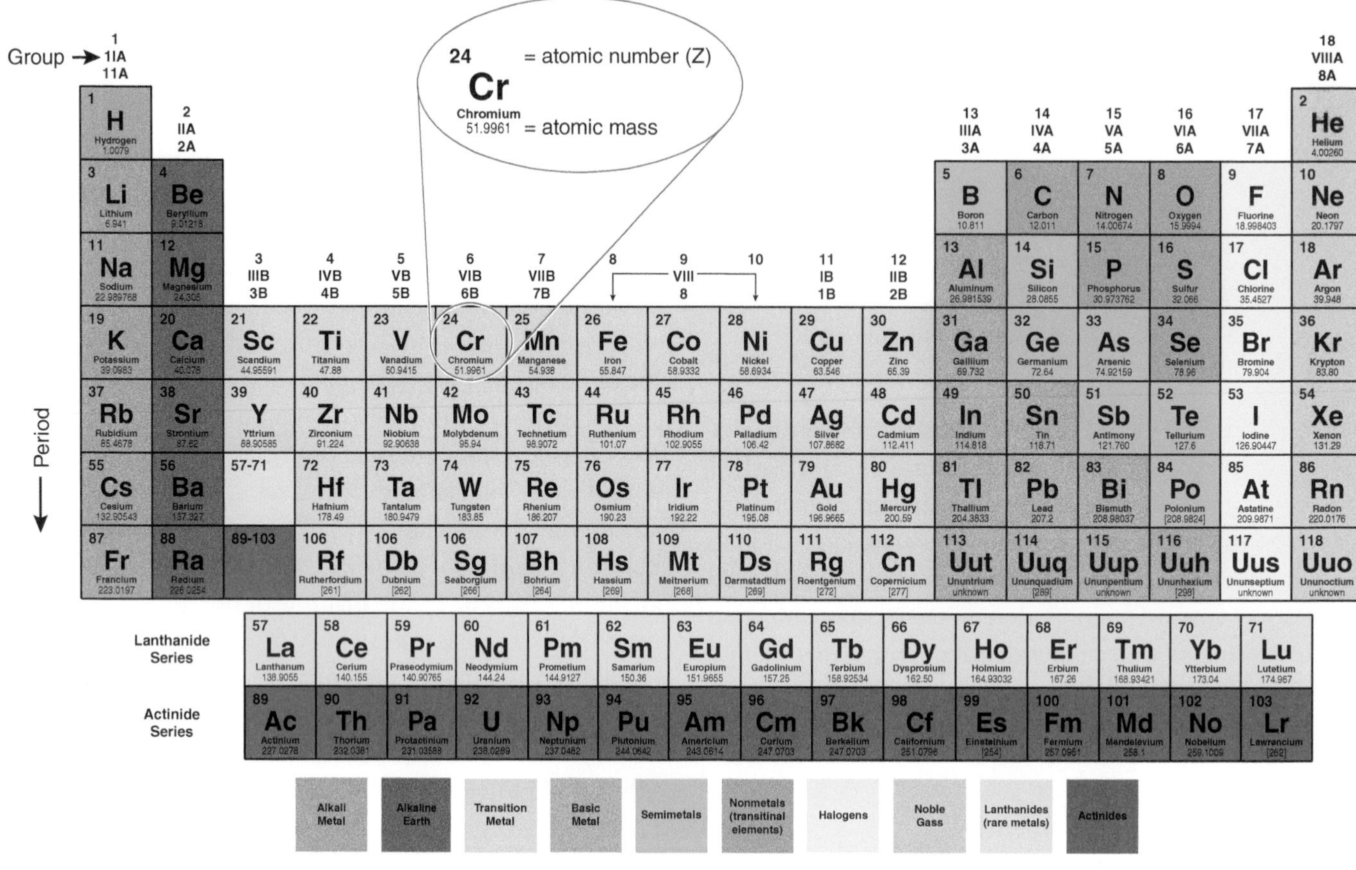

Figure 4.6. **Periodic table.**

vertical groups in the periodic table have the same number of electrons in their outer shell. Their chemical characteristics are similar because the chemical characteristics are determined by the number of electrons in the outer shell.

The number of electrons in the outer shell determines the atoms combining ability or valence. The family of elements represented by sodium, potassium, and rubidium has one electron in the outer shell, and the valence is +1. Each of these elements has a single electron in the outer shell and has chemical characteristics similar to lithium.

Combining Atoms

Up to this point, we have been discussing atoms as singular objects, but as the building blocks of all matter, the atoms must combine in various configurations. How do the atoms become combined, and how do they stay connected to each other? The atoms are combined through chemical bonds, which result in complex matter, like human tissue, to exist. In a previous section, we discussed how molecules are two or more elements that are held together with a strong chemical bond; H"squared"O is a prime example of a molecule. The chemical bonds occur in two primary ways to form complex structures, ionic and covalent bonds.

Ionic bonds occur when two oppositely charged ions are attracted to each other. In order for ionic bonding to happen, an atom must have the ability to either accept an additional electron or to give up an orbital electron to another atom. Remember that an atom that gives up an electron becomes a positively charged ion, while an atom that accepts an electron becomes a negatively charged ion. These charged ions are then attracted to one another and share an orbital electron as seen in Figure 4.7.

Ionic bond. Notice how the positively charged atom is attracted to the negatively charged atom. The two atoms form a chemical bond, which holds them together to form a molecule.

Covalent bonds are based on two atoms sharing an orbital electron, which orbits both atoms. Because the innermost electron shells have a stronger binding energy, the outer shell electrons are more loosely bound to the nucleus, which allows for the electrons to orbit

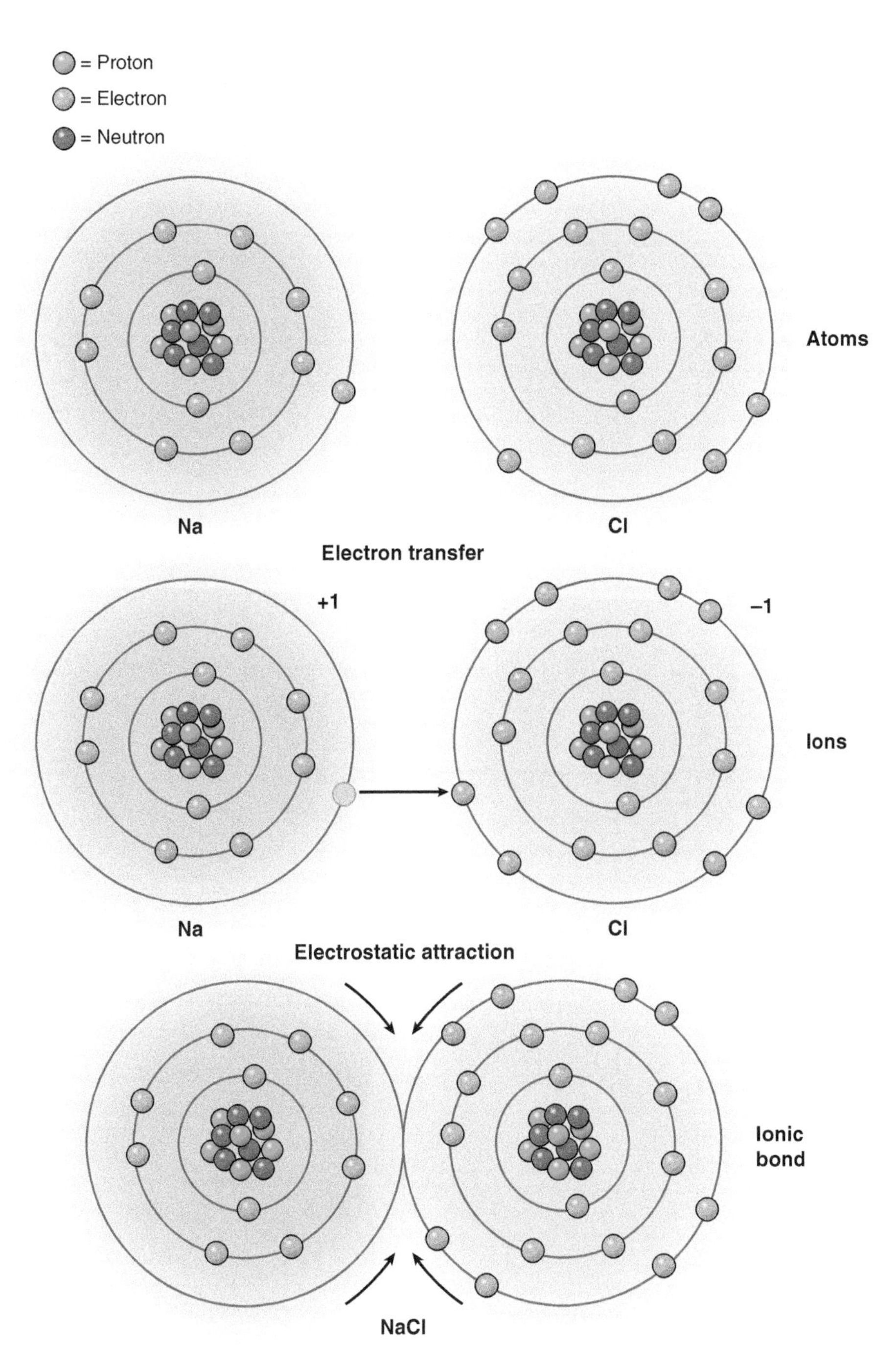

Figure 4.7. Ionic bond.

other atoms. In the covalent bond, the orbital electron first orbits one atom and then orbits the other atom effectively sharing the electron. When two atoms are combined with a covalent bond, the electron orbits in a figure 8 pattern by first orbiting one atom and then the other (Fig. 4.8).

The bonding of various atoms forms molecules, which build complex matter or simple fluids like water. Bonding of atoms is crucial to the existence of plants, animals, and humans.

Atomic Configuration

With the knowledge of atomic mass and atomic number, we will now discuss elements that have been changed and are called the *isos*. This term refers to isotopes, isotones, isobars, and isomers and how each is classified based on the number of protons, neutrons, and electrons. Many elements are composed of atoms with different atomic mass numbers and different atomic masses but identical atomic numbers. The characteristic mass of an element

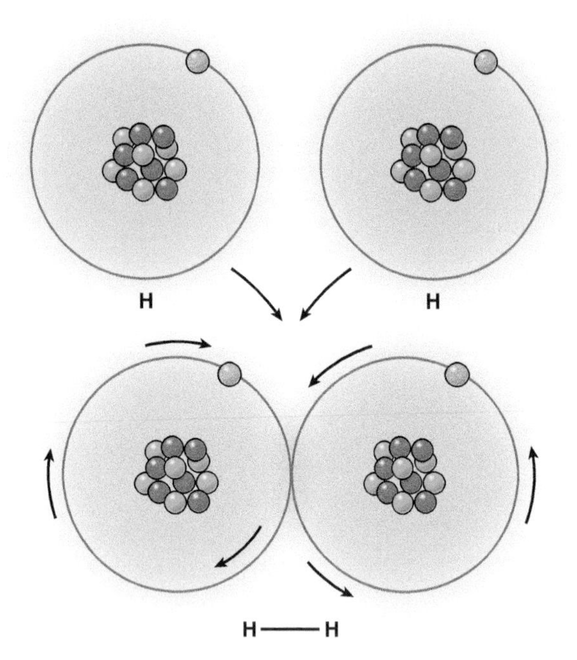

Figure 4.8. **Covalent bond.**

is determined by the number of isotopes and their respective atomic masses.

Atoms of the same element whose nuclei contain the same number of protons but a different number of neutrons are called **isotopes**. Such atoms have different mass numbers. Isotopes have the same chemical characteristics because they all have the same number of outer shell electrons. Most elements have many stable isotopes with varying nuclear configurations, yet the atoms react the same chemically. Calcium has an atomic number (Z) of 20 protons. Naturally occurring calcium consists of seven different isotopes with atomic mass of 40, 42, 43, 44, 46, and 48.

The seven isotopes of calcium are written as:
^{40}Ca, ^{42}Ca, ^{43}Ca, ^{44}Ca, ^{46}Ca, ^{48}Ca

CRITICAL THINKING BOX 4.1

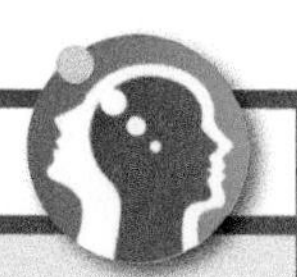

How many protons and neutrons are in each of the isotopes of calcium?

Table 4.4 shows some of the different isotopes of calcium.

Isotones are two elements that have the same number of neutrons and a different number of protons; Chlorine-37 and Potassium-39 both have 20 neutrons but different number of protons. **Isobars** refers to elements whose atoms have the same atomic mass number but a different number of protons but the same total number of nucleons, $_{26}Fe^{58}$ and $_{27}Ni^{58}$ are examples of isobars. The **isomers** are elements with atoms whose number of protons and neutrons are identical but each atom has a different arrangement of the nucleons; this arrangement accounts for the energy differences in the isomers. An example of isomers is technetium-99m (Tc^{99m}) which decays to technetium-99 with the emission of a 140 keV gamma ray. This emission process is very commonly used in nuclear medicine.

To make it easier to remember, the definition focuses on one specific letter in each word: isotope, the p reminds you that the protons stay the same; isotone, the number of neutrons stays the same; isobar, reminds us that the atomic mass number stays the same; and isomer; everything stays the same meaning the number of nucleons has not changed but the energy of each is different.

Radioisotopes

Most isotopes are stable, but some are unstable and spontaneously transform into a different element. Unstable isotopes are termed **radioisotopes** or radioactive isotopes.

TABLE 4.4 **ISOTOPES OF CALCIUM**

Isotope	Atomic Mass (A)	Number of Protons	Number of Neutrons	Abundance %
$^{40}_{20}Ca$	40	20	20	96.941
$^{42}_{20}Ca$	42	20	22	0.647
$^{43}_{20}Ca$	43	20	23	135
$^{44}_{20}Ca$	44	20	24	2.086
$^{46}_{20}Ca$	46	20	26	0.004
$^{48}_{20}Ca$	48	20	28	0.187

Their nuclei have either a deficiency or an excess number of neutrons. Radioactivity is the spontaneous transformation of one element into another element and is accompanied by the release of electromagnetic or particulate radiation. The atomic number of radioactive nuclei changes during the nuclear transformation. The transformation of radioactive nuclei into a different element is also termed radioactive decay. The unit of **activity** is the Becquerel, which is one disintegration per second. The older, conventional unit is the Curie. 1 Ci = 3.7×10^{10} disintegrations per second.

Half-Life

The **half-life** of a radioisotope is the time required to decay one half of the activity of the radioisotope. The half-life depends on the radioisotope. For example, ^{39}Ca has a half-life of 0.8 seconds, the half-life of ^{41}Ca is 8×10^4 years, and the half-life of ^{45}Ca is 2.7 minutes. A sample with an initial activity of 100 mCi of ^{39}Ca will have an activity after time *T* as shown in Table 4.5.

Radioactive Decay

A radioisotope can release different forms of ionizing radiation, which can be either electromagnetic or particulate radiation. X-rays and gamma rays are forms of electromagnetic radiation and differ only in their source or origin. Alpha particles and beta particles are forms of particulate radiation. Gamma rays are the most penetrating of the radiations from **radioactive decay**.

TABLE 4.5 CA-39 RADIOACTIVITY REMAINING AFTER TIME *T*

Time (s)	Number of Half-Lives	Remaining Radioactivity %
0	0	100
0.8	1	50
1.6	2	25
2.4	3	12.5
3.2	4	6.25
4.0	5	3.13

Most radioisotopes emit gamma rays. Gamma rays and x-rays are both electromagnetic radiations and are often called photons. Gamma rays are produced in the nucleus and are useful in nuclear medicine examinations. X-rays are produced through interactions in atomic shells. X-rays are important in radiography because their energy and quantity can be controlled. Due to their low ionization rate in tissue, x-rays are useful for medical imaging procedures.

Alpha Particles

An **alpha particle** is a form of particulate radiation that consists of two protons and two neutrons. It has an atomic mass of 4 and an atomic number of 2. It is identical to the nucleus of a helium atom. Alpha particles are emitted from the nuclei of very heavy elements when they undergo radioactive decay. The alpha particle is very large compared to other types of radiation, but is not very penetrating. They cannot even penetrate the outer skin layer. Because of its size, the alpha particle only travels a short range in matter, only a few millimeters. Alpha particles have no applications in diagnostic radiology.

Beta Particles

A **beta particle** is identical to an electron except for its origin. It has a single negative charge and a mass of 1/2,000 AMU. During beta emission, an electron created in the nucleus is ejected from the nucleus with a considerable amount of kinetic energy and leaves the atom. This results in the loss of a small quantity of mass and one unit of negative electrical charge from the nucleus. At the same time, a neutron converts into a proton. The result is an increase in the atomic number by one, while the atomic mass number stays constant. The nuclear transformation results in the changing of an atom from one type of element into another element.

The beta particle is more penetrating than an alpha particle but less penetrating than a gamma ray or an x-ray. The beta particle can penetrate through several millimeters of tissue. Beta particles are encountered in nuclear medicine applications.

Chapter Summary

1. The Bohr model of the atom consists of a dense positive nucleus surrounded by electrons in shells. The nucleus contains nucleons, which are either protons or neutrons. The proton has a positive charge and an atomic mass of 1 AMU. The neutron has zero charge and an atomic mass of 1 AMU. The atomic number (Z) is equal to the number of protons in the nucleus. The atomic mass (A) is equal to the sum of the neutrons and protons in the nucleus. The electron has a negative charge and a mass of almost zero.
2. Electrons in an atom move in specific orbits. Each orbit or shell has its own binding energy. The binding energy is the energy required to remove an electron from its shell. The shells closer to the nucleus have higher binding energies.
3. Ionization occurs when an electron is removed from an atom. This results in an ion pair made up of one positive and one negative ion. Ionizing radiation consists of electromagnetic and particulate radiations with enough energy to ionize atoms. X-rays and gamma rays are forms of electromagnetic radiation. Alpha and beta radiations are forms of particulate radiation.
4. Elements with similar electron shell structures have similar chemical properties. Isotopes are elements with the same atomic number but different atomic masses. Isotopes have the same chemical properties. The atomic weight of an element is the average of the atomic masses of naturally occurring isotopes.
5. When elements are arranged in order of increasing atomic number, they form the periodic table of elements. The chemical characteristics of the elements are repeated periodically, and elements that lie in the same column of the periodic table have similar chemical properties.
6. Radioisotopes undergo spontaneous transformation. The atomic number and the atomic weight can change during radioactive transformation or decay. The half-life of a radioisotope is the time required for half the material to transform. Radioisotopes can emit electromagnetic radiation, beta particles, or alpha particles. The unit of radioactive decay is the Becquerel or Curie.

Case Study

An x-ray photon with energy of 3.86 keV interacts with an atom of lead.

Critical Thinking Questions

1. The energy is sufficient to remove an electron from which shell?
2. How many keV are required to remove an O-shell electron?
3. What is the maximum number of electrons found in the L shell?

Review Questions

Multiple Choice

1. The Bohr model of the atom consists of a dense __________.
   a. positive nucleus surrounded by a diffuse cloud of negative charge
   b. positive nucleus surrounded by electrons in definite shells
   c. negative nucleus surrounded by a diffuse cloud of positive charge
   d. negative nucleus surrounded by protons in definite shells

2. The electron binding energy is:
   a. the energy of attraction between electrons in the shells
   b. the energy required to remove the nucleus from an atom
   c. the energy required to remove an electron from the nucleus
   d. the energy required to remove an electron from its orbital shell

3. The atomic number is the number of __________ in the nucleus.
   a. protons
   b. neutrons
   c. protons and electrons
   d. protons and neutrons

4. The nucleus of an atom contains which of the following?
   1. Protons
   2. Neutrons
   3. Electrons
   4. Gamma rays
   a. 1
   b. 1 and 2
   c. 2 and 3
   d. 1, 2, and 3

5. The periodic table of elements lists the elements in order of increasing:
   a. atomic number
   b. atomic weight
   c. atomic neutrons
   d. atomic ionization

6. The atomic mass of an element is designated by which letter?
   a. A
   b. M
   c. Z
   d. K

7. Which types of particulate radiation are given off when a radioisotope decays?
   1. Beta
   2. Gamma
   3. Alpha
   a. 1 only
   b. 2 only
   c. 1 and 2
   d. 1 and 3

8. What is the maximum number of electrons of an atom with five orbital shells?
   a. 48
   b. 50
   c. 72
   d. 98

9. Which electron shell has the highest binding energy?
   a. P shell
   b. L shell
   c. K shell
   d. Q shell

Short Answer

1. Explain the difference between alpha and beta particles.

2. List the fundamental particles found in an atom.

3. Define element.

4. Who developed the concept of the atom with the electrons orbiting the atom?

5. What is a compound? Write the chemical equation for water.

6. Explain the half-life of an isotope.

7. Define the octet rule.

8. What is electron binding energy?

9. Could atoms be ionized by changing the number of protons?

5

Electromagnetic Radiation

Objectives

Upon completion of this chapter, the student will be able to:

1. Name the different types of electromagnetic radiation and describe each.
2. Describe the characteristics of electromagnetic waves.
3. Describe the relationships between frequency, wavelength, velocity, and energy of electromagnetic radiation.
4. Define radiation intensity and describe how it varies with distance from the radiation source.
5. Explain the difference between electromagnetic and particulate radiation.
6. Define wave-particle duality and how it relates to x-rays and gamma rays.
7. Discuss ionization and the characteristics of alpha and beta particles.

Key Terms

- amplitude
- electromagnetic spectrum
- frequency
- intensity
- inverse square law
- period
- photon
- wavelength

Introduction

In this chapter, we review the types and characteristics of electromagnetic radiation and the electromagnetic spectrum. Frequency and wavelength have a direct effect on the energy of a wave or particle and will be discussed in detail. Radiographers use the properties of wave-particle duality to produce ionizing x-radiation. A thorough understanding of the intensity of radiation is essential knowledge that a student must possess to work effectively while using only the amount of radiation necessary to make an exposure.

Characteristics of Electromagnetic Radiation

Electromagnetic radiation consists of vibrations in electric and magnetic fields. It has no charge, has no mass, and travels at the speed of light. The waves move in a sinusoidal (sine) waveform in electric and magnetic fields. Electromagnetic radiation is described in terms of the following characteristics:

- Velocity: how fast the radiation moves
- Amplitude: the magnitude of the wave
- Frequency: how many cycles per second are in the wave
- Period: the time for one complete cycle
- Wavelength: the distance between corresponding parts of the wave
- Energy: the amount of energy in the wave
- Intensity: the flux of energy

Velocity

All electromagnetic radiation travels in a vacuum or in air at 3×10^8 m/s (186,000 miles/s), regardless of whether it is in a wave or particle form. Even though this is incredibly fast, light requires some time to travel huge distances. For example, it takes 8 minutes for light from the Sun to reach the Earth. Therefore, velocity is the speed at which the radiation moves.

Amplitude

The **amplitude** of a wave is the maximum height of the peaks or valleys (in either direction) from zero. As the energy of the wave increases, the height of the wave also increases. Figure 5.1 compares the amplitudes of two electromagnetic waves as a function of time. Sine wave A has the largest amplitude as seen in a higher peak with a corresponding higher energy. Sine wave B has a much smaller peak indicating a lower energy wave. Sine waves are variations in amplitude over time. A rope that is moving up and down quickly will cause a vibration along the rope. The rope moves in a sine-wave pattern; upon moving the rope upward it will eventually reach a peak followed by a downward movement that creates a valley. As long as the rope is moving up and down, the sine-wave pattern will be seen.

Frequency

The **frequency** of a wave is the number of cycles that pass a given point per second. One cycle consists of one peak and one valley on the sine wave. The frequency is the number of peaks and valleys occurring each second. The unit of frequency is hertz (Hz), which is one cycle per second. In the United States, electricity has a frequency of 60 Hz, that is, 60 cycles per second. A typical radio wave has 700,000 Hz (700 kHz). A 1,000 Hz is equal to 1 kHz. One megahertz (MHz) is equal to one million (10^6) Hz or cycles per second.

Period

The **period** of a wave is the time required for one complete cycle. A wave with a frequency of two cycles per second has a period of one-half second; that is, one complete wave cycle occurs each half second. Figure 5.2 illustrates the relationship between frequency and period (time) in a sine wave.

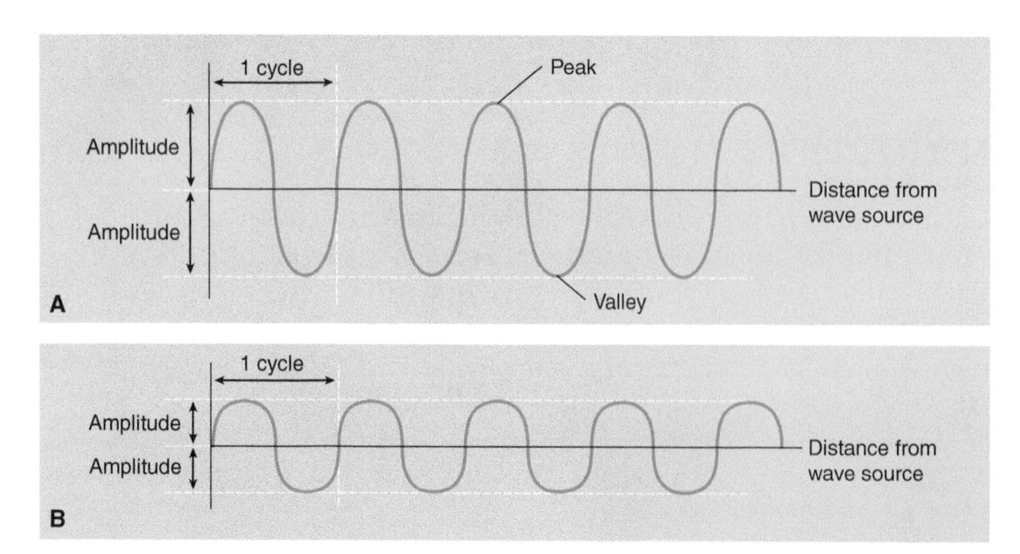

Figure 5.1. (A, B) These two sine waves are identical except for their amplitudes.

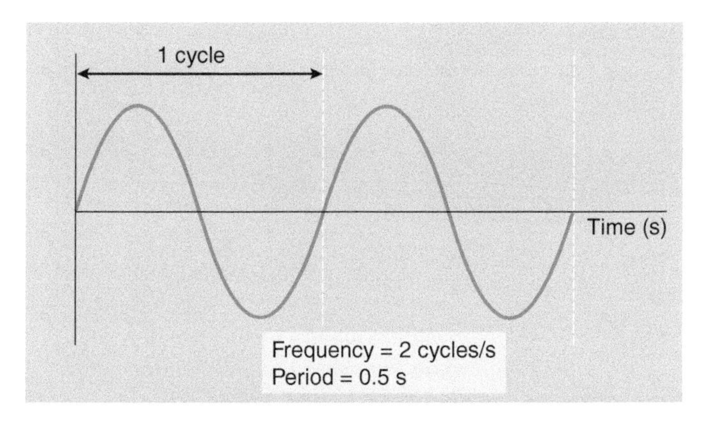

Figure 5.2. The relationship between frequency and period of a waveform.

Wavelength

The distance from one peak to the next peak of a sine wave is the **wavelength** and is represented by lambda (λ). Wavelength is one of the important characteristics in determining the properties of x-rays. Electromagnetic radiation with shorter wavelengths has higher energy and frequencies, which creates greater penetration. Wavelength is measured in meters, centimeters, or millimeters. Figure 5.3 illustrates the relation between wavelength and frequency.

A change in frequency causes a change in wavelength while velocity remains constant. Frequency and wavelength are related, and a change in one factor causes a change in the other factor. The wave is demonstrated with this formula:

$$c = f\lambda$$

where c (velocity) is the speed of light (3×10^8 m/s, in air), f is the frequency, and lambda (λ) is the wavelength. Note that the product of frequency and wavelength must always equal the velocity. Thus, frequency and wavelength are inversely proportional. Therefore, when frequency is increased, wavelength must decrease, and vice versa. For example, if frequency is doubled, the wavelength is halved, and if the frequency is tripled, the wavelength is reduced by one-third.

The equation can be changed to solve for changes in either frequency or wavelength. Variable formulas include

$$f = c/\lambda \quad or \quad \lambda = c/f$$

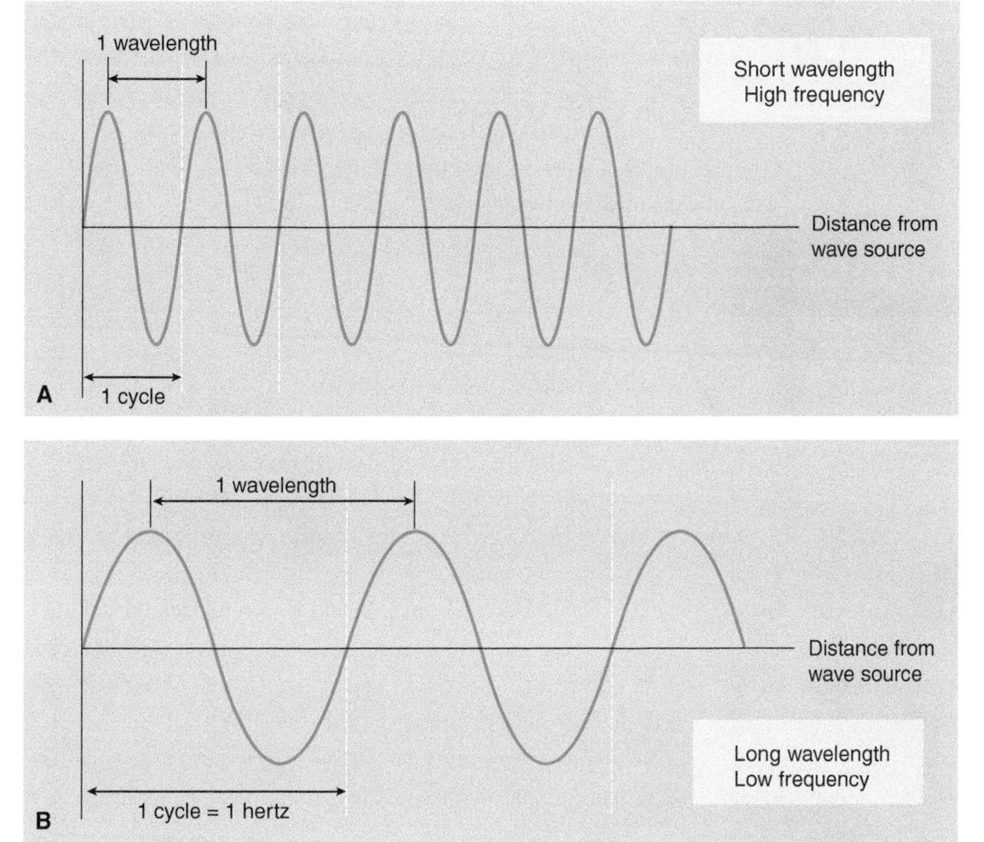

Figure 5.3. (A) Demonstrates the relationship between frequency and wavelength. When a short wavelength is seen, there is a greater number of vibrations. Note how the peaks are closer together. This waveform has high penetrability and represents an x-ray waveform. (B) In the bottom waveform, note the distance between the peaks. As the distance between the peaks increases, the wavelength becomes longer and there are fewer peaks. This waveform has low penetrability.

CRITICAL THINKING BOX 5.1

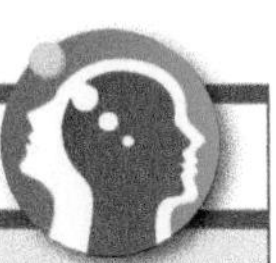

A radio station is broadcasting a signal with a frequency of 27,000 Hz. What is the wavelength of the signal in meters?

CRITICAL THINKING BOX 5.2

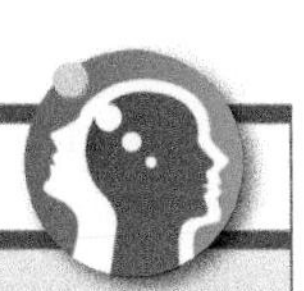

What is the frequency in MHz of a cell phone signal if the wavelength is 333 mm = 3×10^8 m/s?

CRITICAL THINKING BOX 5.3

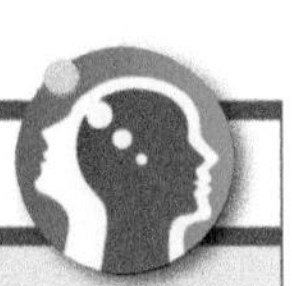

An x-ray beam was produced with 120 kVp and has a frequency of 3.14×10^{19} Hz. Determine the wavelength.

CRITICAL THINKING BOX 5.4

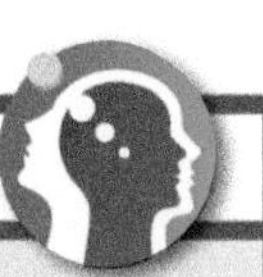

What is the frequency of electromagnetic radiation if the wavelength is 2×10^{-10} m?

Electromagnetic Radiation

thePoint® *An animation for this topic can be viewed at http://thepoint.lww.com/Orth2e*

Types of Electromagnetic Radiation

All electromagnetic radiation consists of simultaneous electric and magnetic waves. These waves are really fluctuations caused by vibrating electrons within the fields. The amount of vibrations of the electrons will determine the frequency and wavelength for the various types of electromagnetic radiations. Electromagnetic radiation has no mass, travels at the speed of light, and carries energy in electric and magnetic waves. Each type of electromagnetic radiation has its own unique frequency and wavelength (Fig. 5.4).

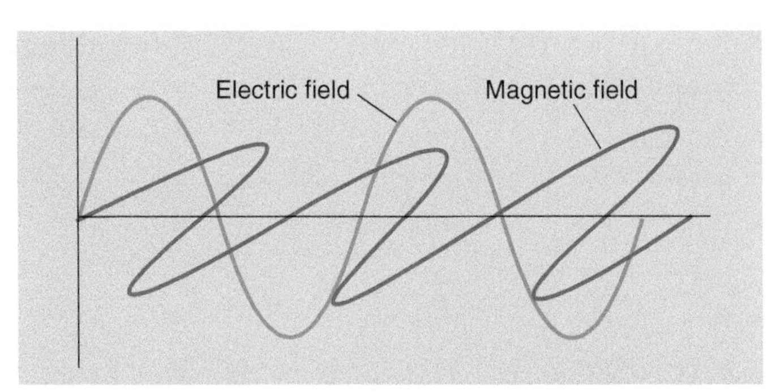

Figure 5.4. **Electromagnetic waveform illustrates the electric and magnetic waves that make up the electromagnetic waveform. Typically, only the electric wave is shown in illustrations.**

Electromagnetic radiation may appear in the form of visible light, x-rays, infrared, or radio waves, depending on its energy. The entire band of electromagnetic energies is known as the **electromagnetic spectrum**.

The electromagnetic spectrum lists the different types of electromagnetic radiations varying in energy, frequency, and wavelengths. The energy of the radiation is measured in electron volts or eV. Figure 5.5 illustrates the different forms of the electromagnetic spectrum from long-wavelength, low-energy radio waves to short-wavelength, high-energy gamma rays. Although Figure 5.5 appears to indicate sharp transitions between the types of radiations, there are no clear boundaries between the various regions in the electromagnetic spectrum.

Radio Waves

Radio waves are long-wavelength, low-energy radiation waves. A radio wave that is 10,000 m in length is equivalent to placing ~92 football fields end to end. Television and radio station broadcasts are identified by transmission frequency, called radiofrequency emissions. Each station transmits on a unique frequency; TIGR might broadcast at 101.9 Hz. Magnetic resonance imaging (MRI) uses the magnetic nuclei of hydrogen atoms in the body. The hydrogen atoms will absorb and emit radio waves of particular frequency. The radio waves are processed by computer programs and an image is produced. Human tissue has an abundant amount of hydrogen that produces a substantial signal, which is then manipulated to produce MR images of various tissues. Cell phones utilize radio

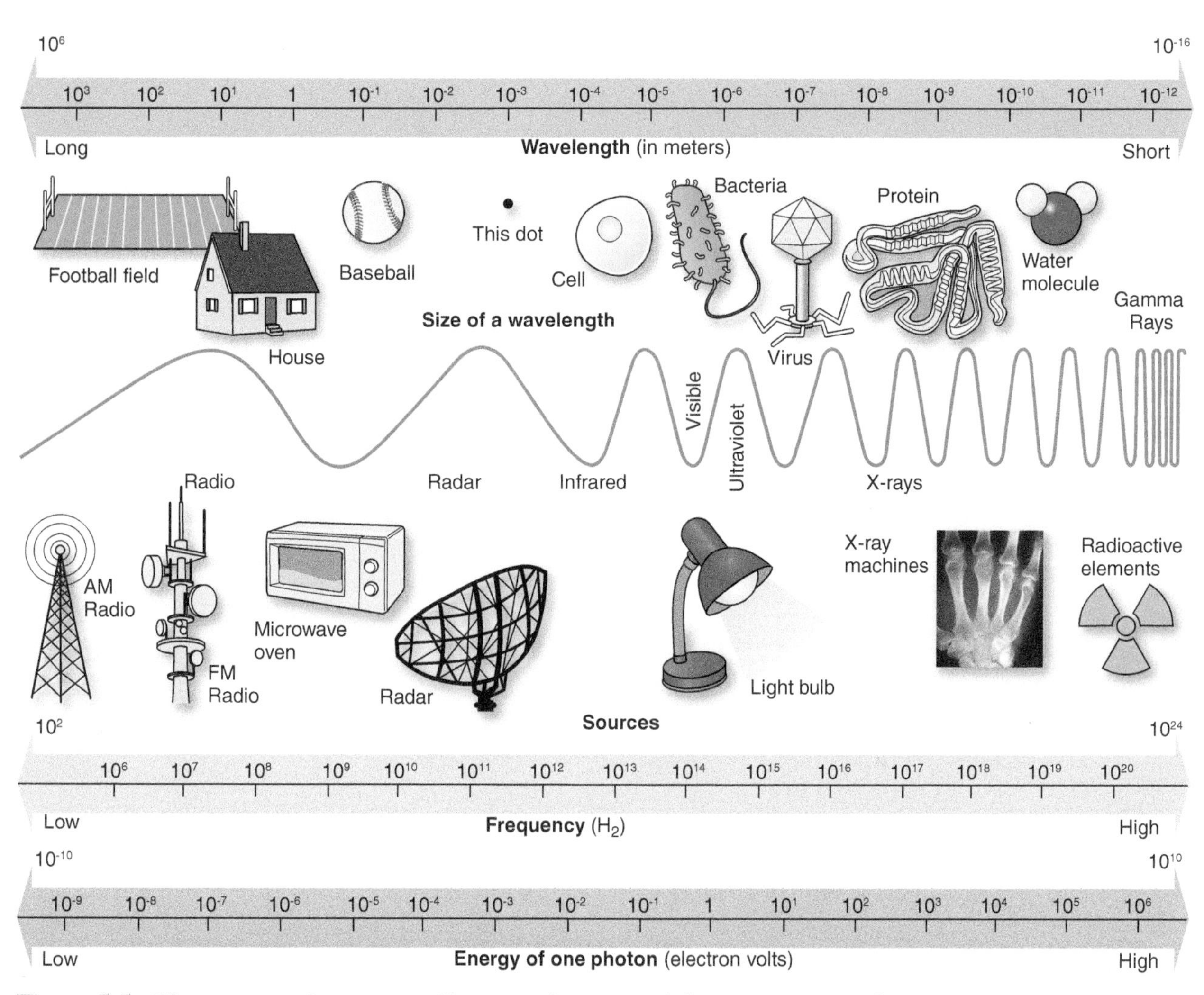

Figure 5.5. **Electromagnetic spectrum illustrates the range of electromagnetic radiation.**

waves to transmit information from one cell tower to another and finally to a cell phone. Television antennae receive the electromagnetic wave from the broadcast station, and the image is displayed on the television screen. Music can be heard because it reaches our ears in the form of a radio wave.

Microwaves

Microwaves have shorter wavelengths and higher energy than do radio waves. Microwaves are used in ovens, in transportation, and by law enforcement officers to monitor the speed of cars. In a microwave oven, the microwave energy forces the water, sugar, and fat molecules in food to rapidly vibrate and release excess energy, thus heating the food. Microwaves are also used for communication and overlap with radio waves on the electromagnetic spectrum. Cell phone signals are carried on microwaves.

Visible Light

Visible light occupies a narrow band in the electromagnetic spectrum, with wavelengths between 10^{-5} and 10^{-6} m. As sunlight passes through a prism, it emerges as a broad range of colors. White light is composed of photons in a range of wavelengths, and as the light is passed through the prism, the wavelengths are separated and grouped into colors, each having a distinct wavelength and energy. The length and energy of the wavelength determines the color. The color red has the longest wavelength and lowest energy. Blue and violet colors have the highest energy and the shortest wavelengths in the visible spectrum. Sunlight also contains infrared and ultraviolet light, which is invisible.

Infrared Light

Infrared light is composed of photons with wavelengths that are longer than visible light. Infrared light has shorter wavelengths and higher energy than do microwaves. Infrared light can heat any substance with radiant heat. For example, you can feel the heat from your toaster, which uses infrared light. The high-energy end of the infrared region is visible and can be seen in the red heating elements of your toaster. Another example of infrared light is the signal from the remote control to the TV; when the buttons on the remote control are pressed, the infrared light is received by the circuitry on the TV and the channels magically change!

Ultraviolet Light

Ultraviolet light is the part of the spectrum just beyond the higher energy of the visible-light region. Ultraviolet light falls on the spectrum between visible light and ionizing radiation (x-rays). Ultraviolet wavelengths range from 10^{-7} to 10^{-9} m. Ultraviolet lights are used in biological laboratories to destroy airborne bacteria. Tanning beds use ultraviolet light bulbs to produce changes in the melanin in the skin thereby creating a tan. Whether the ultraviolet light is natural or from a light bulb, it is believed to be responsible for the majority of sunburn and skin cancer.

X-Rays and Gamma Rays

X-rays and gamma rays are very-short-wavelength, high-frequency, and high-energy radiation. Compared to other types of electromagnetic radiation, the frequency is higher and wavelength is much shorter of x-rays and gamma rays. X-rays and gamma rays also have more energy than visible light. The energy is measured in thousands of electron volts (keV) and is capable of ionization. Ionizing radiation such as x-rays and gamma rays has enough energy to remove an electron from its orbital shell.

The only difference between x-rays and gamma rays is their origin. X-rays come from interactions with electron orbits and are used in the production of medical images. Gamma rays come from nuclear transformations (radioactive decay) and are spontaneously emitted from the nucleus of a radioactive atom. X-radiation is utilized in various industries including for screening baggage in airport security and large crates of merchandise at ports of entry as well as for imaging chest plates the military will use in combat.

The Inverse Square Law

All electromagnetic radiation travels at the speed of light and diverges from the source at which it is emitted. **Intensity** is energy flow per second and is measured in watts/cm^2. The intensity of the radiation decreases with an increase in the distance from the source. This is because the x-ray energy is spread over a larger area. It is called the **inverse square law** because the intensity is inversely proportional to the square of the distance. A simple flashlight can be used to demonstrate the change in a light field when distance changes are made. Hold a flashlight above the floor at a given height. Notice the size of the circle of light and the brightness or intensity of the light on the floor. Now move the flashlight farther from the floor and note how the circle of light becomes larger with the increasing distance. The brightness of the light is lessened, meaning the intensity of the light is less than at the previous distance. Figure 5.6 illustrates

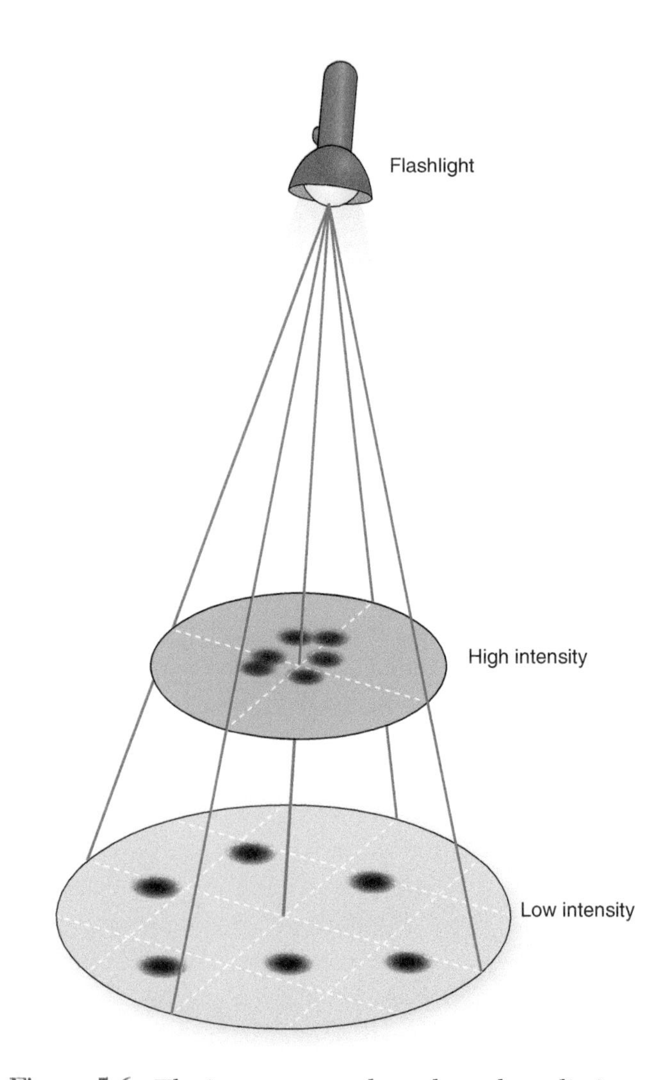

Figure 5.6. The inverse square law relates the radiation intensity to the distance from the source. As distance is increased, the intensity of the radiation is decreased by one-fourth.

how the intensity decreases as the distance from the source increases.

Mathematically, the inverse square law is expressed as follows:

$$\frac{I_1}{I_2} = \frac{(d_2)^2}{(d_1)^2}$$

where I_1, old intensity; I_2, new intensity; d_1^2, old distance squared; and d_2^2, new distance squared. If the distance from the x-ray source is doubled, the intensity is decreased by a factor of 4. That is, the intensity at twice the distance is one-fourth the original value. If the distance from the x-ray source is halved, the intensity is four times greater. The exposure and exposure rate from an x-ray source also follow the inverse square law. To decrease radiation exposure during a fluoroscopic exam, a radiographer needs to increase his or her distance from the x-ray tube. Every step away from the tube decreases the amount of radiation the radiographer will be exposed to.

CRITICAL THINKING BOX 5.5

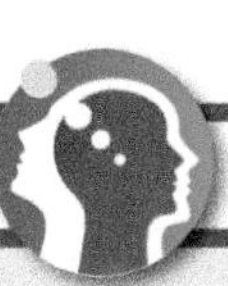

The intensity of radiation at a distance of 2 m from the source is 32 mR/h. What is the exposure rate when the distance is increased to 4 m?

CRITICAL THINKING BOX 5.6

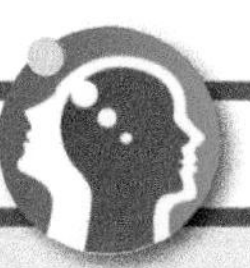

The x-ray intensity is measured at 40 mR/h at 72″. What is the intensity at 36″?

CRITICAL THINKING BOX 5.7

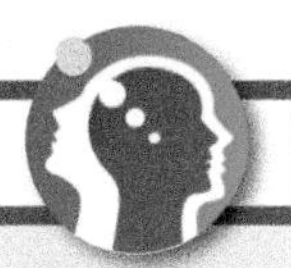

Intensity of radiation at a 40″ SID is 150 mR/h. What is the intensity of radiation when the distance is increased to 80″ SID?

Wave-Particle Duality

Electromagnetic radiation can be characterized as either a wave or particle. This is a phenomenon known as wave-particle duality. When electromagnetic radiation acts as a wave, it has a definite frequency and wavelength. However, when electromagnetic radiation acts as a particle, it is called a **photon** or quanta. German physicist Max Planck described the direct relationship between frequency and energy; as photon frequency increases, so does photon energy. He theorized that electromagnetic radiation exists as bundles of energy or photons and that the energy and frequency of the photons are directly proportional. Planck also identified the relationship between photon wavelength and photon energy as inversely proportional. Thus, high frequency and short wavelength create higher energy. Planck's formula describes the relationship between photon energy and frequency. The constant, h, is the mathematical value used to calculate photon energies based on frequency and is named for Planck. The formula is expressed as:

$$E = hf$$

where E is photon energy in electron volts, h is a conversion factor called Planck's constant (4.15×10^{-15} eVs), and f is the photon frequency.

CRITICAL THINKING BOX 5.8

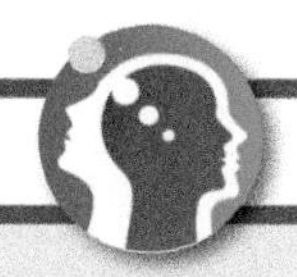

What is the frequency of a 56-keV x-ray photon?

CRITICAL THINKING BOX 5.9

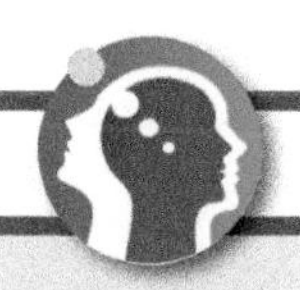

How much energy is found in one photon of radiation during a cell phone transmission of 900 kHz?

CRITICAL THINKING BOX 5.10

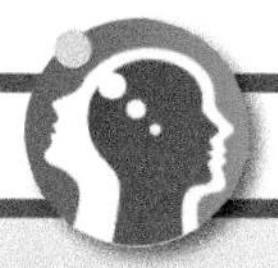

What is the frequency of a 95 keV x-ray?

Chapter Summary

1. Electromagnetic radiation ranges from low-energy, low-frequency, long-wavelength radio waves to high-energy, high-frequency, short-wavelength gamma rays, all of which form an electromagnetic spectrum.
2. Waves are characterized by velocity, frequency, period, wavelength, and amplitude.
3. X-rays act like both waves and particles and have higher energy than do other types of electromagnetic radiation.
4. The inverse square law describes how electromagnetic radiation intensity changes with distance. As the distance increases, the electromagnetic radiation intensity decreases.

Case Study

John is preparing an experiment to explain the inverse square law. He has determined that he needs to accurately demonstrate the effect of changing distance on the amount of radiation reaching the image receptor.

Critical Thinking Questions

1. What are the tools that John needs to complete the experiment?
2. How does the changing distance effect the radiation reaching the image receptor?

Review Questions

Multiple Choice

1. **What is the basic charged particle?**
   a. Electron
   b. Neutron
   c. Volt
   d. Coulomb

2. **The frequency of an electromagnet wave is measured in:**
   a. the height of the wave
   b. the number of cycles per second
   c. the distance between adjacent peaks
   d. the length of time it takes to complete one cycle

3. **X-radiation is part of the __________ spectrum.**
   a. radiation
   b. energy
   c. atomic
   d. electromagnetic

4. **Electrons have __________ electrical charge.**
   a. a positive
   b. a negative
   c. an alternately positive and negative
   d. no

5. The wavelength and frequency of x-rays are __________ related.

   a. directly
   b. inversely
   c. partially
   d. not

6. X-rays have a dual nature, which means that they behave like both:

   a. atoms and molecules
   b. photons and quanta
   c. charged and uncharged particles
   d. waves and particles

7. Wavelength is represented by which Greek letter?

   a. Omega
   b. Lambda
   c. Delta
   d. Zeta

8. When there is an increase in distance from the course, how is the intensity of radiation changed?

   a. The intensity is increased.
   b. There is no change in the intensity.
   c. There is a decrease in the intensity.

9. Planck discovered that as the wavelength became shorter the energy increased.

   a. True
   b. False

Short Answer

1. Which type of electromagnetic radiation has the lowest energy and frequency but the longest wavelength?

2. Describe the change in intensity if the distance between two objects is doubled?

3. How do x-rays and gamma rays differ from each other?

4. If the frequency of a sine wave is decreased, what happens to the wavelength?

5. How is the amplitude of a sine wave related to the energy of the wave?

6. What is the formula for the inverse square law?

7. Which formula is used to describe the relationship between photon energy and frequency?

8. Describe how radio waves are used in MRI.

9. Write the wave formula.

PART II

Creating the X-Ray Beam

6

Electricity

Objectives

Upon completion of this chapter, the student will be able to:

1. Identify the four types of electrical materials.
2. Describe the direction and movement of current flow.
3. Define current, voltage, and electric power and identify their units.
4. Identify Ohm's law and state the relationship between current, voltage, and resistance.
5. Distinguish between alternating and direct current.
6. Describe series and parallel circuits.

Key Terms

- alternating current (AC)
- ampere
- conductor
- current
- direct current (DC)
- electrodynamics
- electromotive force (EMF)
- electrostatics
- insulator
- ohm
- parallel circuit
- potential difference
- power
- resistance
- semiconductor
- series circuit
- superconductor
- voltage
- volts

Introduction

In this chapter, you will learn about electrostatic charges and the laws of electric charges at rest. We will study the movement of electric charges or electricity. An understanding of the underlying principles of electricity and electric current aids in understanding radiologic equipment and image production. In this chapter, we identify different types of electrical materials and define current, voltage, resistance, and electric power. We also discuss the difference between alternating current (AC) and direct current (DC) and how each is used in electrical circuits.

Electrostatics

Electrostatics is the study of stationary or resting electric charges. Another name for stationary charges is static electricity.

As we discussed in Chapter 4, the concept of electric charges can be seen at the atomic level, in positively charged protons and negatively charged electrons. The negatively charged electrons travel around atoms in orbital shells. Loosely bound electrons can be made to jump or move from one object to another object. The most familiar example of this is static electricity. In this chapter, we discuss how the movement of electrons, which are the basic charged particles, can cause electric charges on a larger level. A discussion of electrostatics must begin with an understanding of electric fields and the various forms of electrification.

Electric Fields

An electric field describes the electrical force exerted on a charge. An electric field exists around all electric charges. The electric field is directed away from positive charges and toward negative charges. When two charges are brought near each other, their fields interact. The resulting force of attraction or repulsion depends on the sign of the charges. There is no electric field around neutral objects, however; neutral objects are affected by strongly charged objects.

Electrification

Electrification occurs when electrons are added to or subtracted from an object; therefore, an object can be negatively charged or positively charged. An object having more electrons than another object is considered to be negatively charged. The concept of a positively charged object does not mean the object has only positive charges or protons. We know this is true because atoms have orbital electrons; therefore, a positively charged object has a weaker negative charge. When discussing electricity, it is important to remember that the two objects are being compared, not their actual atomic charges. The three methods of electrification include friction, contact, and induction (Fig. 6.1).

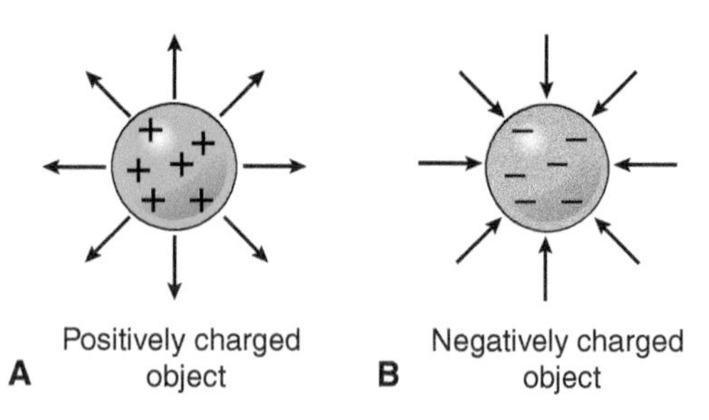

Figure 6.1. **(A) Positively charged object. (B) Negatively charged object.**

Friction

Electrification by friction involves the removal of electrons from one object by rubbing it with another object. A familiar game that children play is to rub a balloon on their hair. Electrons from the hair will be transferred to the balloon causing the balloon to be negatively electrified. When the negatively electrified balloon is placed on a smooth wall, which has a primarily positive charge, the buildup of electrons will allow the balloon to stick to the wall.

Contact

Electrification by contact occurs when two objects touch, allowing electrons to move from one object to another. When an object charged by friction touches an uncharged object, the uncharged object will acquire a similar charge. If the first object is positively charged, it will remove electrons from the uncharged object, causing it to be positively charged. Likewise, if a negatively charged object touches an uncharged object, it will give up some of its electrons, making the second object negatively charged. Therefore, an uncharged body will acquire *the same kind of charge* of the charged body with which it comes in contact.

Electrons move in an attempt to equalize the charged body. An example of this equalization can be seen when a person wearing socks walks across a wool rug and then touches a metal lamp. Electrons from the rug are transferred to the socks and eventually to the body, giving the person a negative charge. Reaching out toward a metal lamp will cause a static discharge to jump between your hand and the metal lamp. The electrons move from a location of a high negative charge to an area of low negative charge. This transfer of excess electrons will neutralize the person (Fig. 6.2).

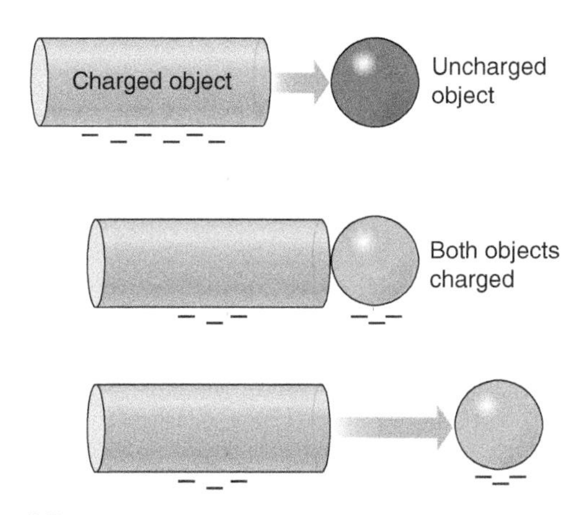

Figure 6.2. **Electrification by contact.**

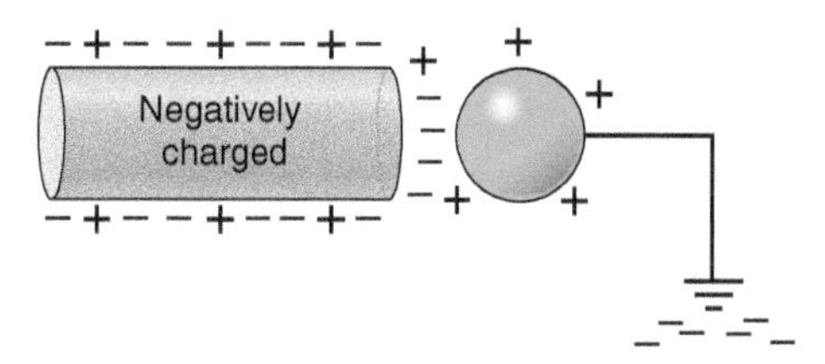

Figure 6.4. **Grounding of electrical charges will allow excess electrons to flow into the Earth. This principle can be used to temporarily magnetize a metal object.**

Induction

Electrification by induction is the process of electrical fields acting on one another without making contact. A charged object has a force field surrounding it, and if this force field is strong enough, it can cause electrification of a weakly charged object. The force field is called an electric field. A neutral metallic object experiences a shift in electrons in the direction toward an opposite charge when brought into the electric field of a charged object. Keep in mind that a neutral object has an equal number of protons and electrons and when acted upon by a strongly charged metallic object, *only the electrons will move*.

As seen in Figure 6.3, a negatively charged bar magnet is brought close to a neutral or uncharged metal ball but does not touch it. Excess electrons from the bar magnet will repel the electrons on the side of the ball that is closest to the bar magnet. This leaves the side of the ball closest to the bar magnet positively charged.

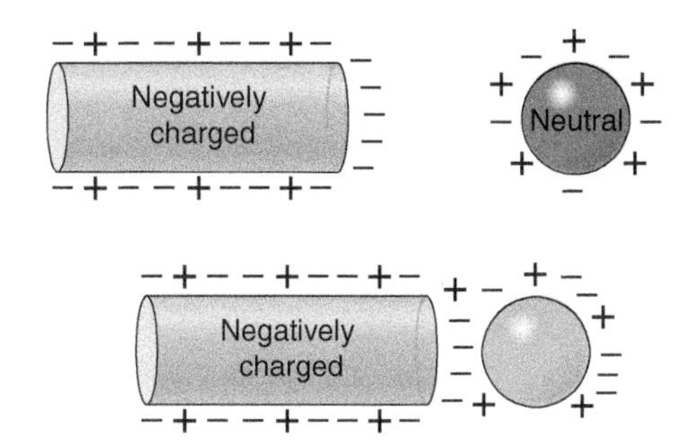

Figure 6.3. **Electrification by induction. The force of one field acting on another field can cause the electrons to either repel or attract each other.**

The reverse occurs when a positively charged bar magnet is brought close to an uncharged metal ball. The electrons from the metal ball are attracted to the positive charge of the bar magnet, thus leaving the side of the ball closest to the bar magnet with a negative charge. In both examples, the electrification by induction is a temporary opposite charge, and the electrons will return to their original positions when the charged object is withdrawn (Fig. 6.3).

Electrification by induction can also be used to semipermanently change the charge of an object. This is accomplished by connecting the end of a metallic object to the ground. The Earth is a huge neutral object and an infinite reservoir of electrons and can be used to neutralize any charged object. In Figure 6.4, a neutral metal ball is connected to the ground. A negatively charged bar magnet is brought close to the neutral metal ball. The forces of repulsion move the negative charges from the side of the metal ball closest to the bar magnet to the opposite side of the metal ball. Because the metal ball is attached to the ground, the excess negative charges will flow to the ground. If the ground connection and bar magnet are removed, the metal ball will remain positively charged. It will retain this charge until the metal ball is attached to the ground at which point the electrons will move up from the ground to neutralize the metal ball.

Unit of Charge

To quantify these electric charges, a basic unit of measure is needed. Although the basic charged particle is the electron, the standard unit of charge is the coulomb. One coulomb is much larger than the charge on an electron. There are 6.3×10^{18} electron charges in one coulomb. Thus, the charge of one electron is 1.6×10^{-19} coulomb.

Electrostatic Laws

Certain physical laws govern how these electrostatic charges interact. The major laws of electrostatics are as follows:

Repulsion-attraction: Like charges repel, and unlike charges attract.
Coulomb's law: The electrostatic force between two charges is directly proportional to the product of their quantities and inversely proportional to the square of the distance between them.
Distribution: Electric charges only reside on the external surface of a conductor.
Concentration: Electric charges concentrate on the surface of a conductor.
Movement: Only negative charges move along solid conductors.

The first law, like charges repel and unlike charges attract, holds true because of the force field surrounding electrical charges. As previously discussed, the force field or lines of force act to repel like charged objects away from each other and to attract opposite charged objects together (Fig. 6.5).

The second law, the force between two charges is directly proportional to the product of their quantities and inversely proportional to the square of the distance between them. Coulomb's law describes the force between two charges. Coulomb's law states that doubling the distance between two charges reduces the force by a factor of 4. Two charges of the same sign, either positive or negative, always have a repulsive force between them. Two charges of opposite signs always have an attractive force between them. The force between two charges increases as the strength of the charge increases. Likewise, the force between the charges increases as the distance between them decreases.

This law is written as follows:

$$F = k\frac{Q_1Q_2}{d^2}$$

where F is the force, k is a proportionality constant, and d is the distance between charges Q_1 and Q_2.

The third law, electric charges reside on the external surface of a conductor, is true because when a metal wire is charged, all the negative charges (electrons) are repelled from each other and therefore move to the outside of the wire leaving the inside of the wire uncharged (Fig. 6.6). This distribution occurs as the electrons attempt to get as far away from each other as possible. In a solid conductor, this occurs on the surface because the surface area is larger, which allows the electrons to be repelled from one another.

The fourth law, electric charges concentrate on the surface of a conductor. Figure 6.7 illustrates how the electric charges will concentrate at the sharpest point on an object. This is also caused by the law of repulsion-attraction. Each negative charge is repelled by other negative charges, which causes the charges to collect at the sharpest curve or point. If enough negative charges collect, they can cause ionization in the air and discharge to the closest point of low concentration in an attempt to neutralize the excess negative charges.

The fifth law states that only negative charges move along solid conductors because the positive charges do not drift in solid conductors. The positive charges or protons are tightly bound inside the atom's nucleus and are not easily moved. The electrons, which orbit the atom, can be easily removed with the appropriate amount of force.

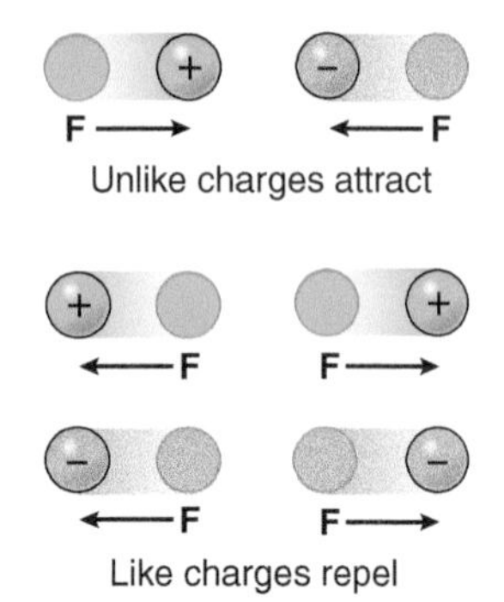

Figure 6.5. The law of attraction and repulsion of electric charges.

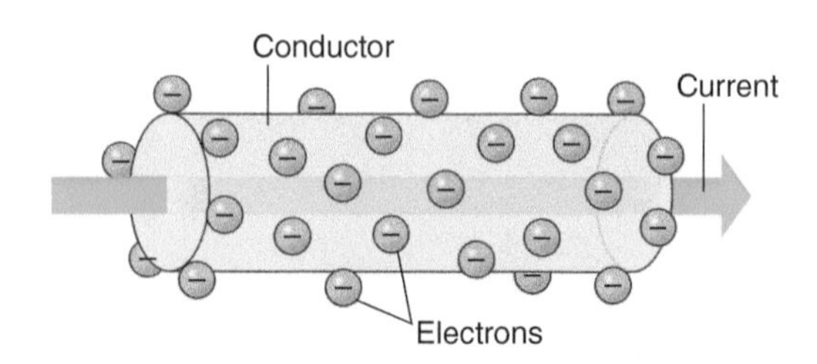

Figure 6.6. Electrostatic law of distribution. Negative charges will reside on the surface of a solid conductor when the conductor is charged.

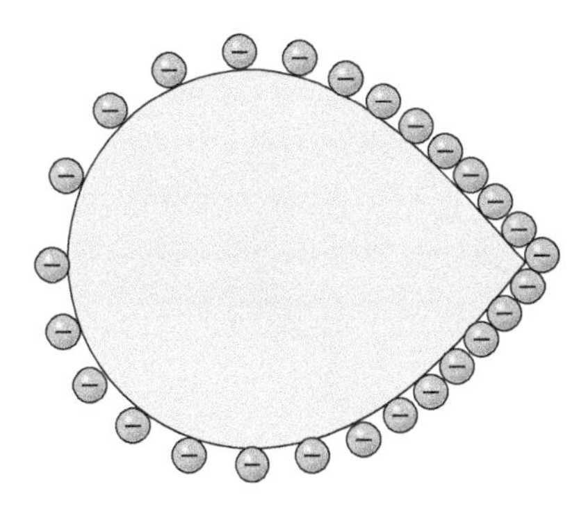

Figure 6.7. **Electrostatic law of concentration. Due to repulsion, negative charges will concentrate to the sharpest point on a curved object.**

These laws are used in radiographic imaging equipment, including image intensifier tubes, x-ray tubes, and image display systems. These systems can only operate through the use of electricity, and electricity cannot exist without utilizing the principles of electrostatics and moving negative charges. Radiographic equipment uses electricity to power equipment and to create, drive, and focus electrons within the x-ray tube and image intensifier tube. These concepts are built upon in subsequent chapters for a comprehensive understanding of the whole process of producing a radiographic image.

Types of Electrical Materials

There are four types of electrical materials: conductors, insulators, semiconductors, and superconductors. Each is discussed in detail below.

Conductors

Because electrons are rotating around the atom in orbital shells, the electrons are able to move freely through a **conductor**. Tap water containing impurities and most metals are good electrical conductors. Copper and silver are very good conductors with copper commonly used in electrical wiring. Electric current will flow easily through conductors.

Insulators

The electrons in an **insulator** are held tightly in place and are not free to move. Rubber, wood, glass, and many plastics are good insulators. Electric current will not flow through an insulator.

Semiconductors

Semiconductors can act as either conductors or insulators, depending on how they are made and their environment. Rectifiers in an x-ray circuit are made of semiconducting material. They conduct electrons in one direction but not in the other direction. Some semiconductors conduct or insulate, depending on surrounding conditions. A photodiode is a semiconductor that is an insulator in the dark but becomes a conductor when exposed to light.

Superconductors

Superconductors are materials that conduct electrons with zero resistance when they are super cooled to very low temperatures. Superconductors are used to produce the magnetic fields in magnetic resonance imaging units. Table 6.1 summarizes the four types of electrical materials.

TABLE 6.1 **FOUR TYPES OF ELECTRICAL MATERIALS**

Type of Material	Characteristics	Examples
Conductor	Electrons move freely	Copper, silver
Insulator	Electrons are fixed; no current can flow	Wood, plastic, glass
Semiconductor	Can be either a conductor or an insulator, depending on the conditions	Silicon, germanium
Superconductor	Zero resistance to low temperatures; current will flow continuously once started	Special metal alloys

Electrodynamics

The study of moving electric charges is called **electrodynamics**. Moving electric charges or electric current can occur in a variety of conditions. Electrons can move in a vacuum, gas, isotonic solution, and metal conductor. Of these, we will focus on the principles necessary for electrons to flow in a wire or metal conductor.

Movement of Electric Charges

Electric charges will move when an electrical potential energy difference exists along a conductor. An electrical potential energy difference occurs when one end of a conductor has an excess of electrons creating a strong negative charge while the other end has a deficiency of electrons and a lower negative charge. When this occurs, electrons will move from the area of excess to the area of deficiency, which causes an electric **current** to flow.

Unit of Current

An electric current is a flow of electrons over a set amount of time. The **ampere** (A) is the unit of current and is defined as one coulomb of electric charge flowing per second (1 A = 1 C/s). The milliampere (mA) is a smaller unit of current; it is equal to 1/1,000 of an ampere (10^{-3} A). Diagnostic radiographic equipment uses a variety of mA units to regulate the number of electrons needed to produce x-ray photons. Different current values are used in different parts of x-ray circuits (Table 6.2).

Direction of Current Flow

When Ben Franklin was working with electricity, he speculated about whether positive or negative charges come out of the battery. Unfortunately, he guessed wrong. He thought that positive charges flow from the positive terminal (the anode) of a battery to the negative terminal (the cathode).

TABLE 6.2 TYPICAL CURRENTS ASSOCIATED WITH THE FILAMENT AND X-RAY TUBE

Location	Current
X-ray filament	2–5 A
X-ray tube	50–800 mA

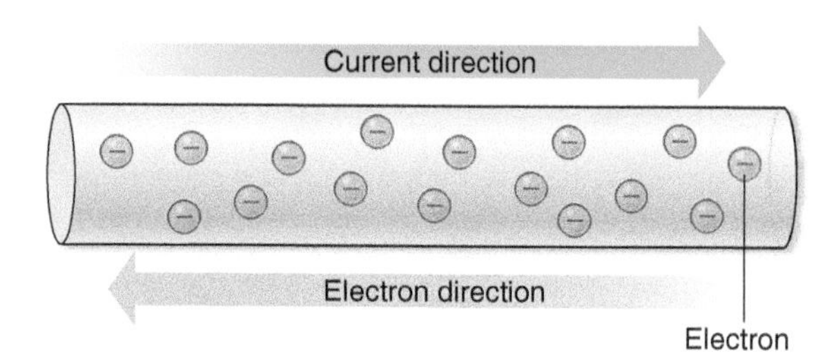

Figure 6.8. **In an electric circuit, electrons flow in one direction and positive current flows in the opposite direction.**

What really happens is that negative charges (electrons) flow from the negative cathode to the positive anode. In practice, all drawings of electric circuits are based on Ben Franklin's theory. We assume that current is flowing from positive to negative, even though we know that electrons are actually flowing in the opposite direction. Figure 6.8 illustrates the direction of current and electron flow in a wire.

Voltage

Voltage is the force or electrical pressure that produces electron movement and current flow. A voltage increase results in an increase in current flow, just as higher water pressure increases the amount of water flow. Electrons flow in response to the difference in pressure or **potential difference** (PD) in the circuit.

Unit of Voltage

The unit of voltage or electrical PD is measured in **volts** (V) and is sometimes called the **electromotive force** (EMF). EMF is the maximum PD between two points on a circuit. Therefore, the force with which electrons move can be described by the terms PD, EMF, or voltage (V). Higher voltages give electrons higher energies. Voltages of 20,000 to 120,000 V are used in x-ray circuits to produce high-energy x-rays. One kilovolt (kV) is equal to 1,000 (10^3) volts.

Resistance

Resistance is the opposition to current flow in a circuit. The unit of resistance is the **ohm** and the symbol is the Greek letter omega (Ω). The composition of the circuit will determine the amount of resistance that is present. There are four factors that affect the amount of resistance in a circuit:

1. Conductive material
2. Length of conductor
3. Cross-sectional diameter
4. Temperature

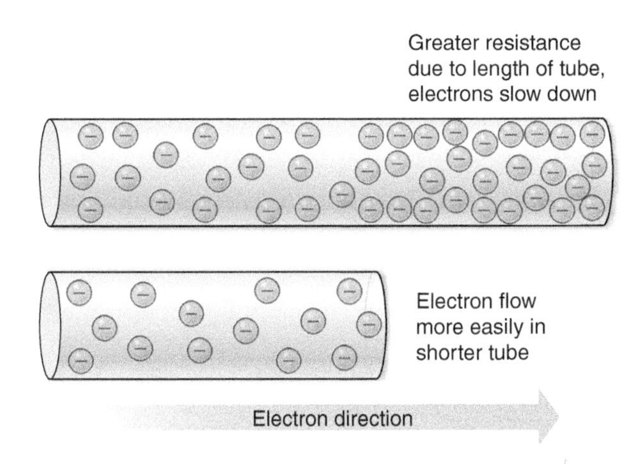

Figure 6.9. **Long pipe = high resistance. Short pipe = low resistance.**

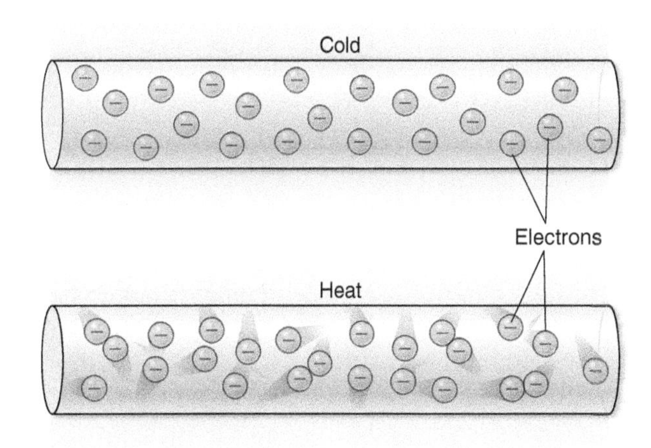

Figure 6.11. **High temperature = more resistance.**

Conductive Material

As previously discussed, the conductive ability of the material will have a direct effect on the flow of electrons. The least amount of resistance is found in a wire that is made of a good conductive material like copper and silver. Although copper does not conduct as well as silver, it is much cheaper and used extensively in electrical circuits.

Length

The length of the conductor is directly proportional to the amount of resistance in the wire. As the length of a conductor increases, so does the resistance. The resistance in a wire is analogous to the flow of water through a pipe. As the water flows, the molecules in the water collide with the molecules in the pipe causing friction to occur, which in turn causes resistance. If the length of a water pipe doubles, the resistance to the flow of water will also double (Fig. 6.9).

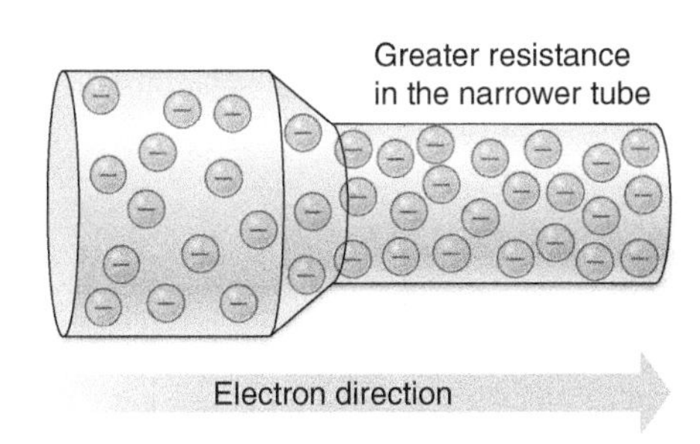

Figure 6.10. **Illustrates the effect of cross-sectional area on resistance.**

Cross-Sectional Diameter

The cross-sectional diameter of the wire is inversely proportional to the resistance. As the cross-sectional diameter doubles, the resistance will be halved. A wire with a large diameter has more area for electron flow and therefore offers a small amount of resistance to the flow of electrons. This principle is utilized when it is desirable to decrease the overall resistance in a wire while maintaining the length of the wire (Fig. 6.10).

Temperature

When electrons flow along a conductor, they collide with other electrons and the wire conductor. All of these collisions create friction, which results in heat being produced. As the heat builds on the conductor, the electrons have collisions with other electrons, which creates more resistance along the conductor. Therefore, higher resistance leads to less current flow (Fig. 6.11).

Ohm's Law

All electricity flowing in circuits has three characteristics: current, resistance, and electromotive force. German physicist Georg Ohm studied the relationships between voltage, current, and resistance. These relationships are expressed mathematically as:

$$V = IR$$

where V, voltage; I, current; and R, resistance. In Ohm's formula, the ampere is abbreviated with an I for intensity. The unit for resistance is the **ohm** and is abbreviated with the Greek letter omega (Ω) or R for resistance. Voltage is the unit for electromotive force or electric potential and is measured in volts. One volt has enough electrical force to push 1 A of current through 1 Ω of resistance. Electrons with high voltage have a high potential energy. When the electron flow is inhibited along a conductor, the resistance in the circuit is high.

Ohm's law states that the voltage (V) is equal to the product of the current (I) flowing through a conductor and the resistance (R) of the conductor. Higher voltage and lower resistance result in higher current flow. As you can see, when one factor is changed, it affects the remaining factors. Using Ohm's formula is easy as long as you know two of the three factors. Figure 6.12 provides a handy tool for determining how to set up the formula based on the factor that is unknown. Notice that V is always on top and never divided into the other factors. If the voltage is not known, cover up the V, which leaves I to be multiplied by R, the amperage times the resistance. Because the amperage is multiplied by the resistance, the voltage is considered to be fixed in value. Amperage and resistance are then inversely proportional because when amperage is increased, the resistance must be decreased if voltage is to remain constant. If resistance is doubled, amperage must be reduced by one-half. As resistance is cut in half, the amperage doubles because it is easier for it to flow in the circuit. When solving for I, the amperage flowing in the circuit, cover up the I and divide the V by the R. Remember the voltage is always divided by the other factor. Now when solving for R, the resistance in the circuit, cover the R, which leaves the V to be divided by the I. As you can see by remembering and setting up the formula according to Figure 6.12, you will be able to determine any variations of the formula.

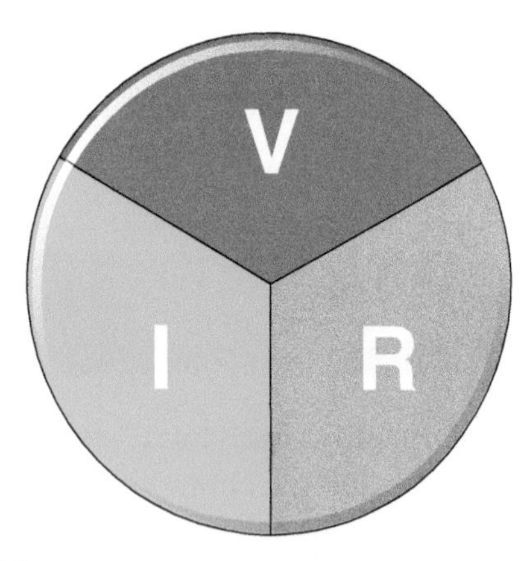

Figure 6.12. **Shows the circle of Ohm. This is an excellent way to remember the various combinations of Ohm's law. The figure shows that $V = IR$ or $I = V/R$ or $R = V/I$. Remember that V is always on top.**

Variations of Ohm's formula are

$$V = IR \quad I = \frac{V}{R} \quad R = \frac{V}{I}$$

CRITICAL THINKING BOX 6.1

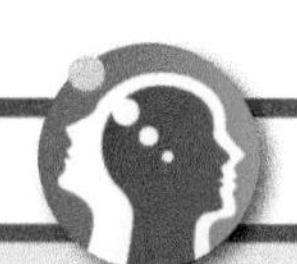

What is the voltage in a circuit if current is 300 A and resistance is 4 Ω?

CRITICAL THINKING BOX 6.2

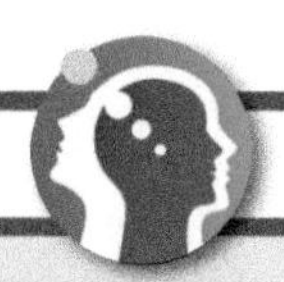

Calculate the current in a circuit with a voltage of 9 V and a resistance of 2 Ω. From Ohm's law, if the resistance and voltage are known, the current can be calculated.

CRITICAL THINKING BOX 6.3

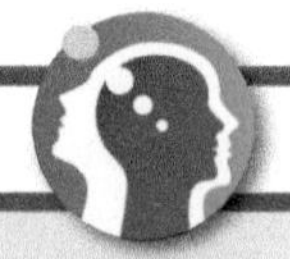

What is the resistance of a circuit if the voltage is 100 V and the current is 5 A?

Electric Power

Electric **power** is measured in watts (W). Power is the rate of energy used and describes the amount of work done or the amount of energy used per second. This is true for both AC and DC circuits. One watt is produced by 1 A of current flowing with an electrical pressure of 1 V. The relationship between power, current, and voltage is

$$P = IV$$

where P, power in watts; I, current in amperes; and V, or potential difference in volts.

The formula can be set up similar to Ohm's law formula. The P stays on top and is never divided by the other variables. The relationships between the factors and the manner in which the factors are multiplied and divided are the same manner as Ohm's formula. Variations of the formula are

$$P = IV \quad I = \frac{P}{V} \quad V = \frac{P}{I}$$

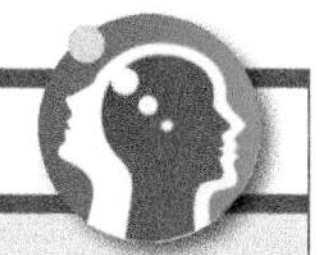

CRITICAL THINKING BOX 6.4

The power expended in a light bulb in a 100-volt circuit with 0.6 A flowing is?

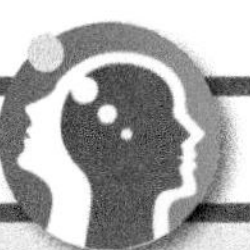

CRITICAL THINKING BOX 6.5

If a mobile x-ray machine operates from a 110-volt wall outlet and is rated at a total resistance of 20 Ω, how much current does it draw during a 1-second exposure? How much power does it use per second?

Direct and Alternating Currents

Electric current describes the amount of electric charge moving through a conductor and is measured in amperes or milliamperes. Current flow is demonstrated by using a sinusoidal or sine waveform. The vertical axis represents the amplitude of the current, while the horizontal axis represents time. The sinusoidal wave is used to demonstrate current flow as either positive flow or negative flow. The two types of electric current are **direct current** (DC) and **alternating current** (AC). In DC circuits, electrons flow in a steady flow in one direction. Batteries and rectifiers produce DC. DC is used in TV sets, microwave ovens, and x-ray tubes.

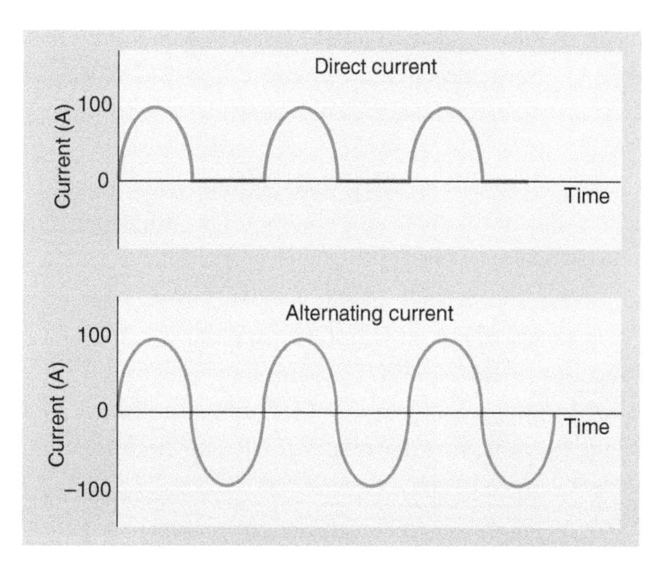

Figure 6.13. **Alternating and direct currents.**

Figure 6.13 is a graph of DC as a function of time. It also demonstrates the sine wave of DC. When the electricity is turned on, the electrons go from a resting state to a moving state. The waveform begins on the line or at zero amplitude because the electrons are at rest. As the electrons begin to move, their potential rises in the positive direction until they reach the maximum potential, which is represented by the peak of the waveform. Once the electrons have reached this peak, they begin to move in the opposite direction with a negative deflection. The electrons will slow down until they again reach zero potential. For DC, the electron flow will continue in this manner until the electricity is turned off.

AC flows half of the time in one direction, and the other half of the time in the other direction. The first half of the AC sine waveform is identical to the DC waveform and consists of positive current flow. During the positive half of the AC sine wave, the current flow begins at zero potential when the electrons are at rest; the electrons begin to rise to the maximum positive potential; the electrons begin to slow down and flow back to zero. At this point, the electrons reverse their motion or change the direction and begin to flow in the negative direction; the electrons flow in the negative direction until they reach the maximum negative potential; the electrons then slow down and flow back to zero. AC waveforms will continue this oscillation as long as a PD exists. The voltage is measured at the peaks of the AC cycle. An AC voltage of 2,000 V is referred to as 2 kVp, where kVp means kilovolt peak.

In the United States, standard AC electric current has a frequency of 60 cycles per second. The duration of the positive half cycle is 1/120 seconds (s). The duration of the negative half cycle is also 1/120 seconds. One cycle per second is also known as one hertz (Hz). AC is used in most electrical appliances. The x-ray machine utilizes AC in the high-voltage circuits. Before we discuss high-voltage circuits, it is necessary to have an understanding of a basic electric circuit.

Electric Circuits

Electric circuits are used to provide a path for electricity to flow. The circuits are constructed of certain elements: a power source, a conductor or wire, a switch, and a resistance. The resistance in a circuit can be as simple as the load on the circuit or as complicated as multiple resistors. The load on a circuit is the thing that requires electricity to operate; a light bulb is a simple example of a load. To light the bulb, the electricity must be turned on, and as long as the electricity is flowing, the light bulb will act as the resistance in the circuit. Figure 6.14 illustrates a circuit with electricity flowing. A battery provides the direct current for the circuit. In order for the electrons to flow across the circuit, the switch must first be closed. This creates a connection between two points on the conductor; another way to think about it is that the wire no longer has any gaps in it but is one continuous wire. With the switch closed, notice how the electrons flow from the negative pole of the battery to the positive pole. As long as the switch remains closed, the electrons will continue to flow. To stop the flow of electrons, the switch is opened, which creates a gap in the wire. Using the light bulb as the example, when the light switch is flipped on, effectively closing the switch in the circuit, the light bulb begins to emit light. The light bulb will continue to emit light until the switch is turned off, effectively opening the circuit.

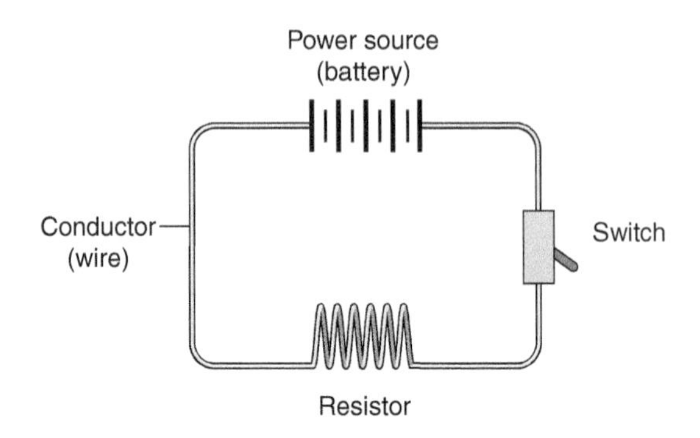

Figure 6.14. Simple electrical circuit illustrating the basic elements needed in a circuit.

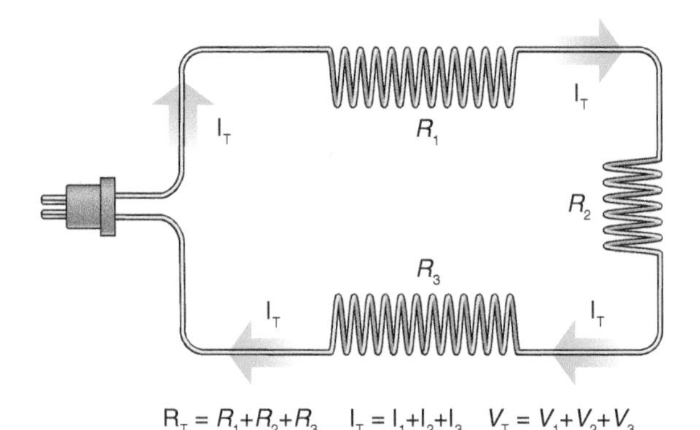

Figure 6.15. Series circuit. Resistors in a series along the main wire of the circuit. Ohm's law applies to the entire circuit and to each part. The current is the same across the whole circuit. The amount of voltage flowing through each resistor will vary depending on the amount of resistance in each resistor.

Series and Parallel Circuits

There are two basic types of electric circuits: a **series circuit** (Fig. 6.15) and a **parallel circuit** (Fig. 6.16). A series circuit is one conductor (wire) along which all circuit elements have been connected. Another way of saying this is the elements are wired in series with each other.

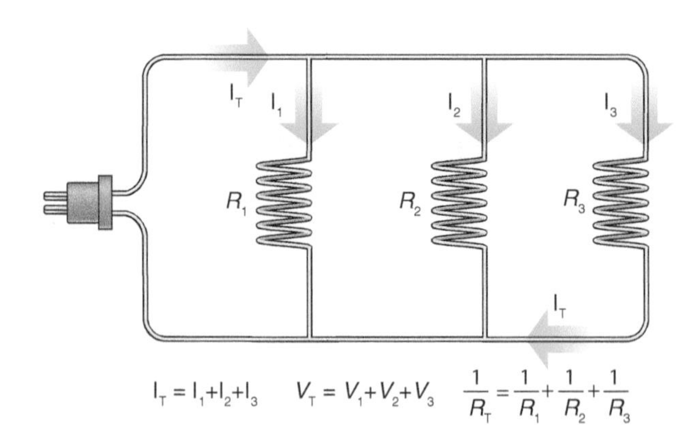

Figure 6.16. Parallel circuit. Resistors in parallel. The resistors create a branch connecting two points on the main wire of the circuit. The voltage is the same across the whole circuit and each branch. The amount of current flowing through each branch is dependent upon the amount of resistance in each branch.

The circuit elements include a power source, a conductor, and resistors. In a series circuit, all circuit elements are on the same conductor. A common example of a series circuit is a string of Christmas lights. Christmas lights, which are wired in series, have one wire that connects each bulb. When one bulb goes out, the whole string of lights goes out. This is because the bulb that goes out acts as a switch that has opened the circuits and disrupted the flow of electricity. Once the bulb is replaced, the string of bulbs will shine once again.

Rules for Series Circuits:

1. The total voltage is equal to the sum of the individual voltages across each circuit element.

$$V_t = V_1 + V_2 + V_3$$

2. Amperage is the same throughout the circuit. Each circuit element has the exact same amperage as the whole circuit.

$$I_t = I_1 = I_2$$

3. The total resistance is equal to the sum of the individual resistances across each circuit element.

$$R_t = R_1 + R_2 + R_3$$

Each of these formulas can be used to determine the voltage, resistance, and current in a series circuit. If you know two factors, the third factor can be determined. Ohm's law formula can be used to solve mathematical equations for series circuits. Figure 6.15 is a schematic of a simple series circuit.

CRITICAL THINKING BOX 6.6

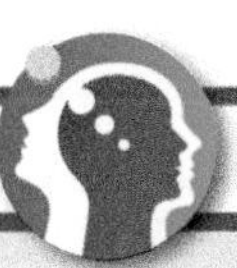

A series circuit has 30 V and 6 Ω of resistance. How much amperage is flowing in the circuit?

CRITICAL THINKING BOX 6.7

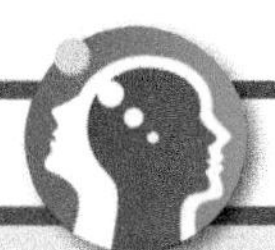

What is the total voltage in a series circuit when resistor 1 has 10 V, resistor 2 has 3 V, and resistor 3 has 1 V?

CRITICAL THINKING BOX 6.8

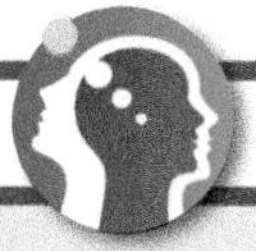

Find the total resistance in a series circuit when there is 10 A flowing and resistor 1 has 20 V and resistor 2 has 10 V?

Parallel circuits contain the same circuit elements as a series circuit except the circuit is wired differently. In parallel circuits, the ends of the elements are connected together and are not part of the main wire. Figure 6.16 illustrates a parallel circuit. Notice the power source and wire that make up the main components. Additional resistors are placed with each end making contact with the main wire. This type of wiring has permits individual sections to continue to operate when one section goes out. Let us consider the string of Christmas lights. To prevent the whole string from going out when one bulb no longer works, the string of lights can be wired in parallel. Each bulb will have two wires, which connects it to the main wire. When one bulb burns out, the remainder of the bulbs remain lit because the flow of electricity has not been disrupted to the whole string.

Rules for Parallel Circuits:

1. The individual voltage through each circuit element is the same and equals the total circuit voltage.

$$V_t = V_1 = V_2 = V_3$$

2. The total amperage is equal to the sum of the individual amperages across each circuit element.

$$I_t = I_1 + I_2 + I_3$$

3. The total resistance is the inverse of the sum of the reciprocals of each individual resistance.

$$1/R_t = 1/R_1 + 1/R_2 + 1/R_3$$

Figure 6.16 is a schematic of a parallel circuit. The resistors are wired in parallel. This design allows the current to divide among the several paths or branches, which results in the total resistance of the circuit being less than that in an individual branch. As more resistors are added in parallel, there is an increase in their total cross-sectional area so that the total resistance decreased. Variations of Ohm's law formula are also used to determine the unknown factor whether it is the voltage, resistance, or current.

CRITICAL THINKING BOX 6.9

Find the total current in a parallel circuit that has 60 V and resistor 1 has 1 Ω, resistor 2 has 2 Ω, resistor 3 has 3 Ω, and resistor 4 has 4 Ω.

CRITICAL THINKING BOX 6.10

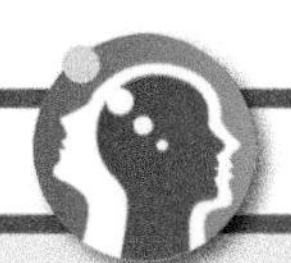

Find the total current in a parallel circuit which has 80 V, resistor 1 has 10 Ω, resistor 2 has 5 Ω, and resistor 3 has 4 Ω.

Chapter Summary

1. Electrons moving through a conductor make up an electric current. Current is the amount of electrons moving in a conductor per second and is measured in amperes or milliamperes. Current flows from the positive to the negative terminal in an electric circuit. Electrons flow from the negative to the positive terminal.
2. Voltage is the electrical pressure or EMF applied to the electrons in the conductor and is measured in volts.
3. Resistance, which is the opposition to current flow, is measured in ohms. Ohm's law, written $V = IR$, states the relationship between voltage, amperage, and resistance.
4. Electric flow is either direct or alternating current. DC flows only in one direction, while AC flow alternates directions. One cycle of AC consists of current flow in one direction for half of the time and in the other direction for the other half of the time. One cycle per second is one hertz.
5. Power is the rate at which energy is used. The equation for electric power is $P = VI$. Power is measured in watts.
6. There are two basic types of circuits: series and parallel circuits. The circuits are used in common electrical items like strings of light or in more advanced radiographic equipment.

Case Study

Liz is designing a circuit for a new radiographic unit. There are many aspects that Liz must think about. Answering the following questions will help her design an appropriate circuit.

Critical Thinking Questions

1. When designing the circuit, which factors must Liz utilize to decrease the total amount of resistance in the circuit?
2. Which type of material will provide the most conduction of the electrons?
3. How do these factors affect Liz's design of the circuit?
4. What type of wire configuration must be used to dissipate heat buildup from electron collisions?

Review Questions

Multiple Choice

1. The unit of electric current is the:
   a. watt
   b. ampere
   c. volt
   d. ohm

2. The unit of electrical potential is the:
   a. watt
   b. ampere
   c. volt
   d. ohm

3. Electrons move from the __________ terminal of a power source to the __________ terminal.
   a. positive to negative
   b. negative to positive
   c. neutral to positive
   d. neutral to negative

4. Which of the following are considered a load on a circuit?
   a. Toaster
   b. Hair dryer
   c. Light bulb
   d. a and b
   e. a, b, and c

5. One kilovolt is equal to __________ V.
   a. 1/1,000
   b. 1/100
   c. 1/10
   d. 1,000

6. Increasing the resistance in a circuit results in a(n):
   a. increase in current
   b. increase in voltage
   c. decrease in current
   d. decrease in voltage

7. As the length of the wire increases, the resistance of the wire:
   a. increases
   b. decreases
   c. stays the same

8. Which of the following factors is inversely proportional to the resistance in a circuit?
   a. Magnetic field strength
   b. Diameter of the conductor
   c. Length of the conductor
   d. Temperature

9. Current that flows first in a positive direction and then in a negative direction is called:
   a. direct current
   b. alternating current

10. What happens in a parallel circuit if one of four branches fails?
    a. Circuit becomes open, and electrons stop flowing.
    b. Circuit remains closed and electrons flow through the remaining branches.
    c. The electrons will only move along the main line of the circuit.
    d. Electrons continue to flow in the open circuit.

Short Answer

1. What unit is defined as the rate of one coulomb per second?

2. List and describe the three components of an electrical circuit.

3. What is a series circuit?

4. A circuit has a potential difference of 78 V and a current of 20 A. What is the resistance in the circuit?

5. Define the four types of conducting materials.

6. When a circuit has 110 V and 9 Ω, what is the amperage flowing through the circuit?

7. What is the resistance in a circuit with 12,000 V and 65 A?

8. How much power was used in a mobile radiographic unit with 220 V and .8 A?

9. Write the Ohm's law formulas.

7

Electromagnetism

Objectives

Upon completion of this chapter, the student will be able to:

1. State the laws and units of magnetism.
2. Identify the different types of magnetic materials.
3. Identify the four types of electrical materials.
4. Describe the direction and movement of current flow.
5. Explain electromagnetic induction: both mutual induction and self-induction.
6. Distinguish the basic principles of operation of generators and motors.

Key Terms

- armature
- bipolar
- commutator rings
- diamagnetic materials
- electromagnetic induction
- ferromagnetic materials
- helix
- magnetic dipole
- magnetic domain
- magnetic field
- magnetic induction
- magnetism
- nonmagnetic materials
- paramagnetic materials
- permeability
- retentivity
- rotor
- slip rings
- solenoid
- stator

Introduction

All radiologic equipment is based on the laws of electricity and magnetism. Thus, an understanding of the underlying principles of electricity and magnetism aids in understanding radiologic equipment and image production. In this chapter, we discuss properties of magnetism, including types of magnetic materials, magnetic fields, and the laws and units of magnetism. Magnetic resonance imaging (MRI) has developed into a diagnostic imaging tool for imaging the body. In radiography, the properties of magnetic induction are used to make the anode rotate in the x-ray tube.

Magnetism

Early man discovered that some rocks seemed to have magical powers. They were called lodestones. Lodestones are natural magnets and attract pieces of iron. **Magnetism** is the ability of a lodestone or magnetic material to attract iron, nickel, and cobalt. This magnetic property is used in medical imaging.

Types of Magnetic Materials

Different types of materials respond differently to magnetic fields. There are four types of magnetic materials:

1. Ferromagnetic materials, which react and are strongly attracted to magnets or a magnetic field
2. Paramagnetic materials, which are slightly attracted to magnets and influenced by a magnetic field
3. Diamagnetic materials, which are weakly repelled by all magnetic fields
4. Nonmagnetic materials, which do not react in a magnetic field

Each of these is discussed in detail below.

Ferromagnetic Materials

Ferromagnetic materials are attracted to a magnet. Ferromagnetic materials include iron, cobalt, and nickel. Ferromagnetic materials' orbital electrons spin in predominantly the same direction. These atoms create tiny magnets called **magnetic dipoles**. When these dipoles form groups of similarly aligned atoms, it forms a magnetic domain. These domains act like tiny magnets inside the material. In the nonmagnetized state, the domains are randomly oriented, so there is no net magnetization. When a ferromagnetic material is placed in a strong magnetic field, the domains align with the external magnetic field. The domains become organized, meaning they all point in one direction. The result is the formation of a permanent magnet. It contains the magnetic properties of each metal to form a strong magnet. Figure 7.1 illustrates how ferromagnetic materials are magnetized by aligning the domains inside the material. Alnico is an alloy made of aluminum, nickel, and cobalt. Alloys are designed to have properties that are easily magnetized. Heating a magnet can destroy its magnetism because heat rearranges the domains into a random orientation, resulting in a loss of permanent magnetism.

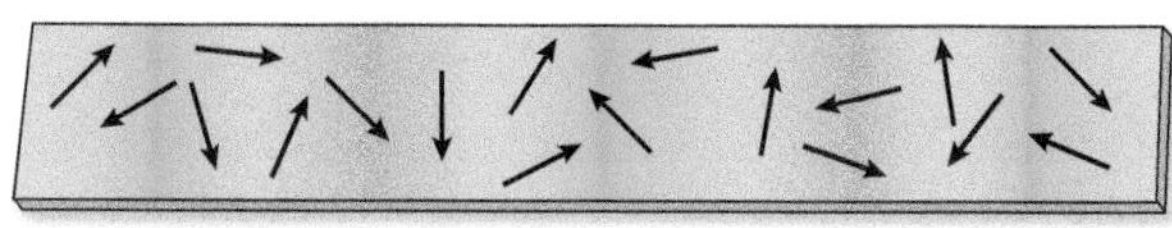

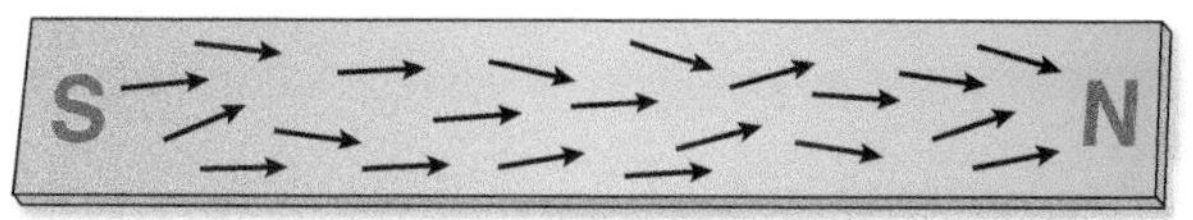

Figure 7.1. **Illustrates the magnetic domain alignment of magnetic and nonmagnetic materials.**

Paramagnetic Materials

Paramagnetic materials are weakly attracted to magnetic fields. When placed in a magnetic field, only some of the domains are aligned in the same direction, which means they cannot be permanently magnetized and do not retain any magnetism after the magnetic field is removed. Aluminum and platinum are examples of paramagnetic materials. MRI contrast agent, gadolinium, is also a paramagnetic material.

Diamagnetic Materials

Diamagnetic materials are weakly repelled by a magnet. Copper, beryllium, bismuth, and lead are examples of diamagnetic materials.

Nonmagnetic Materials

Nonmagnetic materials do not react with magnetic fields. Wood, glass, rubber, and plastics are examples of nonmagnetic materials. In this type of material, there is an equal number of dipoles spinning in both directions; therefore, the material is not attracted to magnetic fields. Materials in the magnetic resonance room must be nonmagnetic.

Magnetic Fields

A **magnetic field** is the space surrounding a magnet or moving electric current in which magnetic forces are detectable. All magnets are surrounded by a magnetic field. A magnetic material placed in a magnetic field experiences a force. This magnetic force will align the domains along the magnetic field. To understand the phenomenon of magnetism, it is important to study

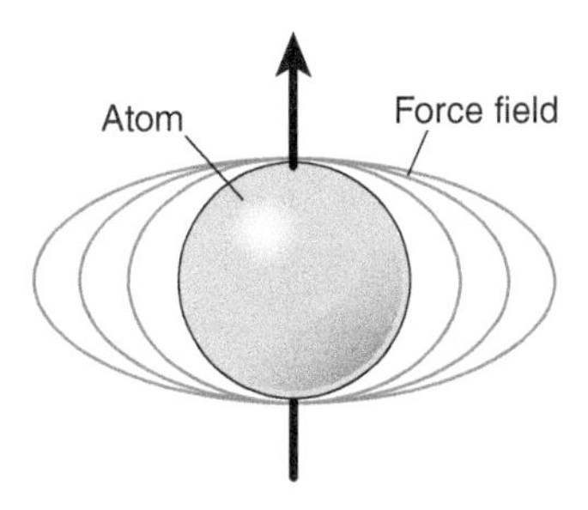

Figure 7.2. **Magnetic field lines around an atom. Demonstrates the path of the magnetic field lines surrounding a magnet.**

atomic structure and the effects of electron movement around a nucleus.

All atoms have orbital electrons, which spin on their axes around the nucleus of the atom. When a charged particle (electron) is in motion, a magnetic force field is created around the particle. This force field moves away from the center of the particle and is perpendicular to the charged particle as represented as field lines. In every magnet, the lines of the magnetic field are in closed loops (Fig. 7.2).

Each atom acts as a very small magnet and is called a magnetic dipole. A group of such atoms with their dipoles aligned in the same direction creates a **magnetic domain**. Atoms having electrons that are all spinning in the same direction will exhibit a net magnetic field.

Typically, magnetic domains are arranged randomly in an object. When the object is acted upon by an external force field, the dipoles will become oriented to the field. If enough of the dipoles become aligned in the same direction, the object will exhibit a strong magnetic field and will then be called a magnet. These force fields are also called lines of force, lines of flux, or the magnetic field. These magnetic field lines flow from the north pole to the south pole on the outside of the magnet. Within the magnet, the field lines flow from the south pole to the north pole. The number and concentration of field lines will determine the strength of the magnet; the stronger the magnetic field, the greater the number of field lines and the more concentrated the field lines are at the poles.

Every magnet is **bipolar**, having two poles: a north pole and a south pole. Breaking a magnet in half produces two smaller magnets, each with a north and a south pole. The pieces of the magnet can be divided multiple times, and every time the pieces will be bipolar. Figure 7.3 illustrates how a magnet that is broken in half will produce two smaller magnets, each with its own north and south poles.

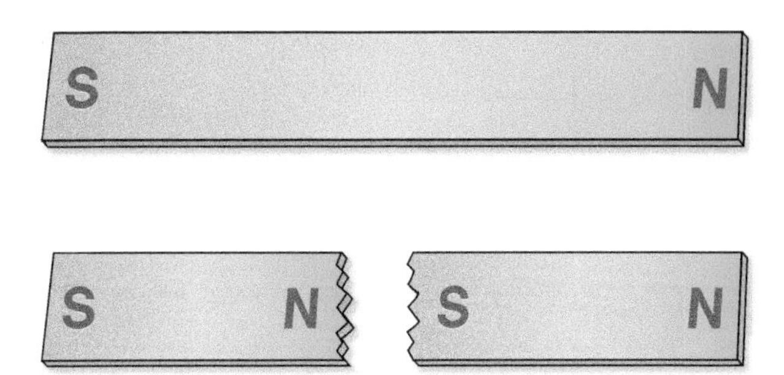

Figure 7.3. **Effect of dividing a magnet into increasing smaller pieces. Each piece, no matter how small, retains the original magnetic properties.**

Laws of Magnetism

The laws of magnetism include the following:

Repulsion-attraction: Like poles repel, unlike poles attract.

Magnetic poles: Every magnet has a north pole and a south pole.

Inverse square law: The magnetic force between two magnetic fields is directly proportional to the product of their magnitudes and inversely proportional to the square of the distance between them.

The first law of magnetism, like poles repel and unlike poles attract, is true because when a magnet is placed in the force field of another magnet it is acted upon by that force field. An example of this law may be seen when the north pole of one bar magnet is placed near the south pole of another bar magnet, their opposite field lines will be attracted to each other. Likewise, when the north poles of two bar magnets are placed close together, the lines of force are in the same direction and will repel each other (Fig. 7.4). It is critical that this law is observed in an MRI department where the strength of the magnet will attract metallic objects and the metal objects will be attracted to or pulled into the magnet.

The second law of magnetism, magnetic poles, states that every magnet has a north pole and a south pole. No matter how many times the magnet is divided, both poles will continue to exist. Perhaps the most dramatic example of this law is the Earth itself, which is actually a giant natural magnet. The Earth spins on an axis and has a magnetic field. Lodestones are ferromagnetic rocks that are natural magnets because their magnetic domains have aligned with the Earth's magnetic field. Two concepts that must be considered with all magnets are **permeability** and

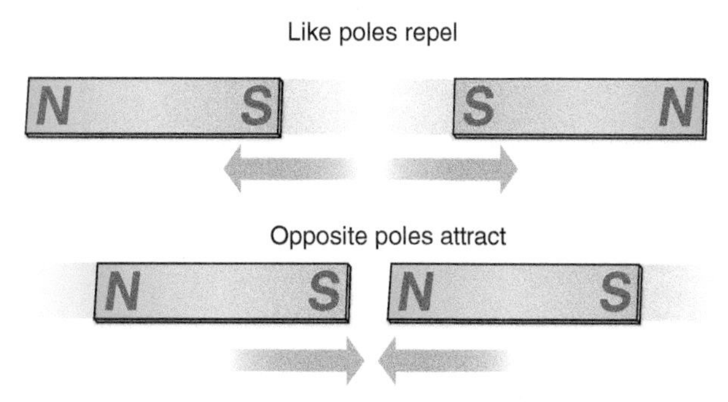

Figure 7.4. **Repulsion-attraction of magnets. When the like poles of two magnets are close to each other, their force fields will repel each other. No matter how hard you try, you will not be able to make the two magnets touch. If you take one of the magnets and turn it so that the opposite pole is now facing the other magnet, their unlike poles will attract each other and the magnets will slam together. It will take a lot of force to separate these two magnets.**

retentivity. Permeability is determined by how easily a material can become magnetized by an external magnetic field. Retentivity is the ability of material to retain its magnetism over time. Most ferromagnetic materials are highly permeable and have low retentivity or retention of the magnetic field. Once magnetized, they will lose the magnetism if tapped outside of the external magnetic field. The tapping causes the magnetic domains to convert back to a random orientation, which renders the material nonmagnetic.

Permanent artificial magnets are made of alloys that are designed to improve retention of the magnetic field. When the alloy is exposed to a very strong magnetic field, the alloy becomes magnetized and tends to remain magnetized for long periods of time. This means that the artificial magnet has high retentivity.

The third law of magnetism, the magnetic force between two magnets decreases as the square of the distance between the magnets increases, is based on the inverse square law used in electrostatics. An example of this law is demonstrated when opposite poles of two magnets are placed within 1 inch of each other. When the force fields of the two magnets influence each other, the magnets will be pulled together. Now take the two magnets and place them 2 inches apart, and if the force fields are strong enough, they may still interact with each other, but first, they must overcome the distance between the magnets. As distance is doubled between two magnetic objects, the attraction will be one-fourth the original attraction.

Magnetic Induction

When an iron bar is brought within the flux lines of a strong magnet, the domains in the iron bar will temporarily align themselves with the flux lines passing through the iron bar. As seen in Figure 7.5, the magnetic field lines will pass through the iron bar causing it to become temporarily magnetized. Soft iron makes an excellent temporary magnet because it is highly permeable, but it will only remain magnetized as long as the magnetic field lines are in place. This process is called **magnetic induction**, and it will work with any ferromagnetic material. When the strong magnetic flux lines are removed, the domains in the iron bar will return to their original random state.

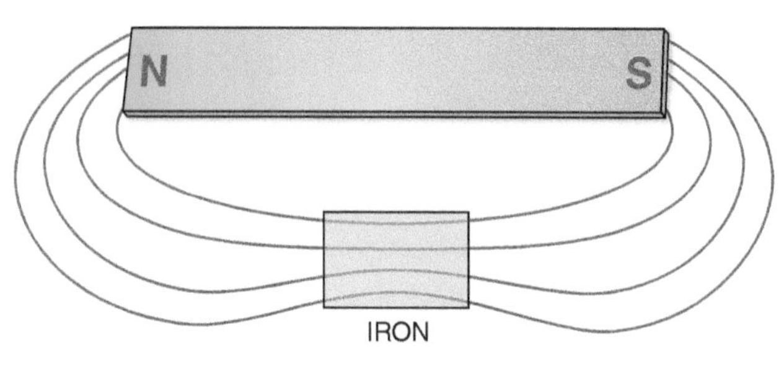

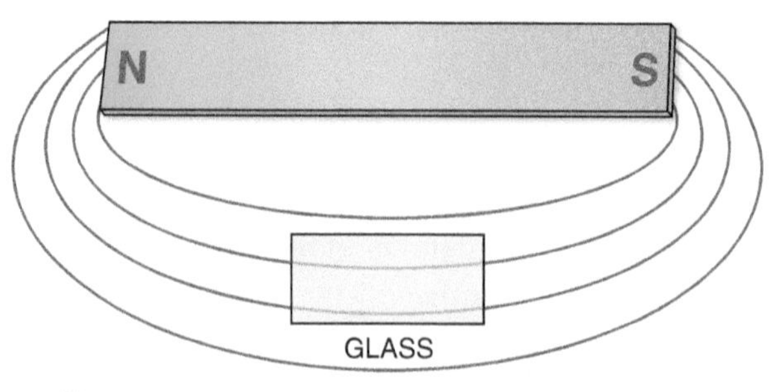

Figure 7.5. **(A) Ferromagnetic material like an iron bar attracts the magnetic field lines. (B) Nonmagnetic material does not affect the magnetic field lines.**

Electromagnetism

Electromagnetism is the branch of physics that deals with the relationship between electricity and magnetism. In the 19th century, scientists studied electricity and magnetism but did not connect the two concepts together. In 1820, Hans Oersted, a Danish physicist, discovered that a magnetic compass needle would turn when placed near a wire carrying direct current. The needle then went back to its normal position when the current was discontinued. He concluded that a magnetic field always surrounds a conductor in which electric current is flowing. His discovery led to the development of motors and generators, which is discussed later in this chapter. Figure 7.6 shows the magnetic field around a current-carrying conductor. The magnetic field is represented by imaginary lines that form circles around the conductor or wire. The accompanying magnetic field is a fundamental property of electric currents. The strength of the magnetic field increases with an increase in the current.

A conductor that is coiled into one or many loops is called a **helix**. When current is supplied to the helix, one end acts as the north pole and the opposite end the south pole of a magnet. When the conductor is coiled in a loop, it forms a helix, and when current is supplied to the helix, it makes a solenoid. Such a helix carrying current is called a **solenoid**. The magnetic fields from different parts of the coil compress together, which increases the magnetic field in the center of the coil. Increasing the current or the number of turns in the coil produces a stronger magnetic field in the center of the coil. This occurs because the magnetic fields will interact with each other, which creates a stronger current flow.

Adding a ferromagnetic material such as iron in the center of the coil also increases the magnetic field strength by concentrating the field through the center of the iron. Figure 7.7 shows how the magnetic field in the center of a coil is increased by adding turns to the coil and adding ferromagnetic material to the center of the coil. The

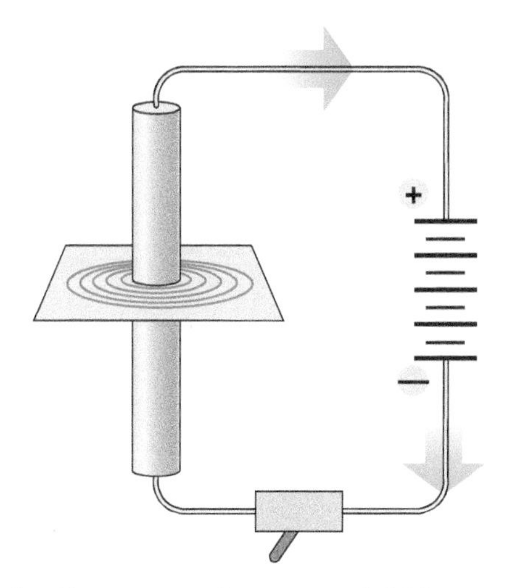

Figure 7.6. Illustration of magnetic field lines around a conductor carrying a current.

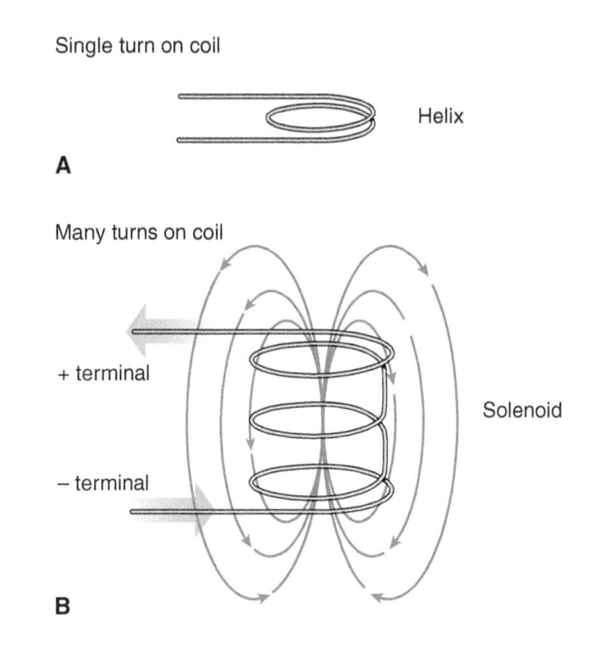

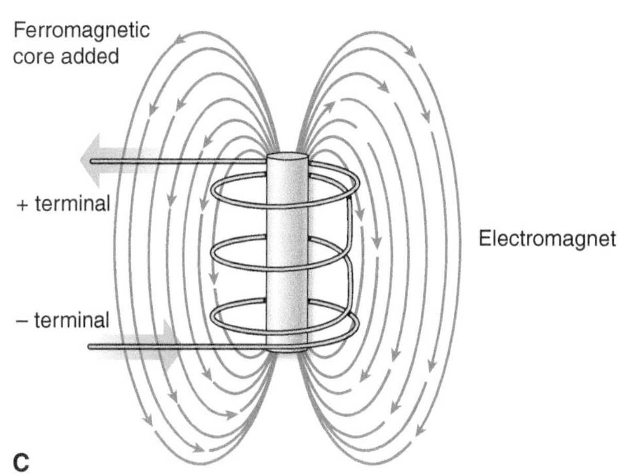

Figure 7.7. (A) Helix. (B) Helix + flowing current = solenoid. (C) Solenoid + iron core = electromagnet.

ferromagnetic iron becomes magnetized, and its magnetic field lines interact with the electric field of the solenoid. This produces a powerful electromagnet, which is utilized in radiographic equipment. The electromagnet will produce electric current as long as the helix is supplied with electricity. Once the electricity is turned off, the electromagnet will no longer produce current because the magnetic field collapses and disappears when the current is shut off. Therefore, an electromagnet is a temporary magnet, which has almost no retentivity.

Electromagnetic Induction

The relationship between current, a ferromagnetic core, and changing magnetic fields is called **electromagnetic induction** and is the basis of transformer operation. A changing magnetic field produces an electric field. This electric field will cause electrons to flow in a conductor. Electromagnetic induction is the production of a current in a conductor by a changing magnetic field near the conductor. The magnetic field must be changing. A steady magnetic field does not induce an electric current.

Closely behind Oersted's discovery, Michael Faraday, a British scientist, performed a series of experiments to find out if the reverse of Oersted's discovery could be true. Faraday found that when a bar magnet is placed next to a conductor, there is no resultant current flow in the conductor. He then moved the magnet and found that when the magnet was moved, the conductor would have current flowing.

Faraday's experiments demonstrated that an electromotive force (*emf*) or voltage can be induced in a conductor in three ways.

One method is to move a magnet near a stationary conductor carrying a current. As the magnet approaches the conductor, the magnetic field around the conductor increases. As the magnet moves away from the conductor, the magnetic field decreases. The change in the magnetic field as the magnet approaches and recedes induces voltage to flow in the conductor (Fig. 7.8).

A second method to induce voltage is by moving a conductor near a stationary magnet. In this case, the magnetic field is stationary and the conductor moves. The relative motion between the magnet and the conductor is the same regardless of which part moves and which is stationary. In either case, voltage is induced in the conductor (Fig. 7.9).

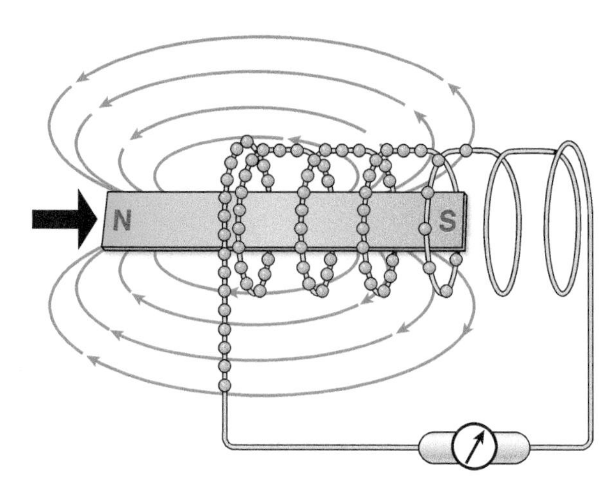

Figure 7.8. **Moving a magnet near a stationary conductor results in current flowing in the conductor.**

A third method of inducing voltage is to hold the conductor stationary and generate the magnetic field with a stationary AC electromagnet. The magnetic field from the electromagnet expands and contracts. This changing magnetic field induces voltage to flow in the conductor (Fig. 7.10). In every case, the change in the magnetic field induces the current. The amount of induced current depends on the strength of the magnetic field and how quickly it is changing.

Faraday's observations are summarized in Faraday's law. The magnitude of the induced *emf* depends on four factors. Maximizing these variables individually or in combination will produce the highest possible voltage

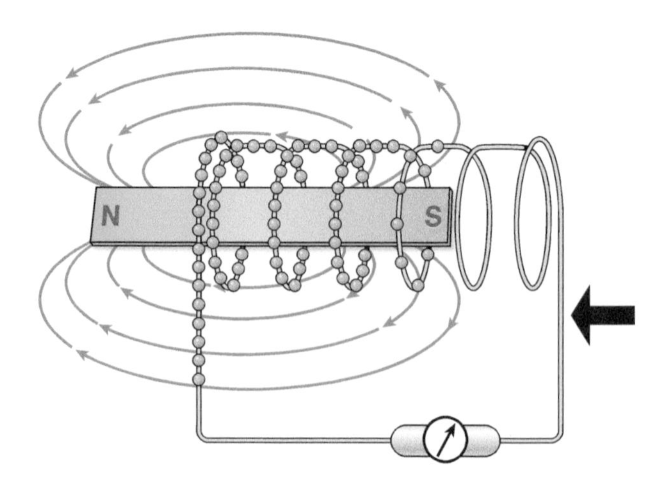

Figure 7.9. **Moving a conductor near a stationary magnet will create current flow in the conductor.**

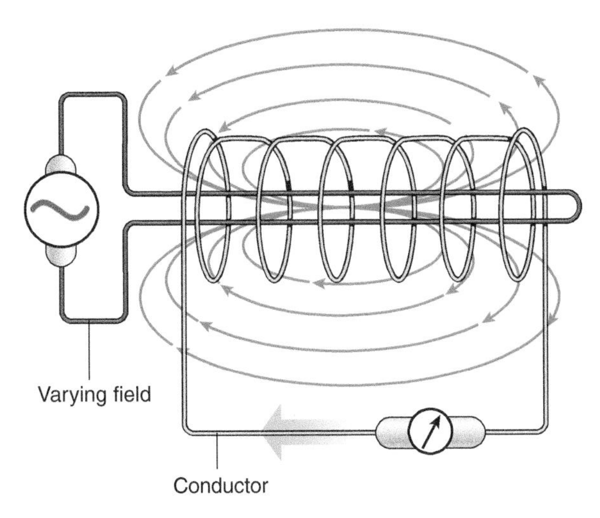

Figure 7.10. **Using an AC electromagnet to induce voltage in a stationary conductor.**

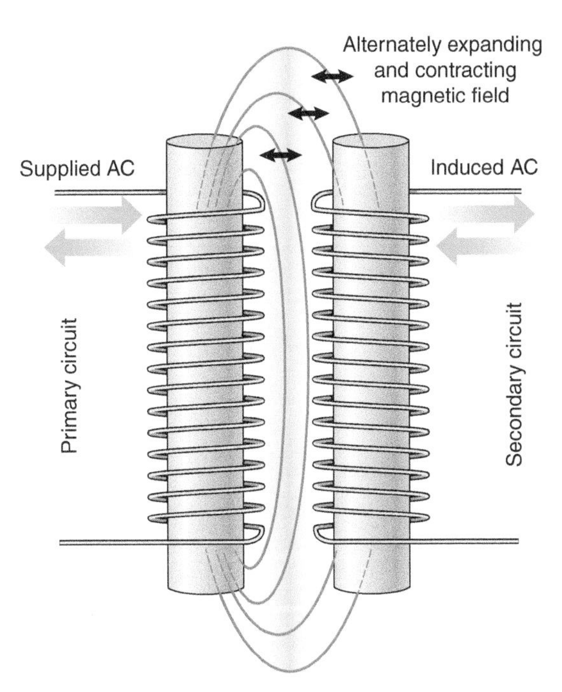

Figure 7.11. **Mutual induction. When the primary coil is supplied with AC, lines of force are induced in the primary coil. These expanding and contracting lines of force then interact with the nearby secondary coil, thereby inducing AC flow in the secondary coil.**

for the materials used in the conductor. These four factors are:

1. The *strength* of the magnetic field. Increasing the magnetic field strength will produce stronger field lines, which will then produce a more powerful *emf* in the conductor.
2. The *velocity* of the motion between field lines and the conductor. As the rate or speed at which the conductor crosses the magnetic field lines increases, a higher *emf* will be produced because more field lines will be crossed per second.
3. The *angle* between the magnetic field lines and the conductor. Magnetic field lines that are at a 90-degree angle to the conductor will produce the greatest amount of *emf* because the conductor is crossing through the maximum number of field lines possible per second.
4. The *number of turns* in the conducting coil. Conductors with more turns or coils will produce greater *emf* because each turn or coil will produce its own *emf*, which will then interact with the other turns, thereby increasing the *emf* even more. The induced *emf* is directly proportional to the number of turns in the coil.

Mutual Induction

Mutual induction occurs when two coils are placed close to each other and a varying current supplied to the first or primary coil induces a similar current flow in the second or secondary coil. AC in an electromagnet produces a changing magnetic field. As the magnetic field lines expand and contract in the primary coil, they are providing the relative motion necessary to induce AC flow in the secondary wire. This is the principle of transformer operation (Fig. 7.11).

Self-Induction

X-ray machines operate by using two forms of electromagnetic induction: mutual induction and self-induction. Heinrich Lenz experimented with *emf* and determined that an induced *emf* always creates a current whose magnetic field moves in the opposite direction of the original *emf*. A phenomenon known as self-induction.

Electromotive force, when produced with the motion of a magnetic field near a conductor, will act or move in reverse of the motion of the original magnetic field. A prime example is when a rare earth magnet is moved into close proximity to a clockwise-rotating copper conductor. As the conductor rotates, its magnetic field lines will expand and act upon the magnet. The magnet will rotate in a counterclockwise direction as seen in Figure 7.12.

Now let us apply this explanation to inducing current. Consider Figure 7.13 where the coil is connected to an AC

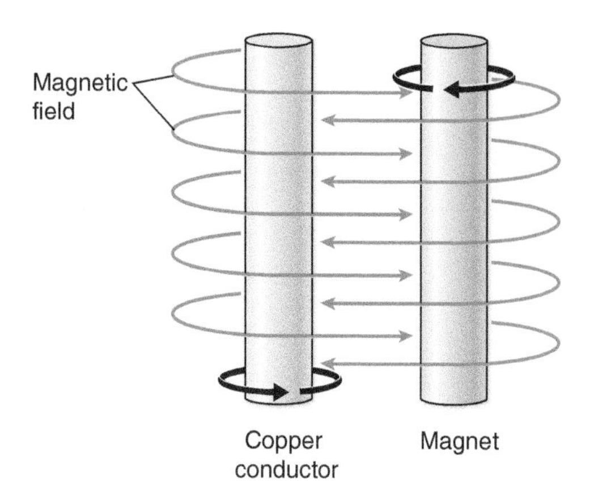

Figure 7.12. **Self-induction. The magnetic field from a conductor will cause a magnet to spin in the opposite direction.**

power source. As the *emf* flows from the power source, the magnetic flux lines will expand outward from the center of the coil. As the magnetic lines move, they "cut" through the turns of the coil. This "cutting" creates or induces current within the same coil. The induced current moves in the opposite direction of the original *emf*. This process will continue as long as the coiled conductor is supplied with AC power. This phenomenon of self-induction is used in the x-ray circuit in the autotransformer. X-ray circuitry and autotransformers are covered in Chapter 8.

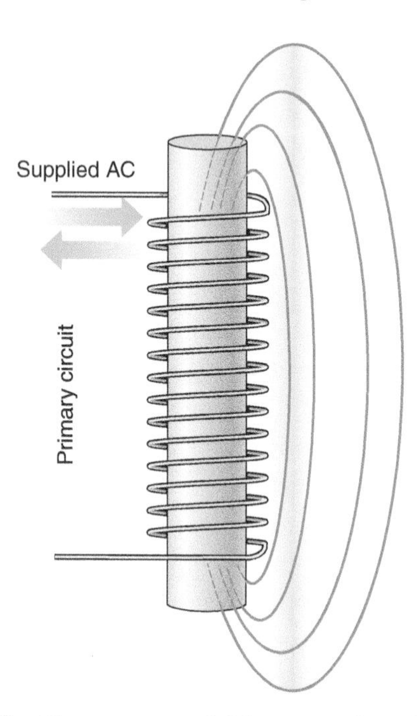

Figure 7.13. **The magnetic field is created in this coil and expands outward from the center of the coil. When the alternating current moves back and forth through the coil, it creates current to be produced. This is another example of self-induction.**

Electric Generators

thePoint® ***An animation for this topic can be viewed at http://thepoint.lww.com/Orth2e***

An electric generator converts mechanical energy into electrical energy. A simple generator is made of a conductor and magnets arranged as shown in Figure 7.14. The conductor is a coil of wire called an **armature**, and the armature is set between the opposing magnetic poles. As the armature is turned by a mechanical method (a crank), an electric current is induced in the armature that is moved through a magnetic field across or perpendicular to the magnetic field lines. In other words, the armature or metal conductor is coming into contact with the magnetic field, when this happens the magnetic field produces an electric current in the armature.

As the mechanical crank continues to turn, the conductor or armature moves parallel to the magnetic field, there is no current induced in the conductor because the magnetic field is not intersecting with the armature. The conductor must cut through the magnetic field lines in order to induce a current.

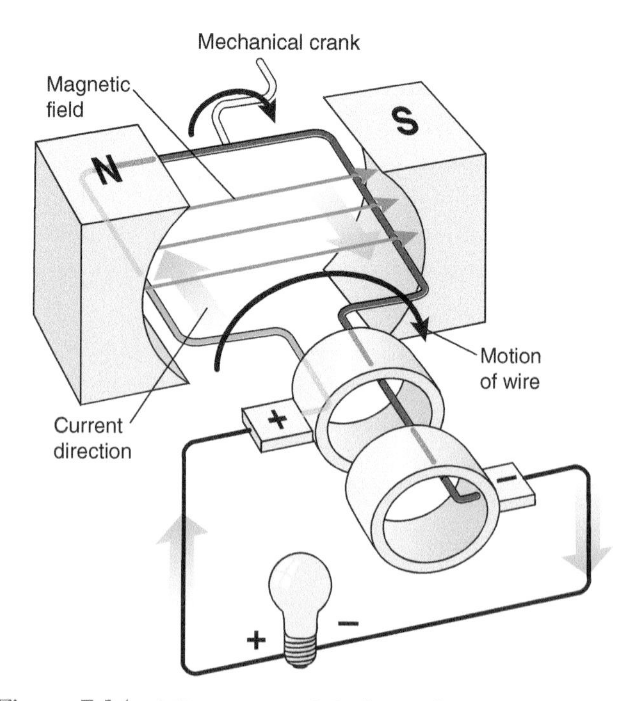

Figure 7.14. **AC generator. Mechanical energy rotates the shaft that is attached to the armature. As the armature rotates through the magnetic fields, it crosses through the magnetic lines of force and produces electric current.**

It is crucial to note the method by which the induced current flows in a circuit. Each end of the armature is connected to a metallic **slip ring**, which allows constant contact with a set of brushes. The slip rings are stationary and allow the armature to rotate within the magnetic fields. The induced current flows from the armature through the slip rings to the brushes and finally through the circuit (Fig. 7.14) to give power to the light bulb. As the armature turns, the induced current will flow in one direction and then in the opposite direction. Thus, this type of generator produces alternating current.

Figure 7.15 illustrates how a coil rotating in a magnetic field produces an alternating current. To understand exactly how the current is induced in the circuit, it is necessary to follow the production step by step. It is important to understand the angle between the armature's motion and the magnetic lines of force between the stationary magnets.

Step A: The armature is parallel to the magnetic field lines, so no current is being produced. This is seen on the sine wave as no current flow when the armature is at 0 degrees.

Step B: As the armature begins to rotate, it will come into contact with the magnetic field; when the armature is at a 45-degree angle, it is intersecting with the magnetic field. At this time, the electric current will be produced, but it is not very strong as seen by the slight upward movement of the sine wave. This is because at a 45-degree angle the magnitude of the emf is rising but has not reached its peak.

Step C: The armature continues to turn until it is at a 90-degree angle to the magnetic field lines. This is the maximum angle that represents the peak of the sine wave or maximum electrical current.

Step D: As the armature rotates more and reaches a 135-degree angle, notice how the sine wave is starting to go down. The induced voltage is beginning to go back toward zero.

Step E: The armature is again parallel when it is at 180 degrees and there is no current being produced. The sine wave is again at zero.

Step F: As the armature begins to move to the 215-degree angle, notice that the sine wave is now under the line; this is the negative portion of the sine wave.

Step G: The armature is not at 270 degrees, which is 90 degrees in the opposite direction from where the sine wave began. At this point, the alternating current is being produced because the armature's motion relative to the lines of force is reversed.

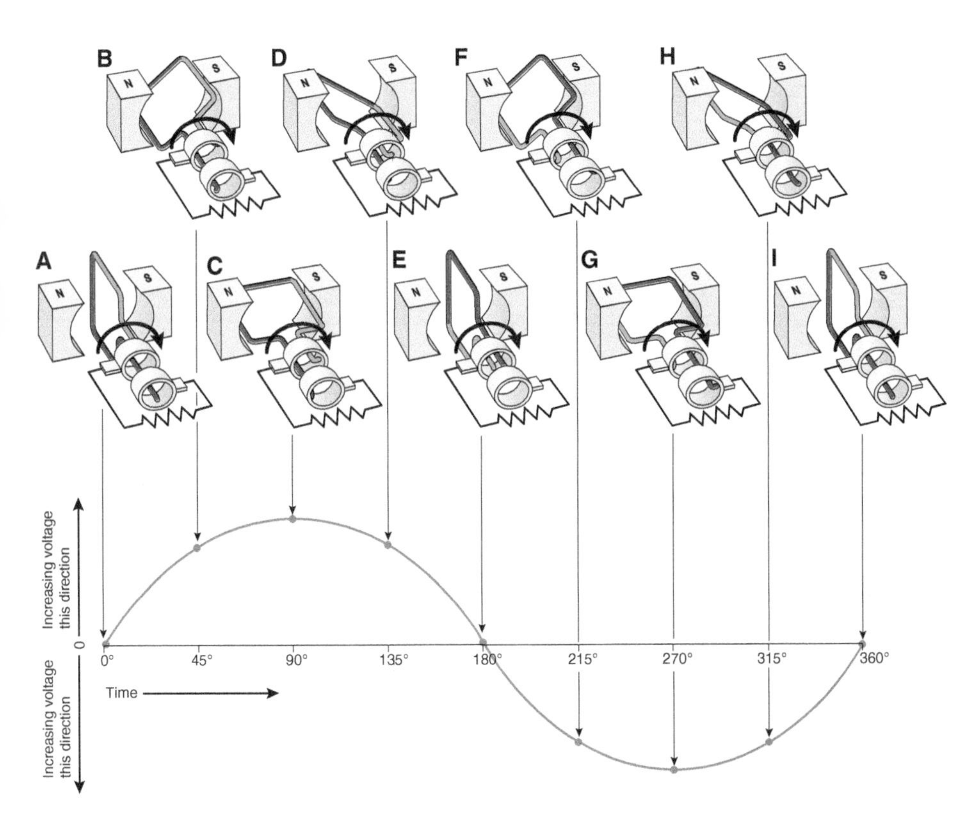

Figure 7.15. **Rotating coil of wire produces an AC. Notice how the placement of the armature in relation to the magnetic field is demonstrated on the sine wave.**

Step H: The armature continues its rotation toward parallel but is still intersecting the magnetic field lines so a lower amount of current is being produced.

Step I: The armature is again parallel to the magnetic field lines and no current is induced. The induced current is an alternating current.

One complete turn from step A to step I represents one complete sine wave or one cycle. This description is based on a single loop of coil; additional loops in the coil increase the voltage induced in the coil because there would be more opportunities for the armature to be intersecting with the magnetic field.

A DC generator utilizes the same design as an AC generator, except that the slip rings are replaced with a **commutator ring**. A commutator ring is a single ring that is divided in half with the halves separated by an insulator. Each half of the commutator ring is connected to one end of the armature. The armature is turned mechanically and moves through the magnetic field lines inducing a current. Although the action of the DC generator is the same as an AC generator (Fig. 7.16, steps A–C), the resulting sine wave is routed differently. In Figure 7.16, step D, the armature has begun to turn toward the second phase of the cycle. As the commutator ring rotates the armature through the magnetic field, the polarity of each half of the ring will alternate. This allows the current to flow first in one direction and then in the reverse direction resulting in current flowing out of the commutator in one direction, notice the orientation of the needle on the gage of the circuit wire. Step E represents the armature as parallel to the magnetic field lines where zero current is induced. The armature will continue to turn and produce direct current where the sine wave is only seen above the line.

Electric Motors

A motor converts electrical energy into mechanical motion. The simple electric motor has the same basic construction as a DC generator, except there is an external power source supplying current to the commutator ring. Electric motors work on the principle of the Magnetism Law of Repulsion and Attraction.

The process of moving the armature through the external magnets field is illustrated in Figure 7.17 and can be described by the following steps:

Step 1: The commutator ring directs the flow of current to the armature, which causes a magnetic field to build around the armature.

Step 2: As the magnetic field of the armature is attracted to the external magnet, the armature will rotate through the external magnet's magnetic field. Notice the direction of the magnetic lines of force flowing from the north pole of the magnet to the south pole.

Step 3: As the armature becomes aligned with the external magnet, the commutator switches the direction

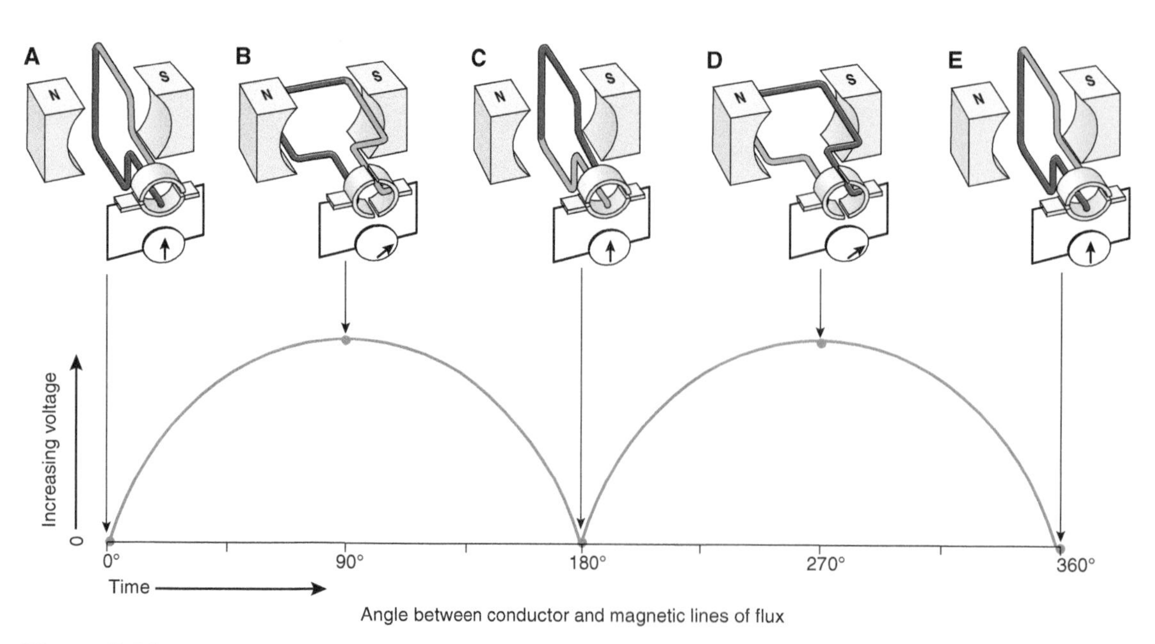

Figure 7.16. DC generator.

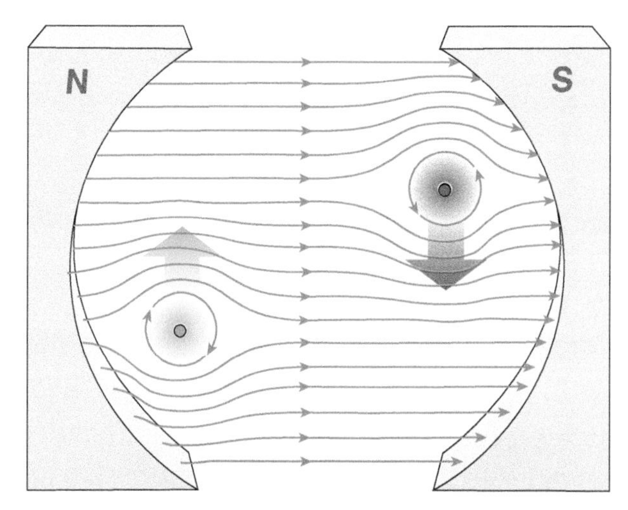

Figure 7.17. **Because the conducting wires of the armature lie within the lines of force from the north and south pole of a horseshoe magnet, when current begins to flow through the armature, the induced lines of force will be attracted downward for the left wire and upward for the right wire. At the same time, the wires will be repelled in the opposite direction (upward for the left wire and downward for the right wire). The result is that the conductor begins to move in the direction of the *arrows*.**

of current flow through the armature, thereby reversing the armature's required alignment. At this point, the magnetic fields of the external magnet and armature are the same, which will cause the armature to be repelled by the external magnet, moving the armature out of the external magnet's field.

Step 4: The armature will rotate 180 degrees toward the other pole of the external magnet because it is attracted to that magnetic field. Essentially, the armature is seeking alignment with that pole, which is the opposite polarity of the armature's magnetic field.

Step 5: As the armature moves into the magnetic field, the commutator will again switch the current flow to force the armature to rotate again.

The result will be that one arm of the armature is "attracted" to the magnetic field, while the other arm is "repelled" away from the magnetic field. This process will continue to keep the armature rotating continuously. These interactions will continue as long as a current is supplied to the armature. Effectively, the armature motion creates the electrical energy that moves a mechanical object. Once the current is turned off, the magnetic field surrounding the armature will collapse and it will no longer move.

Induction Motors

Induction motors are AC motors that operate on the principle of mutual induction. In an x-ray tube, the rotating anode is driven by a **rotor** attached to an induction motor. The components of an induction motor include a rotor and a **stator**. The rotor is in the center of the induction motor and consists of copper bars arranged around a cylindrical iron core. The stator has an even number of stationary electromagnets placed around the rotor. Both the rotor and the anode are sealed inside an evacuated glass envelope. The stator, located outside the glass envelope, is supplied with alternating current, which produces changing magnetic fields by switching the current in each set of electromagnets. As illustrated in Figure 7.18, the electromagnets of the stator are energized in sequence, creating magnetic fields that induce current in the copper bars. As the magnetic fields of the copper bars reach a point, they are equalized with the electromagnets magnetic field, and the next set of electromagnets is activated by the alternating current. This forces the rotor to follow the external magnetic fields of the stator, thereby pulling the rotor to the next position. This sequence continues to occur as long as there is alternating current being supplied to the stator.

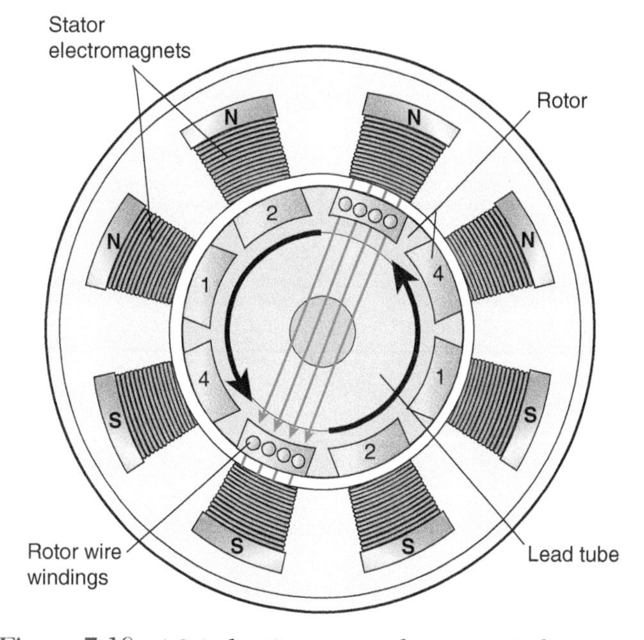

Figure 7.18. **AC induction motor: the rotor windings will move perpendicular to the magnetic lines of flux, in the direction of the *arrows*. The stator electromagnets are supplied with multiphasic current (AC) to activate them in sequential pairs to maintain maximum perpendicular force. As long as the AC is flowing, the rotor will continue to turn.**

Chapter Summary

This chapter has continued to present foundational information that is essential for you to understand the science behind radiology and to prepare you for the later, more applied chapters.

1. Magnetism pertains to the attracting of iron by a magnet or moving electrical current.
2. There are four types of materials (ferromagnetic, paramagnetic, diamagnetic, and nonmagnetic) and their varying degree of attraction to magnets, magnetic fields, the laws that govern magnets, and the units used to measure magnetic flux.
3. Electrons moving through a conductor make up an electric current. Current is the amount of electrons moving in a conductor per second and is measured in amperes or milliamperes.
4. Voltage is the electrical pressure or *emf* applied to the electrons in the conductor and is measured in volts.
5. There are multiple methods that can be used to induce current in a conductor.
6. Generators and motors are used in x-ray equipment.
7. DC electricity always moves electrons in one direction, while AC oscillates the electrons in one direction and then the opposite direction.
8. Devices that use electromagnetic induction require alternating current to keep the magnetic fields moving.
9. Electrical generators convert mechanical energy into electrical energy. Electrical motors convert electrical energy into mechanical energy. Both operate on the principles of electromagnetic induction.
10. Induction motors can be constructed with only coils of wire and use the principles of mutual induction to operate.

Case Study

Sally was given an assignment to design and build an electromagnet for her physics class. She is to research the types of magnetic materials, properties of magnets, and conductors to determine the most efficient design.

Critical Thinking Questions

1. What are the types of magnetic materials and which one is the most suitable for Sally to use?
2. Which properties must Sally consider when deciding on the material with the highest likelihood of becoming magnetized?
3. What are the factors that influence the amount of *emf* that is produced in the circuit?
4. How can the addition of an iron bar into a coiled conductor increase the strength of the voltage that is produced?

Review Questions

Multiple Choice

1. **What is the basic charged particle?**
   a. Electron
   b. Neutron
   c. Volt
   d. Coulomb

2. **Which statement is not one of the laws of magnetism?**
   a. Like poles repel.
   b. Unlike poles attract.
   c. Stronger magnets have larger poles.
   d. The force between magnets decreases with the square of the distance between them.

3. **Which type of magnetic material is weakly repelled by other magnetic fields?**
   a. Diamagnetic
   b. Ferromagnetic
   c. Paramagnetic
   d. Nonmagnetic

4. **The field lines of a magnet flow __________ to the magnet.**
   a. parallel
   b. perpendicular
   c. either parallel or perpendicular
   d. neither is correct

5. **A magnetic domain is best described as:**
   a. the dipoles in a magnetic material are all oriented in the same direction
   b. the spinning of electrons on their axes as they orbit an atom
   c. a group of atoms whose dipoles are aligned in the same direction
   d. the domains in a magnetic material are randomly oriented

6. **Faraday's law states that electrical current will flow through a conductor when it is placed in a __________ magnetic field.**
   a. stationary
   b. moving

7. **Alternating current is required for any device that operates on the basis of:**
   a. self-induction only
   b. mutual induction only
   c. electromagnetic induction

8. **The three types of diamagnetic materials are:**
   a. copper
   b. beryllium
   c. iron
   d. a and b
   e. b and c

9. **When the north pole of one magnet is placed close to the south pole of another magnet, the magnets will:**
   a. be repelled from each other
   b. be attracted to each other
   c. be pushed apart

Short Answer

1. **Describe the change in intensity if the distance between two magnified objects is doubled.**

2. **Describe the third law of magnetism.**

3. Which magnetic material is not affected by a magnetic field?

4. Explain how a magnetic domain can cause an object to behave like a magnet.

5. Describe retentivity as it relates to magnetic materials.

8

X-Ray Unit Circuitry

Objectives

Upon completion of this chapter, the student will be able to:

1. Identify single-phase, three-phase, and high-frequency waveforms.
2. Describe the relationship between current and voltage in the primary and secondary sides of step-up and step-down transformers.
3. Identify the components of a typical x-ray circuit and their purpose.
4. Describe the purpose and operation of a rectifier.
5. Describe the operation of a transformer.
6. Define voltage ripple.
7. Explain the components of the control console and how each is used during an exposure.

Key Terms

- anode
- autotransformer
- cathode
- half-wave rectification
- high-frequency generator
- rectifiers
- ripple
- shell-type transformer
- single-phase circuits
- step-down transformer
- step-up transformer
- three-phase circuit
- transformers

Introduction

X-ray circuits convert electric energy into x-ray energy. Knowledge of the components of an x-ray circuit will assist the radiographer in detecting and correcting problems with the technical settings used to produce the x-ray image. X-ray circuits generate x-rays using transformers that convert low voltage (100 to 400 volts [V]) into high voltage (thousands of volts called kilovolts). X-ray circuits utilize transformers to change the voltage, rectifiers to convert alternating current (AC) into direct current (DC), and autotransformers to select the milliamperes and kilovolts peak applied to the x-ray tube. X-ray circuits were previously referred to as x-ray generators. However, the term generator used in this context has nothing to do with the generators described in Chapter 7, which are used to generate electric currents. Combining this information with correctly setting the control console will result in the radiographer producing exposures with the minimum amount of radiation necessary to produce a quality image.

Basic X-Ray Machine Circuit

The material from previous chapters has formed a foundation of knowledge that will culminate in the discussion of the basic x-ray machine circuit. The main circuit is composed of three sections: the control console, the high-voltage circuit, and the x-ray tube. Components of the high-voltage circuit include the high-voltage transformer, the step-down transformer, and the **rectifiers**. Each of these types of **transformers** is necessary to produce the appropriate amount of voltage and amperage needed to produce x-rays.

The power plant provides the incoming line voltage that is used throughout the hospital. This incoming line voltage tends to fluctuate based on current usage, and when coupled with the large amounts of electricity used in a hospital, the incoming voltage is unreliable. The equipment in the imaging department must have consistent voltage supplied to it; this is accomplished with a line voltage compensator. The purpose of the line voltage compensator is to maintain a constant voltage to the equipment. In modern equipment, this is done automatically in the circuit. The result of the line voltage compensator is consistent voltage, which allows radiographers to set reliable radiographic techniques with confidence. The following sections will describe the equipment that is used to confidently set exposure factors.

thePoint® *An animation for this topic can be viewed at http://thepoint.lww.com/Orth2e*

Transformers

Transformers are devices that use the properties of electromagnetism, which are essential to operate x-ray equipment. Radiographic equipment uses AC and operate by electromagnetic induction. Transformers are the portion of the x-ray circuitry that transforms voltage and current into higher or lower intensity. A transformer makes use of Faraday's law and the ferromagnetic properties of an iron core to efficiently raise or lower AC voltages. It cannot increase the power in the circuit, so if voltage is raised, the current is proportionately lowered and vice versa.

In a sinusoidal wave, as the AC moves from positive to negative and back again, the flow of electrons causes a magnetic field to continuously build and collapse around the wire carrying the AC. This action combined with the principles of mutual induction and Ohm's law provides the basic functions of a transformer. Figure 8.1 illustrates the components of a basic transformer: primary coil, secondary coil, and ferromagnetic core.

An AC supplied to the primary coil changes the magnetic field around the coil. The changing magnetic field from the primary coil, or input circuit, induces a current in the secondary coil, or output circuit. This is the principle of mutual induction. The magnetic fields surrounding the primary and secondary coils will continue to expand and collapse, thereby causing mutual induction in each coil. The input circuit voltage and current on the primary coil will differ from the output circuit voltage and current on the secondary coil.

The secondary coil of a transformer can be linked to the primary coil by an iron core to improve its efficiency. The iron core acts as an electromagnet when current is supplied to the primary coil. When the magnetic fields of the primary coil interact with the iron core, the iron core will then produce a magnetic field. This magnetic field will then interact with the primary and secondary coils, thereby increasing the amount of mutual induc-

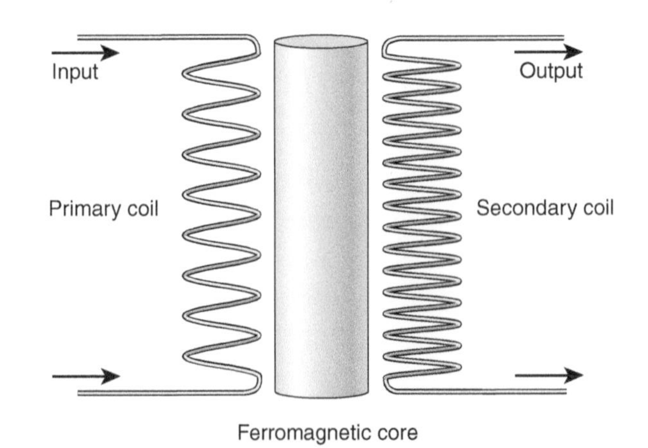

Figure 8.1. Components of a simple transformer.

tion and ultimately increasing the amount of current flowing in the secondary coil. Just as Faraday discovered it would do!

The transformer is used to change the amount of voltage and current in an AC circuit. The key principle is that when the secondary coil has more turns or windings than does the primary coil, the change in voltage is directly proportional in the secondary coil. Imagine the secondary coil has twice as many windings as the primary coil; the induced voltage in the secondary coil would be doubled. This is called a step-up transformer for voltage. The voltage in the secondary coil of a transformer is related to the voltage in the primary coil by the transformer law for voltage:

$$V_s / V_p = N_s / N_p$$

where V is the potential difference in volts, N is the number of turns of wire in the coil, p is the primary coil, and s is the secondary coil. The turns ratio, N_s/N_p, is the ratio of the number of turns in the secondary coil to the number of turns in the primary coil.

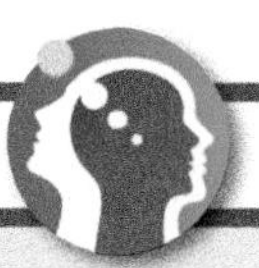

CRITICAL THINKING BOX 8.1

If a transformer is supplied with 120 V and has 200 turns of wire in the primary coil and 40,000 turns of wire on the secondary coil, what will be the resultant voltage in the secondary coil? What is the turns ratio?

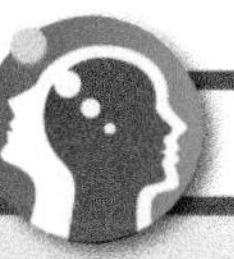

CRITICAL THINKING BOX 8.2

There are 140 turns on the primary side of a transformer and 20,000 turns on the secondary side of a transformer. What is the turns ratio for this transformer?

The output voltage in the secondary coil depends on the turns ratio and on the primary voltage. Increasing the number of turns in the secondary coil of a transformer increases the output voltage and decreases the output current. You are likely thinking that the transformer law defies the law of conservation of energy. Remember that you cannot increase voltage without something decreasing. Theoretically, the power will remain constant, which means that when resistance is fixed, the amperage must decrease anytime there is an increase in voltage. According to Ohm's law, the induced voltage and current in the transformer coils are inversely related: higher voltages in the secondary coil are accompanied by lower currents or amperage in the secondary coil. This occurs because the power output of the transformer cannot exceed the power input. When the secondary voltage is higher than the primary voltage, the secondary current must be less than the primary current. If the secondary voltage is lower than the primary voltage, the secondary current is higher than the primary current.

Transformers are used to change voltage; however, Ohm's law is in effect, and the effect of the transformer on voltage, amperage, and number of turns in the coil can be determined by combining the transformer law with Ohm's law. Remember, the change in current is inversely proportional to the ratio of the number of turns in the primary coil to the number of turns in the secondary coil. The following formulas demonstrate the combination of these two laws:

$$\text{Transformer law for current } I_s / I_p = N_p / N_s$$

$$\text{Transformer law for voltage and current } I_s / I_p = V_p / V_s$$

where I is amperage, V is voltage, N is the number of turns, p is the primary coil, and s is secondary coil.

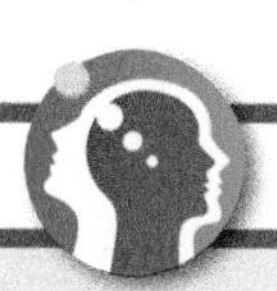

CRITICAL THINKING BOX 8.3

The turns ratio in a filament transformer is 0.175. There is 0.6 A of current flowing through the primary coil. What will be the resultant filament current?

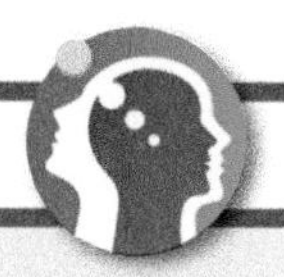

CRITICAL THINKING BOX 8.4

There are 130 turns on the primary side of a transformer and 80,000 turns on the secondary side. If 220 V of AC are supplied to the primary winding, what is the induced voltage in the secondary winding?

When working with transformers, it is helpful to remember that voltage and the number of turns are directly proportional, while voltage and amperage are inversely proportional. Therefore, the amperage and number of turns also have an inverse relationship. In a step-up transformer, the voltage is increased and the amperage must decrease to keep the power constant. Conversely, a step-down transformer will decrease voltage from the primary coil to the secondary coil, with a corresponding increase in amperage. The amount of increase or decrease in voltage is directly related to the number of primary and secondary turns. Therefore, a step-up transformer will have more turns in the secondary coil, which means higher voltage and lower amperage. A step-down transformer will have fewer turns in the secondary coil than the primary coil, which provides a lower voltage and higher amperage in the secondary coil. As you can see, when voltage changes, amperage must have a corresponding change to keep power equal.

Types of Transformer Cores

There are many different ways to build a transformer to improve efficiency, and each has a different type of core configuration. Various types of cores have been designed and used, but there was a lack of efficiency in producing voltage. The closed core transformer was designed to use layers of iron to form the ferromagnetic core. Layering the iron sheets helped to reduce energy losses, which resulted in greater efficiency. The closed core is shaped in a square with the primary and secondary windings on opposite sides. This configuration will confine the magnetic field lines to the core resulting in the field lines making a continuous loop. The design directs the field lines from primary core to secondary core, which results in a significantly higher increase in field strength. The **shell-type transformer** uses a central iron core with both the primary and secondary windings wrapping around the iron core. The primary and secondary windings are heavily insulated to prevent the bare wires from touching each other. Placing the wires around the iron core decreases the distance between the coils, which allows for maximum mutual induction to occur (Fig.8.2). In modern x-ray equipment, most transformers are the shell type.

Autotransformers

Autotransformers work on the principle of self-induction. Incoming power goes to the autotransformer first, which then directs the flow of power to the rest of the x-ray circuit. The incoming line voltage is controlled by the autotransformer, which has the capability of varying the voltage. The function of an autotransformer is to provide a variety of voltages for input to the step-up and step-down transformers.

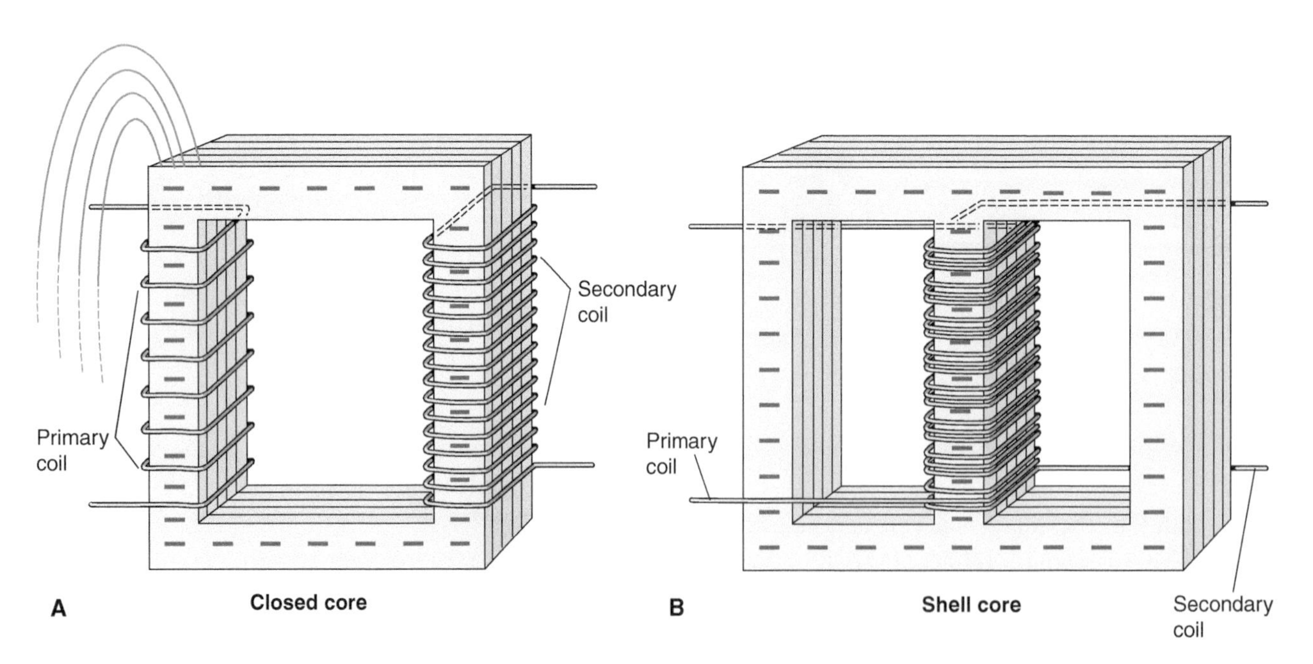

Figure 8.2. Types of transformer cores: (A) closed core and (B) shell type.

An autotransformer has an iron core with only one coil, which serves as both primary and secondary transformer windings. This single winding has a number of connections along its length. The connections on the primary side conduct the line voltage to the autotransformer. In an x-ray circuit, the output of an autotransformer is used to change the voltage in the primary coils of the step-up transformer. The secondary side has output connections, which are attached at different points along the coil. Different output voltages are obtained by selecting one of the output taps, thereby changing the input voltage to the step-up transformer. Through the process of induction, the voltage received and the voltage produced are directly related to the number of turns that were tapped. The number of turns selected is adjustable and moving the contactor to tap more or fewer turns on the secondary side varies the ratio from secondary to primary (Fig. 8.3). Varying the voltage to the step-up transformer allows for changes to the output voltage. As an example, if the input voltage of the autotransformer is 220 V and the output tap is selected for half the voltage, the resultant voltage to the primary coil would be 110 V. The autotransformer law is the same as the transformer law, and the formula is used in the same manner.

Step-Up Transformers

A step-up transformer converts a lower AC voltage into a higher AC voltage and is also called the high-voltage transformer. Step-up transformers have more turns in the secondary coil than in the primary coil (Fig. 8.4). The output voltage of a step-up transformer is higher than the input voltage, and the output amperage is always less than the input amperage. Step-up transformers are used to supply high voltages to the x-ray tube. Figure 8.5 illustrates the input voltage and amperage on the primary

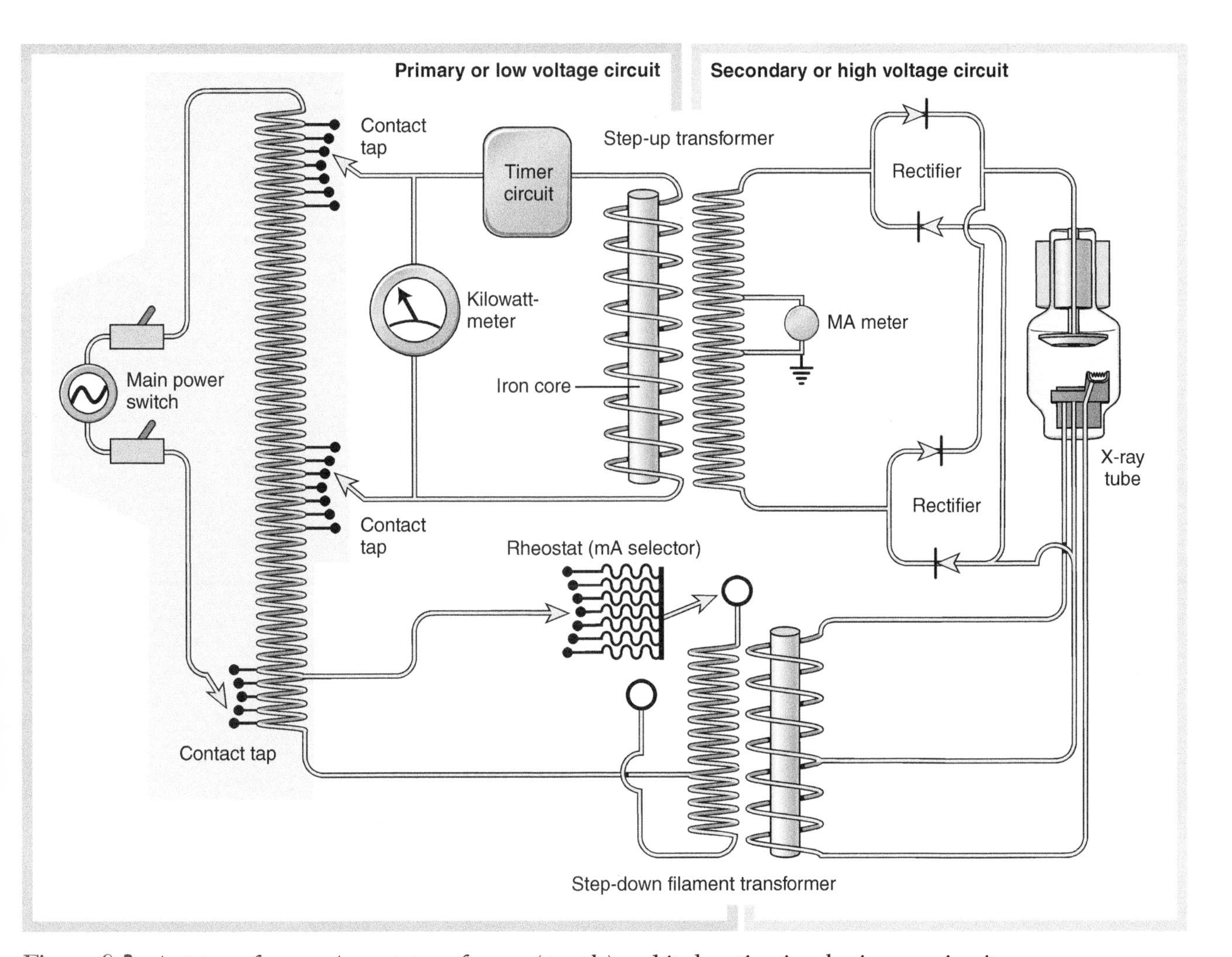

Figure 8.3. **Autotransformer. An autotransformer (*purple*) and its location in a basic x-ray circuit.**

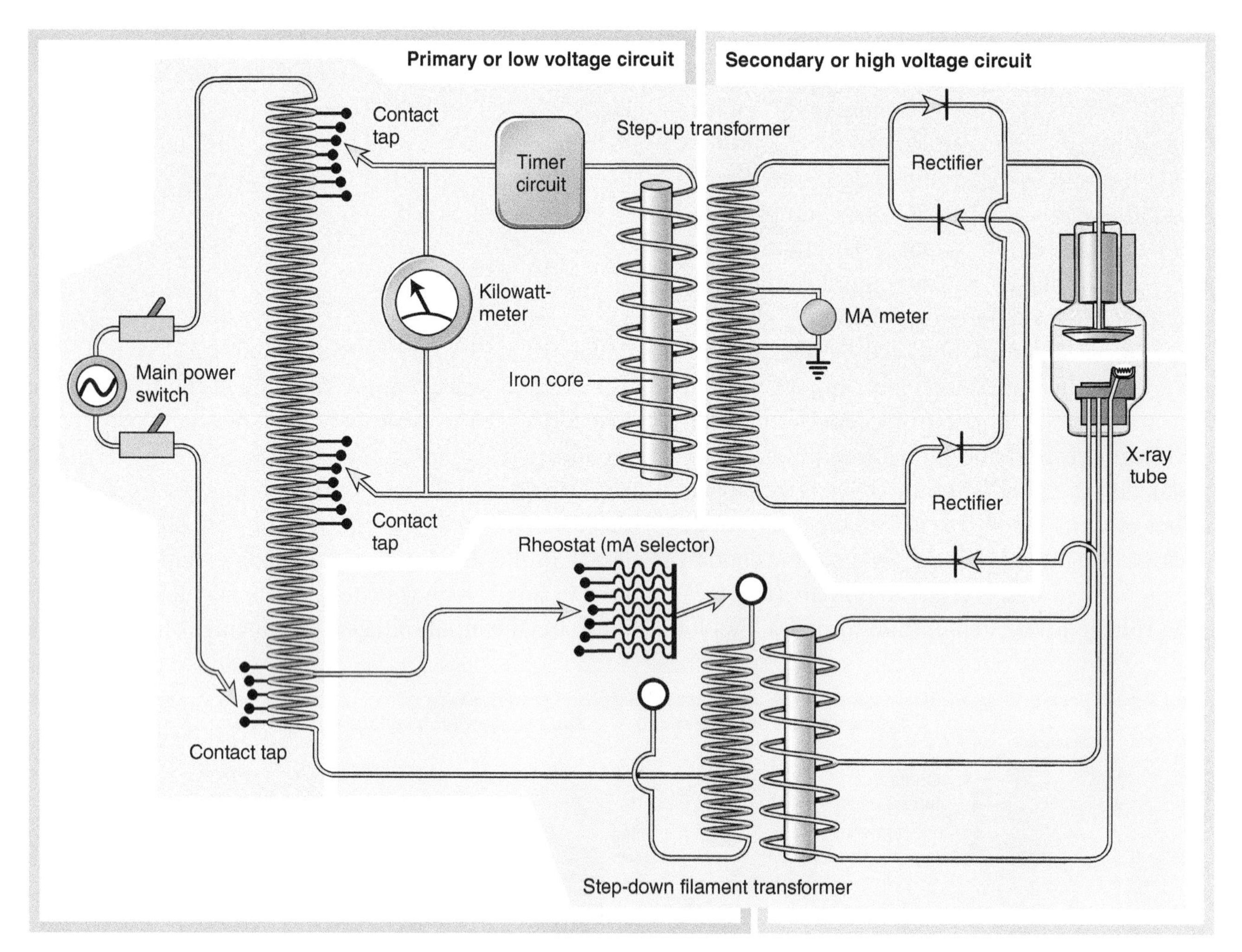

Figure 8.4. Step-up transformer. A step-up transformer (*purple* and *green*) and its location in a basic x-ray circuit.

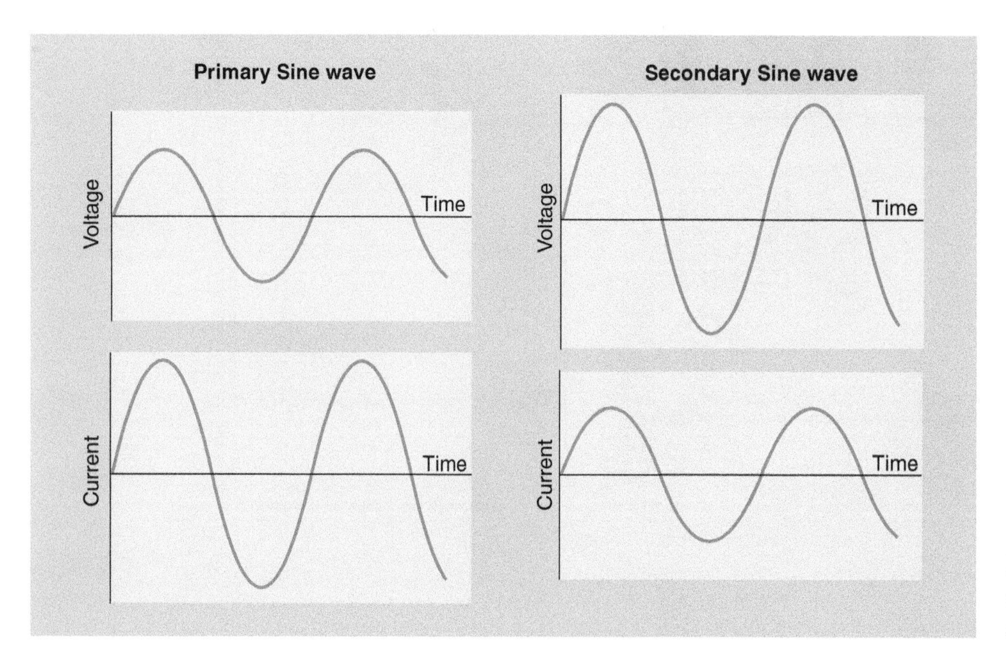

Figure 8.5. Voltage and current on the primary and secondary sides of a step-up transformer.

side as it is coming into the x-ray unit. Notice that in the output side, an increase in voltage has a corresponding decrease in amperage. This occurs due to Ohm's law, which states that as voltage is increased there must be a corresponding decrease in amperage. Remember these changes are inversely proportional to each other.

X-Ray Unit Circuits

Figure 8.4 is a general illustration of a basic x-ray circuit. There are three individual circuits in the x-ray unit: the primary circuit, secondary circuit, and filament circuit. Each section has specific components that play a rather important part in the production of a beam of x-radiation. The circuits work together to supply the x-ray tube with the correct amount of voltage and amperage for a given exposure.

Primary Circuit

The primary circuit is the first circuit in the series of circuits. The power plant provides incoming line voltage, which has fluctuations that when combined with the usage of power at the hospital result in an inconsistent voltage. A line voltage compensator measures the incoming voltage and automatically compensates by adjusting the autotransformer slightly up or down. A circuit breaker is another component that protects the unit. When the circuit has an overload or short circuit in any part of the system, severe damage and heating can occur. The circuit breaker will kick off and stop the flow of electricity, which could potentially damage delicate electronic components in the circuit.

There are two circuits, which utilize the incoming line voltage: the primary circuit and filament transformer. Most of the voltage is used in the primary circuit, and a small amount is used in the filament circuit. The primary circuit is the autotransformer, which is composed of one coil, which has both primary windings and secondary windings. The autotransformer is an adjustable transformer, which is controlled by the kilovoltage peak selector on the control console. When the radiographer selects a given kVp setting, the autotransformer determines the number of turns on the secondary side that will be part of the circuit element and the resultant kVp. This autotransformer is sometimes called the kVp selector, and its purpose is to provide voltage that will be increased by the step-up transformer to produce the kilovoltage selected at the operating console. A prereading voltmeter is used to read out the kVp. The meter measures the amount of voltage selected from the autotransformer before it is stepped up. The meter readout is located on the control console and demonstrates what the kVp will be when it reaches the x-ray tube. The kVp meter is seen in Figure 8.4.

The step-up transformer is the dividing line between the primary and secondary circuits. The primary coil is in the primary circuit and the secondary coil is in the secondary circuit. This transformer is not adjustable like the autotransformer and increases voltage by certain amounts. An exposure timer is located in this section because it is easier to control low voltage than a very high voltage. There have been several types of timers used in an x-ray circuit. A synchronous timer was the first type of timer used and is based on a synchronous motor. The motor was designed to turn a shaft at exactly 60 revolutions per second, which controls the on and off switches in the circuit. An electronic timer is a sophisticated and highly accurate device that is commonly used today. This timer is based on the time it takes to charge a capacitor through a variable resistor. As soon as the capacitor receives its preprogrammed charge, the exposure will be terminated. Automatic exposure control (AEC) devices are also used to determine the amount of exposure that is necessary to produce a diagnostic image. AECs have ionization chambers, which are selected based on the anatomy to be imaged. When the AEC has received the correct amount of electric charge, the exposure is terminated. AECs are discussed in further detail later in the chapter.

Secondary Circuit

The secondary circuit begins on the other half of the step-up transformer and induces a secondary voltage that is higher than the primary voltage. The high-voltage transformer has a turns ratio between 500:1 and 1,000:1. Transformers operate on AC, which means the waveform on both sides of the high-voltage transformer is an unrectified sinusoidal wave. In Figure 8.6, the primary and secondary sine waves are seen. The only difference is that the amplitude for the current is much higher in the secondary sine wave. The primary sine wave is measured in volts, while the secondary sine wave is measured in kilovolts. The primary current is measured in amperes,

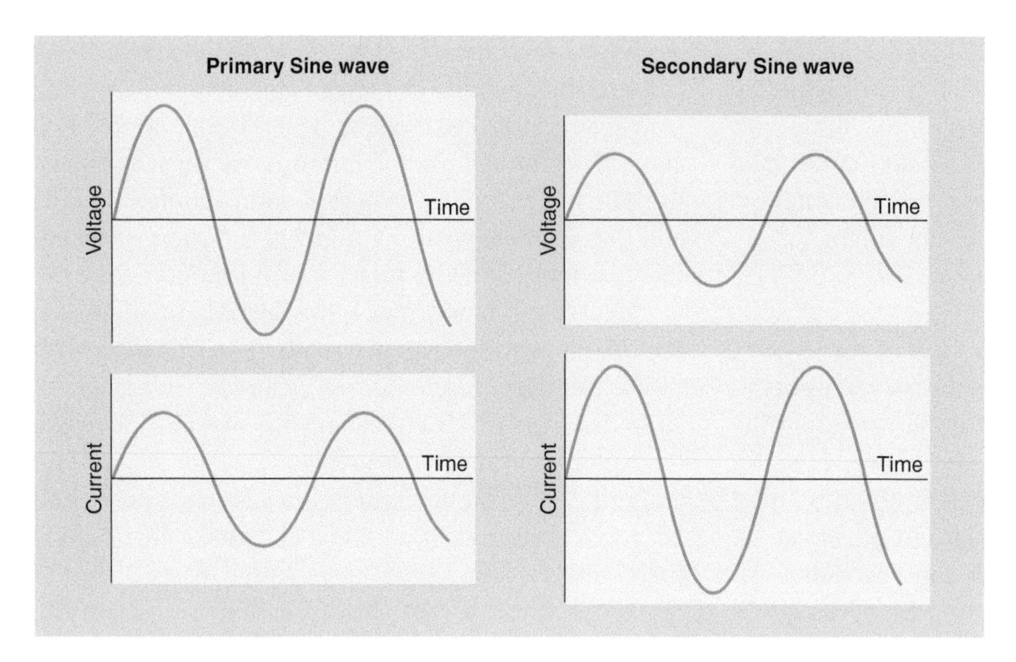

Figure 8.6. **Voltage and current on the primary and secondary sides of a step-down transformer.**

while the secondary current is measured in milliamperes. The secondary circuit includes a milliampere meter to monitor current going to the x-ray tube.

In the general x-ray circuit, AC is necessary to induce voltage, which allows transformers to operate properly. However, the x-ray tube would receive severe damage if it were exposed to AC. The x-ray tube requires DC, which moves electrons in only one direction. In order to change the AC to DC, the electrons must go through a bank of rectifiers in the rectification process.

Rectification

The current from a common wall electrical outlet is 60 Hertz (Hz) AC. This current changes 120 times per second; however, the x-ray tube requires DC. There must be a final step to convert the AC to DC. Rectifiers are solid-state devices that allow current to flow in only one direction. They are used to convert high-voltage AC from the secondary side of the step-up transformer to high-voltage DC, which is applied to the x-ray tube. Current flows from the positive terminal of the x-ray tube, which is called the **anode**, to the negative terminal of the x-ray tube, which is called the **cathode**. Although current is said to flow from positive to negative, in an x-ray tube, electrons actually flow from the cathode to the anode or negative to positive. X-ray tubes must operate with DC, which will only allow electron flow from the cathode side of the x-ray tube to the anode side of the tube. If AC were permitted, electrons would flow from the anode side to the cathode side resulting in damage to the fragile filament.

Modern solid-state diodes have two semiconducting crystals; one is a p-type crystal (positive) and the other an n-type crystal (negative). The p-type crystal has holes in the outermost shells of its molecules, and the holes can be made to drift or move. The n-type crystal has loosely bound electrons that are free to flow. The diode is constructed by connecting the two crystals at the n-p junction with each side connected to a wire conductor as seen in Figure 8.7. When electricity is applied to the wire conductor on the side of the n-type crystal, the crystal's electrons will be repelled toward the n-p junction.

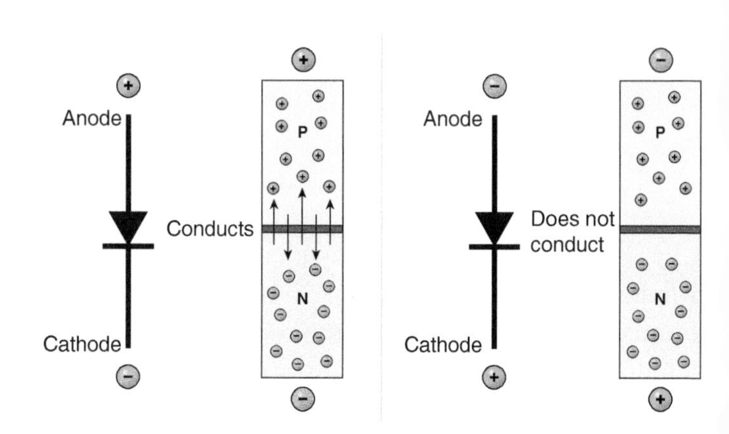

Figure 8.7. **Solid-state rectifier with n-type and p-type crystals connected at the n-p junction. Note the change in polarity in the rectifier, which results in conduction and nonconduction phases.**

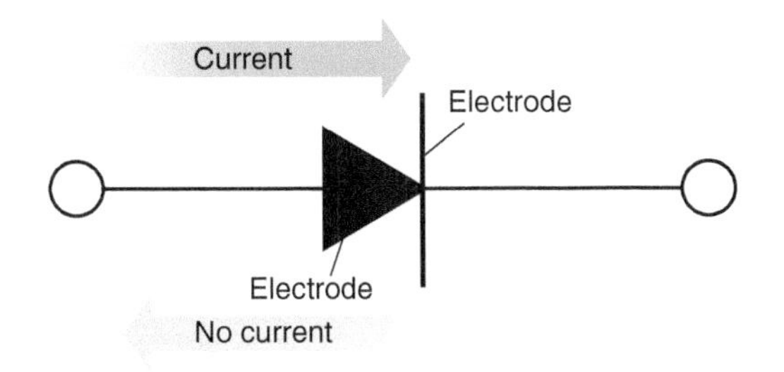

Figure 8.8. **This symbol for a diode represents the flow of current through a rectifier. The current flows easily out of the point of the electrode. The other electrode blocks the flow of current.**

The holes on the p-type crystal drift or move toward the n-p junction in response to the positive charge on the wire connected to the p-type crystal. The electrons will fill the holes and move across the junction in response to the potential difference that exists at the n-p junction. As long as this process is occurring, the solid-state diode will conduct electricity. When the AC cycle reverses the negative electricity flows to the p-type crystals and the positive electricity flows to the n-type crystals, the solid-state diode will not conduct electricity. This occurs because the holes and electrons are attracted to opposite ends of the crystals; as long as no potential difference exists, the electricity will be blocked. Therefore, the solid-state diodes are rectifiers because they conduct electricity in only one direction. The symbol for a rectifier is seen in Figure 8.8. To use the symbol to determine current flow, notice the triangle shape in the middle. The current will flow with the direction of the point of the triangle, and electrons flow against the direction of the point.

Half-Wave Rectification

Half-wave rectification uses two rectifiers in the electronic circuits to convert AC to DC. During the positive portion of the sine wave, the rectifier allows the electric current to flow through the x-ray tube in the correct way. During the negative half of the sine wave, the solid-state diodes are used to effectively suppress or block the negative portion of the AC sine wave. Figure 8.9 demonstrates the resultant wave pattern where there is a series of positive pulses separated by gaps when the negative current is not conducted. The resultant waveform shows the current is flowing in only one direction. This type of rectification is called half-wave rectification. The positive portion of the sine wave is utilized to produce pulsating DC with 60 x-ray pulses per second.

Full-Wave Rectification

Full-wave rectification uses at least four rectifiers in the electronic circuit.

Figure 8.10A shows the arrangement of four rectifier diodes, which are color coded to show which pair is in use during each half of the cycle. During the positive half of the AC waveform, the red diodes are activated and the green diodes block electron flow. As the electrons flow from the negative side to the red and green diodes, the green diode is not able to conduct the electrons in that direction. The electrons must go through the red diode to reach the x-ray tube.

After the electrons flow through the x-ray tube, they run into the other set of red and green diodes. Only the red diode is positioned to conduct the electrons, and they flow to the positive side of the transformer, completing the circuit.

During the negative half of the AC cycle as seen in Figure 8.10B, the green diodes are activated, while the red diodes are not. Notice how the polarity of the x-ray tube does not change, the cathode is always negative and the anode is always positive even when the induced secondary voltage alternates between positive and negative.

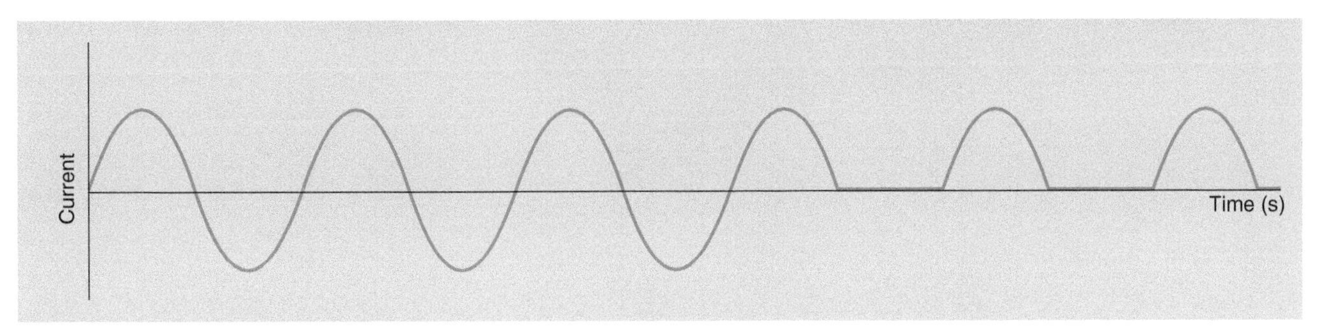

Figure 8.9. **Half-wave rectification. Notice how the negative half is not used and results in gaps between each positive wave.**

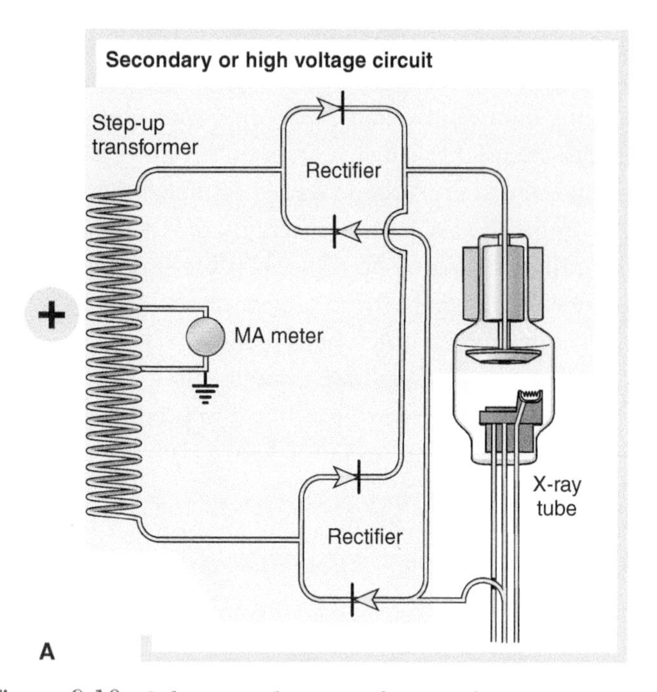

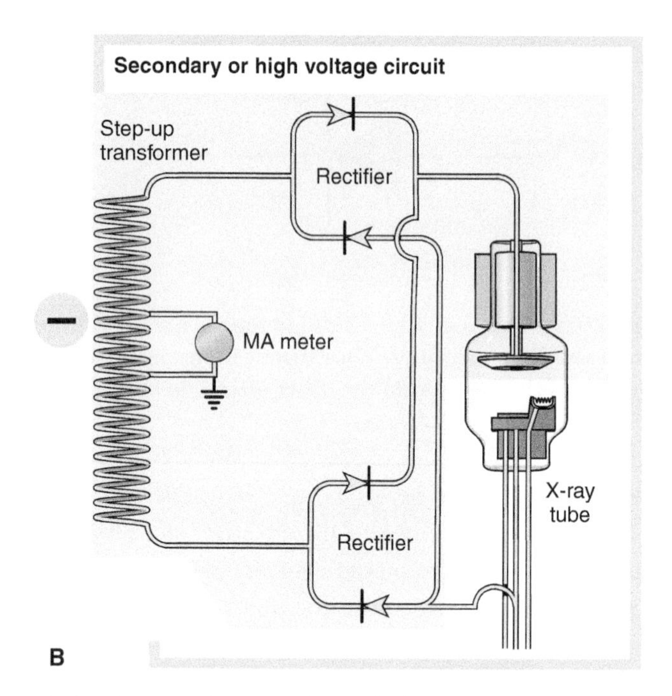

Figure 8.10. **Schematic diagram of a typical x-ray circuit. The rectifier diode pairs are color coded because they operate together in each half of the cycle. (A) During positive half of wave form the red diodes are activated to allow electron flow. (B) During the negative half of the wave form the green diodes are activated to allow electron flow.**

Notice that the output voltage passes through the x-ray tube from cathode to anode during each phase. The output current waveform shown in Figure 8.11 shows that the negative part of the AC sine wave is inverted to a positive wave. With full-wave rectification, the positive flow remains the same, but the negative portion is converted to positive current flowing in only one direction, or DC. This produces a more uniform pulsating DC sine wave, which starts at zero and fluctuates to a maximum voltage and then returns to zero. This is called "ripple," and when the voltage starts at zero and ends at zero, there is a 100% **ripple**, which is seen in single-phase full wave.

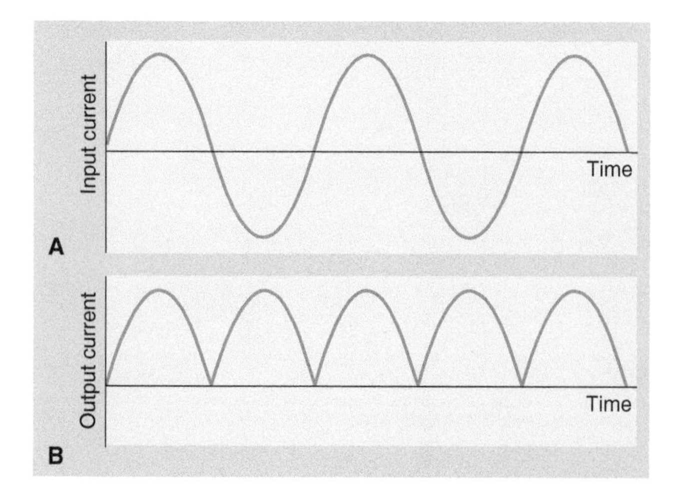

Figure 8.11. **Output current for full-wave rectified circuit.**

Single-Phase Power

Single-phase circuits use single-phase power that results in a pulsating x-ray beam. This pulsation is caused by the alternating change in voltage from zero to maximum potential 120 times each second in a full-wave rectified circuit. The x-rays produced when the voltage is near zero are of little diagnostic value as their energy is too low to adequately penetrate the tissue. The solution to this problem was to develop a method for using three simultaneous voltage waveforms out of step with one another.

The AC shown in Figure 8.12 is a single-phase current. With a 60-Hz supply of electricity, the voltage will reach zero two times in each cycle resulting in the voltage

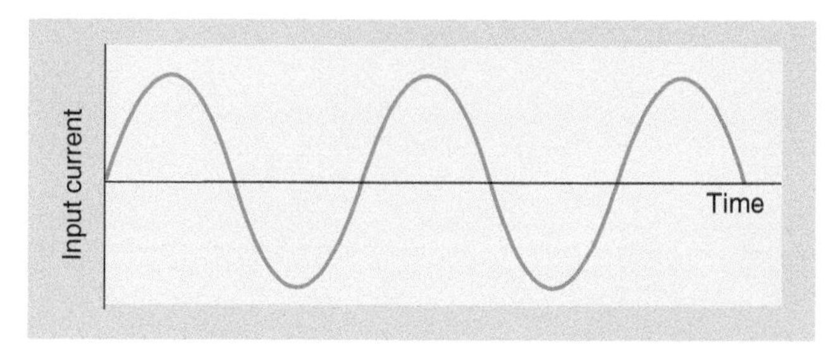

Figure 8.12. **Single-phase current.**

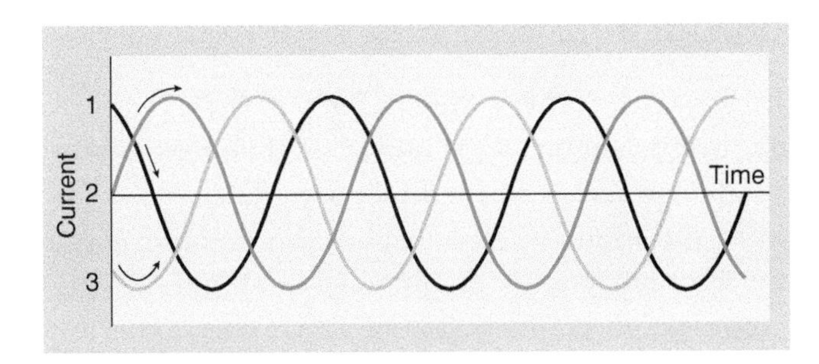

Figure 8.13. **Current flow of a three-phase circuit. Note how the waves are out of step, which prevents the sine wave from reaching zero.**

turning off and on 120 times per second. This type of current is very inefficient and modern equipment will not operate with single-phase current. By adding more circuit elements, it is possible to add two more phases to form a **three-phase** circuit. The major advantage of a three-phase circuit is that the current and voltage are more nearly constant, which results in more efficient x-ray production (Fig. 8.13).

Three-Phase Power

The solution of using three AC waveforms at the same time required engineers to figure out how to synchronize the waveforms. The three-phase six-pulse circuit requires six rectifiers to produce six usable pulses per cycle. The addition of two more circuits will create a total of three waveforms. Each wave is generated and then phased so that each pulse is 120 degrees out of phase or out of step with the other waves. Essentially, each wave is out of step by one-third. Notice how the overlapping waveforms result in a waveform that never reaches zero, thereby providing an overall increased voltage. The resultant waveform is seen in Figure 8.13 and will produce 360 pulses per second. Table 8.1 presents the number of rectifiers used in different forms of x-ray circuits.

The pattern of the waveform is called a *ripple*. Ripple measures the amount of variation between maximum and minimum voltage. Because most x-ray production occurs when the applied voltage is at maximum, the percent ripple provides a good indication of how much variation there is in the x-ray output. As we have discussed, when the voltage is increased, there are more x-rays produced. At higher voltages, more x-rays are produced and the x-rays are more penetrating. There is an increase in amperage in the circuit because more current is flowing. This means there is an increase in the quality and quantity of the x-ray beam. For a given exposure, the amount of remnant radiation reaching the plate or cassette is doubled when changing from a single-phase circuit to a three-phase circuit. Therefore, the technique can be cut in half and still maintain adequate exposure to the detector. The changes in techniques can either be a reduction in mAs by one-half or the kVp can be decreased to 15%. It is preferable to reduce the mAs because it will greatly decrease radiation dose to the patient.

By adding additional components, it is possible to further improve efficiency by producing 3-phase, 12-pulse voltage. The number of pulses is increased from six to twelve per cycle for a total of 720 pulses per second. This provides a more constant voltage waveform. Increasing the number of pulses in the waveform by using a 3-phase, 12-pulse circuit results in a waveform that maintains a nearly constant high voltage. Figure 8.14 demonstrates

TABLE 8.1 RECTIFIERS USED IN X-RAY CIRCUITS

Type of Circuit	Number of Rectifiers
Single phase, full wave	2 or 4
Three phase, six pulse	6
Three phase, twelve pulse	12

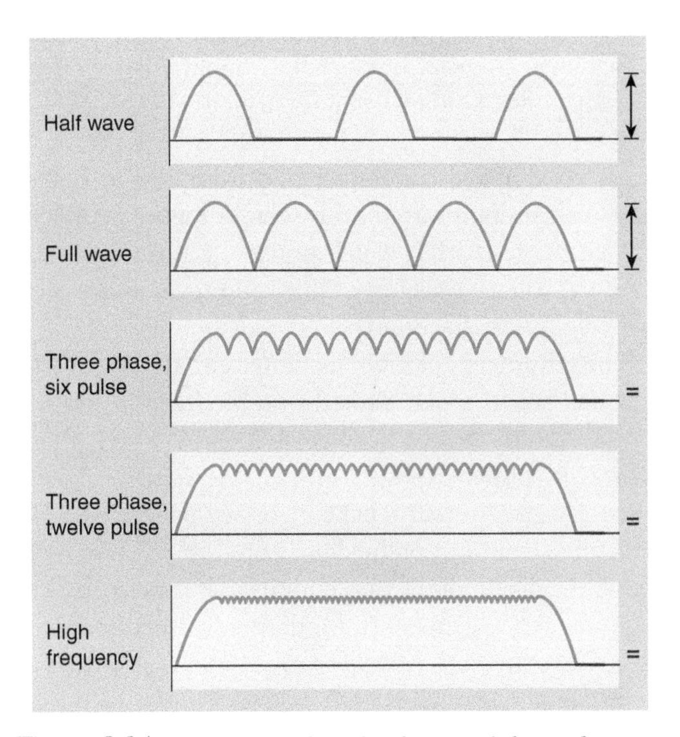

Figure 8.14. **Evolution of single-phase and three-phase waveforms.**

TABLE 8.2 THE AVERAGE VOLTAGE AND AMOUNT OF RIPPLE OF X-RAY CIRCUITS

Type of Circuit	Average % of set kV	Percent Ripple
Single phase	1/3 of set kV	100
Three phase, six pulse	91	14
Three phase, twelve pulse	97	4
High-frequency generator	~100	<1

the evolution from single-phase and three-phase waveforms with no rectification and rectified three-phase waveforms. Notice how the voltage becomes more consistent with the three-phase six-pulse waveform. The 100% ripple seen in the full-wave–rectified circuit decreases to about 14% ripple in the three-phase six-pulse system. The ripple was further decreased to about 4% in the three-phase twelve-pulse circuit. The overall effect of increasingly more sophisticated electronics is that the x-rays are produced anywhere from 87% to 100% of the kVp selected at the console for three phase six pulse to 96% to 100% for three phase twelve pulse (Table 8.2).

High-Frequency Generator

The efficiency of three-phase twelve-pulse systems led to the next advancement in transformer design: **high-frequency generators**. Transformers operate more efficiently at higher frequencies because the coupling between the primary and secondary windings is more effective. High-frequency circuits convert the input waveform from 60 Hz to a higher frequency ranging from 500 to 25,000 Hz. The resultant waveform is seen in Figure 8.14. The voltage ripple is <1%, which provides a nearly constant potential voltage waveform, which improves image quality while further lowering patient radiation dose.

The advantages of high-frequency circuits are smaller size, less weight, and improved x-ray production. The mA stations can be as high as 800 to 1,200 mA, which allows for much shorter exposure times. This is advantageous when imaging pediatric patients or any patient who has difficulty breathing or holding still. Table 8.1 demonstrates the evolution of x-ray circuits from single-phase to high-frequency generators. Modern computed tomography (CT) scanners have high-frequency circuits mounted in the rotating gantry. High-frequency circuits with their lightweight transformers make spiral CT practical. Most x-ray units installed today have high-frequency circuits.

Filament Circuit

The filament circuit is the final step in the x-ray circuit. Referring to Figure 8.15, notice the filament circuit is directly connected to the main x-ray circuit at a point before the input voltage reaches the autotransformer. The filament circuit incorporates a **step-down** transformer, which produces an output voltage that is lower than the input voltage. In a step-down transformer, the number of turns or windings on the secondary coil is less than the number of turns on the primary coil. Step-down transformers are used to supply high current to the tube filament. The filament circuit has a rheostat, a type of resistor, which varies current resistance and acts as a variable milliampere (mA) selector. When the radiographer selects the mA (current) on the control console, the rheostat determines the amount of resistance required for the mA selection. Since a rheostat is a variable resistor, it can apply less resistance to accomplish a large or high mA selection or more resistance for a lower mA selection.

The filament circuit contains a filament ammeter, which measures the amount of amperage. It is critical to control the amount of amperage that is crossing the filament in the x-ray tube. The filament step-down transformer is used to decrease the incoming line voltage from 15 to 5 V and 3 to 5 amperage range to heat the x-ray tube filament. The filament is made of two small wires, which are heated to boil off electrons for the exposure. If the filament is heated too much, damage can occur, so it is crucial that the filament ammeter accurately measure the amperage used in the circuit.

The filament circuit produces a sine wave in which the input and output voltages and currents are the same as a step-down transformer sine wave seen in Figure 8.7. The output voltage sine wave has less amplitude compared to the incoming line voltage. Conversely, the output current has much greater amplitude, which demonstrates the increase in amperage.

Control Console Operation

The first step in producing an x-ray exposure is selecting the technical factors necessary for the exposure. Radiographers use the various components on the control console to set appropriate factors. The control console components include the kVp, time and mA selectors, and the AEC circuit.

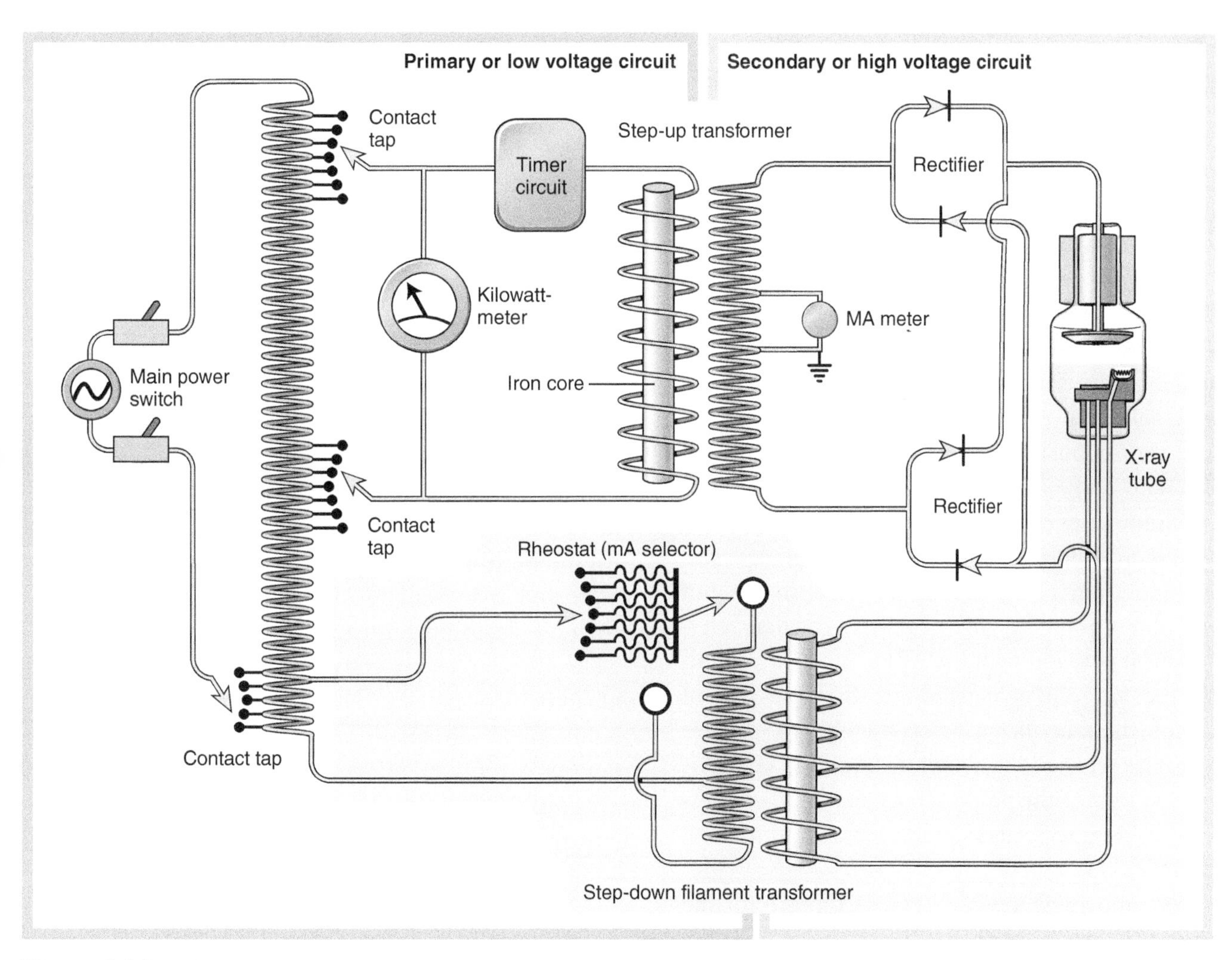

Figure 8.15. **Filament circuit. A filament circuit (gold) and its location in the basic x-ray circuit.**

kVp and mA Selectors

The control console allows adjustments to be made in the amount of kVp set for an exposure. There are two types of kVp controls: major kVp and minor kVp. The major kVp adjustment allows the radiographer to quickly select larger kVp settings to accommodate thicker anatomy, while the minor kVp adjustment allows for smaller kVp changes to "fine tune" the kVp setting. The radiographer can use these two controls to more precisely select the required kilovolt peak. The kVp determines the quality or penetrability of the x-ray beam. Remember that the **step-up** transformer is used to increase the incoming line voltage to thousands of volts. To accurately measure the amount of kVp in the circuit, a prereading kVp meter is placed between the autotransformer and the step-up transformer. This meter allows for a readout to be displayed on the control console for the purpose of monitoring the voltage in the circuit.

The mA selectors are used to set the amount of milliamperes, which will cross from the cathode to the anode in the x-ray tube. The setting controls the temperature of the filament, which is responsible for burning off electrons from the filament, and the temperature is controlled by the current in the filament circuit. The filament ammeter measures the amperes in the circuit. When the current increases, the filament becomes hotter and more electrons will be released from the filament wires in a process called thermionic emission. The filament operates at currents of 3 to 5 A. The rheostat results in fixed mA stations that provide tube currents of 100, 200, or 300 mA or higher.

Timing Circuits

Timing circuits shut off the high voltage to terminate the x-ray exposure after a selected exposure time. The timer opens a switch to cut off the high voltage from the x-ray tube and stop x-ray production. Exposure times are selected from the control panel to control the amount of x-rays produced. Short exposure times should be selected to minimize patient motion artifacts, while longer exposure times are used when blurring of anatomic structures are desirable.

Automatic Exposure Control Circuits

In addition to kvp, mA, and timer controls, many x-ray units also have a device that measures the amount of radiation reaching the image receptor. This device is commonly called an AEC. The purpose of an AEC is to achieve more consistent exposures, reduce repeated exposures, and reduce radiation exposure to patients. The first automatic exposure terminating device that measured light emitted from a fluorescent screen was called a phototimer. This device is no longer in use, but the term "phototiming" is still widely used when referring to exposures made with an AEC. An AEC circuit measures the amount of radiation leaving the patient and turns off the x-ray beam when the correct amount of radiation has reached the detector. The AEC circuit is calibrated to produce the proper image density regardless of patient size. Figure 8.16 illustrates the operation of an AEC circuit.

The AEC unit provides the correct exposure for the anatomic part to be imaged. At the control panel, the exposure mA and time can be selected independently, or the milliampere-time (mAs), which is the combination of milliamperes and time, can be selected, in which case the control circuits choose the highest mA and the shortest time allowed. The AEC detector is placed between the patient and the image receptor.

In operation, the AEC circuit acts as the timer for the x-ray circuit. Radiation is detected by ion chambers or solid-state devices, which generate electrical charges. The electrical charges reach preset levels and signal the operating console to terminate the exposure. The AEC circuit still requires the radiographer to set the mA and kVp correctly, although some units automatically select the highest mA allowable in order to reduce the exposure time and reduce the effects of patient motion.

Typical AEC systems have three rectangular-shaped detectors placed roughly at the corners of a triangle. Figure 8.17 shows a picture of an image receptor holder with the position of the AEC detectors indicated. AECs are located in the wall bucky and table bucky, which provide more flexibility for using the equipment.

The three detector cells can be selected to operate individually, in pairs, or all together, depending on the examination and patient orientation. A vast majority of examinations utilize the center detector. The AEC unit must initially be calibrated when installed and anytime there is a change in the image receptors that are used by the facility. Positioning the anatomic area of interest is critical to allow the proper amount of radiation to be detected through the part under examination.

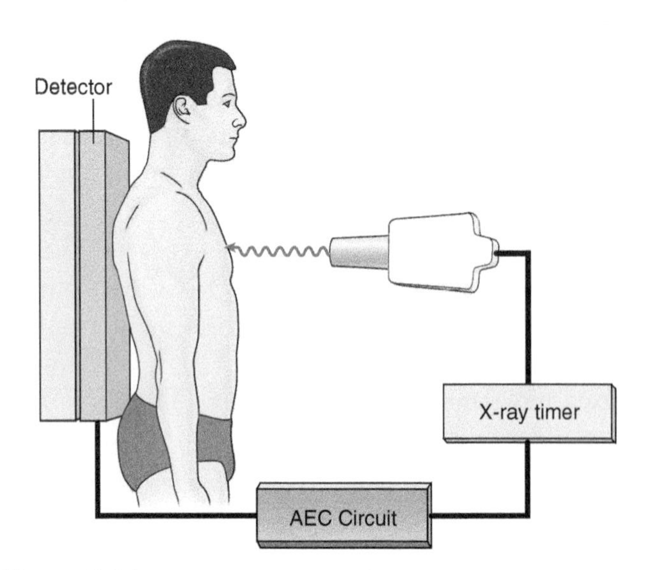

Figure 8.16. **AEC. Notice that the AEC is positioned behind the patient.**

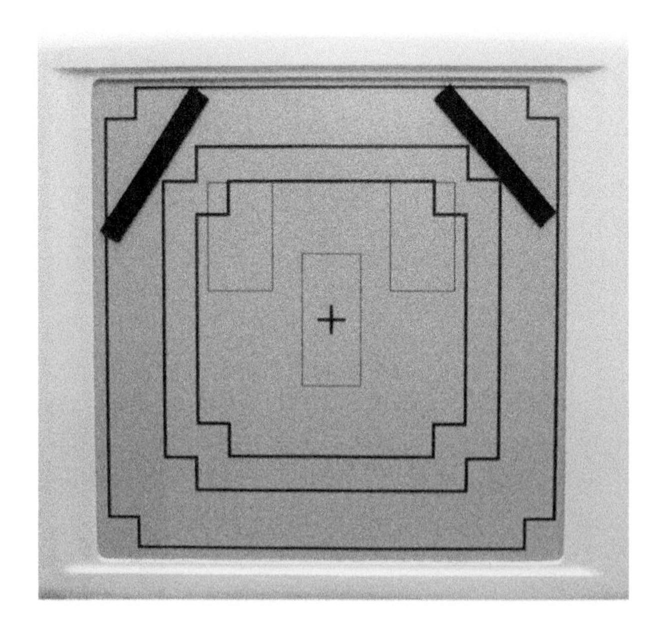

Figure 8.17. **Photograph of an image receptor (vertical Bucky) with the outline of the AEC cell locations indicated.**

AEC units have a provision for adjustments to give the radiographer a way of modifying the overall density on the image. Each adjustment step produces approximately a 30% change in density.

Backup Timer

The backup timer terminates the exposure when the backup time is reached. The electronic timer is set to 1.5 times the expected exposure time as a backup timer in case the AEC fails to terminate the exposure. If the x-ray beam does not reach the AEC detectors, excess radiation could reach the patient and the tube could be damaged. This could happen if the x-ray beam and the detectors were not aligned. The backup timer terminates the exposure before the tube limits are exceeded. These precautions are meant to protect the patient and the x-ray tube.

Chapter Summary

1. X-ray circuits convert low-voltage AC input to high-voltage DC, which is applied to the x-ray tube.
2. The kVp selector is an autotransformer that changes the input to the step-up or high-voltage transformer.
3. The mA selector is an autotransformer that changes the input to the step-down transformer to control the filament current.
4. The ratio of the number of turns on the secondary to the number of turns on the primary is called the turns ratio. A transformer with a turns ratio >1 is a step-up transformer; the output voltage is greater than the input voltage. A transformer with a turns ratio <1 is a step-down transformer; the output voltage is less than the input voltage.
5. Rectifiers are composed of two semiconducting crystals that control the flow of electricity in the high-voltage circuit.
6. Ripple is a measure of the variation between the maximum and minimum voltage. Circuits with low ripple produce a more constant x-ray output. Three-phase and high-frequency x-ray circuits have less ripple and produce more constant output than single-phase x-ray circuits but do not change the maximum voltage.
7. Automatic exposure detectors are placed between the patient and the image receptor to terminate the x-ray exposure when the proper image density is reached. Selection of the proper combination of detector cells is based on the examination and patient orientation. The backup timer prevents damage to the x-ray tube if the AEC circuit does not terminate the exposure before the tube limits are reached.

Case Study

Bill is assisting his imaging department in deciding which type of x-ray equipment would meet their needs. He has researched three-phase 6-pulse, three-phase 12-pulse, and high-frequency generators in his quest to find the best equipment for the procedures the department performs.

Critical Thinking Questions

1. What is the percentage of ripple for each type of circuit?
2. What type of transformer will be used by the equipment?
3. What component changes the incoming line voltage into usable voltage in the x-ray tube?
4. How is the filament protected from damage?

Review Questions

Multiple Choice

1. The automatic exposure control circuit:

a. terminates the x-ray beam when the proper exposure is reached
b. measures the amount of radiation striking the patient
c. measures the amount of radiation leaving the cathode
d. turns off the filament cooling circuit when the proper exposure is reached

2. A rectifier in an x-ray circuit:

a. prevents positive charge from reaching the anode
b. converts AC to DC
c. prevents excess grid bias on the anode

3. A transformer can operate only on:

a. AC
b. DC

4. An x-ray tube can operate only on:

a. AC
b. DC

5. An autotransformer functions as a(n):

a. line voltage compensator
b. kVp or mA selector
c. filament transformers
d. automatic exposure controller

6. Which type of transformer has a square-shaped ferromagnetic core and a primary and secondary coil?

a. Closed core
b. Shell type
c. Air core
d. Open core

7. What does ripple measure on a sine wave?

a. Total tube voltage
b. Variation between maximum and minimum mA
c. Variation between maximum and minimum voltages
d. Total mA

8. What is the output voltage of a transformer with a primary voltage of 150 V and with 500 turns on the primary and 400,000 turns on the secondary?

a. 20,000 V
b. 120,000 V
c. 250,000 V
d. 400,000 V

9. The transformer that has a single winding that acts as both the primary and secondary windings is called a(n):

a. autotransformer
b. step-down transformer
c. step-up transformer

10. A transformer with more turns in primary winding than in secondary winding would be expected to:

    a. increase the voltage and decrease the amperage
    b. increase the voltage and increase the amperage
    c. decrease the voltage and decrease the amperage
    d. decrease the voltage and increase the amperage

11. What is the turns ratio if the number of windings on the primary coil is 800 and the number of windings on the secondary coil is 600,000?

    a. 400
    b. 750
    c. 375
    d. 650

12. If a transformer is supplied with 700 V to the primary coil and has 400 turns of wire on the primary coil and 60,000 turns of wire on the secondary coil, what will be the kilovoltage in the secondary coil?

    a. 105,000
    b. 4.6
    c. 0.0046
    d. 105

Short Answer

1. List the four main components of the control panel.

2. What is the purpose of the filament step-down transformer?

3. Write the transformer law formula for current and voltage.

4. Describe the process of mutual induction.

5. Describe a rectifier and how it changes AC to DC.

6. What is the relationship between the number of coils in a winding and the amount of voltage and amperage that is produced?

7. Define full-wave rectification.

8. Compare a single-phase circuit to a three-phase six-pulse circuit.

9. Describe how an AEC operates.

9

The X-Ray Tube

Objectives

Upon completion of this chapter, the student will be able to:

1. Identify the construction of the x-ray tube.
2. Describe the process of producing a beam of x-radiation.
3. Explain the materials used to construct an anode.
4. State the function of the rotating anode.
5. Define thermionic emission.
6. Describe the line focus principle.
7. Explain how the anode heel effect can be used in radiography.
8. Define and calculate anode heat units.
9. Recognize allowed and forbidden tube heat loads.

Key Terms

- actual focal spot
- anode
- anode angle
- anode heel effect
- cathode
- effective focal spot
- filament
- focal spot
- focal track
- focusing cup
- leakage radiation
- line focus principle
- off-focus radiation
- rotating anode
- rotor
- SID
- space-charge effect
- thermionic emission

Introduction

This chapter covers the components, operation, and limitations of x-ray tubes.

The x-ray tube is one of the most important components of the x-ray machine. The sole purpose of the x-ray tube is to produce an x-ray beam. It is necessary for radiographers to understand the construction of the x-ray tube and the role each component plays in the production of the x-radiation. For each exposure, the radiographer must select the kVp, mA, and time on the control panel. All these settings control the actions that take place in the tube. The radiographer must also understand the effect these selections have on the amount of heat production for each exposure and the potential harm that can occur with improper selections that result in excessive heat within the tube.

X-Ray Tube

thePoint® *An animation for this topic can be viewed at http://thepoint.lww.com/Orth2e*

The major components of the x-ray tube are the cathode, anode, rotor/stator, glass or metal envelope, tube port, and tube housing. The tube components are sealed inside an evacuated (vacuum) glass or metal envelope. The vacuum allows the electrons to travel freely from the negative cathode to the positive anode. A thorough discussion of each component follows along with discussion for utilizing safe practices to extend the life of the x-ray tube.

Tube Housing

The tube housing is a solid, mechanical support for the x-ray tube and high-voltage cable connectors. The housing is a lead-lined metal structure that guards against electrical shock. In the early days of radiography, the threat of electrocution was a very real hazard for radiographers and physicians using the tubes. In modern times, electrocution is still an issue for anyone using the x-ray equipment. The high-voltage cables are delivering thousands of volts to the x-ray tube; poor connections or cracked insolated wiring is a real concern. The metal housing also prevents damage to the tube caused by rough handling of the equipment.

When a beam of x-rays is produced, 99.5% of the energy is emitted as heat from the x-ray tube and into the housing. Within the tube housing, the x-ray tube is surrounded by oil, which helps to insulate the tube and to dissipate the heat. A fan is often used to transfer the heat from the housing to the room air by convection (Fig. 9.1). The fans help to circulate air around the housing to further dissipate heat.

During the production of the x-ray beam, the x-rays are produced isotropically, which means they are emitted in all directions. The portion of the x-ray beam that is emitted through the target window of the tube housing is known as the primary beam. The target window allows for the maximum amount of x-rays to be transmitted with very little absorption of the x-ray beam. The housing protects against electric shock and absorbs leakage radiation emitted outside the x-ray beam. The **leakage radiation** is a source of unnecessary exposure for the radiographer and patient. Regulations require that the leakage radiation through the tube housing be <100 mR/h at 1 m from the tube.

Because there is high voltage present in the tube, a radiographer must be cautious when handling the equipment. The tube housing can become quite hot with extended periods of use. Another caution that is a concern is the high-voltage cables. These are not meant to be used as handles to maneuver the tube into various horizontal, vertical, or angled positions. There is a potential hazard to the radiographer and potential damage to the equipment if not properly handled.

The x-ray tube is a vacuum tube with two electrodes: the cathode and the anode. These components are housed

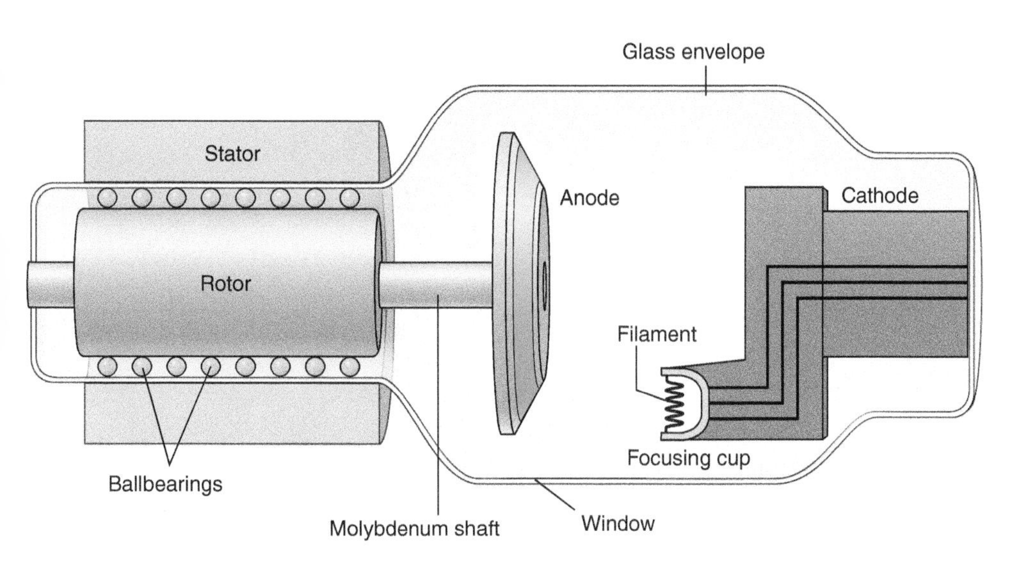

Figure 9.1. Components of a typical x-ray tube.

in an evacuated envelope where all the air is removed from the envelope creating a vacuum. The envelope also provides some insulation from electrical shock, which may occur because of the high voltage within the tube, and it dissipates the heat that builds up in the tube during an exposure. The heat is dissipated into the oil bath that surrounds the envelope.

There are two basic types of envelopes: glass and metal. The glass envelope is made of Pyrex glass, which is able to withstand the tremendous heat produced during an exposure. One disadvantage to the glass envelope is that tungsten can be evaporated from the filament wire during an exposure. When this happens, the evaporated tungsten metal particles will coat the inside of the glass envelope; this deposition occurs most frequently in the middle of the envelope. The evaporated tungsten can affect the electrons as they flow from the cathode to the anode. This coating can result in electrons arcing, which leads to tube failure.

Modern x-ray tubes are commonly designed with a metal envelope. Using a metal envelope eliminates tungsten vaporization, which coats the inside of the envelope thereby prolonging tube life. The metal envelope avoids the buildup from happening because there is a constant electrical potential between the electrons in the tube current and the envelope. Another advantage of the metal envelope is the reduction of off-focus radiation. The metal envelope will attract the projectile electrons that are not part of the electron cloud and will conduct them away from the anode.

Cathode

The **cathode** is the negative electrode of the x-ray tube. The function of the cathode is to produce a thermionic cloud, conduct the high voltage to the space between the cathode and anode, and focus the electron stream as it speeds toward the anode. The cathode contains the filament or filaments, focusing cup, and wiring for filament current.

Filament

The purpose of the **filament** is to provide projectile electrons for acceleration to the positively charged anode. The filament, a coil of tungsten alloy wire, is heated to boil off electrons. Tungsten is the material of choice because it has a high atomic number (Z = 74), it has a high melting point (6,200°F or 3,400°C), and it resists vaporization. Thorium is a metal that can be added to the tungsten to increase the efficiency and extend the life of the filament. The filament is connected to the filament circuit that provides a voltage, which varies from 6 to 10 V and variable current up to 1,200 mA. Changes in the filament current, termed milliamperes (mA), produce changes in the filament temperature. This causes a change in the number of projectile electrons boiled off the filament in a process called **thermionic emission**. Thermionic emission causes electrons to boil off the filament wire and to form a thermionic cloud. Remember that the electron cloud will only flow from the cathode to the anode at the time when the tube voltage is applied between the electrodes. Upon complete depression of the exposure switch, the tube voltage is applied, and the electron cloud is driven toward the anode target where x-ray photons are produced. An increase or decrease in the mA will affect the number of projectile electrons striking the anode, which changes the number of x-rays photons produced.

The control panel of diagnostic x-ray tubes offers the selection of either the large filament or the small filament. This is called a dual-focus system as illustrated in Figure 9.2. The size of the focal spot is determined by the size of the filament coil. The large filament is typically 1.5 to 2 times longer than the small filament. The small filament is ~1 cm in length. Only one filament

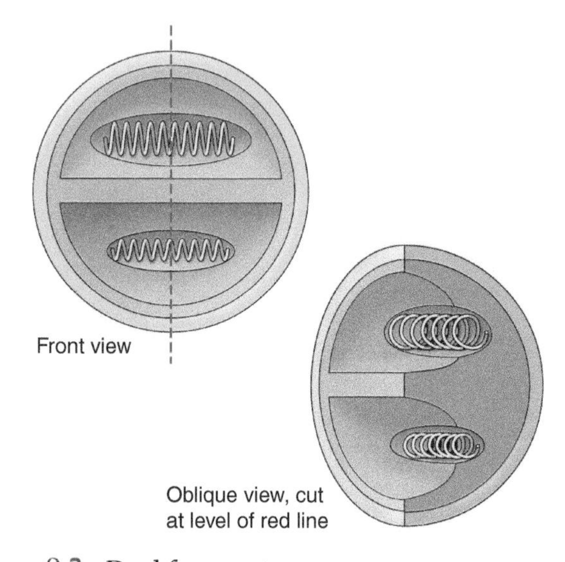

Figure 9.2. **Dual-focus system.**

can be energized at one time. The large filament is used when high x-ray production is needed for thicker anatomical parts. The larger filament produces a larger focal spot to distribute the heat over a larger area on the focal track, which allows higher tube currents without damaging the anode. The smaller filament produces a small focal spot when sharper images or better spatial resolution is required for smaller anatomical parts. Lower tube currents are used with small focal spots. Large filaments typically produce 0.4- to 1.2-mm focal spots, and small filaments produce focal spots of 0.1 to 0.5 mm. Focal spot size is determined automatically by selecting larger or smaller mA stations or manually by the focal spot size selection.

Filament Current

Upon turning on the x-ray machine, a low current flows through the filament to warm and prepare it for the high mA necessary to form a thermionic cloud. The filament has two wires going into it on the top and one wire leaving it on the bottom (Fig. 9.3). The filament current is responsible for heating the filament up to the temperature that corresponds to the mA station selected for the exposure. The current flows into and through the filament before flowing out of the filament, the current flows through one wire. The second wire entering the filament carries the tube current from the high-voltage main circuit. This wire supplies enough charge to force the electrons boiled off of the filament to "fly" across the tube to bombard the anode. The energy of the voltage is carried across the tube to the anode by the electron stream. Once the anode is bombarded, the energy does not stop there and must continue on a path to exit the anode. What is the "path" the electrons must follow? To answer this question, remember that the anode is connected to the positive side of the high-voltage circuit by a wire. The strong attraction of the electrons to the positive charge on the wire will cause the electrons to flow down the anode shank and to exit on the wire connected to the anode.

The x-ray tube has fixed mA stations of 100, 200, 300, and so on to provide the necessary milliamperage for a multitude of various exposures. When sufficient mA is applied, the electrons begin to build up into a cloud around the filament; this is called a space charge. The electrons reach a point where their negative charges begin to oppose the emission of additional electrons in a phenomenon called **space-charge effect**. The space-charge effect limits x-ray tubes to maximum mA ranges of 1,000 to 1,200. When the filament current is high enough for thermionic emission, a small increase in filament current results in a large increase in tube current.

Focusing Cup

The **focusing cup** is made of nickel and molybdenum with two depressions that contain the filaments. Electrons with their negative charge tend to diverge in a wide pattern because of electrostatic repulsion. A low negative charge on the focusing cup surface forces the electron cloud into a narrow beam. When the large voltage is applied between the cathode and anode, the projectile electrons form a tight stream as they are accelerated toward the anode. The anode region where the projectile electrons strike is called the **focal spot**. Figure 9.4 demonstrates the focusing action of a typical dual-focus cup.

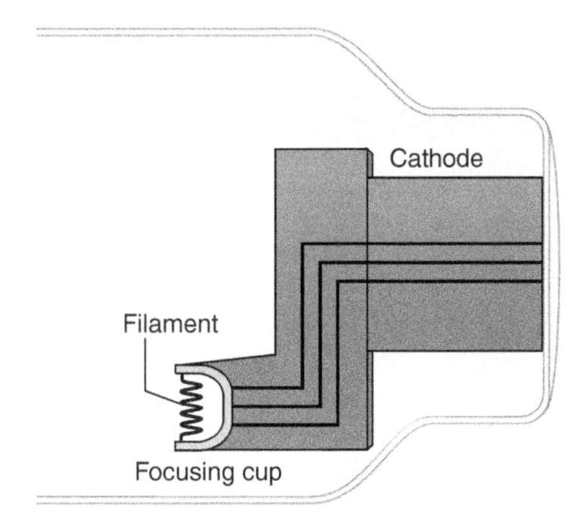

Figure 9.3. **Wires supplying current to the filament and completing the circuit for the electricity to leave the filament.**

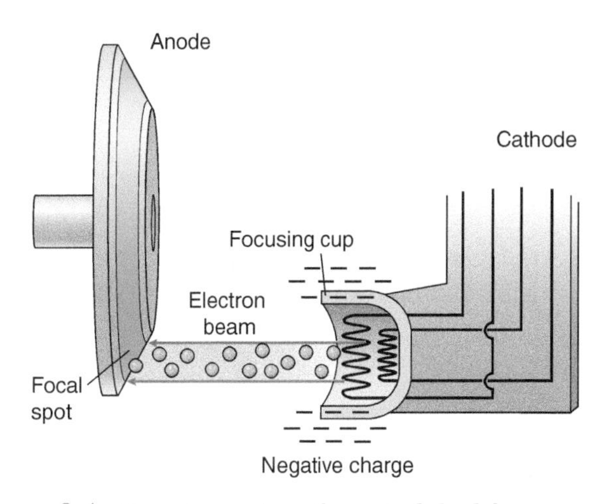

Figure 9.4. **Focusing action of a typical dual-focus cup.**

Anode

The positive electrode in the x-ray tube is the **anode**. This electrode carries a high positive potential difference relative to the negatively charged cathode. The anode is located on the positive side of the x-ray tube and it has three functions: (1) it serves as a target surface for high-voltage electrons from the filament and is the source of x-ray photons; (2) it conducts the high voltage from the cathode back into the x-ray circuitry; and (3) it serves as the primary thermal conductor in the tube. The anode is a beveled disk, which is mounted on a rotor supported by bearings in the x-ray tube insert. The positive anode contains the focal spot, the area where the projectile electrons strike the anode and deposit their energy. When the projectile electrons hit the anode, more than 99% of the electron energy is deposited in the anode as heat. Only about 1% of the projectile electron energy is converted to x-ray photons. The tremendous amount of heat that is produced with each exposure has the potential to damage the anode. To avoid heat damage, exposures using large tube current and the length of time for the exposure must be limited. We will discuss the concept of heat buildup in the tube later in the chapter.

Anode Materials

The target or focal spot on the anode can reach temperatures >3,000°C during an x-ray exposure. The anode must be made of a material with a high melting point to prevent damage. The target is a metal that abruptly decelerates and stops electrons, which allows for the production of x-rays. The material chosen should have certain properties:

1. A high atomic number, which has a high conversion efficiency for electrons into x-rays
2. A high melting point so that the large amount of heat released during an exposure causes minimal damage to the anode
3. A high heat conduction ability to remove heat rapidly away from the anode

In stationary anodes, the target area was pure tungsten because the atomic number of 74 results in production of diagnostic-range photons. There are tremendous temperatures created with each x-ray exposure, and tungsten's high melting point allows it to withstand normal use and operating temperatures. Tungsten also conducts heat very well, which helps the anode cool down more rapidly. Heat from the focal spot is carried to the anode stem by conduction. Anode heat is transferred from the anode to the walls of the tube housing. The housing walls are cooled by convection of room air, which may be increased by fans mounted on the housing.

In addition to tungsten, molybdenum and graphite are layered under the tungsten target. Molybdenum (Z = 42) also has a high melting point of 2,620°C and can store two times the amount of heat than tungsten. Both molybdenum and graphite are less dense metals than tungsten, which makes it easier to rotate the anode without increasing wear to the bearings.

The addition of 5% to 10% of rhenium (Z = 75, melting point 3,170°C) to tungsten greatly reduces damage by increasing tungsten's ability to avoid cracking at high temperatures. Rhenium alloys are used in the focal track because it ensures high-quality constant exposures, which lengthens tube life. Tungsten-rhenium alloys, which melt at 3,400°C, are commonly used as the target focal track material in anode construction. As seen in Figure 9.5, a thin layer of tungsten-rhenium alloy is used; this prevents distortion of the metal that may occur from the differences in thermal expansion of each metal.

Anode Configurations: Stationary and Rotating

The original tubes used by Roentgen and into the 1900s featured a stationary anode consisting of a tungsten insert embedded in copper. Copper was used as the

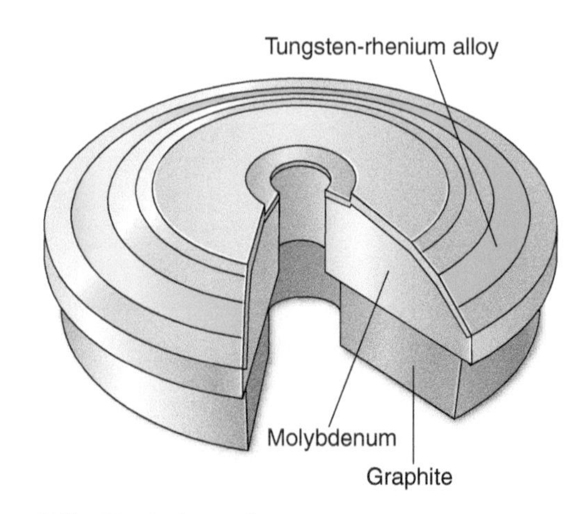

Figure 9.5. **Typical anode construction.**

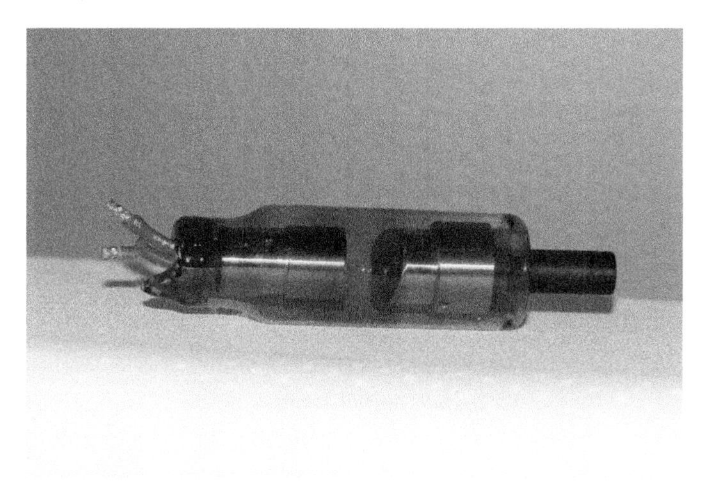

Figure 9.6. **Stationary anode.**

mechanical support structure for the tungsten and for its ability to efficiently conduct heat away from the tungsten target. The stationary anode had a small area for the focal spot, which limited the amount of tube current that could be used and the length of time for x-ray production (Fig. 9.6). These limitations made it very challenging to produce x-rays with high tube currents without causing damage from the excessive temperature in the anode. As the equipment design progressed and it became necessary to use higher tube currents for diagnostic radiography, the stationary anode was replaced with an anode, which rotates and dissipates heat more efficiently.

The **rotating anode** consists of a target, stem, and rotor. Rotating anodes spread the heat produced when the electrons bombard a focal track (Fig. 9.7) rather than concentrating the energy in a single spot on the anode surface as seen with stationary anodes. Modern rotating anodes have a higher heat loading capability and have a higher

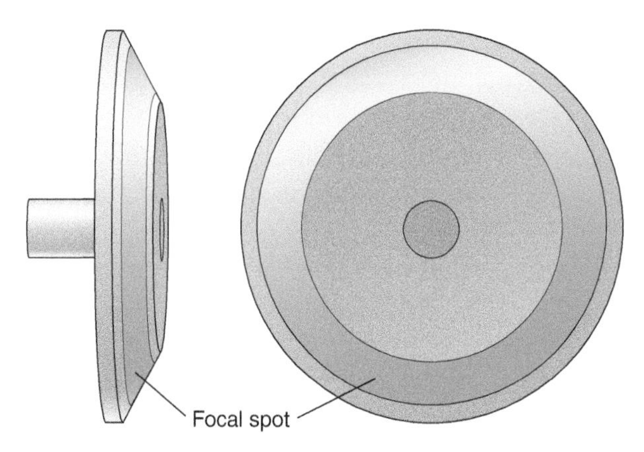

Figure 9.7. **Focal spot on anode.**

x-ray intensity output. The design spreads the heat over a larger area permitting exposures using much larger tube currents and extended exposure time. Most anodes rotate from 3,000 to 3,600 revolutions per minute (rpm) while high-speed tubes have anodes that rotate up to 10,000 rpm with 3-phase circuits. The anode rotation speed changes the anode heat capacity for greater heat dissipation.

The anode is rotated by using an induction motor, which was discussed in Chapter 7. The anode, stem, and rotor are sealed inside an evacuated tube as seen in Figure 9.8A. The stem is made of molybdenum and connects the anode to the rotor. Molybdenum is a strong metal with low heat conductivity, which prevents the anode heat from reaching and damaging the **rotor**. The rotor is made of a copper cylinder and is seen in the stem of the x-ray tube. The rotor assembly is supported by high-strength ball bearings in the x-ray tube insert that allow the rotor to spin smoothly. To allow for smooth rotation and long tube life, the ball bearings are lubricated with powdered silver paste and placed between the copper cylinder and the supporting mechanism. The

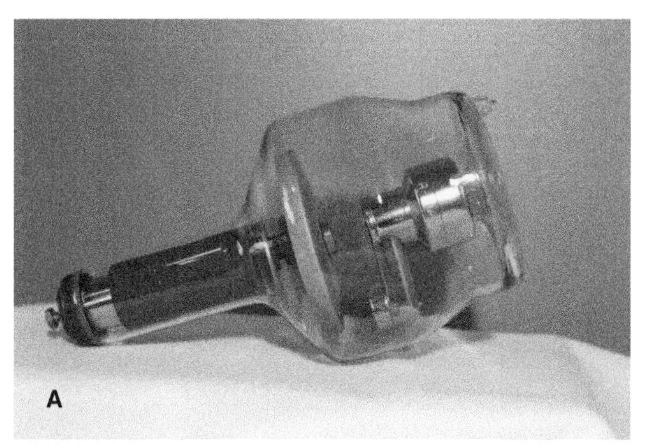

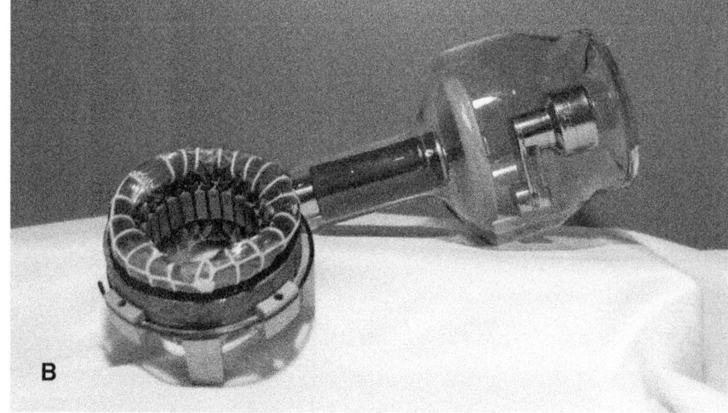

Figure 9.8. **(A) Stator and x-ray tube. (B) Stator with x-ray tube inserted.**

copper cylinder is drilled out in specific locations to perfectly balance it so that is will rotate smoothly. Rotor bearing damage is a major cause of tube failure.

A stator is a ring of electromagnets that surrounds the rotor and is mounted on the outside of the glass envelope (Fig. 9.8B). Alternating current (AC) passes through the stator windings and produces a rotating magnetic field that causes each electromagnet to fire in sequence so that the magnetic field around the electromagnets rotates. The strong, constantly moving magnetic field interacts with the rotors copper cylinder, inducing electricity to circulate in the copper cylinder. The copper cylinder becomes magnetized, and according to Lenz's law, the induced current flows in the opposite direction to the original current in the stator. These two opposing magnetic fields cause the rotor to spin in synch with the stator. At the time the exposure switch is depressed, there is a short delay (1 to 2 seconds), which allows the rotor to reach maximum speed. A "whirring" sound is heard while the rotor is spinning up to speed. Once the maximum speed has been reached, the x-ray unit will allow the tube to be energized and an exposure to be made. After the exposure is complete, the rotor will begin to slow down; a similar "whirring" sound will be heard. Because the bearings are so perfectly balanced, the slowing process could take several minutes. The induction motor is automatically run in reverse, which creates a braking effect and slows the rotor to a stop in ~1 minute.

Remember that each time the exposure switch is depressed, the induction motor is energized which brings the anode up to speed. At the same time, the filament is also heating up to the temperature necessary for an exposure. The "prep" phase of the exposure encompasses this delay until the tube is ready for the exposure. At the correct time, the "exposure-ready" light is lit on the control panel; there is typically an audible click, which signals the anode is up to speed. An experienced radiographer becomes familiar with the sounds the tube makes during all phases of creating an exposure: prep, exposure, and slow down of the anode. The two-step process of making an exposure typically occurs with a two-position switch or two separate buttons on the control panel, which allows the radiographer to rotor or "prep" for some time before making the exposure. This practice is useful in situations when the exposure must be precisely timed to create an image with the least amount of movement by the patient. When imaging pediatric patients or patients on a mechanical ventilator, it is often necessary to time the exposure to the breathing pattern of the patient. By "rotoring" and carefully watching the patient, an exposure can be made at the appropriate time. This is not a practice that should be used extensively as it causes unnecessary wear and tear on the anode stem bearings and burning of the filament.

Target Area

The portion of the anode where the high-voltage electron stream will impact is called by the following names: the target, the focal spot, or the focal track. The target area is where the electron stream strikes the anode, decelerates, and stops, which produces x-ray photons. Stationary anodes have a focal spot, which is a fixed area on the surface of the target. In the rotating anode, the circular path that will be bombarded with the electron beam is called the **focal track**. As illustrated in Figure 9.9, the stationary anode has the one area of impact, while the rotating anode has the focal track. In the rotating anode, the focal spot size will not change, but the actual area bombarded by the electrons is constantly changing, which creates the focal track or path where the electrons will strike. The focal track allows the heat to be distributed over the entire path, which increases the heat loads produced by higher exposure factors. Radiographic equipment uses the rotating anode to image the body, while the stationary anodes are used in dental radiography and are limited to exams of small anatomic structures like teeth.

The anode is a beveled disk, which has a steep angle in respect to the horizontal electron stream. Anode angles typically range from 7 to 20 degrees with 12-degree angles being the most common. The **anode angle** affects the effective focal spot size, tube output intensity, and x-ray field area projected toward the patient.

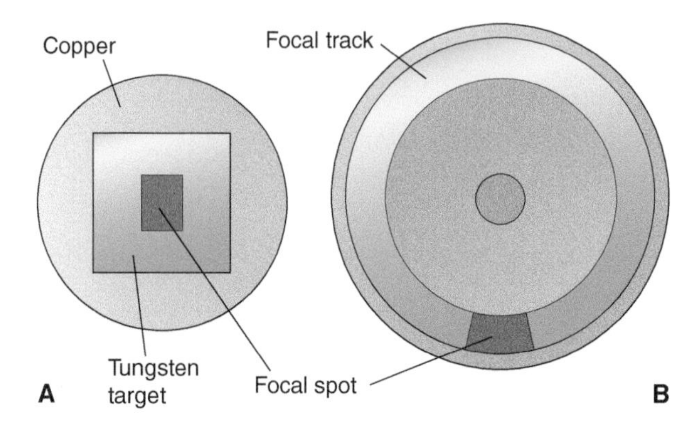

Figure 9.9. **(A) Stationary anode front view showing fixed focal spot. (B) Rotating anode front view showing focal track and focal spot.**

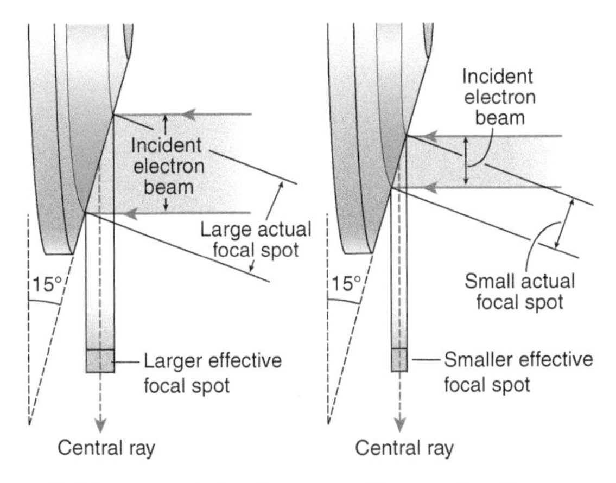

Figure 9.10. **Actual focal spot. Effective focal spot.**

Two terms we must discuss are actual focal spot and effective focal spot. **Actual focal spot** is used to describe the actual area on the focal track that is impacted. The actual focal spot is determined by the length of the filament and the width of the focusing cup depression. The **effective focal spot** describes the area of the focal spot that is projected out of the tube in a downward path and toward the object being imaged (Fig. 9.10), in other words primary radiation. Because of the angle of the anode, the effective focal spot is always smaller than the actual focal spot.

Line Focus Principle

The **line focus principle** states that by angling the anode target, a large actual focal spot can be maintained while a smaller effective focal spot is created. If the target were angled to 45 degrees, the size of the actual and effective focal spot would be identical; this would do nothing to improve the sharpness of the resultant image. Smaller focal spot sizes produce sharper images that are critical especially when imaging tiny bones. Figure 9.11 illustrates how reducing the anode angle reduces the effective focal spot size while maintaining the same target area on the anode surface (actual focal spot). The smaller target angle results in a smaller effective focal spot size and better detailed images.

Anode Heel Effect

The **anode heel effect** produces an intensity variation in the x-ray beam between the cathode and anode sides of the x-ray field. This causes a variation in image density or image receptor exposure from the anode side to cathode side, where the radiation intensity is greater on the cathode side. The anode heel effect occurs because of the geometry of an angled anode target. The target angle creates an oblique plane and the x-rays emitted toward the anode side must pass through more anode material than the x-rays emitted toward the cathode side. The resultant x-ray intensity is decreased toward the anode side of the tube.

Figure 9.12 illustrates how x-rays emitted toward the cathode side of the x-ray tube pass through less anode material than x-rays emitted toward the anode side of

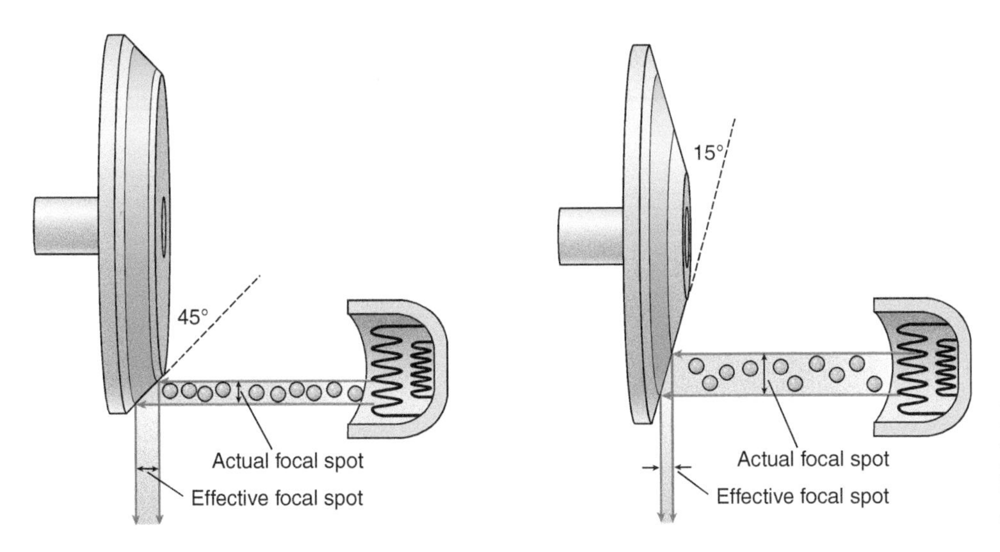

Figure 9.11. **Use of the line focus principle to obtain an effective focal spot that is smaller than the actual focal spot.**

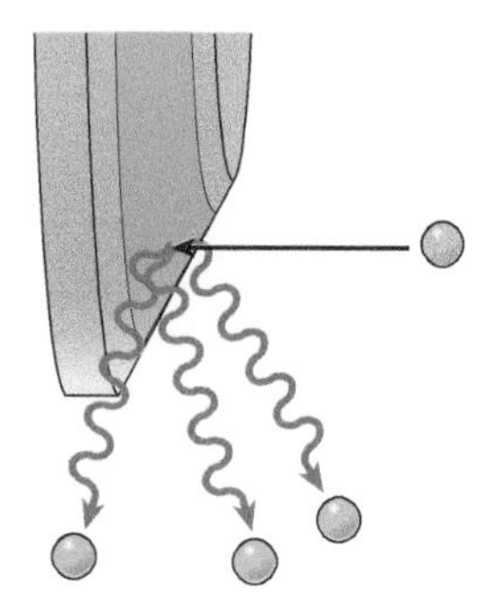

Figure 9.12. **High-speed electron impacts focal spot and produces x-ray photons.**

the field. The anode heel effect can produce intensity variations of more than 40% between the anode and cathode sides of the field (Fig. 9.13). The anode heel effect is more noticeable with (1) smaller anode angles, (2) larger field sizes, and (3) shorter source to image receptor distances (**SIDs**).

Smaller field sizes and a larger SID reduce the anode heel effect. The anode heel effect is applied in clinical situations to achieve a more uniform density when there is a large variation of body thickness across the x-ray field. The anode is recognized as the "head" end of the table to more fully utilize the anode heel effect to the best advantage. The cathode side of the tube is placed over the thicker or denser body part. An example of this would be imaging the thoracic spine in an AP projection. The cathode side would be placed over the lower thoracic spine with the anode toward the upper thoracic area to produce a more uniform density of the entire thoracic spine.

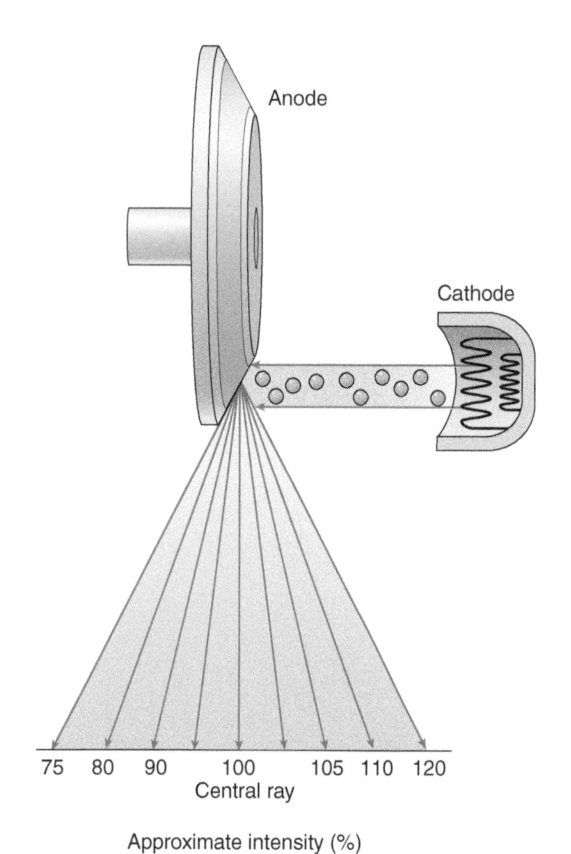

Figure 9.13. **Approximate intensity of x-ray beam.**

Off-Focus Radiation

Off-focus radiation consists of x-rays produced at locations outside of the focal spot. It occurs when projectile electrons strike other parts of the anode away from the focal spot. These electrons cause low-intensity x-ray photons over the entire anode causing radiographic images to have geometric blurring, reduce image contrast, and expose the patient's tissue outside the intended imaging area (Fig. 9.14). Most off-focus

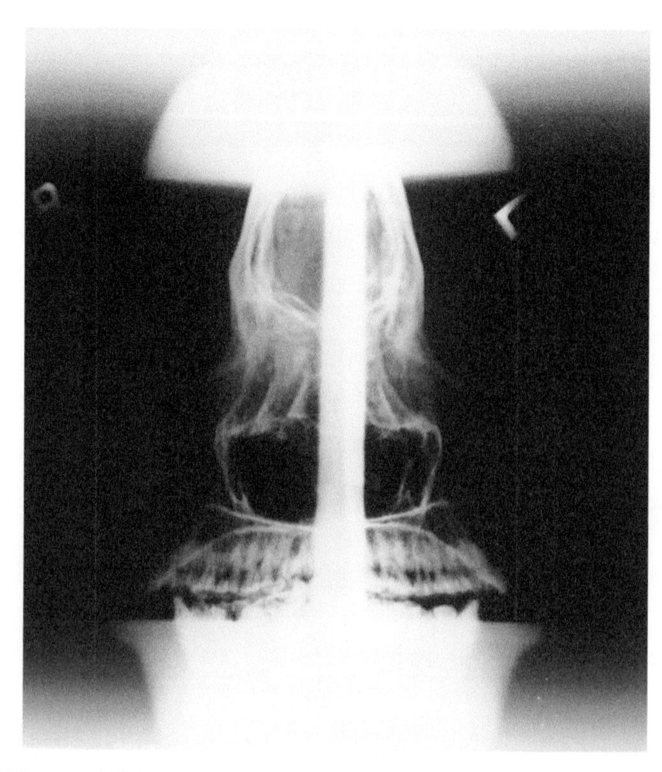

Figure 9.14. **Effect of off-focus radiation.**

radiation is attenuated by the tube housing and the first-stage collimator located near the window of the tube housing.

X-Ray Tube Failure

There are several causes for an x-ray tube to fail; most are from thermal characteristics of the tube. Tremendous amounts of heat are generated with each exposure, and the heat must be dissipated quickly for the tube to continue to operate. As tubes are used over the course of many years, the tungsten from the filament tends to burn off, and it builds up on the glass envelop and window area. When sufficient amounts of tungsten is coating the glass, electricity can arc down the metal, which cracks the glass and causes abrupt failure. Another cause of failure is related to the excessive heat transferred down the anode stem to the ball bearings. Prolonged exposures lasting 1 to 3 seconds cause the anode to become extremely hot, and the anode may glow red hot. Between exposures, heat is dissipated by radiating out to the oil bath, while some heat is conducted down the anode stem to the rotor assembly. The excessive heating will eventually warp the ball bearings, and their shape will become imperfectly round. This leads to a grinding noise and wobbling of the rotor that eventually throws the focal tract of the anode off center and tube efficiency drops significantly.

A third cause of tube failure is the cumulative effect of heat on the focal track. Over time, the focal track will become rough with microcracks and pits in the anode surface. The pitting is caused by the electron stream bombarding one area on the anode for an extended time. The pitting is an area of irregularity on the anode surface and will result in extreme loss of image sharpness. This is a reason to cease use of the tube. A final cause of tube failure is damage to the filament. Using high milliamperage settings for prolonged periods will cause excessive heating where tungsten is vaporized from the filament, which causes the filament wire to become thinner over time. Eventually, the filament will break from the heat load resulting in abrupt tube failure. A radiographer must remember to use the lowest mA station possible to produce a diagnostic image. Using safe practices will prevent damage and will extend the life of the tube.

Tube Rating Charts and Cooling Curves

Each radiographic unit has a set of charts that help the radiographer use the x-ray tube within a set of acceptable exposures to avoid damage to the x-ray tube. The three types of tube rating charts are:

1. Radiographic tube rating charts
2. Anode cooling curves or charts
3. Housing cooling charts

Radiographic Tube Rating Charts

Tube rating charts are designed to guide the radiographer in determining the maximum technical factor combination that can be used without overloading the tube. Each filament of each tube has a unique tube rating chart to assist in plotting milliamperes, kilovoltage, and time for an exposure. Each chart plots the kilovoltage on the y-axis and exposure time in seconds on the x-axis. The various mA stations are plotted within the chart, and any exposure with a combination of kVp and time that falls below the mA station is considered safe. If an exposure is made with a combination of kVp and time that falls above the mA station, the exposure is unsafe and may result in sudden tube failure (Fig. 9.15). An x-ray unit has a built-in safety control that will not allow an unsafe exposure. A warning message of "Tube Overload"

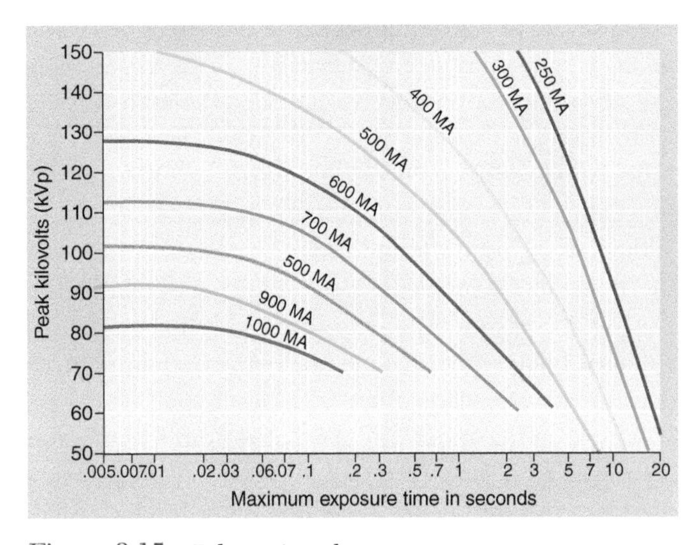

Figure 9.15. Tube rating charts.

or similar message along with an audible beep will alert the radiographer to an improper combination of kvp, mA, and time.

Each system has a series of charts based on filament size, anode rotation speed, target angle, and voltage rectification (single phase, 3 phase, or high frequency). The radiographer should use the correct chart for the unit, and when the tube is replaced, the new chart should be reviewed as it may be different from the original chart.

CRITICAL THINKING BOX 9.1

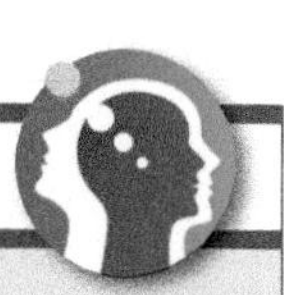

Referring to Figure 9.15, which of the following sets of exposure factors are safe and which are unsafe?

a. 700 mA, 0.3 second, 90 kvp
b. 400 mA, 3 seconds, 95 kVp
c. 900 mA, 0.05 second, 90 kVp
d. 1,000 mA, 0.007 second, 80 kVp
e. 500 mA, 0.6 second, 115 kVp

Anode Cooling Curves

The anode has limited capacity to store heat. The heat is dissipated into the oil bath and tube housing. Exams where prolonged use or multiple exposures are made in rapid succession can exceed the heat capacity of the anode. These practices should be limited, but there are fluoroscopy exams where it is necessary to produce several images per second to adequately visualize structures. But how can the radiographer perform these exams while taking care to minimize heat exposure to the anode? The use of anode cooling curves provides the radiographer with the tools that are needed to avoid damage to the tube. Anode cooling curves or charts allow the calculation of the time necessary for the anode to cool enough for additional exposures to be made. The heat deposited in the anode by the projectile electrons depends on the mA, kVp, and exposure time. Exposures with higher applied voltages, higher tube currents, and longer exposure times deposit more heat on the anode focal spot. The heat deposited in the anode and dissipated from the anode is measured in heat units (HU). HU are calculated using the kVp, mA, time, and generator factor for each unit. The generator factor is used to compensate for the type of generator that powers the unit: single phase, 3 phase, or high frequency. The number of HU is obtained by using the following formulas for a single-phase generator:

$$\text{HU} = \text{kVp} \times \text{mA} \times \text{time} \times 1(\text{generator factor})$$

CRITICAL THINKING BOX 9.2

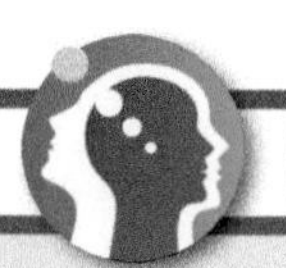

What is the heat load in HU from a single-phase exposure with technical factors of 125 kVp, 200 mA, and 0.3 second?

Modern equipment using 3-phase and high-frequency generators produce more heat per exposure because of the different electrical waveform utilized by x-ray circuitry. The use of these types of generators must be factored into the equation for determining HU. The generator factor for 3 phase equipment is 1.35, and 1.40 is the generator factor for high-frequency equipment. The HU formula for each is expressed as:

$$3\,\text{phase}: \text{HU} = \text{kVp} \times \text{mA} \times \text{time} \times 1.35$$
$$\text{High-frequency}: \text{HU} = \text{kVp} \times \text{mA} \times \text{time} \times 1.40$$

CRITICAL THINKING BOX 9.3

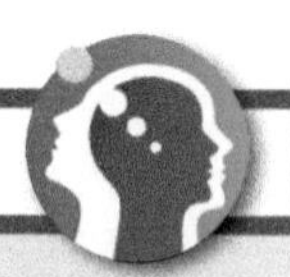

What are the HU produced if the exposure is made with a high-frequency circuit, 100 kVp, 200 mA, and 0.1 second?

CRITICAL THINKING BOX 9.4

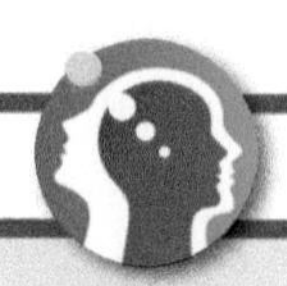

Five abdominal images are exposed with a phase circuit using 85 kVp and 135 mAs. What are the total HU generated?

Modern x-ray circuits have safety controls to prevent multiple exposures with no cooling between exposures. It is essential to wait between multiple exposures to allow the anode to cool if each exposure is near the maximum heat capacity of the anode. Many x-ray circuits will prevent additional exposures from being made until the anode has had sufficient time to cool. Figure 9.16 represents an anode cooling curve with a maximum heat capacity of 350,000 HU. The chart is used to determine the amount of time it will take for the anode to completely cool after an exposure. The initial cooling is quite rapid, but as the anode cools, the rate of cooling slows down. For example, a cup of steaming hot chocolate is placed on the counter at room temperature of 70°F. There is a vast difference between the hot chocolate temperature and room temperature, and the hot chocolate will begin to dissipate its heat rapidly. As the hot chocolate cools down, there is less heat to dissipate; therefore, the cooling process slows down. The initial steep slope of the anode cooling curve represents this phenomenon; notice how the slope becomes less steep and broader as the anode cools over time.

To determine the amount of time for the anode to cool completely, the radiographer must first plot the amount of time that corresponds with the HU produced for a given exposure. Subtract that number from the maximum amount of time that is needed to completely cool the anode. On Figure 9.16, the maximum amount of time is 15 minutes for the anode to cool completely.

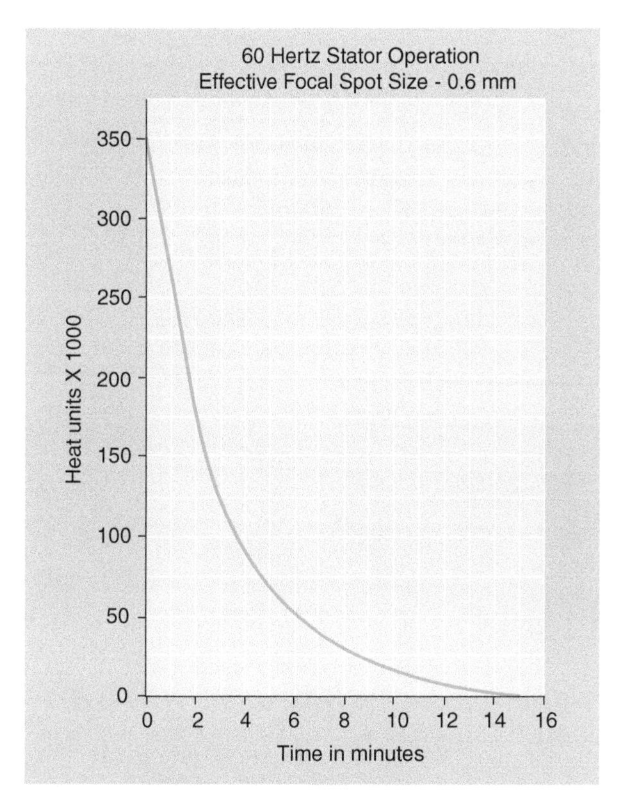

Figure 9.16. **Anode cooling curve.**

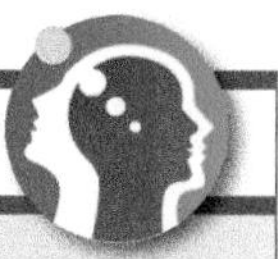

CRITICAL THINKING BOX 9.5

A fluoroscopic exam produces 100,000 HU in the anode in a few seconds. Calculate the amount of time required for the anode to cool completely.

Using the chart in Figure 9.16, plot the HU delivered and subtract this from the maximum amount of cooling time.

Another use for the anode cooling curve is to determine if a set of exposures will overload the anode. During fluoroscopic procedures, it may be necessary to produce multiple sets of exposures, which will heat the anode for an extended period of time. To avoid damage to the anode, the radiographer can determine the amount of time that must lapse between exposures to allow the anode to cool sufficiently for the next set of exposures. Remember that the anode does not have to cool completely before the next set of images are obtained, but rather a fraction of time may be all that is needed.

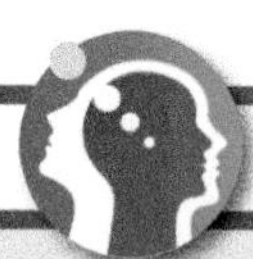

CRITICAL THINKING BOX 9.6

An initial heat load of 350,000 HU was produced for a series of exposures. Using the anode cooling curve in Figure 9.15, calculate the length of time it will take for the anode to cool before another series of exposures can be made totaling 100,000 HU.

Housing Cooling Charts

The housing cooling charts for the x-ray tube allow the calculations to determine how long it will take to cool the housing before additional exposures can be made. The charts are very similar to anode cooling charts and are used exactly the same way. In all actuality, the anode will overheat long before the tube housing overheats. The tube housing has a forced-air fan to dissipate the heat that has built up on the tube housing.

Tube Failure and Warm-Up Procedures

An x-ray tube costs about the same as a full-size new car. It is important to extend the life of the tube by properly warming up the tube before beginning clinical exposures. Tubes fail because of heat damage, either to the bearings or to the anode surface. Excessive heat can cause filament failure, bearing damage, and anode cracks. Proper tube warm-up will extend the tube life. Figure 9.17 shows an anode after a heat-induced crack split the anode into two pieces.

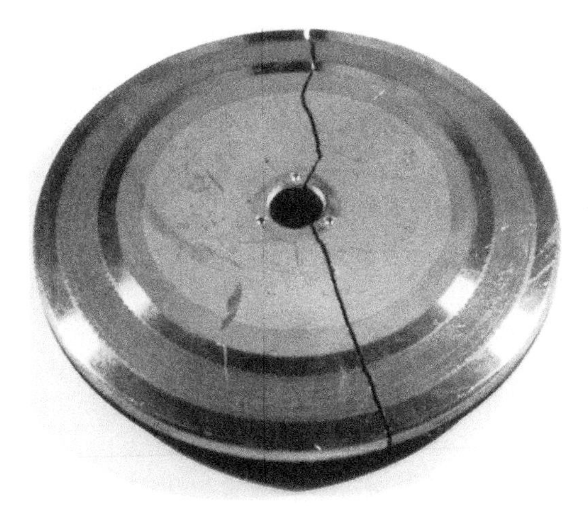

Figure 9.17. **Anode damage from not properly warming anode.**

Proper warm-up exposures eliminate anode cracking by spreading the heat over the entire target surface. A proper warm-up procedure uses at least a 1-second exposure to include many rotations of the anode during the exposure. A very short exposure on a cold anode concentrates the heat on a fraction of the anode surface. This can cause uneven thermal expansion of the anode and may crack the anode. A typical warm-up procedure would consist of two 70 kVp with several low mA long exposures and 2-second exposures. Tube warm-up procedures should be performed whenever the x-ray tube has not been used for several hours.

While the x-ray unit is on, it remains in the standby mode with a filament current of a few amperes keeping the filament warm and ready to be heated to its operating temperature. Just before the exposure is made, the anode begins rotating, and the filament is heated to operating temperature by the boost current. This is termed the prep stage of exposure. A safety circuit prevents exposure prior to the anode reaching full rotation speed. The boost current raises the filament temperature to begin thermionic emission. The boost current is present while the exposure switch is activated. Maintaining the tube in the boost mode or prep stage after the x-ray exposure is completed can significantly shorten tube life by burning out the filament. The exposure switch should be released as soon as the exposure is completed. The standby mode does not shorten tube life.

Heat is the primary cause of tube failure. Heat increases rotor bearing wear and damages the anode surface. When tube bearings begin to fail, they emit a grinding noise noticeable after every exposure.

Chapter Summary

1. The negative cathode of the x-ray tube contains the filament. Thermionic emission from the heated filament produces projectile electrons, which are accelerated to the positive anode.
2. The positive anode is a disk-shaped structure constructed of a high atomic number alloy with high thermal conductivity and a high melting point.

3. The anode and cathode are contained in an evacuated glass tube surrounded by an oil bath inside a metal housing. The oil bath provides electrical insulation and cooling.
4. The projectile electrons stop in the anode and produce x-rays photons. More than 99.5% of the electron energy is converted to heat in the anode; the remainder is converted to x-ray photons.
5. X-ray tubes utilize rotating anodes to distribute the heat around a circular track on the anode surface.
6. The line focus principle uses an angled anode to spread the heat over a larger area (the actual focal spot) while still maintaining a smaller effective focal spot.
7. The heel effect causes different x-rays intensities at the cathode and anode ends of the tube that limit the useful field size. The heel effect is caused because some of the x-rays are produced below the anode surface. These x-rays are attenuated as they leave the anode. The intensity at the anode end is less than at the cathode end of the field.
8. Heat units (HU) are the product of the kVp, mA, and exposure time. HU depend on the focal spot size and the type of x-ray circuit used. It is important to extend the tube life by following proper warm-up procedures. Heat limit curves demonstrate the safe and unsafe exposure regions for tubes. There are separate curves for the large and small focal spots.

Case Study

Mark is performing a barium study on a patient. During the exam, the high-frequency x-ray machine stopped producing the x-ray beam because the maximum amount of heat units, 350,000, was used during fluoroscopy. Mark needs to produce seven more images using 100 kVp and 250 mAs.

Critical Thinking Questions

1. What is the formula to determine heat units?
2. How many heat units will this set of exposures produce?
3. Using the anode cooling curve in Figure 9.16, how long must the anode cool before the additional exposures can be made?

Review Questions

Multiple Choice

1. The anode heel effect is described by which of the following?

a. It causes greater radiation intensity on the cathode side.
b. It occurs because x-rays produced inside the cathode are attenuated.
c. It depends on mA and kVp.
d. It is reduced by dual focal spots.

2. Which best describes the line focus principle?

a. Makes the focal spot appear larger than it really is
b. Makes use of an angled cathode structure
c. Produces x-ray lines on the image
d. Spreads the heat over a larger part of the anode

3. The purpose of the cathode focusing cup is to:

a. alter the filament size
b. group the electrons for their passage to the anode
c. regulate the anode rotation speed
d. increase the heat capacity of the tube

4. Most x-ray tubes have two filaments for which reasons?

a. Because the second filament can be used as a spare when the first burns out
b. Provides two focal spot sizes
c. Allow for cooling of the filament by alternating exposures
d. Improve tube cooling by sharing the heat between the two filaments

5. The anode heel effect is more pronounced:

a. further from the focal spot
b. with a large focal spot
c. with a small cassette
d. with a small target angle

6. Which metal is used on the target of the anode?

a. Molybdenum
b. Rhenium
c. Graphite
d. Tungsten-rhenium alloy

7. The __________ is used to determine the maximum combination of technical factors an x-ray machine can handle.

a. anode cooling curve
b. housing cooling chart
c. tube rating chart
d. all of the above

8. Which best describes thermionic emission?

a. The point where an electron's negative charge begins to oppose the emission of additional electrons.
b. The electrons boil off the filament and form a cloud, which is propelled toward the anode.
c. Photons that were not produced at the focal spot.
d. The electrons boil off the anode prior to impacting the cathode.

9. Which of the following is not a reason to use tungsten in an x-ray tube?

a. Tungsten has a high melting point.
b. It has a relatively high atomic number.
c. It efficiently dissipates heat that was produced during the exposure.
d. It doubles the heat loading capacity of the anode.

10. Which metal is combined with tungsten to form an alloy for the anode target track?

a. Rhenium
b. Graphite
c. Molybdenum
d. Copper

Short Answer

1. Describe the type of radiation that does not contribute diagnostic information to the image but rather results in unnecessary exposure to the patient and radiographer.

2. Define the anode heel effect, and describe how it can be used to the radiographer's advantage.

3. What is the purpose of having two filaments?

4. Explain line focus principle.

5. Briefly describe how to use a tube rating chart.

6. What is the focusing cup?

7. Define leakage radiation.

8. List the parts of the cathode.

9. Why is the filament embedded in a focusing cup?

10. Define an x-ray photon.

10

X-Ray Production

Objectives

Upon completion of this chapter, the student will be able to:

1. Describe the Bremsstrahlung x-ray production process.
2. Describe the characteristic x-ray production process.
3. Explain the effect of kVp and filtration on beam quality.
4. Identify the information contained in an x-ray spectrum.
5. Explain the effects of kVp, mA, filtration, x-ray circuit waveform, and anode material on the x-ray emission spectrum.

Key Terms

- Bremsstrahlung interactions
- characteristic cascade
- characteristic interactions
- incident electron
- inherent filtration
- keV
- kVp
- x-ray beam quality
- x-ray beam quantity

Introduction

This chapter covers the two x-ray production processes that take place in the anode, the Bremsstrahlung interactions and characteristic interactions. The amount and energy distribution of the x-rays photons from these interactions are different and influence the appearance of the final image. This chapter describes the two interactions and the effect on the x-ray beam by changes in the kVp, mA, filtration, x-ray circuit waveform, and anode material.

X-Ray Production

Filament projectile electrons produced by thermionic emission in the cathode are accelerated by the high voltage to the anode; the filament electrons will penetrate to a depth of 0.5 mm and interact with the tungsten target atoms. The atoms are mostly composed of empty space and move very rapidly; the projectile or incident electrons may pass through numerous atoms before finally interacting with an atom. The incident electrons may interact with orbital electrons or the nucleus. Once the incident electrons have struck the anode target area, either bremsstrahlung interactions or characteristic interactions occur. Every exposure that is made results in thousands of interactions that occur at the same time. Remember that a great amount of heat (~99%) is produced with each exposure. The diagnostic range is 30 to 150 kVp as selected at the control panel. When kVp is set lower than 70 kVp, all interactions will be brems interactions. When kVp is above 70 kVp, ~85% of the interactions produced are brems with the remaining being characteristic interactions.

The kinetic energy of the incident electrons is converted into heat and x-ray energy. Most of the projectile electron energy is converted into heat energy; only about 1% is converted into electromagnetic energy or x-rays. The interaction that will occur depends on the electron kinetic energy and the electron binding energy of the electron shells.

Bremsstrahlung Interactions

thePoint® ***An animation for this topic can be viewed at http://thepoint.lww.com/Orth2e***

Bremsstrahlung is the German word for "braking or slowing down radiation." Bremsstrahlung, also referred to as "brems," is radiation that is produced when incident electrons are slowed down or decelerated in the anode. **Bremsstrahlung interactions** occur when the **incident electron** interacts with the force field of the nucleus. The protons in the nucleus have a very strong positive charge, which the negatively charged incident electrons are attracted to. The incident electron must have enough energy to penetrate the orbital shells of the atom. When the incident electron gets close to the nucleus, the powerful nuclear force field is much too great for the incident electron to penetrate. The force field makes the incident electron slow down or "brake" and then causes the incident electron to change directions. As the electron slows down, it will lose kinetic energy that is emitted as an x-ray photon. The x-ray photon will have the same energy as the lost kinetic energy.

The bremsstrahlung interaction produces x-rays with different energies because the incident electrons are slowed down at different rates. Projectile or incident electrons that pass very close to the nucleus of the anode target atoms produce higher-energy x-ray photons than do those that pass further away. The amount of kinetic energy that is lost is dependent upon how close the incident electron gets to the nucleus. When the incident electron is farther away from the nucleus, very little kinetic energy will be lost, resulting in a low-energy bremsstrahlung x-ray photon. When the incident electron is closer to the nucleus, more kinetic energy is lost, resulting in a higher-energy bremsstrahlung x-ray photon (Fig. 10.1).

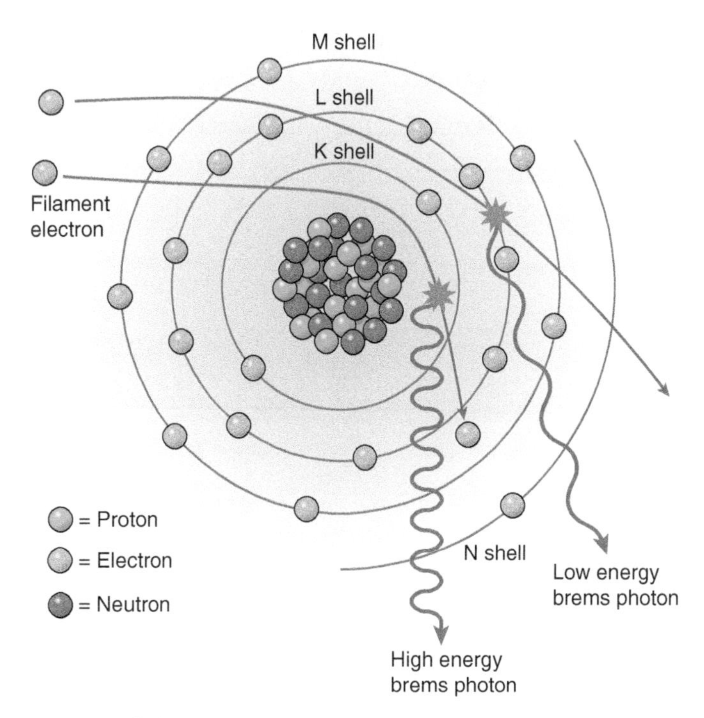

Figure 10.1. Demonstrates projectile electrons producing bremsstrahlung radiation of different energies. The distance the electron is from the nucleus when it "breaks" determines the energy of the brems radiation.

These incident electrons have the ability to interact with many target atoms and to cause many bremsstrahlung interactions. In other words, the bremsstrahlung x-ray photons can vary from maximum kVp selected (incident electron passes very close to nucleus and loses all its energy) to almost zero (incident electron passes at a great distance and loses almost no energy). For example, when a radiographer selects 80 kVp at the control panel, the incident electrons have kinetic energies up to 80 keV. The incident electrons can lose all, none, or any amount of kinetic energy in the bremsstrahlung interaction, which means that the x-ray photons produced can have any amount of energy up to the maximum amount of energy selected. The energy of a brems photon is determined by subtracting the energy of the incident electron as it leaves the atom from the energy it had when it entered the atom. For example, an incident electron with 80 keV of energy enters an atom and passes very close to the nucleus. As the incident electron slows down and changes directions, it leaves the atom with 25 keV. The brems photon energy is 55 keV (80 keV − 25 keV = 55 keV). This represents just one brems photon, which was produced during the exposure. The average energy of one brems photon is one-third of the kVp selected. As the incident electron interacts with an atom, it will continue to move as long as it has kinetic energy. Each interaction the incident electron has with other atoms will decrease the kinetic energy of the incident electron until the electron has no more kinetic energy and drifts away to join the current flow.

Characteristic Interactions

thePoint® *An animation for this topic can be viewed at http://thepoint.lww.com/FosbinderText*

The second type of interaction that occurs when the projectile electron strikes the anode is the **characteristic interaction**. Characteristic interactions occur in a tungsten anode when the projectile electron passes near an orbital electron; the negative energy from the projectile electron ejects the orbital electron from its orbit causing a vacancy in that orbital shell. The orbital electrons consist of potential energy while they are revolving around the nucleus. When an electron is ejected from its shell, some potential energy is given up. According to the law of conservation of energy, this potential energy does not disappear but merely changes into another form of energy. When a projectile or incident electron has sufficient energy to remove an orbital electron from an inner electron shell, a vacancy is created and the atom becomes unstable. The atom attempts to return to its normal state by the movement of higher-energy electrons dropping into shells that have a vacancy. Orbital shells fill from the shell nearest the nucleus outward. As each shell is filled, the potential energy lost is converted into a characteristic x-ray photon.

In diagnostic x-ray tubes with tungsten alloy anodes, the most common transition is from the L shell to the vacant K shell. However, it is possible to have the K shell filled by electrons from shells further from the nucleus. As the L-shell electron fills the K-shell vacancy, a vacancy is created in the L shell. The M shell will lose an electron to the L shell and so on. This transition of electrons between shells creates a process called a **characteristic cascade**, which can produce many x-ray photons for each electron that leaves the atom (Fig. 10.2). The characteristic photon is named for the shell being filled regardless of where the electron started from. Only K-shell vacancies from high–atomic number elements produce characteristic x-ray photons with high enough energy to be useful in diagnostic radiology. K-characteristic x-ray photons produce a discrete spectrum, meaning that only x-rays with the characteristic energies are present. The characteristic interactions created at the anode target are called primary radiation.

A tungsten atom has 74 electrons orbiting in six shells. The K shell has the highest binding energy because it is the closest to the nucleus. The filament electron must have sufficient energy to remove the K-shell electron. The filament electron may interact with any of the atoms electrons, but medical imaging primarily focuses on the interactions that create the highest energies because these are most useful in imaging. To produce K-characteristic x-ray photons, the K-shell orbital electron must be removed. The electron binding energy of the K-shell tungsten atom is 69.5 **keV**. If a filament electron with 55 keV of kinetic energy strikes a K-shell electron, it will not remove the

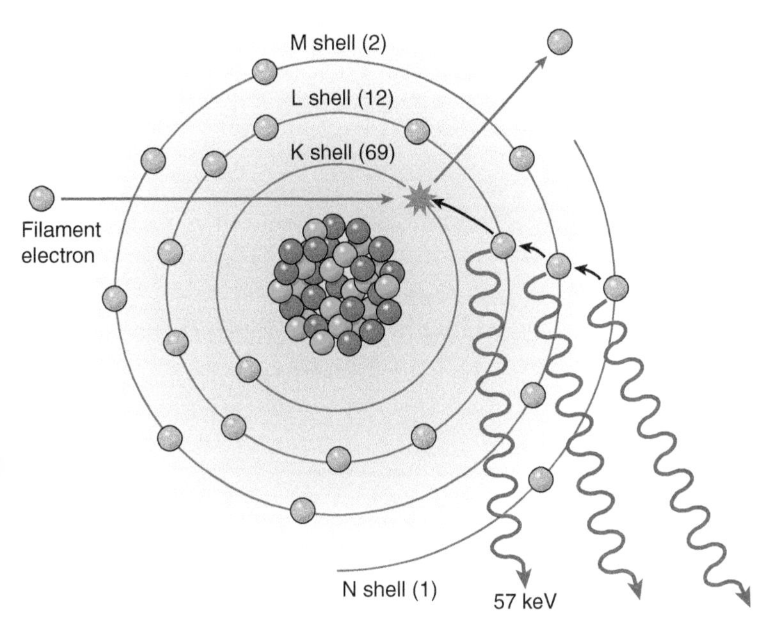

Figure 10.2. **Illustrates the filling of a tungsten K-shell vacancy with an L-shell electron. Note how the outer-shell electrons will fill inner-shell vacancies. The excess energies are released as characteristic x-ray photons in a cascade effect.**

K-shell electron because there was not sufficient energy to make that happen. This type of interaction results in the K-shell electron absorbing the filament electron's energy and emitting it as heat. This process will occur anytime there is not sufficient kinetic energy to remove an orbital shell electron. The filament electron will continue to have interactions with orbital electrons until it has lost all of its kinetic energy, at which point it will drift away to fill an orbital shell vacancy in another atom or it joins the current flow. On the other hand, if the filament electron had 120 keV of energy, it would easily remove the K-shell electron, and the characteristic cascade would take place. But how much energy would the K-characteristic photon have? To answer this question, the energy of the filament electron is subtracted from the binding energy of the K-shell electron. The result is that a characteristic x-ray emitted has an energy of 120 – 69.5 = 50.5 keV. Table 10.1 provides the binding energies for each shell of the tungsten atom.

TABLE 10.1 TUNGSTEN BINDING ENERGIES

K shell	69.5 keV
L shell	12.1 keV
M shell	3 keV
N shell	1 keV
O shell	0.1 keV
P shell	0.008 keV

CRITICAL THINKING BOX 10.1

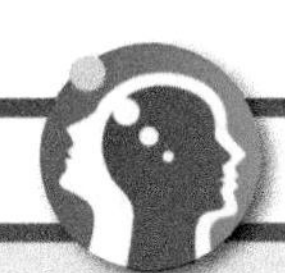

To determine the characteristic photon energy, you need to know the binding energies of the shells. Remember, the filament electron must possess kinetic energy equal to or greater than the shell binding energy to remove the electron from its orbit. The characteristic photon energy is equal to the difference in binding energy of the shells involved in the interaction.

Example

A filament electron removes a K-shell electron, and an electron from the L-shell fills the vacancy. Use Table 10.1 to determine the resultant characteristic photon energy.

K-shell binding energy =
L-shell binding energy =

What is the keV of the K-characteristic photon?
An M-shell electron then drops into the vacancy in the L-shell. Determine the L-characteristic photon energy.

L-shell binding energy =
M-shell binging energy =

What is the keV of the L-characteristic photon?

X-Ray Beam Properties

The x-ray beam is characterized by various properties that describe how the beam was produced and how the beam interacts with matter. The discussion of bremsstrahlung and characteristic photons must be furthered with the discussion of beam quality and beam quantity. A skilled radiographer will apply these concepts when deciding on the kVp and mAs factors selected at the control panel.

Beam Quality

X-ray beam quality refers to the penetrating ability of the x-ray beam. The selection of **kVp** at the control panel directly affects the penetrating power of the x-ray beam. Penetration refers to the x-ray photons that are transmitted through the body and strike the image receptor. It is important that some x-rays reach the image receptor to create dark areas while other x-rays do not pass through the body creating light areas on the image. If there is no penetration of the x-ray beam through the patient, an image will not be produced. Atoms with higher atomic numbers improve the quality of the beam because higher-energy brems and characteristic photons will be emitted. Brems photons are produced when atomic nuclei are larger and have a stronger positive charge to pull the projectile electron with greater force results in greater slowing of the electron. The lost kinetic energy is greater, which creates a higher-energy brems photon to be emitted. In regard characteristic interactions, the larger atomic nuclei have higher binding energies in the orbital shells. There is a greater difference between binding energies of the shells, which creates a higher-energy characteristic photon. Beam quality depends on the average x-ray energy of the x-ray beam, which is mainly controlled by the kVp setting. When kVp is increased, the beam's penetrating ability also increases; the same relationship is true if the kVp is decreased. High-energy x-ray beams are considered to be high-quality or hard beams. Low-energy x-ray beams are then low-quality or soft beams.

Beam quality is also affected by filtration of the beam. Filtration removes low-energy photons, which effectively increase the average energy of the beam. A way to consider this relationship is the effect on a student's grade when the two lowest quiz scores are removed; the average grade will increase. Table 10.2 provides a summary of the factors and how changes in each affect beam quality.

TABLE 10.2 **FACTORS THAT AFFECT BEAM QUALITY**

Increase In	Effect on Quality
kVp	Increases
Filtration	Increases

Half-Value Layer

The **half-value layer** (HVL) is defined as the amount of material required to reduce the x-ray beam intensity to one-half its original value. The HVL is affected by the amount of kVp and filtration in the beam. The lower-energy, less penetrating x-ray photons are removed from the beam, so the exit beam is more penetrating and has a higher-average energy than the entrance beam. This removal of "soft" x-ray photons results in a hardening of the beam, which increases the ability of the x-ray photons to penetrate tissue. At diagnostic x-ray energies, the HVL of soft tissue is ~4 cm. As the x-ray beam passes through four centimeters of tissue, the x-ray intensity is reduced to one-half its original value. The HVL describes the x-ray beam quality or penetration of the beam (Fig. 10.3).

Beam Quantity

X-ray beam quantity or the amount of x-ray photons in the beam is directly related to x-ray beam intensity. Recall that intensity is a measure of the amount of x-ray energy flowing through an area each second. Intensity

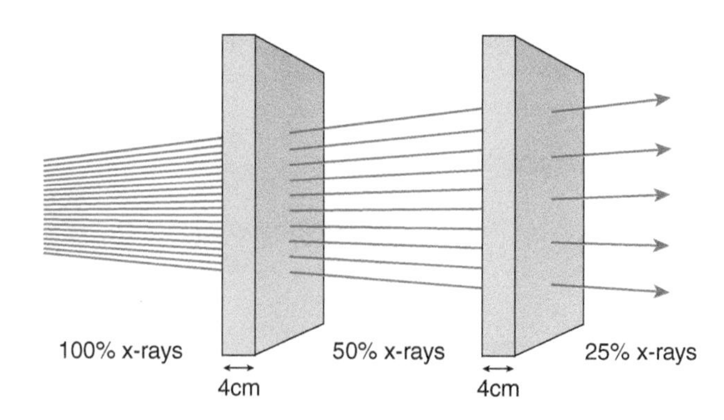

Figure 10.3. **Demonstrates how two HVLs reduce the intensity of the x-ray beam to one-quarter of its original value.**

depends on the number and energy of x-ray photons in the beam. The intensity of the beam is affected by mAs, kVp, distance, and filtration. mAs controls the number of electrons burned off the filament and available to produce x-ray photons. X-ray beam quantity is directly proportional to the mAs setting. mAs is the radiation dose to the patient, and the amount of mAs used for each exposure must be considered so that only the correct amount of mAs is used. When the mAs setting is doubled, there will be two times the amount of radiation produced. This correlates to a doubling of radiation dose to the patient. This practice must be carefully monitored by the radiographer especially when imaging larger anatomic areas or obese patients.

kVp controls the number and energy of x-ray photons, which affects beam quantity. This is not a directly proportional relationship because of the inherent energy in the x-ray beam. The kinetic energy in the filament electron increases significantly when kVp is changed. The kinetic energy is converted to heat and x-ray photons; greater kinetic energy increases the number of x-rays produced. Therefore, a small change in kVp has a large effect on exposure to the image receptor. In fact, when kVp is increased by 15%, there is two times the exposure to the image receptor. This principle is most effectively used when imaging larger anatomic areas or obese patients. Remember that kVp is the penetration of the beam, and higher kvp is needed for many exams on obese patients. To keep the radiation dose at a minimum, the radiographer should increase the kVp by 15%, which doubles the amount of x-ray photons in the beam. This works very well for larger patients. IF the kVp were doubled, the intensity or quantity of the beam would increase by four times; this effectively provides four times the radiation dose to the patient.

The inverse square law applies to the quantity of photons in the beam. Remember that the inverse square law states that beam intensity is inversely proportional to the square of the distance. When distance or SID is reduced by one-half, the original intensity will increase by four times. As previously discussed, when the SID is lower, the beam will not diverge as much; therefore the x-ray photons are more condensed in a smaller area. The more condensed the photons are, the higher the intensity will be. This obviously affects the amount of radiation dose to the patient.

CRITICAL THINKING BOX 10.2

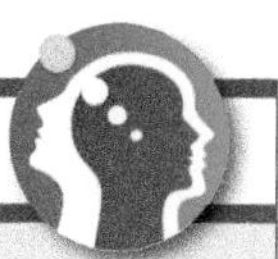

Determine the intensity of the x-ray beam at 36 inches if the intensity is 7R at 72 inches.

CRITICAL THINKING BOX 10.3

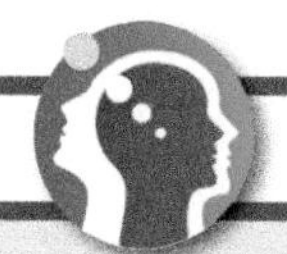

A beam has an intensity of 16R at 30 inches. At what distance will the intensity be 4R?

Types of Filtration

There are two types of filtration of the x-ray beam: inherent and added filtration. Filtration of the useful x-ray photons provided by the permanently installed components of an x-ray tube housing assembly, and the glass window of an x-ray tube is called **inherent filtration**. The inherent filtration of a general x-ray tube is ~0.5 mm Al equivalent. As the tube ages, inherent filtration tends to increase because some of the tungsten metal in the filament and target is vaporized and becomes deposited on the inside of the window.

A very thin sheet of aluminum is placed between the protective tube housing and the collimator; this is called added filtration. The additional sheet of Al filters all x-ray energies emitted from the anode, but a greater number of the low-energy photons are absorbed compared to the higher-energy photons. The result is an x-ray beam of higher energy with greater penetrability, which provides for better quality. Therefore, added filtration reduces the radiation dose to the patient. Table 10.3 is a summary of the factors that affect beam quantity.

TABLE 10.3 **FACTORS THAT AFFECT BEAM QUANTITY**

Increase In	Effect on Quantity
mAs	Increases
kVp	Increases
Distance	Decreases
Filtration	Decreases

X-Ray Emission Spectrum

The x-ray emission spectrum uses graphs to demonstrate the x-ray beam. Bremsstrahlung and characteristic interactions have their own graph to illustrate the emission spectrum for each. Characteristic photons have a discrete emission spectrum, while Bremsstrahlung photons have a continuous emission spectrum. The graphs are a simple tool that illustrates the nature of each beam and the effects of the various influencing factors. The intensity or quantity is represented by the area under the curve; the average energy is indicated by the peak of the curve. The *x*-axis is the x-ray energy, and the *y*-axis is the number of photons produced.

The characteristic or discrete emission spectrum illustrates photon energies, which are limited to a few exact values as seen in characteristic photons. To review, characteristic photons are produced when outer shell electrons fill inner shell vacancies in atoms, and the photon energy is determined by the difference in the shells involved. Remember that the characteristic photon is named for the shell that is filled. On the graph, there are bars for each shell representing the energy variations of the photons. There is a bar for the K-characteristic photons produced when the L-shell electrons fill the K shell, a bar for when the M-shell electrons fill the K shell and so on. The bars along the *x*-axis represent the different energies of the photons even though each is a K-characteristic photon. The graph also includes bars for the L characteristic, M characteristic, etc. Notice the energy bars in Figure 10.4. The lowest-energy bars are not labeled because they are not of diagnostic value. The height of the bars along the *y*-axis represents the number of photons of that type.

Anode Target Materials

Figure 10.4 represents the spectrum for a tungsten target; remember tungsten or a tungsten-rhenium alloy is the most commonly used material in the anode because tungsten has an atomic number of 74, and rhenium has an atomic number of 75. These dense atoms have lots of orbital electrons that the filament electrons will strike. Materials with higher atomic numbers equate to increased efficiency of the interactions and the production of more x-ray photons. Remember that K-characteristic x-ray photons contribute to the image.

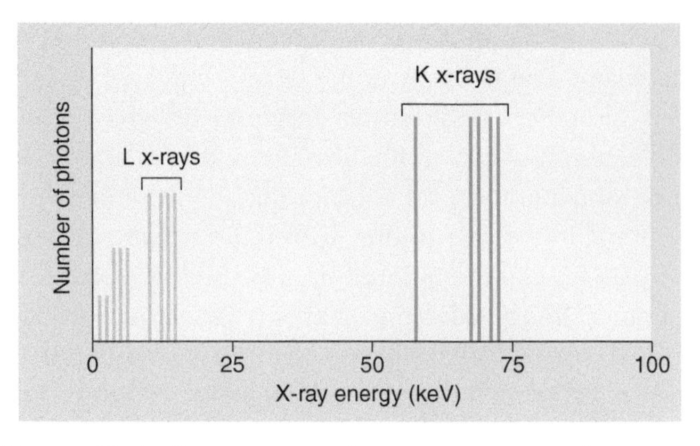

Figure 10.4. Demonstrates the average energy of characteristic x-rays from a tungsten anode. Also called discrete emission spectrum because x-rays are emitted only at discrete energy levels based on the differences between shell binding energies.

The discrete or sharp peak on the graph represents the characteristic radiations from tungsten. The position of the sharp peaks indicates the energy of the characteristic x-rays. Starting on the right side of the graph, all characteristic x-ray photons resulting from L to K transitions have an energy of 57 keV. This is the predominant characteristic or discrete photon from tungsten. A less likely transition would be an M-shell electron filling the K-shell vacancy. M to K transitions produce photons with 66 keV. N to K transitions produce photons with 68 keV, while O-shell electron transitions to the K shell may occur and produce photons with 69 keV. When plotting these energies on the graph, it is seen that the K-characteristic photons have an energy range of 57 to 69 keV. The L-characteristic x-ray photon energies are similarly plotted. Their energy range is ~9 to 12 keV. The transitions further out from the L-characteristic photons are not worth plotting as they are of such low energy that they are filtered out and do not contribute to the radiographic image.

A plot of the number of bremsstrahlung x-ray photons as a function of their different x-ray energies is known as an x-ray spectrum. It plots how many x-ray energies there are from zero to the peak electron energy. The maximum x-ray energy produced by the bremsstrahlung interaction is equal to the energy of the projectile electrons, and that is why it is called kVp or peak kilovoltage. The bremsstrahlung interaction produces a continuous spectrum of x-ray energies; that is, there are no sharp peaks or valleys in the curve (Fig. 10.5).

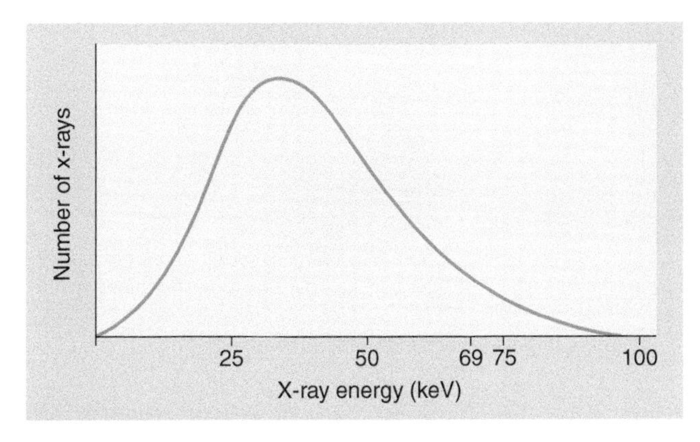

Figure 10.5. **Bremsstrahlung emission spectrum. Continuous emission spectrum from a tungsten or tungsten-rhenium target.**

The smooth curves represent the Bremsstrahlung portions of the x-ray production curve. Low-energy x-rays are filtered out or stopped before they reach the patient. The dotted line shows an unfiltered x-ray spectrum, which would be observed at the anode surface. All x-ray tubes have added filtration to absorb low-energy x-rays. These lower-energy x-rays cannot penetrate through the patient and would not contribute any information to the x-ray image but will contribute to patient dose. The average energy of the x-ray beam depends on many factors.

Anode materials produce different characteristic x-ray energies and various amounts of bremsstrahlung radiation. Tungsten alloy anodes are used in most diagnostic x-ray tubes, although molybdenum anode tubes are used in mammography. Tungsten has 57, 66, 68, and 69 keV characteristic x-ray energies, and molybdenum has 17 and 19 keV characteristic x-rays. Molybdenum anodes are used in mammography because their characteristic x-rays provide good contrast for breast imaging. The smooth curves represent the bremsstrahlung portions of the x-ray production curve, and the discrete or sharp peaks represent the characteristic radiations from tungsten and molybdenum. The position of the sharp peaks indicates the energy of the characteristic x-rays. In addition to the anode material, the four other factors that can influence the x-ray spectra are shown in Table 10.4.

kVp

There are two energies associated with x-ray production. One is the energy of the individual x-ray photons; the other is the energy of the projectile electrons, which is determined by the voltage applied to the x-ray tube.

TABLE 10.4 **FOUR ADDITIONAL FACTORS THAT INFLUENCE THE X-RAY SPECTRA**

kVp	The applied voltage controls the projectile electron energy, the intensity, the maximum, and the average energy of the x-ray beam. Changing the kVp does not change the energy of the characteristic x-rays.
mA	The mA controls the number of projectile electrons striking the anode and the intensity of the x-ray beam.
Beam filtration	Beam filtration influences the intensity and average energy of the x-ray beam by filtering out low-energy photons.
Circuit waveform	The waveform influences the intensity and the average energy of the x-ray beam.

The energy of the individual x-ray photons is measured in kiloelectron volts (**keV**) and is distributed from zero to the maximum energy of the projectile electrons. The voltage applied to the x-ray tube is known as kilovoltage peak (**kVp**) and is equal to the energy of the projectile electrons. Figure 10.6 shows that an applied voltage of 70 kVp produces an x-ray spectrum with a maximum energy equal to 70 keV with an average x-ray energy of 23 keV.

Changes in the applied kVp affect the average energy and the maximum energy of the x-ray beam. When kVp is increased, the penetration of the beam also increases, this is essential for more dense or high-atomic number tissues like bone. Dense tissue is better visualized on the

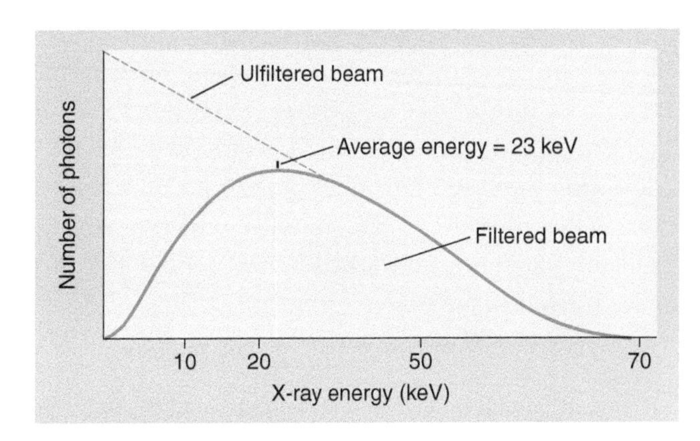

Figure 10.6. **Demonstrates the number of x-ray photons with different energies in the x-ray beam emitted from the anode.**

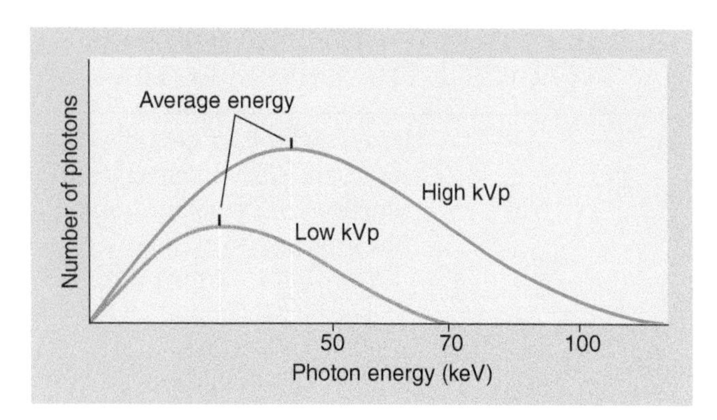

Figure 10.7. **Shows the x-ray spectra resulting from exposures at 70 and 110 kVp. Note how the curve shifts to the right or high-energy side when higher kVp is used.**

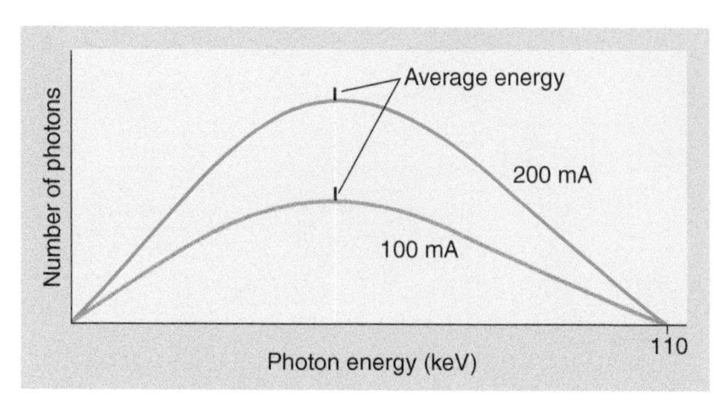

Figure 10.8. **Illustrates the increase in x-ray quantity when the mA is increased from 100 to 200 mA. The increase in mA results in a proportionate increase in the amplitude of the x-ray spectrum at all energies.**

image when a higher quality beam is used. The quantity of photons in the beam also changes with higher kVp because bremsstrahlung production increases with increasing projectile electron energy.

Figure 10.7 shows the x-ray spectra resulting from exposures at 70 and 110 kVp. The curve shifts to the right when higher kVp is selected. This results in the end point of the curve extending farther to the right, which represents the addition of high-energy photons to the beam. Consider a forest of trees of varying heights; if taller trees were added, the average height of the forest would go up. Likewise, increasing the kVp setting to produce higher-energy photons will increase the average kilovolts in the beam. The x-ray intensity or area under the curve, the average energy, and the maximum energy all increase when the kVp is increased.

This increase in energy reflects a nearly doubled amount of energy. More x-rays are being emitted at all energy levels, and this causes more density to appear on the image. Many radiographers use this process to decrease the amount of mAs used during an exposure. The rule of thumb that is used is called the 15% rule, which states that an increase in kVp of 15% is equivalent to doubling the mAs. This phenomenon occurs because the x-ray beam has more penetrability, which means that less of the radiation is absorbed by the patient and more radiation reaches the image receptor.

mAs

The milliamperage, exposure time, and the product of their total are directly proportional. Changes in mA change the quantity but not the energy (quality) of the x-ray beam. Changing the mA, time, or mAs does not change the average energy or the maximum x-ray beam energy. Notice in Figure 10.8 the photon energy lines on the graph start and stop at exactly the same points; the only difference in the two curves is in the number of x-ray photons produced. The number of x-ray photons is exactly twice as much for the 200 mA setting when compared to the corresponding point on the 100 mA curve. The quantity of the x-ray beam is directly proportional to the mA; doubling the mA doubles the quantity of the photons in the x-ray beam. The number of characteristic x-ray photons increases with increasing mA, but the characteristic x-ray energy does not change. Referring to the graph, notice that the peak for each curve is at exactly the same average energy or kVp; this occurs because the same kVp setting was used, but the mA settings are different.

Time has the same effect on x-ray production as mA. Increasing the time increases the number of x-ray photons reaching the patient and the image receptor but does not change the quality or penetration characteristic of the x-ray beam.

Filtration

When an x-ray beam is produced, there is a wide range of energies and wavelengths; the beam can be called polyenergetic or heterogeneous. The purpose of filtration is to remove low-energy x-ray photons before they strike the patient; this is an effective method for decreasing radiation dose to the patient. The filter is made of thin sheets of aluminum or other metal attached between the collimator and the tube housing. Adding 2.0 mm aluminum

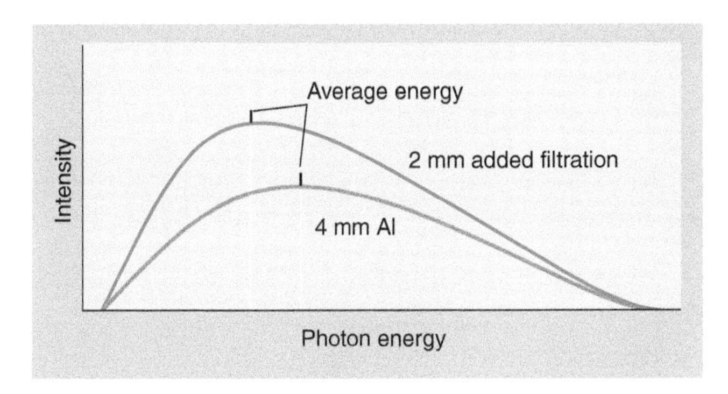

Figure 10.9. **Illustrates the change in the x-ray spectrum resulting from added filtration.**

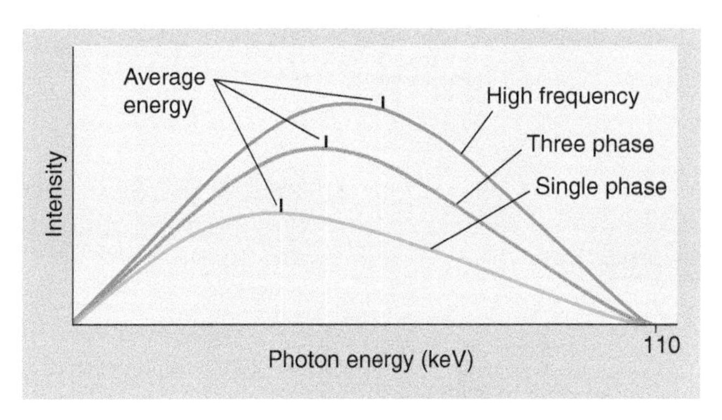

Figure 10.10 **An x-ray spectrum from single-phase, three-phase, and high-frequency x-ray circuits. Note how the average energy and intensity are increased with three-phase and high-frequency circuits.**

filtration removes all photons whose energy is <5 kV; in the graph, this is demonstrated by the starting point of the curve being shifted to the right (Fig. 10.9). When an additional 0.5 mm filter is used, even more low-energy photons are absorbed and prevented from leaving the x-ray tube. As seen in the graph, the starting point of the curve moves further to the right indicating that no x-rays with <10 kV are emitted.

It is interesting to note that the maximum energy of the beam has not changed with the addition of filters. However, because the starting point of the curve has been shifted to the right, the average energy of the beam has also shifted to the right. Therefore, adding filtration increases the average x-ray energy of the beam. The added filtration improves the penetrability of the beam by hardening the beam while decreasing the quantity of photons in the beam.

Generator Type

X-ray production depends on the type of x-ray generator used and the resultant circuit waveform. There are different types of circuits utilized for various x-ray equipment, such as single-phase, three-phase, and high-frequency circuits. As seen in Figure 10.10, the x-ray photons produced are low at the start and end of the wave form with the highest energy at the peak. Electricity flows in a sine wave from zero energy to maximum peak and back to zero energy. This is demonstrated on the graph where all three types of generator energies can be compared. Three-phase and high-frequency generators have minimal ripple effect in the wave because of the overlap of three waveforms. The minimal ripple effect means that this type of generator can maintain a higher-average voltage. At very high voltages, the average approaches the peak kilovolts allowed. The waveform keeps x-ray production high so that a greater number of higher-energy x-ray photons can be produced. Three-phase and high-frequency circuits that allow for more constant voltage result in higher-intensity and higher-average energies for the same mA and kVp settings. All modern x-ray equipment utilizes high-frequency circuits.

Chapter Summary

1. X-rays are produced by either the bremsstrahlung interaction or the characteristic interaction. Bremsstrahlung x-rays are produced when the projectile or incident electrons are slowed down or stopped in the anode.
2. Approximately 90% of diagnostic x-rays are produced by the bremsstrahlung process.
3. Characteristic x-rays are produced by transitions of orbital electrons that fill vacancies in atomic shells. The characteristic x-ray energy depends on the anode material.

4. An x-ray emission spectrum is a plot of x-ray intensity as a function of x-ray energy. The energy of individual x-rays is measured in keV.
5. The kVp is the voltage applied to the x-ray tube. The average energy of the x-ray beam is one-third of the maximum energy in the beam.
6. The x-ray emission spectrum depends on the kVp, mA, time, filtration, and x-ray circuit waveform.
7. Increasing the kVp increases the quality or penetrability of the beam, the average beam energy, and the maximum energy.
8. Filtration removes low-energy x-ray photons; each four centimeters of filtration will decrease the number of x-ray photons by one-half.
9. Increasing the mA increases the quantity but does not change the energy of the beam.
10. Increasing the filtration decreases the quantity or number of photons and increases the average beam energy.
11. Changing from single- to multiphase x-ray circuits increases the quantity and the average energy of the x-ray beam but does not change the maximum energy of the beam.

Case Study

Figure 10.7 demonstrates the x-ray spectrum that resulted from two exposures, one at 70 kVp and the other at 110 kVp.

Critical Thinking Questions

1. What is the main factor that changed the maximum energy of the beam?
2. How does this factor affect the average and maximum energies?
3. How does it change the appearance of the curves in the graph?
4. What change in energy occurs when the factor is decreased?

Review Questions

Multiple Choice

1. **The bremsstrahlung process produces x-rays when:**
   a. projectile electrons are stopped in the cathode
   b. a vacancy in an electron orbit is filled
   c. a vacancy in the nucleus is filled
   d. projectile electrons are slowed down and change direction in the anode
2. **Characteristic radiation is produced when:**
   a. electrons are stopped in the cathode
   b. a vacancy in an electron orbit is filled
   c. a vacancy in the nucleus is filled
   d. electrons are stopped in the anode

3. About ________% of the electron energy is converted to x-ray energy.

a. 1
b. 10
c. 25
d. 99

4. The x-ray tube filtration filters out which of the following?

a. low-energy electrons
b. high-energy x-ray photons
c. high-energy electrons
d. low-energy x-ray photons

5. The energy of the photon is known as the:

a. kVp
b. keV

6. Interactions that produce x-rays in the anode include:

1. coherent
2. Compton
3. bremsstrahlung
4. pair production
5. characteristic

a. 1, 3, and 5
b. 2 and 4
c. 3 and 5
d. 1, 2, 3, 4, and 5

7. The quality of the beam is primarily determined by:

a. mA
b. kVp
c. focal spot size
d. target angle

8. An atom of tungsten has shell binding energies of K shell 69, L shell 12, M shell 3, and N shell 1. Incident electrons must have an energy of at least ________ keV to produce K-characteristic x-rays from tungsten.

a. 50
b. 70
c. 67
d. 58

9. A technologist can control the quantity of x-rays striking the patient by adjusting the:

a. mA
b. kVp
c. mA and kVp
d. mA, kVp, and anode material
e. mA, kVp, rectification, and anode material

10. The maximum kinetic energy of an incident electron accelerated across an x-ray tube depends on the:

a. atomic number (Z) of the target
b. size of the focal spot
c. kilovoltage
d. type of rectification

11. Eight centimeters of filtration is placed into the path of the primary x-ray beam. How much is the intensity of the x-ray beam decreased?

a. 95%
b. 50%
c. 10%
d. 25%

Short Answer

1. Define and explain the 15% rule.

2. Using Figure 10.2, calculate energy of the characteristic x-ray if the K-shell electron is replaced by an L-shell electron.

3. Which type of interaction produces diagnostic x-rays?

4. Identify the factors that have an effect on the x-ray spectrum, and describe how the spectrum is affected by each factor.

5. Describe the characteristic interaction.

6. The majority of electron energy in the x-ray tube is converted to which form of energy?

7. Describe the bremsstrahlung interaction.

8. Explain what the characteristic cascade is.

9. What is an incident electron?

10. Explain how the x-ray circuit influences the production of x-rays.

PART III

Image Production

11

X-Ray Interactions with Matter

Objectives

Upon completion of this chapter, the student will be able to:

1. Describe the x-ray interactions of coherent scattering and Compton scattering.
2. Explain the photoelectric effect.
3. State how backscatter radiation is determined.
4. Discuss the difference between a photoelectron and a Compton scattered photon.
5. State the importance of the atomic number and how it relates to the photoelectric effect.
6. Differentiate between pair production and photodisintegration.

Key Terms

- annihilation radiation
- backscatter radiation
- coherent scattering
- Compton scattering
- pair production
- photodisintegration
- photoelectric effect
- photoelectron
- radiopaque

Introduction

There are five ways that x-rays interact with matter: coherent scattering, Compton scattering, photoelectric effect, pair production, and photodisintegration. Compton scattering and the photoelectric effect are the two interactions that are important in creating the radiographic image. The student will also learn about two processes that occur at extremely high energy levels. These are not used in radiography, but the student must be aware of their potential harm to the patient.

Types of X-Ray Interactions

The five x-ray interactions possible in tissue are

1. coherent scattering
2. Compton scattering
3. photoelectric effect
4. pair production
5. photodisintegration

These interactions take place between the x-ray photons and the target atoms in the tissue. Only the photoelectric and Compton interactions are important in diagnostic radiology.

Coherent Scattering

thePoint® *An animation for this topic can be viewed at http://thepoint.lww.com/Orth2e*

Coherent scattering, also called classical or Thompson scattering, occurs when a low-energy incident x-ray photon interacts with a strongly bound orbital electron causing the electron to become momentarily excited and vibrate. With this interaction, the atom does not lose an orbital electron and does not become ionized but merely excited. The excited atom is unstable, and to regain stability, it immediately releases the excess energy as a scattered x-ray photon with the same energy and wavelength as the incident photon. As seen in Figure 11.1, the incident x-ray photon is moving in a straight line when it interacts with the target atom. The resultant coherent scattered photon changes direction as it leaves the target atom. Notice how the wavelength of the incoming photon and the scattered photon are identical; the term *coherent* is used to signify that the energies of both photons are the same. This interaction occurs with low-energy x-ray photons below the diagnostic range and is not important in diagnostic radiology. British physicist J.J. Thomson discovered this interaction, which is named after him.

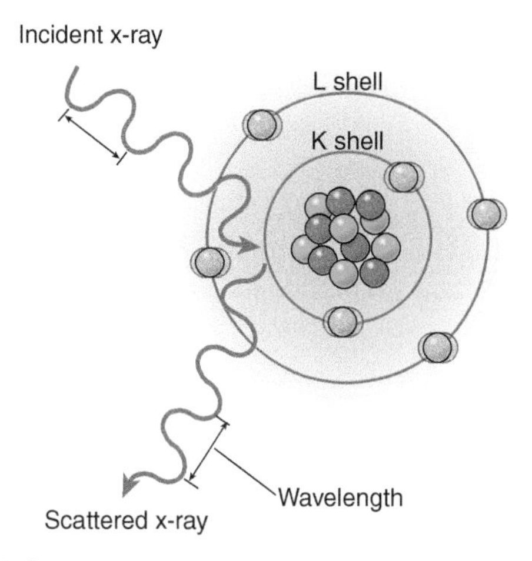

Figure 11.1. **Illustrates coherent scattering, which does not produce ionization. Classical scattering occurs when an incident photon interacts with an orbital electron and excites the electron. The x-ray photon does not lose any energy but changes direction and leaves the atom.**

Compton Scattering

thePoint® *An animation for this topic can be viewed at http://thepoint.lww.com/Orth2e*

In **Compton scattering**, the incident x-ray photon interacts with a loosely bound outer-shell electron. During the interaction, a portion of the x-ray photon's energy is absorbed by an electron. The ionized atom ejects the electron as a recoil or Compton electron. The remaining photon energy is reemitted as a Compton scattered photon, which can travel in a random direction or scatter. The energy of the incident photon is shared between the recoil electron and the Compton scattered photon. The Compton scattered photon has lower energy and longer wavelength than does the incident photon (Fig. 11.2).

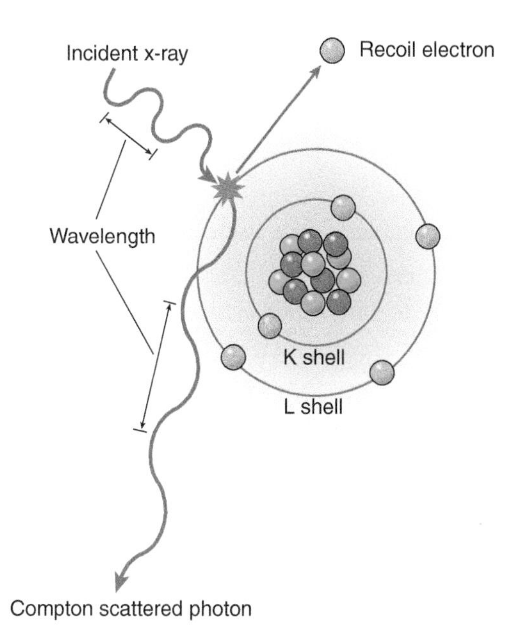

Figure 11.2. **Illustrates Compton scattering of an incident x-ray by an outer-shell electron.**

American physicist Arthur Compton discovered this interaction, which is named for him.

The energy of the Compton scattered photon is equal to the difference in energy between the incident photon and the energy of the recoil electron. The energy of the recoil electron is equal to its binding energy plus the kinetic energy it acquires when leaving the atom. The Compton interaction is represented by the following formula:

$$E_I = E_S + E_B + E_{KE}$$

where E_I is the energy of the incident photon, E_S is the energy of the Compton scattered photon, E_B is the electron binding energy, and E_{KE} is the kinetic energy of the ejected electron.

CRITICAL THINKING BOX 11.1

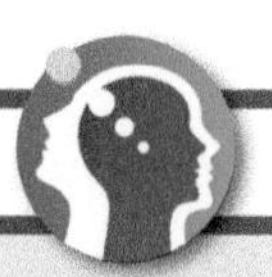

A 35-keV x-ray photon ionizes an atom of iodine by ejecting an M-shell electron that has a binding energy of 1.07 kV with 16 keV of kinetic energy. What is the energy of the Compton scattered photon?

During the Compton interaction, the majority of the energy is divided between the Compton scattered photon and the recoil electron. The Compton scattered photon (originally called the incident x-ray photon) retains most of its energy with a portion going to the recoil electron. The Compton scattered photon and recoil electron may have enough energy to go on to ionize other atoms in the tissue until they ultimately lose all their energy. The Compton scattered photon may be absorbed photoelectrically with an atom, or it may exit the patient and expose the image receptor. The recoil electron loses its kinetic energy through interacting with orbital electrons. Eventually, the recoil electron will fill a vacancy in an electron shell.

Compton scattered photons can be scattered in any direction up to 180 degrees. The angle of deflection is influenced by the energy of the incident x-ray photon. At a deflection of 0 degrees, no energy is transferred because the incident photon does not change its path from the original direction. As the deflection increases to 180 degrees, more energy is given to the recoil electron, and less energy stays with the scattered photon. When a scattered photon is deflected 180 degrees, it will be scattered back in the direction of the incident photon; it is called **backscatter radiation**. Backscatter radiation can cause optical densities on the radiographic image, which decreases image quality. The backscatter radiation deposits unwanted exposure on the image receptor and is called radiation fog. The increase in radiation fog causes a decrease in radiographic contrast. Methods for reducing backscatter radiation are discussed later in the text.

As the x-ray energy increases, the probability of Compton scattering decreases. Of the affects, which do occur, more of them will be projected toward the image receptor, which means the image receptor will receive more scatter radiation with an increase in kVp.

Compton scattering is not determined by the atomic number of the atom involved in the interaction. During radiographic examinations of larger areas of the body, more tissues are irradiated due to the larger field sizes; this produces more Compton scattering. The scatter radiation emitted from the patient is the primary cause of occupational exposure for the radiographer. Fluoroscopic examinations pose a serious radiation hazard due to the large amount of radiation that is scattered from the patient. This is why it is crucial for the radiographer to wear a lead apron, thyroid shield, and gloves during all fluoroscopic examinations.

Photoelectric Effect

thePoint® *An animation for this topic can be viewed at http://thepoint.lww.com/Orth2e*

In the **photoelectric effect** or interaction, the incident x-ray photon is completely absorbed by an inner-shell electron. The orbital electron absorbs all the photon energy, which causes the electron to speed up in its orbit to the point where the electron is "flung" out of orbit, just like a rock is flung out of a slingshot. The photoelectric effect is "all or nothing" meaning all photon energy must be given up for the electron to be ejected. The ejected electron is called a **photoelectron**. The photoelectron has kinetic energy that is equal to the difference between the incident x-ray photon and the binding energy of the inner-shell electron. This is shown mathematically in the equation:

$$E_I = E_B + E_{KE}$$

where E_I is the energy of the incident photon, E_B is the binding energy of the electron, and E_{KE} is the kinetic energy of the photoelectron. For the interaction to occur, the incident photon needs an energy that is equal to or slightly greater than the binding energy of the orbital electron. Table 11.1 shows the atomic number, K-shell, and L-shell electron binding energy for elements common in the body and commonly used in radiography. Most of the atoms in tissue are very low atomic number elements and have very low K-shell binding energies. Carbon atoms have a K-shell binding energy of 0.3 keV and only need a very low-energy incident photon to remove them from their orbit. During this interaction, the resultant photoelectron will be released with kinetic energy almost equal to the energy of the incident photon. Iodine is a higher atomic number atom that is used during special radiographic procedures. The K-shell binding energy of iodine is 33 keV, and it will require a higher energy incident photon to remove the K-shell electron from its orbit compared to the carbon atom.

When the electron is removed from the atom, it causes the atom to become ionized. The vacancy in the K shell will be filled with an electron from the L shell, M shell, or a free electron. Filling the inner-shell vacancy produces characteristic x-ray photons. Characteristic photons from tissue elements (carbon, nitrogen, and oxygen) have very low energies. They are called secondary radiation and act like scatter radiation. Most characteristic x-rays from the tissue do not exit the patient because of their extremely low energies (Fig. 11.3). The final result of the photoelectric effect is the complete absorption of the incident photon. There is no exit radiation after a photoelectric interaction. The photoelectric effect produces the lighter densities on conventional x-ray images.

TABLE 11.1 ATOMIC NUMBER AND ELECTRON SHELL BINDING ENERGIES OF RADIOGRAPHICALLY IMPORTANT ELEMENTS

Element/ Material	Atomic Number	K-Shell Binding Energy	L-Shell Binding Energy
Biological elements			
Carbon	6	0.28 kV	0.022 kV
Oxygen	8	0.54 kV	0.042 kV
Calcium	20	4.04 kV	0.438 kV
Contrast Agents and Shielding			
Iodine	53	33.2 kV	5 kV
Barium	56	37.4 kV	6 kV
Tungsten	74	69.6 kV	12 kV
Lead	82	88 kV	16 kV

CRITICAL THINKING BOX 11.2

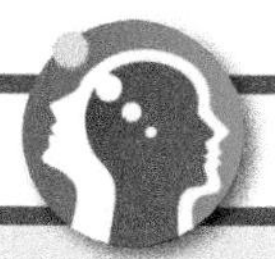

A 95 keV x-ray photon interacts with a barium atom. What is the kinetic energy of the photoelectron?

What is the energy of the characteristic x-ray photon when an L-shell to K-shell transition occurs? (Use Table 11.1 to discover the binding energies of barium.)

The photoelectric effect increases with higher atomic number (Z) atoms. Atoms with higher atomic numbers have higher electron binding energies. Bone (Z 13.8) absorbs more photons than muscle (Z 7.4) because of its higher atomic number. The attenuation of bone is four times greater than the attenuation of muscle at an x-ray energy of 40 keV (Fig. 11.4). Barium (Z 56) and iodine (Z 33) are used as contrast agents because of their high atomic numbers. Structures containing these **radiopaque** contrast agents appear lighter or brighter on conventional radiographic images.

The photoelectron loses energy quickly by interacting with other atoms and eventually becomes absorbed by a vacancy in an orbital shell. The photoelectron does not leave the body but remains in the tissue. This absorption of the photoelectron has a direct effect on the radiographic image because the photoelectron does not reach the image receptor. This means that there is a white or very light gray area on the image. In areas where there are fewer photoelectric interactions, there will be other shades of gray from medium to dark. Remember that all the shades of gray are what allows us to see the radiographic image.

CRITICAL THINKING BOX 11.3

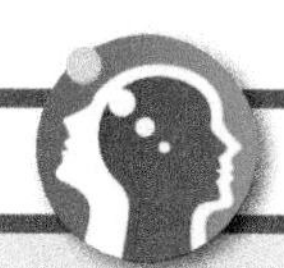

Using Figure 4.3, determine the kinetic energy of the photoelectron that results when a 65 keV x-ray photon interacts with an iodine atom.

Now determine the energy of the characteristic x-ray photon when an L-shell to K-shell transition occurs.

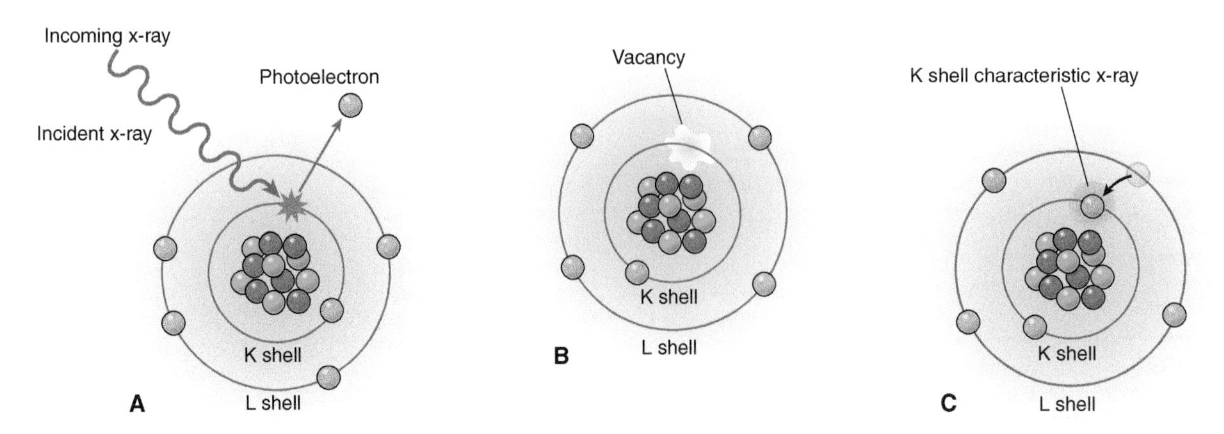

Figure 11.3. **(A–C) The photoelectric effect resulting in vacant electron holes being filled with electrons from higher shells, cascade effect.**

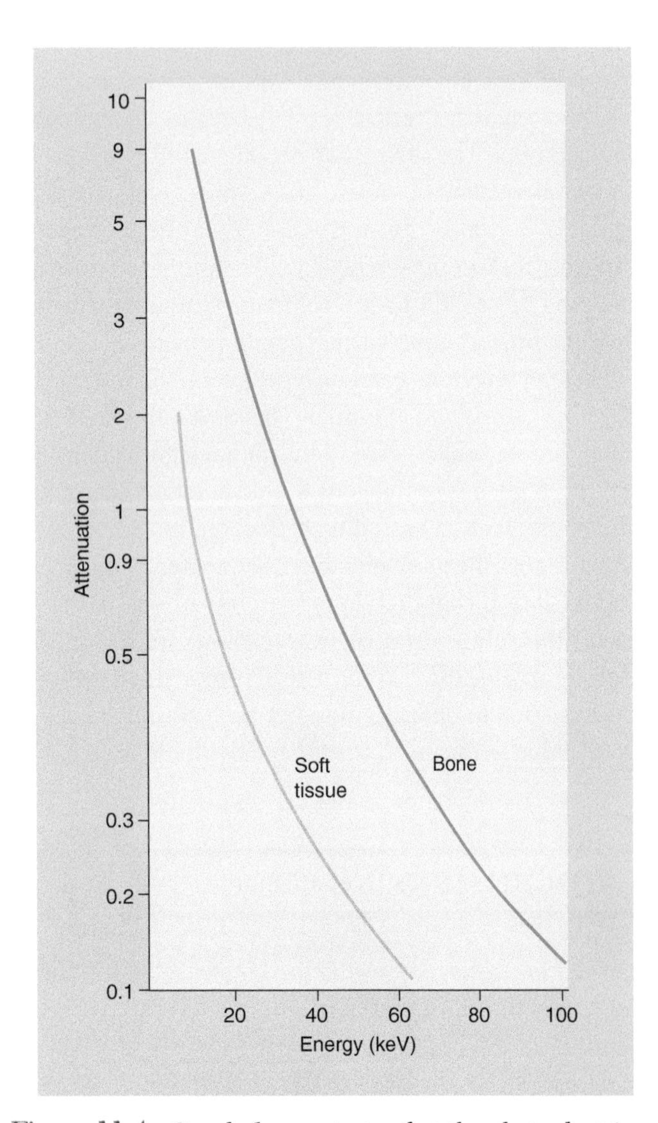

Figure 11.4. **Graph demonstrates that the photoelectric effect is greater in bone than in muscle.**

Pair Production

thePoint® ***An animation for this topic can be viewed at http://thepoint.lww.com/Orth2e***

An incident x-ray photon with energy of at least 1.02 MeV will pass through the orbital electrons to come very close to the nucleus of the atom. The strong nuclear field will interact with the x-ray photon so much that the x-ray photon will disappear. In its place, one positive electron (positron) and one negative electron will equally share the incident photon energy (Fig. 11.5); this is called **pair production**. In pair production, the incident x-ray photon is transformed into two particles, a positron and a negative electron, each having 0.51 MeV of energy. If the incident x-ray photon energy is >1.02 MeV, the excess energy will be given equally to each particle in the form of kinetic energy. Both particles will leave the atom. The negative electron undergoes multiple interactions and loses energy through excitation and ionization to eventually fill a vacancy in an orbital shell.

The positron is an "unnatural" particle that travels around until it finally unites with a free electron, and the mass of both is converted into energy in a process called **annihilation radiation**. During the annihilation event, the positron and electron are both destroyed, and their energy is converted into two x-ray photons that travel out of the atom in opposite directions. Pair production does not occur at diagnostic radiology energies but is important in nuclear medicine and positron emission tomography.

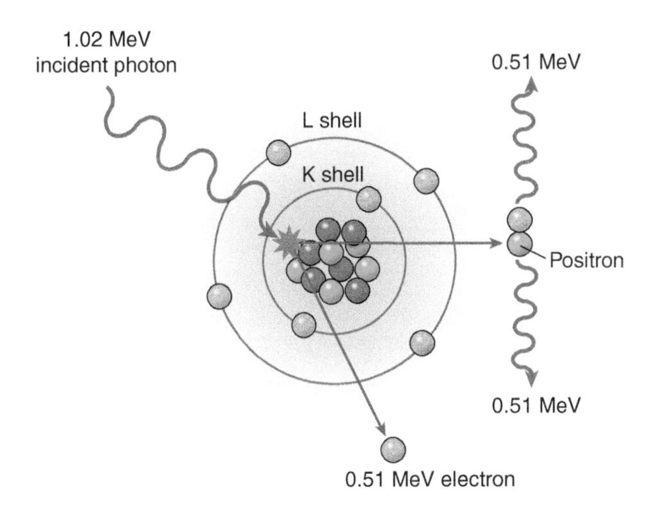

Figure 11.5. **Pair production occurs with x-ray photons having an energy of 1.02 MeV or greater. Upon interaction with the nuclear force field, the photon disappears, and two oppositely charged electrons take its place.**

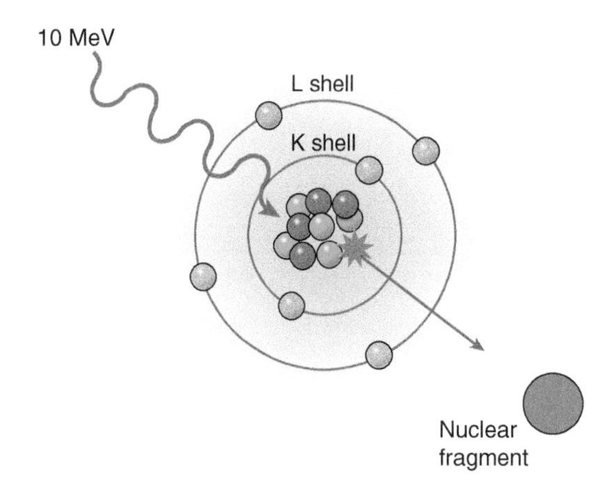

Figure 11.6. **Illustrates the emergence of a nuclear fragment after the incident photon has gone through the process of photonuclear disintegration.**

Photodisintegration

thePoint® *An animation for this topic can be viewed at http://thepoint.lww.com/Orth2e*

In **photodisintegration**, the incident x-ray photon has enough energy (>10 MeV) to bypass the orbiting electron and nuclear field to directly impact the atomic nucleus. When the incident x-ray photon strikes the nucleus, it gives up all its energy to the nucleus; this interaction excites the nucleus and makes it unstable. The excited nucleus then immediately emits a nuclear fragment or particle as a proton, neutron, or alpha particle (Fig. 11.6). Both pair production and photodisintegration require extremely high-energy x-rays and are not utilized in diagnostic radiology.

Chapter Summary

1. Of the five possible types of interactions in tissues, only the photoelectric and Compton interactions are important in diagnostic radiology.
2. The photoelectric effect results in complete absorption of the incident x-ray photon. Photoelectric effects decrease with increasing x-ray energy and increase with increasing atomic number (Z).
3. Compton scattering changes the direction and energy of the x-ray photon. Compton scattering contributes to the loss of contrast on the image and to occupational dose.
4. Photoelectric interactions are most important at lower x-ray photon energies, and Compton scattering is more important at higher x-ray energies.
5. Coherent scattering occurs when low-energy x-ray photons interact with an atom and then the photon changes direction to leave the atom.
6. In pair production, the high-energy x-ray photon comes close to the nucleus of an atom but does not directly interact with the nucleus.
7. Photodisintegration is the process whereby a high-energy x-ray photon directly strikes the atom's nucleus. A nuclear fragment or particle then results from the interaction.

Case Study

During the photoelectric effect, the incident x-ray photon is completely absorbed by the atom. The energy from the photon is transferred to an inner-shell electron causing ionization of the atom and a resultant ejected electron.

Critical Thinking Questions

1. How far will the photoelectron travel in tissue?
2. What happens when the inner-shell vacancy is filled?
3. What will eventually happen to the photoelectron?
4. How does the photoelectric effect change the radiographic image?

Review Questions

Multiple Choice

1. What is(are) the product(s) of Compton scattering?

a. Electron
b. Recoil electron and scattered x-ray photon
c. Electron and positive electron
d. Scattered x-ray photon

2. Compton scattering is responsible for which of the following?

a. Production of scatter radiation that degrades image contrast
b. Increases contrast in radiographic images
c. Produces x-ray photons in the rotating anode
d. Is more important at lower energies

3. Which best describes the photoelectric interaction?

a. Involves changes in energy and direction
b. Involves complete absorption of the photoelectron
c. Involves complete absorption of the incident x-ray
d. Requires at least 1.02 MeV energy

4. Materials or tissues that attenuate small amounts of x-ray photons are called:

a. radiopaque
b. radiolucent

5. The interaction that involves no loss of energy or ionization is:

a. coherent
b. photoelectric
c. pair production
d. Compton
e. photodisintegration

6. Photodisintegration produces a __________ when the incident photon energy is __________.

a. nuclear fragment, deflected
b. scattered electron, partially absorbed
c. scattered photon, completely absorbed
d. nuclear fragment, completely absorbed

7. During pair production, the resulting electrons have how much energy?

a. 0.44 MeV
b. 0.51 MeV
c. 0.36 MeV
d. 0.15 MeV

8. Which x-ray interaction is the most hazardous to the patient and radiographer?
   a. Photoelectric
   b. Coherent scattering
   c. Photodisintegration
   d. Compton scattering

9. When the ejected photoelectron leaves an inner-shell vacancy, which type of x-ray photons are produced?
   a. Bremsstrahlung
   b. Characteristic
   c. Coherent
   d. Compton

Short Answer

1. In which interaction is a secondary electron found?

2. Photodisintegration involves incident photon energies equal to or greater than __________.

3. Describe backscatter.

4. A 50 kV x-ray photon undergoes a Compton interaction with an L-shell electron in a calcium atom. The recoil electron flies away with 7 kV of kinetic energy. Determine the energy of the Compton scattered photon.

5. Write the formula for the photoelectric effect, and explain why it is used.

6. Describe the coherent scatter interaction.

7. X-ray photon interaction with the force field of the nucleus produces __________.

8. Is there an increase or decrease in Compton scattering if the incident photon energy is increased?

9. An incoming x-ray photon interacts with the K-shell of an atom of iodine. How much energy does the x-ray photon possess when the Compton scattered photon has 52.8 kV and the recoil electron has 4 kV of kinetic energy?

12

Beam Attenuation

Objectives

Upon completion of this chapter, the student will be able to:

1. Describe the factors that affect absorption of x-ray photons.
2. Explain the process of beam attenuation.
3. State the factors that affect beam attenuation.
4. Identify the factors that make up subject contrast.
5. Distinguish between differential absorption, scatter radiation, and transmission of x-ray photons.
6. Explain the effect of scatter radiation on the radiographic image.
7. State how fog affects the image.
8. Define remnant radiation.

Key Terms

- absorption
- beam attenuation
- differential absorption
- exit radiation
- fog
- radiolucent
- radiopaque
- remnant radiation
- scattering
- subject contrast
- tissue density
- transmission

Introduction

X-ray photons entering a patient can be absorbed, scattered, or transmitted. When an x-ray photon is absorbed in a patient, all of the energy is transferred to the patient's tissue. Scattering changes the x-ray photon direction and reduces its energy. Scatter contributes to radiographic fog and reduces image contrast. Transmitted x-ray photons pass through the patient without interaction and form the radiographic image. Most diagnostic x-ray photons are absorbed or scattered. Only about 1% of the x-ray photons are transmitted through the patient without any interaction. Radiation leaving the patient is termed exit or remnant radiation. Exit radiation consists of transmitted and scattered x-ray photons. Throughout the chapter, the student will learn about each of these concepts and how they occur during an x-ray exposure.

Differential Absorption

Differential absorption is a process where some of the x-ray photons are absorbed photoelectrically while other x-ray photons pass completely through the patient. *Differential* is a term that means the varying anatomic parts will absorb the primary beam in different amounts because of their own unique atomic number. Tissues with higher atomic numbers will absorb greater amounts of the primary beam than will tissues filled with air. Bone is a dense tissue that absorbs x-ray photons, while lung tissue, which is filled with air, is less dense resulting in lower x-ray beam absorption. It is this varying amount of absorption of the x-ray beam that creates an image of the anatomic structures of interest (Fig. 12.1).

Beam Attenuation

Beam attenuation is the removal of x-ray photons from the primary beam. Beam attenuation occurs when the x-ray beam passes through anatomic tissue and loses some of the x-ray photon energy. This results in the beam having fewer x-ray photons. Beam attenuation results from the photon interactions with the atomic parts of the tissue. There are two processes that occur during beam attenuation: absorption and scattering.

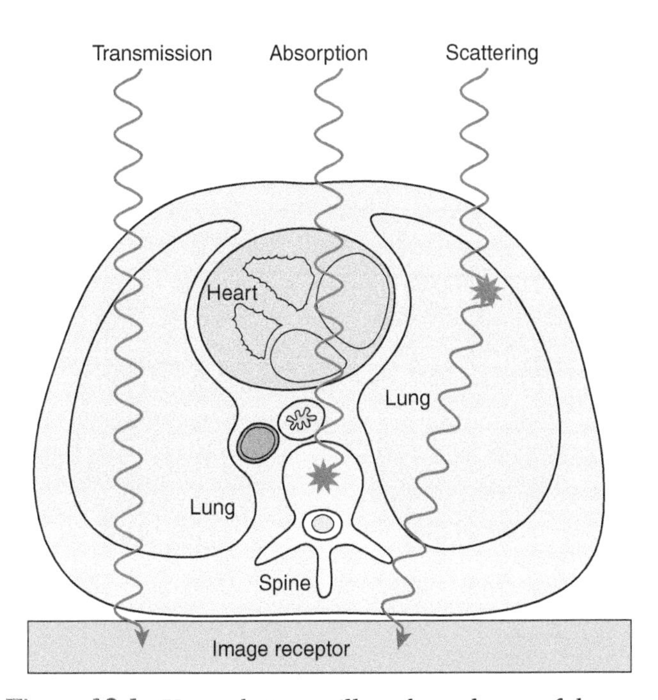

Figure 12.1. X-ray photons will go through one of these processes: absorption, scatter, and transmission.

Absorption

Upon interacting with tissue, some x-ray photons will experience complete energy loss and will remain in the tissue, and this is called **absorption**. The potential for total absorption depends on the energy of the incoming x-ray photon and the atomic number of the tissue. Total absorption occurs when an x-ray photon has enough energy to eject an inner-shell electron. Because the x-ray photons are absorbed, they will not reach the image receptor. Tissue structures that completely absorb the x-ray photons appear as light areas or low-density areas on the radiographic image; these structures are said to be radiopaque.

Scattering

Scattering occurs when some of the x-ray photons are not absorbed but have interactions with atomic structures and lose some of their energy. The incoming x-ray photon loses some of its energy when it interacts with an outer-shell electron; the interaction results in the electron being ejected from its orbit. The low-energy x-ray photon changes direction and may leave the anatomic part to strike the image receptor (Fig. 12.2). Scatter or secondary radiation does not provide useful information

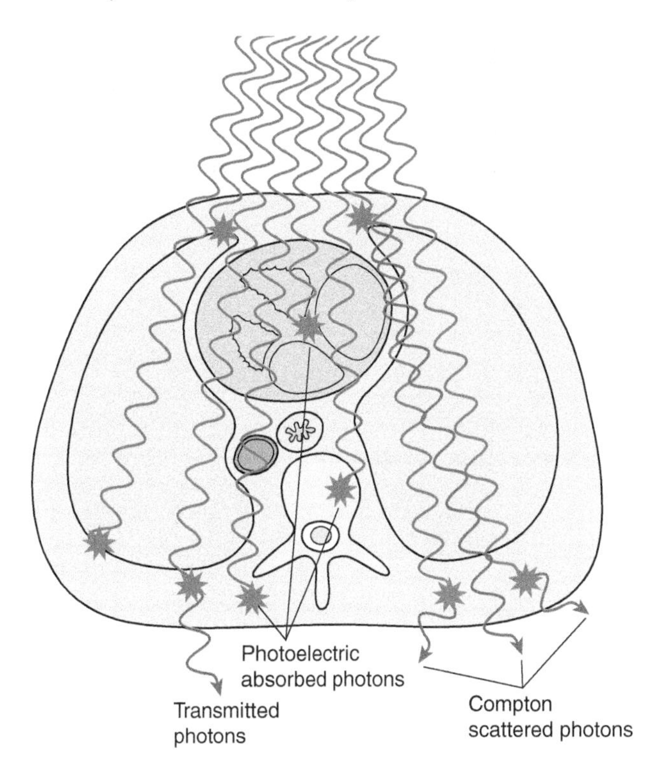

Figure 12.2. (A) Transmission: X-ray photon that penetrates through the body to strike the image receptor. (B) Photoelectric absorption: X-ray photons that are absorbed by tissue. (C) Compton scatter radiation: X-ray photons that become scatter radiation.

to the image receptor. When the scatter radiation remains in the anatomic structure, it contributes to the radiation dose to the patient. If the scattered radiation were to leave the patient but not strike the image receptor, it could contribute to the radiation dose to anyone close to the patient.

Transmission

Some of the remaining photons in the x-ray beam will pass completely through the patient (**transmission**) without interacting with the anatomic structures (Fig. 12.1). These x-ray photons then strike the image receptor and do contribute valuable information to the image. Tissues that are filled with air are called **radiolucent** because the x-ray beam passes through the tissue to strike the image receptor. These x-ray photons appear as dark shades or high-density areas on an image. The combined effects of absorption and transmission are necessary to demonstrate the anatomical area of interest. Without the varying shades created by these processes, there would be no radiographic image.

Factors Affecting Beam Attenuation

The amount of x-ray beam attenuation is dependent on these four factors:

1. Tissue thickness
2. Tissue type (atomic number)
3. Tissue density
4. X-ray photon energy

Tissue Thickness

In Chapter 10, we discussed half-value layer and the effect on the x-ray beam when placing material in the path of the beam. The same concept is also true for anatomic tissue. As the tissue thickness increases, more x-ray photons are attenuated, by either absorption or scattering. X-ray photons are attenuated exponentially, and for every 4 cm of tissue thickness, there is approximately a 50% reduction in the number of x-ray photons in the beam (Fig. 12.3).

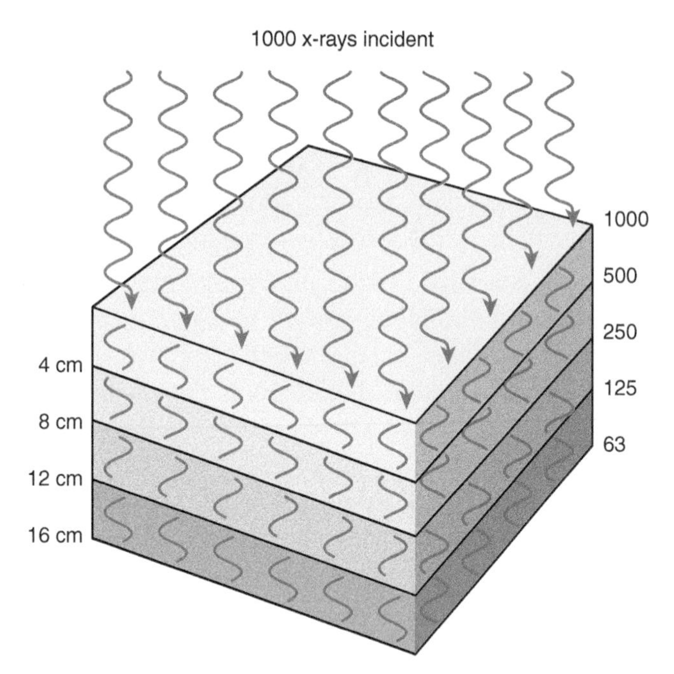

Figure 12.3. **Illustrates the effect tissue thickness has on the exponential attenuation of the x-ray beam as it passes through the body.**

More x-ray photons are attenuated by 20 cm of the tissue than by 16 cm of the tissue. The rule is the thicker the anatomic part, more x-rays are needed to create the radiographic image. Likewise for thinner parts, fewer x-rays are needed to produce the image. Technologists must learn to make adjustments in technical exposure factors (mAs and kVp) to compensate for various tissue thicknesses. A general rule radiographers follow is to change technical factor settings by a factor of 2 for every 4 cm change in part thickness. As discussed in Chapter 10, a 15% increase in kVp will result in doubling the mAs or increasing the mAs by a factor of 2. When a patient's abdomen is 4 cm thicker than an average patient, the kVp must be set 15% higher or the mAs doubled to compensate for the thicker part. The opposite is true if the body part is 4 cm thinner than average where the kVp would be decreased by 15% or the mAs would be halved.

Tissue Type

Tissues or materials with higher atomic numbers (Z) have higher attenuation values. Table 12.1 presents the atomic number of some tissues and materials common in diagnostic radiology. Air, iodine, and barium are contrast materials often introduced into the body

TABLE 12.1 ATOMIC NUMBER OF MATERIALS IMPORTANT IN RADIOLOGY

Type of Substance	Density (g/cm³)	Atomic Number
Human Tissue		
Lung	0.32	7.4
Fat	0.91	6.3
Muscle	1.0	7.4
Bone	1.9	13.8
Contrast Agents		
Air	0.0013	7.6
Iodine	4.9	53
Barium	3.5	56
Other		
Lead	11.4	82

to improve image contrast. Each is used because their atomic numbers or their densities are significantly higher than the surrounding body tissues. Substances that are highly attenuating are termed **radiopaque** and easily absorb x-ray photons. Bone, barium, and iodine are examples of radiopaque substances. Structures that absorb more x-rays are represented on the radiographic image as light (bright) areas. As stated previously in this chapter, substances having low attenuation values are termed radiolucent. Air, bowel gas, and lung tissue are relatively radiolucent and are easily penetrated by x-ray photons. The lungs are a combination of air spaces and tissue with a density between air and muscle. Radiolucent structures are represented as dark areas on the radiographic image.

Tissue Density

Tissue density refers to how closely packed the atomic particles are in a tissue. Density of a body part is measured in grams per cubic centimeter (g/cm³). X-ray photon attenuation is increased in dense tissue. Air or gas has the lowest density in the body. Muscle and fat have similar atomic numbers (Z numbers) but differ in the compactness of the atoms. Because the atoms in muscle are more compact, muscle is more dense than fat. Overall, the attenuation of 1 cm of muscle is >1 cm of fat. Bone has an atomic number nearly twice the atomic number of muscle. When considering types of tissue, remember that bone is more dense than muscle, which is denser than fat, which is more dense than air. Table 12.1 lists the densities of some body tissues and materials important in radiology.

X-Ray Photon Energy

X-ray photons with higher energies (short wavelengths and high frequency) have greater penetration and lower attenuation values. Higher-energy x-ray photons have less differential absorption because they are more penetrating. Higher-penetrating x-ray photons typically do not interact with tissue and are transmitted through the body to strike the image receptor. Changing the x-ray photon energy by changing the kVp will alter the penetration of the x-ray beam. Lower-energy x-ray photons (longer wavelengths and lower frequencies) have higher attenuation and lower penetration values. These low-energy x-ray photons are more likely to interact with tissue and to scatter if not absorbed. Attenuation is increased with low-energy x-rays and decreased with high-energy x-rays (Table 12.2).

TABLE 12.2 FACTORS AFFECTING BEAM ATTENUATION

Factor	Beam Attenuation	Absorption	Transmission
Tissue Thickness			
Increasing thickness	Increases	Increases	Decreases
Decreasing thickness	Decreases	Decreases	Increases
Tissue Type (Z number)			
Increasing Z number	Increases	Increases	Decreases
Decreasing Z number	Decreases	Decreases	Increases
Tissue Density			
Increasing density	Increases	Increases	Decreases
Decreasing density	Decreases	Decreases	Increases
X-Ray Photon Energy			
Increasing energy	Decreases	Decreases	Increases
Decreasing energy	Increases	Increases	Decreases

Higher-energy x-ray photons also produce more Compton scattering than do lower-energy x-ray photons because Compton scattering predominates at higher x-ray energies. This combination of less differential absorption and more scattering results in less subject contrast at higher energies. Subject contrast depends on the average energy of the x-ray beam. Increasing the average energy of the x-ray beam by increasing the kVp or increasing beam filtration lowers the subject contrast.

Remnant Radiation

Remnant or exit radiation is made up of transmitted and scattered x-ray photons. As previously discussed, differential absorption (varying amounts of transmitted and absorbed radiation) creates the radiographic image. Scatter exit radiation (Compton interactions) that reaches the image receptor does not add any diagnostic information to the image. In fact, scatter radiation creates unwanted exposure to the image that results in more density on the image called **fog**. There are methods that reduce the amount of scatter radiation that reaches the image receptor, and these will be discussed later in the text.

Subject Contrast

Differential absorption provides subtle differences in attenuation. These differences represent all the different types of tissue as well as tissue thicknesses in the body. The remnant x-ray beam is made up of these differences in radiation intensity between the various tissues in the body and is transmitted to the image receptor to form an accurate representation of the body's structures (Fig. 12.4). **Subject contrast** is a result of the absorption characteristics of the tissues that are seen as multiple shades of gray on the radiographic image.

Upon reviewing the image, it is noticed that there is greatest subject contrast between bone and soft tissue. Figure 12.4A shows a chest x-ray that demonstrates great subject contrast or high contrast. Notice the lung tissue is seen as darker shades of gray while the ribs and spine are much lighter shades of gray. This degree of high contrast is necessary to adequately visualize anatomic structures in the thorax. Figure 12.4B demonstrates an image of the abdomen. Notice that in the abdomen, there are many shades of gray compared to the chest x-ray. Abdomen images require low contrast to best visualize the soft tissues and organs in the abdomen. If all images had high subject contrast, a lot of tissues would not be visualized. A skilled technologist is able to properly set technical factors that will image the body part with the correct subject contrast.

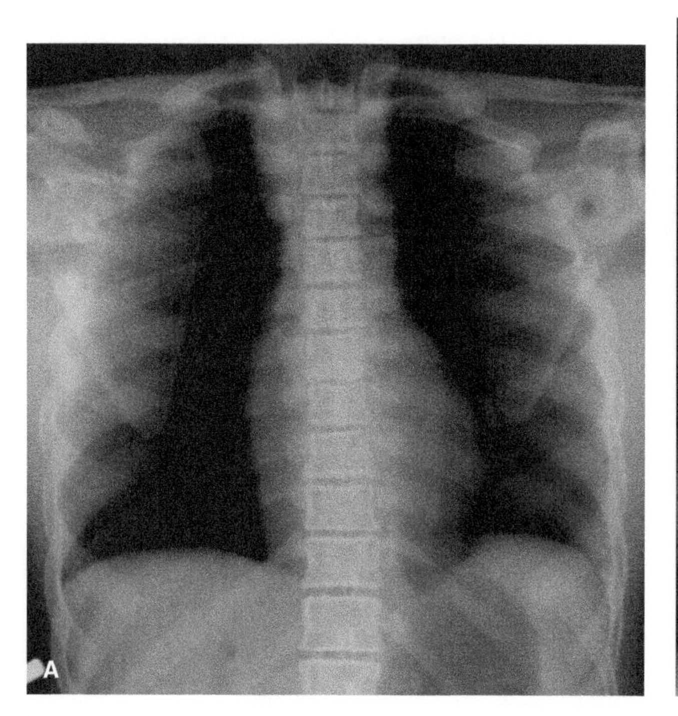

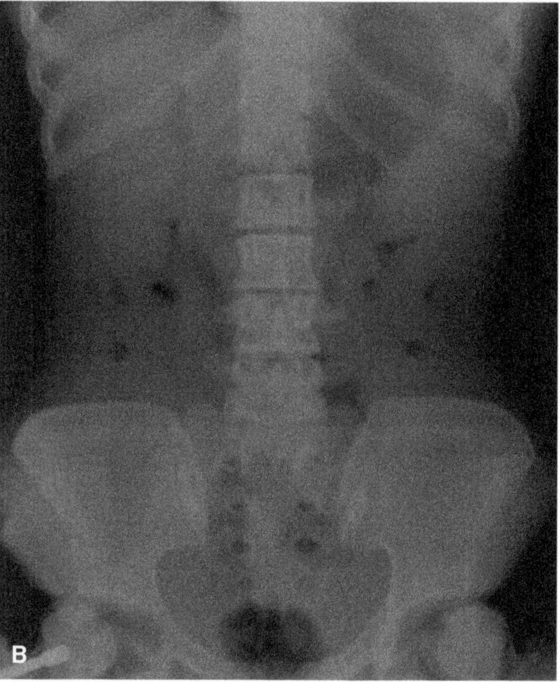

Figure 12.4. **(A) Chest image demonstrating high subject contrast. (B) Abdomen image shows many shades of gray or low subject contrast.**

Scatter

Scatter is radiation that has undergone one or more Compton interactions in the body. As kVp is increased, the percentage of Compton interactions also increases, and the result is an increased amount of scatter reaching the image receptor. The presence of scatter reduces radiographic contrast because the scatter increases the film fog that results in a long scale of gray. Grids are devices used to absorb and reduce the scatter before it reaches the film, thereby increasing contrast. Grids are used when imaging with a high kVp; low kVp imaging does not produce the high percentage of Compton interactions and does not require a grid to absorb the scatter before it reaches the film.

Contrast Agent

The vessels and organs are soft tissue structures with similar densities and are not easily visualized on a radiographic image. To make these structures visible, a substance with a higher density must be used. Adding a higher atomic number contrast agent to vessels or organs in the body increases the differential absorption and results in body structures becoming more visible. Iodine and barium are commonly used as contrast agents because they have high atomic numbers and high densities. Introducing barium into the intestines and introducing iodine into the kidneys are examples of the use of contrast agents in radiology. Barium and iodine are radiopaque substances that absorb the x-ray photons. The increased attenuation makes the structures containing the contrast agent appear lighter than the surrounding tissues and increases subject contrast. The differences in subject contrast between the soft tissue and the structure filled with the barium or iodine allow us to visualize the outline of the vessel or organ. Air is also used as a contrast agent. Air also increases differential absorption because its lower density increases transmission through the air-filled structures. Air is a radiolucent contrast agent, which allows us to visualize lung tissue as well as the ribs and mediastinum outline. Air increases subject contrast and provides a short scale of contrast to better visualize structures.

Chapter Summary

1. X-rays entering a patient can be transmitted, absorbed, or scattered.
2. Attenuation is the combination of absorption and scattering. Attenuation depends on energy, tissue material (atomic number), tissue thickness, and tissue density.
3. Beam attenuation occurs when the primary x-ray beam loses energy as it interacts with tissue.
4. The image is a result of differential absorption of the primary x-ray photons, which interact with various tissue types in the anatomic area of interest.
5. Subject contrast is the difference between various anatomic tissues and their abilities to absorb radiation. It is subject contrast that makes it possible to visualize the structures of the body on the image.
6. Subject contrast is influenced by tissue thickness differences, tissue type, atomic number, tissue density, x-ray beam energy and kVp, contrast media, and scatter.
7. Scatter radiation that reaches the image receptor does not add any useful information to the image but does create fog or unwanted exposure on the image.

Case Study

The remnant or exit beam is composed of photons, which have been transmitted through the thorax. The resultant image demonstrates various types of tissues and structures that become visible on the final image.

Critical Thinking Questions

1. How do the variations in tissue density influence the image?
2. What is the importance of differential absorption?
3. What is subject contrast and why is it necessary?
4. Why does the thorax image demonstrate high subject contrast?

Review Questions

Multiple Choice

1. List the tissues in order of increasing x-ray attenuation:

1. Bone
2. Lung
3. Soft tissue
4. Fat

a. 1, 2, 3, 4
b. 2, 4, 3, 1
c. 4, 3, 2, 1
d. 4, 2, 3, 1

2. Tissues with a lower atomic number have greater:

a. attenuation
b. absorption
c. transmission
d. tissue thickness

3. What percent of an incident x-ray beam is transmitted through a patient?

a. 1%
b. 10%
c. 50%
d. 90%

4. Which type of tissue will attenuate the greatest number of x-ray photons?

a. Fat
b. Muscle
c. Lung
d. Bone

5. Materials or tissues that attenuate large amounts of x-ray photons are called:

a. radiopaque
b. radiolucent

6. Exit radiation is made up of which of the following?

1. Scattered radiation
2. Transmitted radiation
3. Absorbed radiation

a. 1 and 2 only
b. 1 and 3 only
c. 2 and 3 only
d. 1, 2, and 3

7. A scattered photon would create __________ on the image.

   a. gray
   b. low density
   c. fog
   d. high density

8. Assume the average thickness of an abdomen is 30 cm. What adjustment in technical factors is needed for an abdomen measuring 34 cm thick?

   a. Decrease kVp by 10%.
   b. Double the original mAs setting.
   c. Increase kVp by 15%.
   d. a and b
   e. b and c

9. Which materials are used to improve the visualization of soft tissue and vessels?

   a. Barium
   b. Iodinated contrast agents
   c. Oxygen
   d. a and b
   e. a and c

10. High-energy x-ray photons have which of the following?

   a. The ability to penetrate through the part to reach the image receptor
   b. Sufficient energy to prevent them from interacting with tissue
   c. Long wavelength and low frequency
   d. a and b
   e. a, b, and c

11. __________ tissues or structures are filled with air and do not absorb x-ray photons.

   a. Radiopaque
   b. Radiolucent

Short Answer

1. Define attenuation.

2. How does the atomic number of tissue affect absorption?

3. Explain backscatter radiation and its effect on the radiographic image.

4. What is the relationship between tissue type and differential absorption?

5. Why are iodinated contrast agents used to visualize soft tissues?

6. How do variations in tissue density influence the image?

7. Explain the importance of differential absorption.

8. What is subject contrast and why is it needed?

9. Why does the thorax image demonstrate high subject contrast?

13

Radiographic Image Characteristics

Objectives

Upon completion of this chapter, the student will be able to:

1. Explain the importance of density for image quality.
2. List and describe the regions of the characteristic curve.
3. Explain sensitometry and how the characteristic curve is constructed.
4. Identify the optical density of a radiographic film.
5. Identify the factors that make up radiographic contrast.
6. Explain the image characteristics of speed, contrast, and exposure latitude.
7. Describe the difference between long-scale and short-scale contrast images.
8. Differentiate between high- and low-contrast images.
9. Describe the differences of size and shape distortion.
10. Explain the principles of magnification radiography.
11. Define the factors that affect image detail.
12. Discuss appropriate techniques to prevent motion.

Key Terms

- base plus fog (B + F)
- characteristic curve
- densitometer
- distortion
- elongation
- exposure latitude
- film contrast
- film speed
- foreshortening
- geometric factors
- gray scale
- involuntary motion
- log relative exposure
- long scale contrast
- magnification
- optical density
- penetrometer
- radiographic contrast
- radiographic density
- recorded detail
- sensitometer
- sensitometric curve
- sensitometric strip
- sensitometry
- short scale contrast
- shoulder region
- size distortion
- spatial resolution
- speed
- straight-line region
- toe region
- voluntary motion

Introduction

In this chapter, we address the film characteristics that affect the final radiographic image. A quality radiographic image will accurately represent the anatomic area of interest with the correct scales of gray, which are necessary to visualize the different tissues in the body. To ensure a quality image is produced, one must perform sensitometric tests periodically to make certain that the film obtains the optimal density levels. The characteristic curve contains information gathered from the sensitometric tests on the speed, contrast, and exposure latitude of a film. The various characteristics are plotted on a graph, which makes it easy to determine if there are any areas of concern. It is important for the student to understand how changes in the film characteristics can change the appearance of the x-ray image.

Radiographic film is becoming obsolete in the radiology department; however, many foundational principles are still factors in producing a quality image. The factors of recorded detail and distortion are just as important as the characteristic curve.

Image Characteristics

The visualization of the anatomic structures and their accurate portrayal on the radiographic image is the hallmark of a quality image. There are many factors that must be considered when producing a radiographic image. Image characteristics of **radiographic density**, **optical density**, and diagnostic range must all be in the acceptable parameters for a quality image to be produced. In addition, the visibility of recorded detail will be achieved when there is a balance between density on the image and the contrast seen between the structures on the image.

Density

Radiographic film is exposed to the x-ray beam and then processed with various chemicals, which results in deposits of black metallic silver that is seen as density. The various densities seen on the film are the result of beam attenuation of the anatomic tissues. Radiographic density is the amount of overall blackness produced on the processed image. The goal is to have the perfect balance of density on the image: enough density to properly visualize the anatomic area of interest. An image that is too dark has excess density, which will inhibit the ability to adequately visualize the anatomy. On the other hand, when the image is too light, it lacks sufficient density to visualize the anatomy.

Each image must be critically evaluated to determine whether there is sufficient density for the part that was imaged. When the radiographer determines the image lacks the correct amount of density, he or she must determine the reason for the density error. After careful consideration, the technical factor will be changed and a repeat image will be obtained. It takes experience and viewing many radiographic images for a radiographer to develop the problem-solving skills that are necessary to determine and correct errors. The factors that affect the density of the image are discussed in Chapter 14.

Optical Density

Optical density (OD), often called image density or simply density, describes the degree of darkness or blackening of the x-ray image. The amount of density can be measured to find the exact amount of density on the processed film. OD is a precise measurement that compares the incident light intensity on the film (I_o) to the light intensity transmitted through the film (I_t) (Fig. 13.1). Technically, it should be called *transmitted density* because it is a measure of the light transmitted through the transparent-base film. The optical density formula is:

$$\mathrm{OD} = \log_{10}\left(\frac{I_o}{I_t}\right)$$

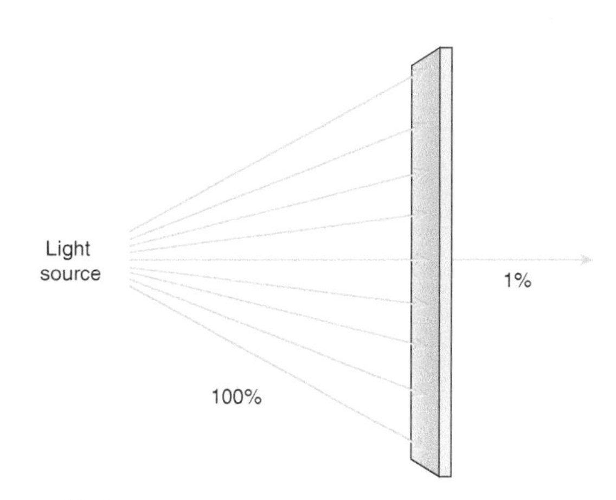

Figure 13.1. **Shows the transmission of light through a film that transmits 1% of the incident light and has an OD of 2.**

where I_o is the incident light intensity and I_t is the transmitted light intensity. OD is a logarithmic function that allows for a broad range of values to be expressed by small numbers. Diagnostic films in radiology have optical densities in the range of 0 to 4. An optical density of 0 is an area that appears clear, and an optical density of 4.0 is a very dark or black area on the processed film. An OD of 0 means that 100% of the light photons were transmitted through the film. When 50% of light is transmitted, the OD is equal to 0.3, and when 25% of light is transmitted, the OD equals 0.6.

A logarithmic scale base 10 is used to demonstrate that for each 0.3 change in optical density, the percentage of light transmitted will change by a factor of 2. Referring to Table 13.1, notice that as the OD number increases, the percentage of light transmitted through the film decreases. This occurs because as the OD number climbs, there is an increasing amount of density on the film, which is blocking the light from being transmitted through the film. Darker films have smaller transmission values and higher optical density values.

TABLE 13.1 RELATIONSHIP OF OPTICAL DENSITIES TO PERCENTAGE OF LIGHT TRANSMISSION

Percent of Light Transmitted (I_t/I_o)	Fraction of Light Transmitted (I_t/I_o)	Optical Density ($\log I_o/I_t$)
100	1	0
50	½	0.3
32	8/25	0.5
25	¼	0.6
12.5	1/8	0.9
10	1/10	1
5	1/20	1.3
3.2	4/25	1.5
2.5	1/30	1.6
1.25	1/80	1.9
1	1/100	2
0.5	1/200	2.3
0.32	2/625	2.5
0.125	1/800	2.9
0.1	1/1,000	3
0.05	1/2,000	3.3
0.032	1/3,125	3.5
0.01	1/10,000	4

CRITICAL THINKING BOX 13.1

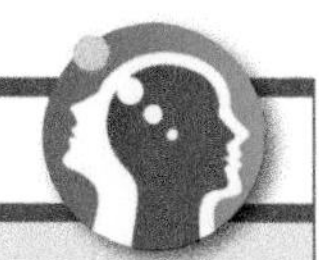

The soft tissue on an abdomen radiograph transmits 36% of the incident light. What is the optical density?

Using Table 13.1, it is easy to determine that with an OD of 1.0, only 10% of light is transmitted through the film and there is a corresponding opacity of 10. If the OD number was increased to 1.3, the percentage of light transmitted through the film would be 5% or one-half. This change means that less light was transmitted through the film, so the opacity of the film is doubled to 20. This demonstrates that changes of 0.3 increments in OD numbers represent a doubling or halving in opacity.

Diagnostic Range

Although optical densities can range from 0 to 4, the diagnostic range for general radiography is ~0.25 to 2.5. This range is located between the extreme low and high densities produced on a radiograph. Many radiographic images can show anatomy patterns in the 0.5 to 1.25 OD. This is toward the low end of densities, and the image may not contain enough density to visualize anatomy. Images with very high OD will have anatomy present on the image, but it is very dark and difficult to see on a standard view box. These "burned-out" images can be held up to a hot light to view the anatomy, but this is not a good practice to follow because it indicates an overexposure of radiation to the image as well as the patient.

The Reciprocity Law states that on a radiographic image, the OD is proportional to the total exposure (mAs) on the film at the time of the exposure and independent of the length of time required to make the exposure. The given radiation dose delivered to the radiographic film primarily determines the amount of OD that is created on the film during processing. The intensity of the exposure is a measurement of the energy and amount of x-ray photons reaching a given area of the film. An increase in exposure intensity correlates to an increase in optical density. The opposite is true for decreasing the exposure intensity.

In film-screen radiography, the final radiographic image cannot be manipulated to change the densities on the film. The skilled radiographer must choose the proper exposure intensity to create the appropriate range of optical densities on the film. Producing the appropriate optical density is critical to producing a quality radiographic image that precisely demonstrates the anatomy of interest.

Image Contrast

Image contrast is the difference in density between two areas on the image. It is the radiographic quality that allows the radiographer to identify different areas of anatomy. When there is no difference in contrast within an image, the human eye will not be able to visualize the image; likewise, if there are minimal differences in contrast, very little information will be available. Image contrast is the result of differences in attenuation of the x-ray photons with various tissues in the body; the density of the tissue will affect the amount of attenuation. Contrast is one of the most important factors in producing a quality diagnostic image.

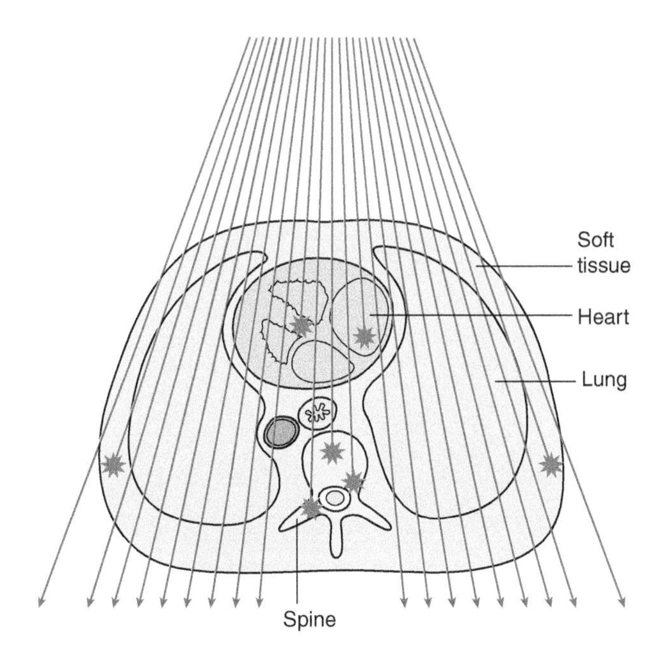

Figure 13.2. Subject contrast depends on different amounts of exit radiation in adjacent areas, which is called *differential absorption*. Subject contrast describes how different areas of a patient attenuate x-ray photons differently.

Radiographic Contrast

When a good quality radiograph is placed on a view box, the variations in OD are easily seen. These density differences between two areas on the image refer to an image's **radiographic contrast**. Radiographic contrast is made up of the total amount of contrast acquired from both the subject contrast and image receptor contrast. Subject contrast describes the amount of exit radiation through different tissues of the body. Image receptor contrast is inherent in the type of radiographic film and intensifying screen that are used to record the range of tissue densities. Image contrast is the difference in OD between different areas on the film. Figure 13.2 illustrates how bone, soft tissue, and lung tissue have different amounts of exit radiation and different subject contrast. When there are no differences in contrast within an image, the human eye will not be able to visualize the image; likewise, if there are minimal differences in contrast, very little information will be available.

Long-Scale and Short-Scale Contrast Images

Radiographic images are described by their scale of contrast or the range of densities that are visible within the image. The number of densities from black to white on a radiographic image is an indication of the range of the scale of contrast. A radiograph with few densities but great variations among them is said to have high contrast or a **short scale** of gray. A radiograph with many densities but little variation between them is said to have low contrast or a **long scale** of gray. When considering the amount of contrast on an image, the radiographer must determine if a short or long scale of gray is most appropriate for the anatomy to be imaged. The terms long scale and short scale describe the number of different densities between black and white on the image. Figure 13.3 shows a step wedge of graduated thickness to illustrate how higher kVp examinations penetrate greater thicknesses and produce long-scale contrast images. Lower kVp examinations penetrate fewer thicknesses and have only a few steps between black and white and so produce short-scale contrast images.

When the primary beam penetrates through tissue with adjacent densities, which have great differences in contrast, the image is described as high contrast. The image will have few shades of gray. A short-scale contrast image has fewer steps between black and white and is a high-contrast image. The human eye can easily distinguish this difference. Low-kVp examinations produce short-scale contrast images. This is the preferred scale

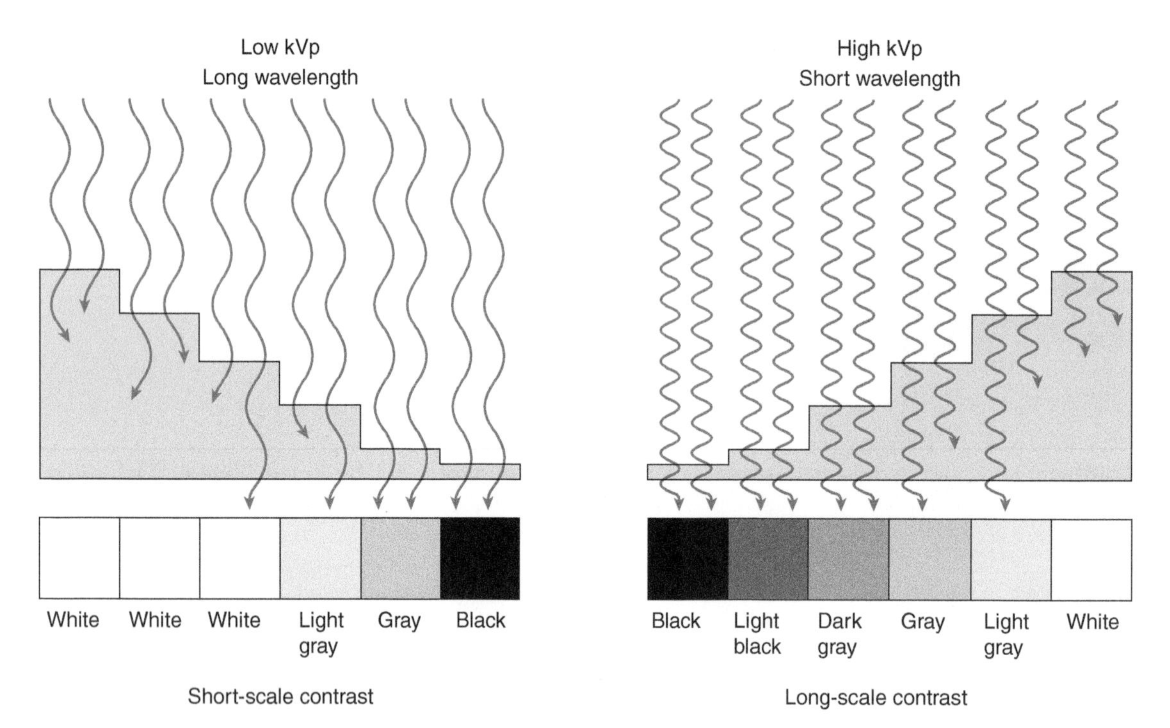

Figure 13.3. **An increase in the thickness of the step wedge decreases the number of x-ray photons reaching the film. Notice the wavelength of the photons for low kVp versus high kVp. Higher-kVp photons have more energy and a short wavelength, which allows more photons to pass through the step wedge.**

of contrast when imaging bony anatomy as this best demonstrates the fine trabecular markings and fractures (Fig. 13.4). A zebra is a great example of high contrast because it has black and white stripes.

Imaging the abdomen requires a long scale of gray because the anatomy of the abdomen is comprised of soft tissue and vital organs with minor density differences. These images will have few differences in contrast because the differences between adjacent densities are small; this is referred to as a long-scale contrast image, which has many steps between black and white and is a low-contrast image. Using higher kVp will produce more shades of gray, which will allow for better visualization of abdominal anatomy. A herd of elephants is an excellent example of a long **gray scale**; each elephant will have a slightly different shade than other elephants; however, they are all some shade of gray.

Figure 13.5 demonstrates three abdomen images. Image A has the lowest contrast, which is obscuring the outlines of soft tissue organs like the kidneys and liver. Image B demonstrates optimum contrast because the soft tissue of the abdomen is clearly visible, and it is easy to distinguish the borders of the kidneys, liver, and psoas muscles. Image C has the highest contrast, which is excellent for spine imaging, but the outlines of the organs and edges of the abdomen are not visible.

Table 13.2 provides a comparison of high contrast and low contrast and the terms used to describe both. It is critical for the radiographer to have an excellent understanding of the scales of gray, how each is produced, and which scale is appropriate for specific anatomy.

Sensitometry

Sensitometry is the study of the relationship between the intensity of the radiation exposure to the radiographic film and the degree of blackness produced after processing. In other words, it is the measurement of a film's response to processing and different amounts of light. Radiographers use sensitometry to evaluate the characteristics of film and film-screen combinations. Manufacturers design radiographic film and film-screen combinations to be capable of responding to the different intensities of radiation used during an exposure. Because there are such vast differences in tissues, film and film-screen combinations

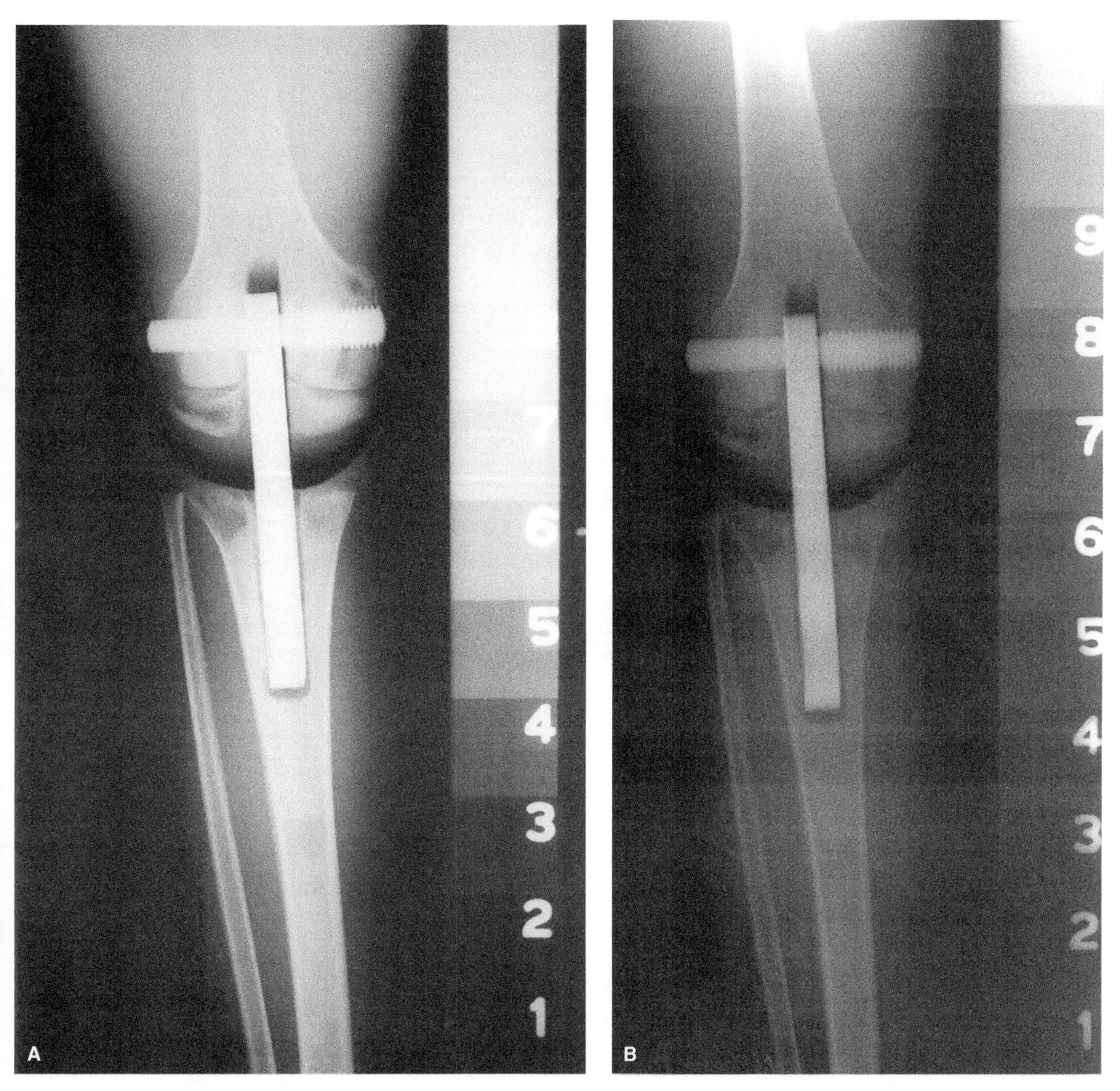

Figure 13.4. Change in subject contrast produced by a change in average x-ray beam energy, demonstrated by radiographs of an anteroposterior knee phantom. (A) Demonstrates a shorter scale of contrast, which is preferred for imaging bone. (B) Demonstrates a longer scale of gray, which obscures the bony markings.

have been developed for specific anatomical areas. For a given exposure, film designed to image the chest will respond differently than extremity film. A skilled radiographer must understand how the film-screen combinations are used to image the different areas of the body. Using the incorrect film-screen combination will undoubtedly result in a nondiagnostic image, which would require a repeat exposure to the patient.

Sensitometry is also used to evaluate the performance of automatic film processors. The automatic processor influences the density and contrast visible on the radiograph. An automatic processor that is not functioning within manufacturer specifications will result in an image that is degraded. Their performance is evaluated with sensitometric methods, which are covered in Chapter 16.

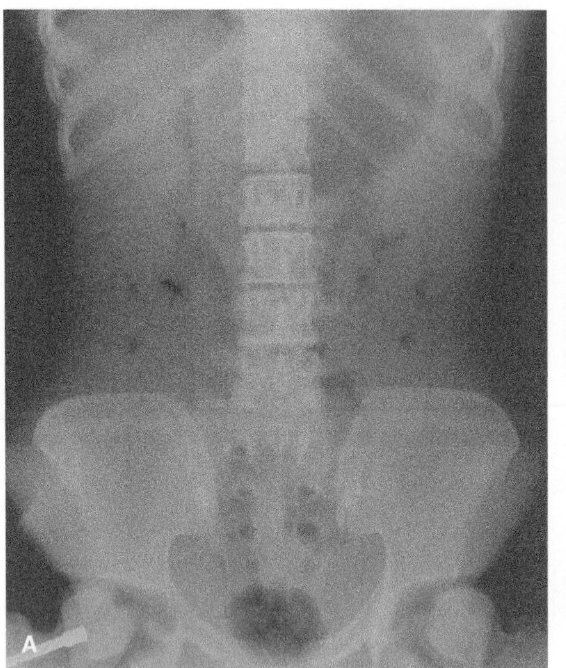

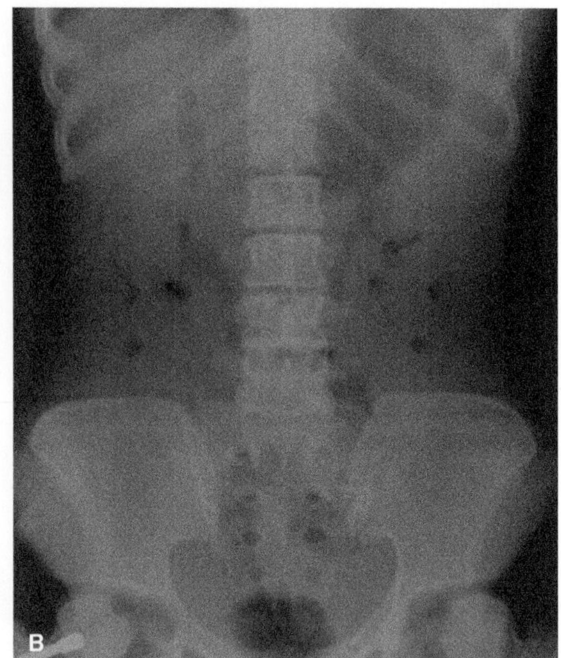

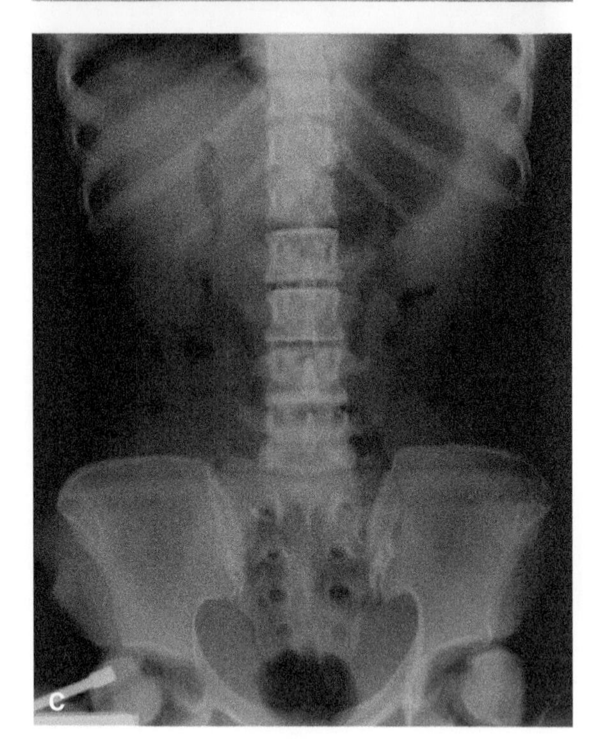

Figure 13.5. **(A) Low contrast hides soft tissue structures. (B) Optimum contrast allows visualization of abdomen structures. (C) High contrast is not effective for soft tissue structures.**

TABLE 13.2 **TERMS USED TO DESCRIBE CONTRAST**

Low Contrast	High Contrast
Many shades of gray	Few shades of gray
Decreased or low contrast	Increased or high contrast
High kVp	Low kVp
Long scale of contrast	Short scale of contrast

Sensitometric Equipment

There are several pieces of equipment that are needed to evaluate the relationship between the intensity of radiation exposure and the density produced after processing. There are two methods that will produce a radiographic image that can then be evaluated. Following is a discussion of the methods and equipment necessary for each.

Penetrometer

A **penetrometer** is a series of increasingly thick, uniform absorbers typically made of aluminum or tissue-equivalent plastic and is known as a step wedge (Fig. 13.6). When exposed to radiation, the penetrometer produces a step-wedge pattern on radiographic film. Because of the large number of variables in generating an x-ray beam, the range of densities produced in the step-wedge pattern can be affected. The unreliability of the penetrometer method led to the development of equipment that could produce consistent step-wedge densities every time.

Sensitometer

A **sensitometer** is designed to expose the film to a reproducible, uniform light through a series of progressively darker filters or optical step wedges (Fig. 13.7). After processing, the image formed by the sensitometer is seen as a series of steps progressing from clear to black and is called a **sensitometric strip**. Figure 13.8 shows an example of a step-wedge pattern produced by a sensitometer. The sensitometer is the preferred device because it reproduces

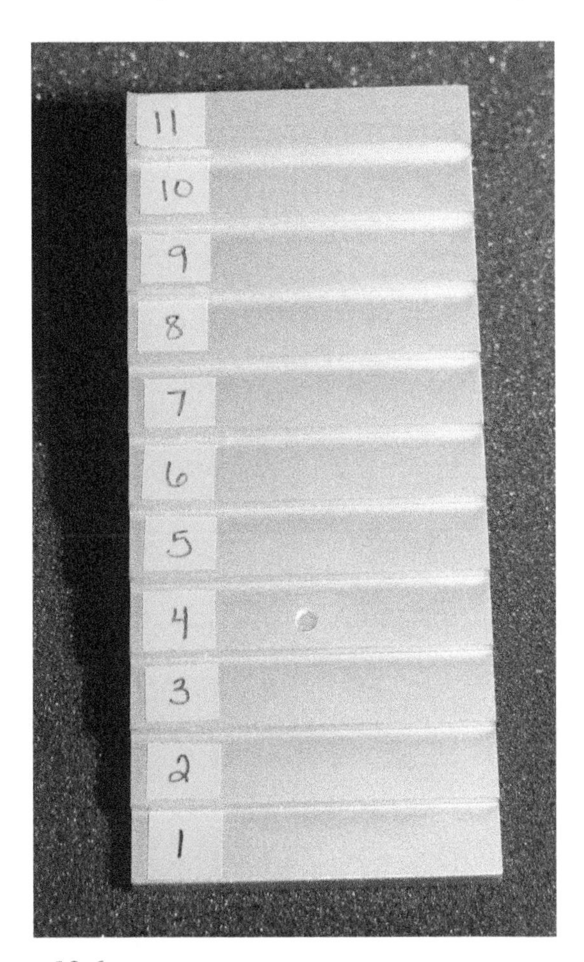

Figure 13.6. Penetrometer.

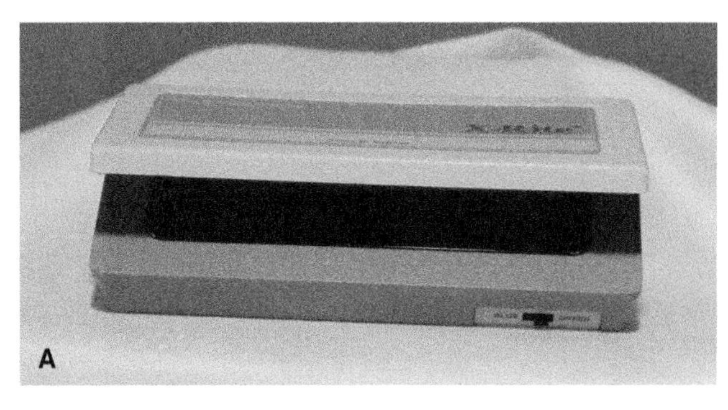

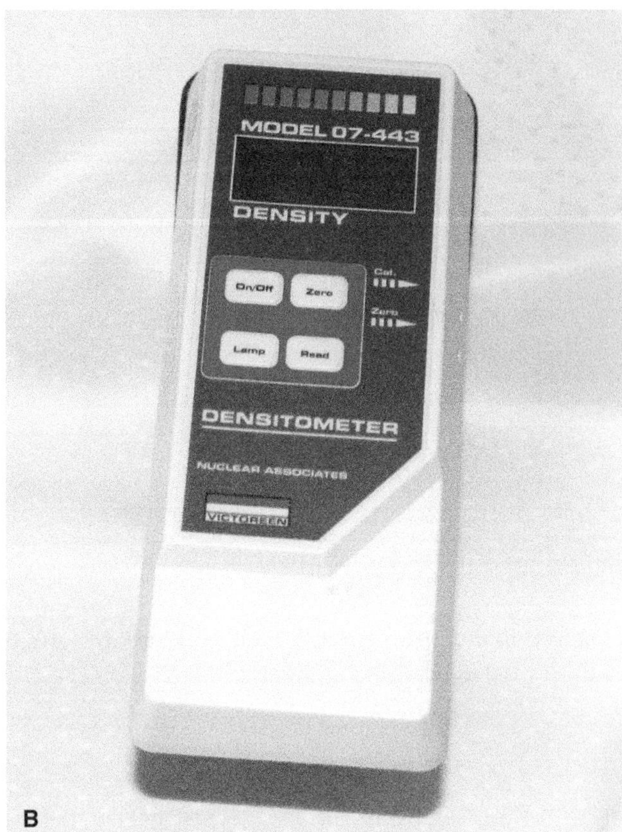

Figure 13.7. (A) Sensitometer. (B) Densitometer.

the same amount of light each time it is used. Factors that might cause the intensity of the x-ray beam to fluctuate are controlled by the circuitry that provides the exact quantity of power each time the sensitometer is used.

Densitometer

A **densitometer** measures the blackness or density of the step-wedge increments in units of optical density. Darker films have higher optical densities, while lighter areas will have lower OD. The densitometer consists of a calibrated light source and a light detector. The sensitometric strip is placed between the light source and light detector, and the amount of light transmitted through each step is

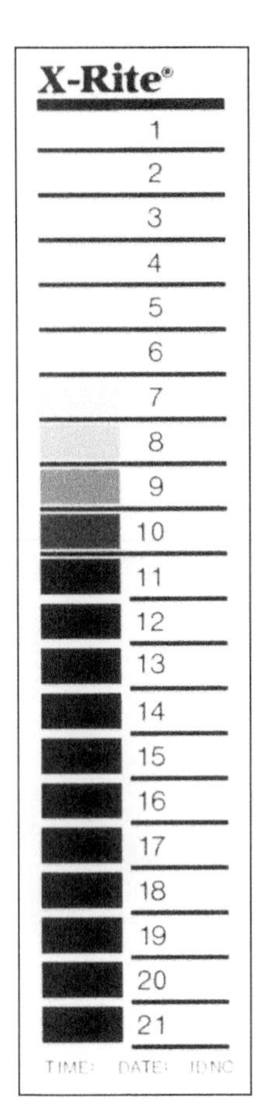

Figure 13.8. **Gray scale image produced by the sensitometer.**

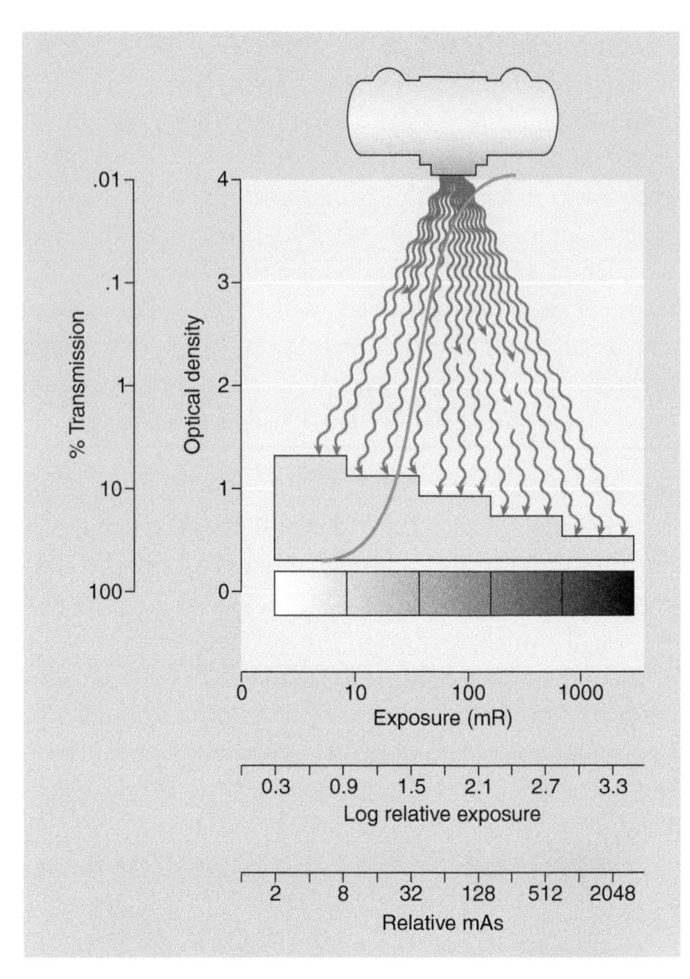

Figure 13.9. **Log relative exposure. The LRE exposure value represents the change in exposure by a factor of 2 with a 0.3 change in LRE. Notice the corresponding change in relative mAs when the LRE increases by 0.3.**

measured to calculate the OD. The OD measurements are then plotted on the **characteristic curve**.

Characteristic Curve

The individual densities on the sensitometric strip are graphed on semilogarithmic paper to produce a representation of the curve that shows the characteristics of the radiographic film. A plot of the optical density as a function of the logarithm of the exposure is called the characteristic curve. The characteristic curve shows the **speed**, contrast, and latitude of a particular film. The characteristic curves are also known as the **sensitometric**, D log E, Hurter & Driffield, or H&D curves.

Log Relative Exposure

Radiographic film is sensitive over a broad range of exposures. Each type of radiographic film will produce its own unique characteristic curve. Keep in mind that we are interested in the intensity of the exposure and the change in optical density over each exposure interval. The **log relative exposure** (LRE) is plotted on the horizontal axis (x).

When considering the intensity of radiation exposure, a constant factor must be used; the increments used are either doubling or halving of an exposure. For each doubling or halving change in the amount of light transmitted, a 0.3 change in OD occurs. The LRE scale demonstrates that the intensity of the exposure will change by a factor of 2 with a 0.3 change in OD. Using Figure 13.9, it is easy to identify that the relative mAs value of 8 has an LRE 0.9 and the relative mAs value of 16 has an LRE 1.2. This concept is demonstrated throughout the LRE scale on the characteristic curve.

Characteristic Curve Regions

Figure 13.10 shows a typical characteristic curve. The characteristic curve demonstrates the relationship between the intensity of radiation exposure on the horizontal axis (x) and the resultant optical densities on the vertical axis (y). The three regions of the characteristic

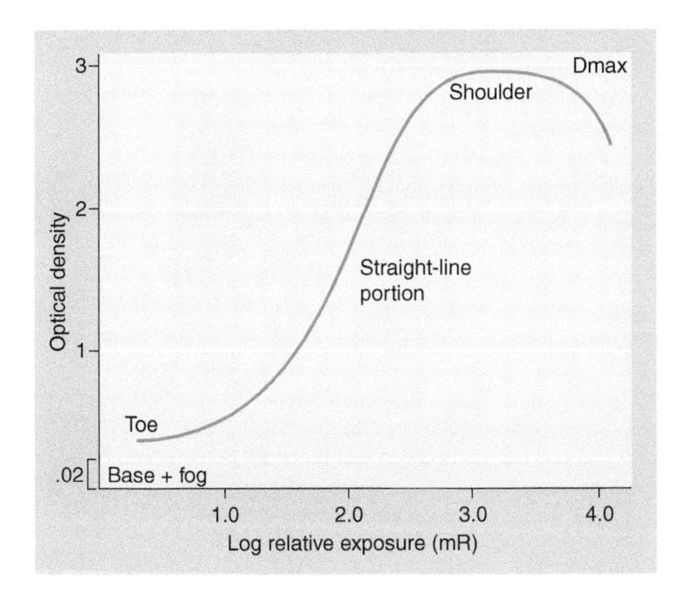

Figure 13.10. **Characteristic curve demonstrating the various regions.**

curve are the base plug fog, **toe region**, **straight-line region**, and **shoulder region**. The position and shape of each region on the curve can vary a great deal and is dependent on the type of radiographic film used.

The **base plus fog** (B+F) region describes the initial film density before exposure to x-ray photons. Base density is inherent in the base of the film and is attributed to the polyester support base and the tint that is added to make viewing more pleasing to the eye. Fog may be caused from exposure to background radiation, heat, and chemicals during storage. Fog density also comes from the development process but adds no useful information. The optical density in the film base before processing is 0.1. Processing typically adds OD 0.1 in fog density. The total base plus fog should not exceed OD 0.2. In the toe region, only a few of the silver halide crystals have been exposed. The toe region represents the area of low exposure levels. The optical density in the toe region ranges from 0.1 to 0.2. When the changes in exposure begin to have a greater effect on optical density, the shape of the curve changes along the *x*-axis. The **straight-line region** of the curve demonstrates a linear relationship between optical density and the logarithm of the relative exposure (log relative exposure). The straight-line region is where the diagnostic range of densities are produced. The optical density of the straight-line region ranges from 0.25 to 2.5.

In the **shoulder region** of the curve is the highest point of the characteristic curve and represents the region where all the silver halide crystals are completely covered in silver atoms and cannot accept any more. A point has been reached where changes in exposure intensity will no longer affect optical density. The shoulder region represents the area of high exposure levels and is called D_{max}. The optical density in the shoulder region is >2.5. Additional exposure will result in less density because the silver atoms will become ionized again, which will reverse their charge and cause them to be repelled resulting in the loss of optical density. This process is called solarization, and it is utilized in the design of duplication film.

Film Speed

Film speed describes the ability of an x-ray film to respond to low x-ray exposure. A low exposure of 1 mR can be detected with a film-screen combination. Speed is determined by the film's sensitivity to a given exposure, and the speed indicates the amount of optical density produced. The position of the toe will determine how soon the straight-line portion will begin, which is also an indication of the speed of the film (Fig. 13.11).

The speed point of a film describes the exposure required to produce an optical density of 1 above base plus fog. This point is called the speed point. The speed point marks the optical density within the straight-line region of the characteristic curve. The speed point serves as a standard method for indicating the speed of the film. Figure 13.11 is a characteristic curve for two radiographic films each with a different speed point. Film A requires less exposure to produce OD, and the curve is

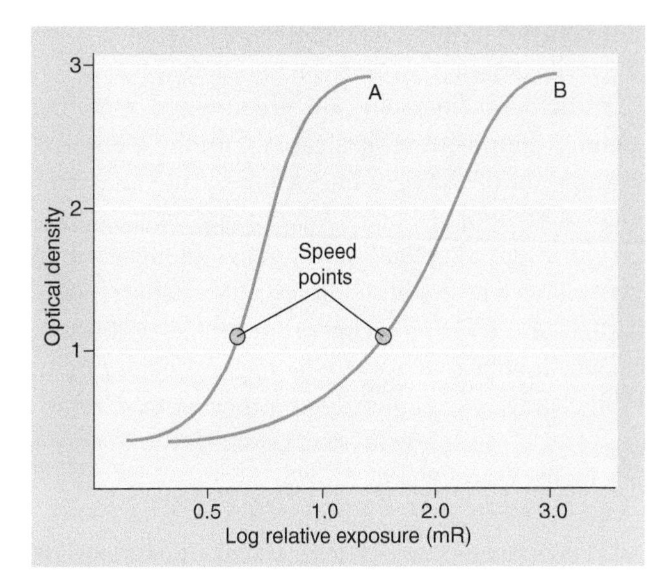

Figure 13.11. **Shows the characteristic curves for two films with different speeds. Film A is faster, and film B is slower. Film A is faster than film B because it requires less exposure to achieve an OD of 1 above the base plus fog level.**

positioned to the left (closer to the *y*-axis). Film B requires more exposure to produce OD and is positioned to the right on the graph. Film B is a slower speed film that is less sensitive to exposure than Film A. If Film A were two times as fast as Film B, A would require half the mAs required by B. The speed exposure point is the log exposure that produced the speed point for a given film. This can be plotted on the characteristic curve by drawing a line from the speed point on the log exposure (*x*-axis). Film A has a speed exposure point of 0.6, which is faster than Film B speed point of 1.5. In radiography, the speed of the film is expressed in numbers relative to 100; this is called par speed. Numbers higher than 100 refer to fast or high-speed image receptors. In sensitometry, 1 above base plus fog is used to determine the speed of the film. The speed is measured in reciprocal roentgens (1/*R*):

Speed = 1 / Exposure in roentgens to produce an OD of 1 above base plus fog

CRITICAL THINKING BOX 13.2

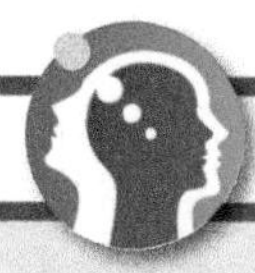

What exposure is required to produce OD of 1 above B+F on a 400 speed film?

Film Contrast

Film contrast or image contrast is the difference in optical density between two areas in the image. The contrast of a particular radiographic film is controlled by the manufacturer. Film contrast is measured on the steepness of the slope on the straight-line region of the characteristic curve at the speed point. Comparing the slope of the curve provides a method of evaluating the level of contrast produced by the film. Films with exposures between OD 0.25 and 2.5 exhibit contrast in the diagnostic range. Films with optical density in the toe or shoulder portion of the characteristic curve demonstrate a loss of contrast (Fig. 13.12). Films with steeper straight-line portions have higher contrast (Fig. 13.13).

Various methods can be used to specify image contrast. The average gradient of the slope is most commonly used. The average gradient is determined by drawing a straight line between two points on the characteristic curve at ODs 0.25 and 2 above B+F.

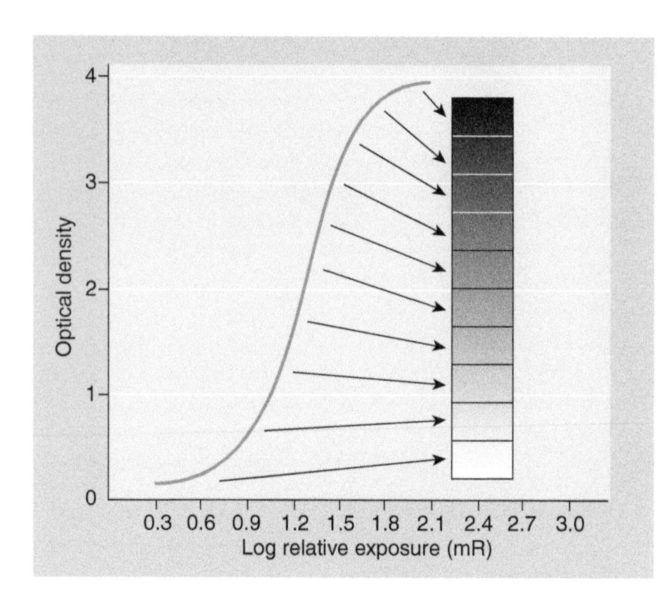

Figure 13.12. Contrast is reduced when an exposure results in densities that lie in the toe or shoulder regions. The radiographer must control exposure factors to produce optical densities in the diagnostic range.

Exposure Latitude

Exposure latitude describes the range of exposures that produce an acceptable radiograph with densities in the diagnostic range or straight-line region of the characteristic curve. Films can have wide or narrow latitude. Latitude and contrast are inversely related, meaning that as contrast increases latitude will decrease.

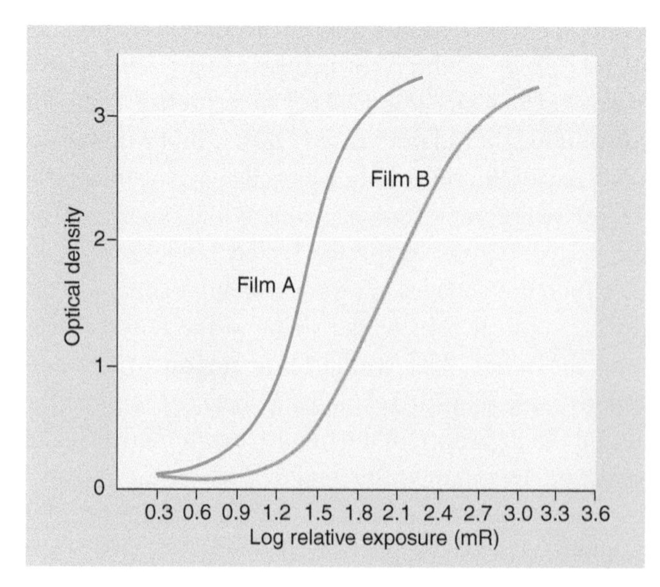

Figure 13.13. Comparison of film contrast. Film A has higher contrast because it has a greater slope of the straight-line portion.

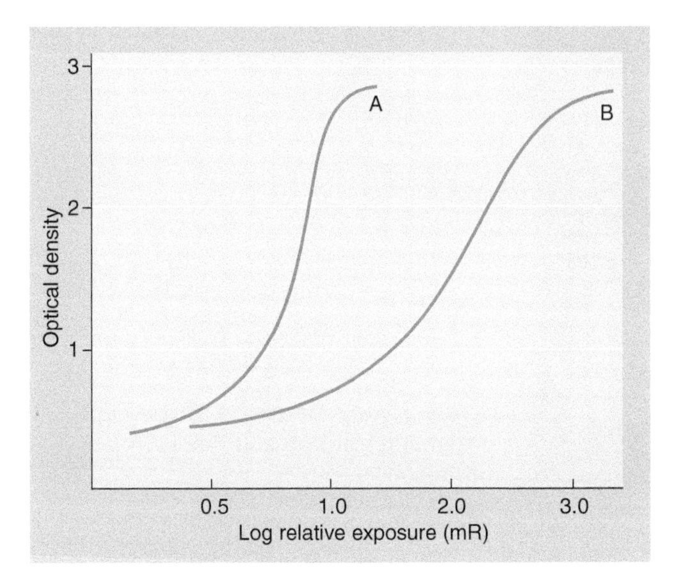

Figure 13.14. Characteristic curves of films having different latitude values.

Wide-latitude images are termed long gray scale contrast or low contrast and produce images with high-kVp setting. They produce acceptable images over a greater range of technical factors. There is more margin of error in the mAs settings with wide-latitude images. Conversely, an image with a narrow latitude requires the mAs and kVp to be set close to the optimal settings and are caused by using low kVp. Narrow-latitude images are termed short gray scale contrast or high contrast, and there is less margin of error with the mAs and kVp settings. Figure 13.14 demonstrates the characteristic curves of films with the wide and narrow latitudes.

Film A has a narrower latitude and a higher contrast than film B. Films with narrow latitudes have a steeper slope, which indicates high-contrast images. Film B has a wider latitude and produces lower-contrast images. Generally, higher-speed films have higher contrast and narrower latitude; slower-speed films have lower contrast and wider latitude.

Recorded Detail

The appearance of the radiographic image is governed by two primary **geometric factors, recorded detail** and **distortion**. Recorded detail is the degree or amount of geometric sharpness of an object recorded as an image. The recorded detail in an image is easy to evaluate and adjust if you understand what constitutes recorded detail. Recorded detail is also referred to as definition, sharpness, spatial resolution, or simply as detail. In this section, we will discuss the properties that affect recorded detail and distortion (Table 13.3).

Spatial Resolution

Detail, image sharpness, and **spatial resolution** are terms used to describe the sharpness of the image and how well the system images adjacent small structures such as the edges or borders of structures that appear in hairline fractures. Detail is defined as the smallest separation of two lines or edges that can be recognized as separate structures on the image. An image with adequate detail will demonstrate even the smallest parts of the anatomy, which will allow the radiologist to visualize all the structures possible for a diagnosis.

The degree of sharpness or spatial resolution is determined by line pairs per millimeter (lp/mm). A high-contrast resolution phantom, which has lead strips of different widths and interspaces, is used to produce the resolution test pattern (Fig. 13.15). The radiographer evaluates the test pattern to determine which of the smallest lines are separated from one another while being easily discernable. The speed of the film determines the number of lines and

TABLE 13.3 SUMMARY OF FACTORS THAT AFFECT RECORDED DETAIL AND DISTORTION

Factor	Patient Dose	Magnification	Film Density
Film speed	Decrease	Unchanged	Increase
Patient thickness	Increase	Increase	Decrease
Focal spot size	Unchanged	Unchanged	Unchanged
SID	Decrease	Decrease	Decrease
OID	Unchanged	Increase	Unchanged
mAs	Increase	Unchanged	Increase
Exposure time	Increase	Unchanged	Increase
kVp	Increase	Unchanged	Increase

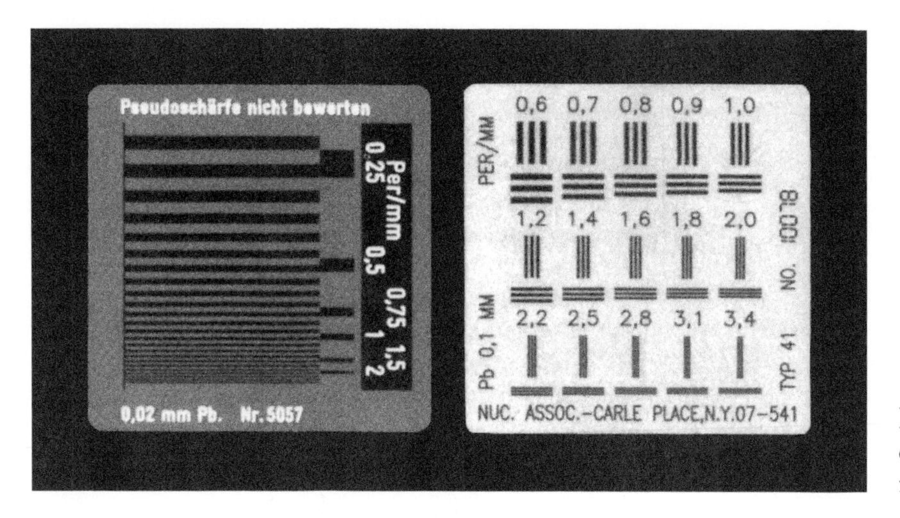

Figure 13.15. **Illustrates the concept of spatial resolution and line pairs per millimeter.**

spaces that are seen. Very fast screens can resolve 7 lp/mm, while fine-detail screens can resolve 15 lp/mm. High-speed screens have low spatial resolution, and fine-detail screens have high spatial resolution. The human eye is able to discern ~10 lp/mm. Therefore, imaging systems with better resolution can resolve more line pairs per millimeter.

Distortion

Distortion is the misrepresentation of an object. This misrepresentation is known as either size or shape distortion based on the distance of an object from the imaging receptor or source device. Distortion reduces the visibility of detail and resolution in an image. The radiographer must be familiar with normal radiographic anatomy to assist in evaluating the diagnostic quality of the image. Careful evaluation of the image typically reveals that the distortion is directly related to positioning. The radiographer must pay attention to using the proper source-to-image receptor distance (SID), tube placement in relation to the anatomical part, proper central ray location, and accurate positioning of the part of interest to ensure that minimal distortion occurs.

Magnification

Magnification or **size distortion** results from the represented object appearing larger on the final radiographic image. The majority of imaging procedures require the smallest amount of magnification possible; however, there are limited situations when magnification is necessary. An example would be performing a magnified image of the scaphoid bone to identify hairline fractures (Fig. 13.16). As routine practice, magnification of a body part should be kept to a minimum to avoid masking other structures. Magnification is controlled by using the maximum SID possible for the examination and positioning the body part to minimize object-to-image receptor distance (OID).

Size distortion is seen in a radiographic image as magnification. The magnification of an object is determined by the magnification factor, which is the ratio between the SID and the source-to-object distance (SOD). The degree of magnification is mathematically represented by:

$$mF = \frac{SID}{SOD}$$

where mF is the magnification factor. Images that are formed with small SOD values and short SID values have larger magnification factors (Fig. 13.17). The SOD is the OID minus the SID. An object midway between the image plane and the source has a magnification factor of 2. A magnification of 1 means the image is the same size as the object. This occurs when the object is in contact with the image receptor.

CRITICAL THINKING BOX 13.3

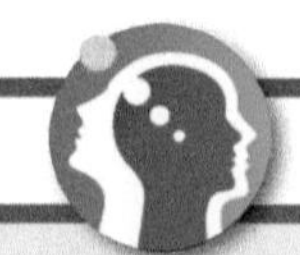

What is the magnification of an image taken at 40-inch SID with a 32-inch SOD?

CRITICAL THINKING BOX 13.4

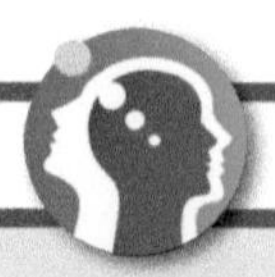

If the SID is 72 inches and the OID is 4 inches, what is the magnification factor? First you need to determine SOD.

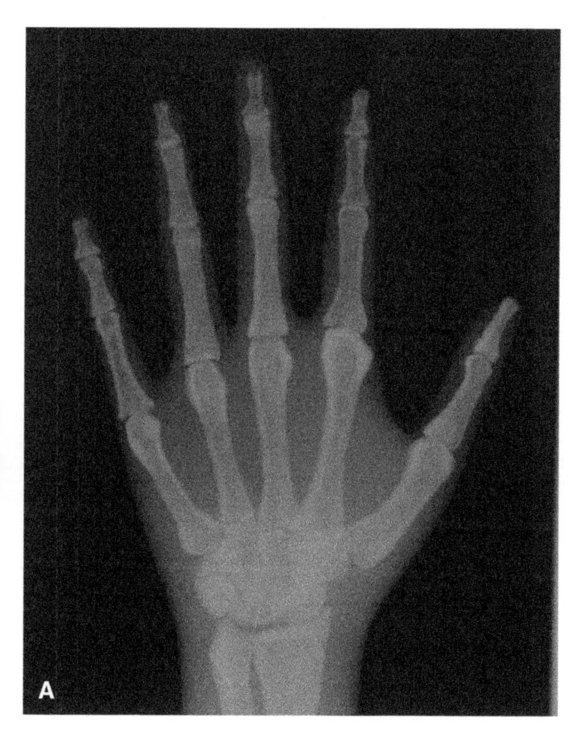

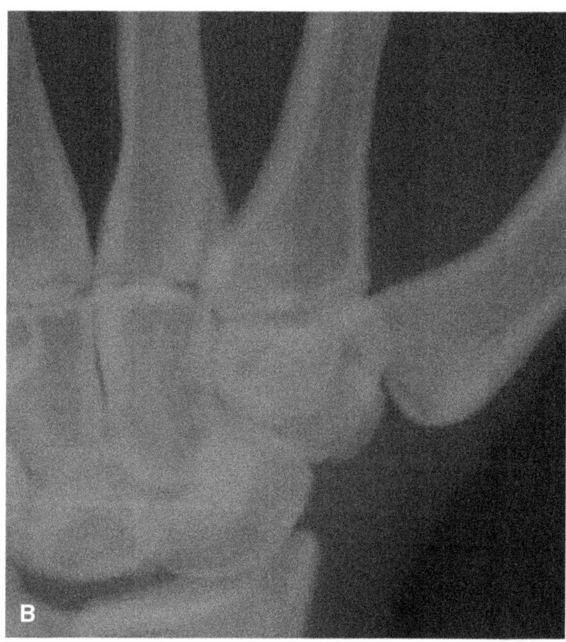

Figure 13.16. **Magnification size distortion of scaphoid bone. (A) Routine PA hand image at 40-inch SID. (B) Decreasing the SID will cause magnification of the anatomy.**

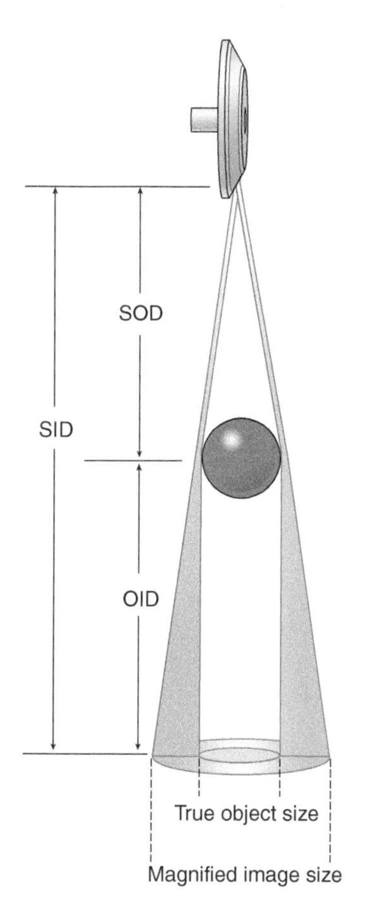

Figure 13.17. **Shows magnification and its relationship between the true object size and the image size.**

Magnification occurs with an increase in OID. As OID increases, SOD must decrease to maintain the normal size of the structure. SOD is inversely proportional to SID; therefore, decreasing SOD increases the magnification factor. An example of this is the thoracic spine. In an anteroposterior projection, the thoracic spine is placed very close to the image receptor. When the thoracic spine is positioned in a lateral projection, the spine is further away from the image receptor yet closer to the x-ray tube or source. As seen in the next examples, objects that are closer to the source have a higher magnification factor.

CRITICAL THINKING BOX 13.5

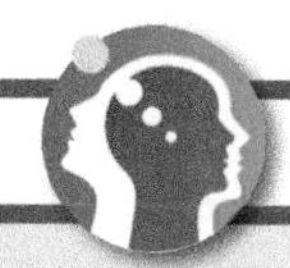

An AP image of the thoracic spine was taken at a 40-inch SID and a 3-inch OID. What is the magnification factor?

CRITICAL THINKING BOX 13.6

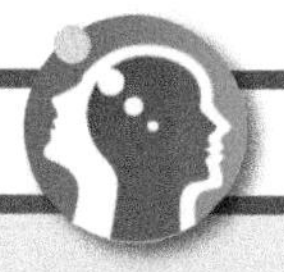

A lateral image of the thoracic spine was taken at a 40-inch SID with a 15-inch OID. What is the magnification factor?

In radiography, the SID is a known factor and can be accurately measured. The SOD can be estimated fairly accurately when a radiographer has a good basis in human anatomy. The magnification factor allows for the calculation of the actual size of the structure, which can be calculated using the following formula:

$$O = \text{Image size}\left(\frac{\text{SOD}}{\text{SID}}\right)$$

where O is the object size, SOD is source-to-object distance, and SID is source-to-image receptor distance.

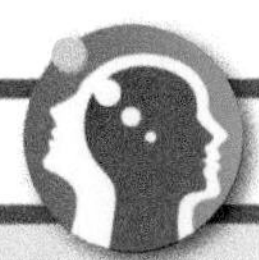

CRITICAL THINKING BOX 13.7

What is the size of an object imaged at a 40-inch SID with a 10-inch OID if the image measures 2.4 inches on the radiograph?

SID/OID

The distances between the x-ray source or focal spot (SOD), object (OID), and image receptor (SID) are all critical pieces that affect the amount of recorded detail. As represented in Figure 13.18, SOD + OID = SID. When OID is reduced, the resolution is improved, and when OID increases, the resolution is degraded. For this reason, the affected side or part of interest is typically placed as close as possible to the image receptor. Upon reviewing an image, if an improvement in detail is needed, the first factor to consider is OID. The minimum OID is used to improve detail.

The OID can also be minimized by performing an exam on the tabletop instead of in the Bucky. Extremity exams are performed with the part of interest directly placed on the image receptor. Although this works well for imaging anatomy <10 cm thick, it does not work well for parts larger than 10 cm thick, which require a grid. For such anatomy, the radiographer must consider the surface supporting the anatomy and the image receptor. The Bucky tray may be as much as 4 inches below the tabletop, which would significantly increase the OID and cause a loss in detail.

Routine radiographic protocols have been established to use a 40-inch or 100-cm SID for the majority of examinations. This SID represents the amount of distance necessary to project the accurate size of the anatomical part onto the image receptor. For extremity and abdominal images, the 40-inch SID works exceptionally well; however, when imaging with a horizontal beam, a 72-inch SID is used when the OID is excessive. Chest imaging has been performed at 72-inch SID for many years to reduce the size of the heart shadow, and the lateral cervical spine image also uses a 72-inch SID to correct for the excessive OID of the spine to the image receptor.

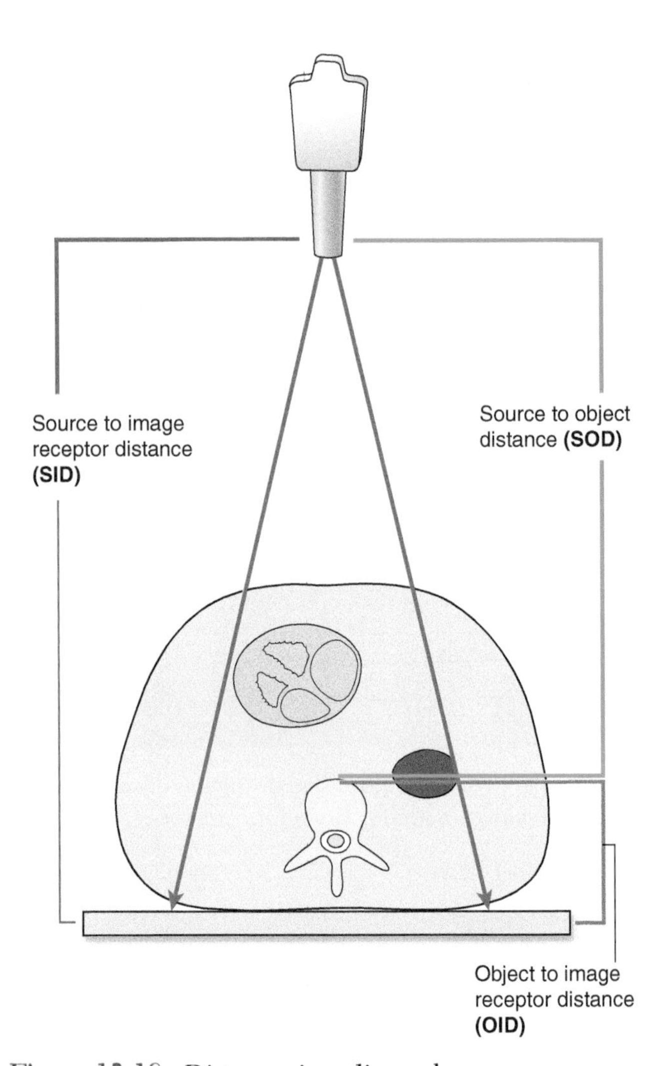

Figure 13.18. **Distances in radiography.**

The majority of body parts have a certain amount of OID over which the radiographer has limited control. The SID must be maximized to decrease the magnification created by the OID. Radiographic examinations of body parts with large OID, such as the lateral sternum and lateral cervical spine, use a large SID when possible to provide the most accurate representation of the actual size of these structures on the radiographic image.

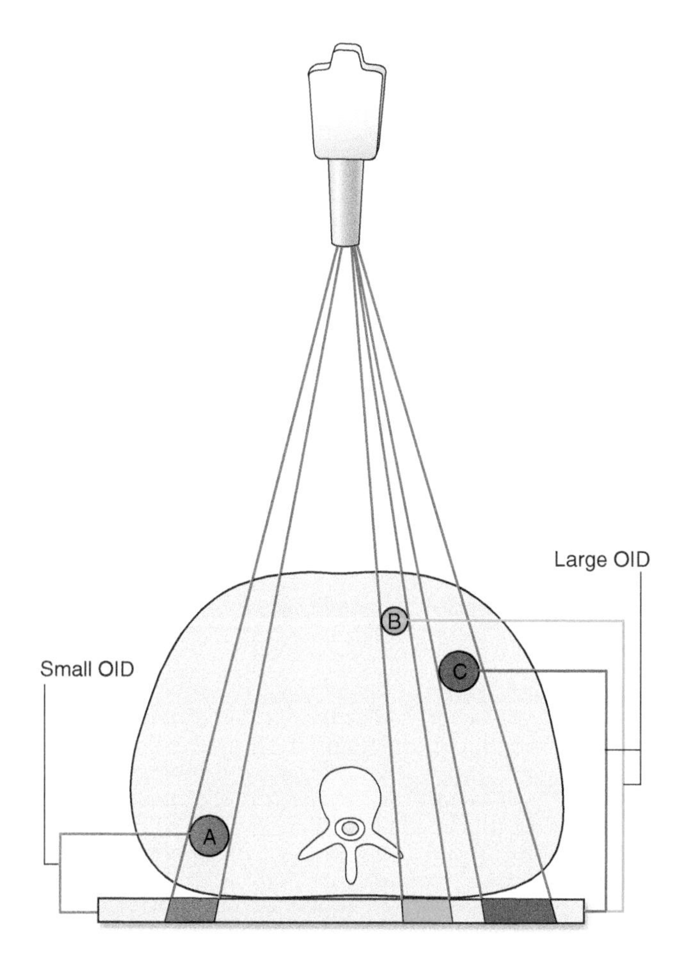

Figure 13.19. **Demonstrates the effect of OID on image size magnification. Structures A and C are the same size, but due to their OID, their projected images are of significantly different sizes. Structure B is significantly smaller than C; however, their sizes appear identical because of B's greater OID.**

OID also plays a critical role in magnification and resolution. Figure 13.19 demonstrates two relationships of OID: location in the body and size of the part. As seen in this cross-sectional image, each anatomical structure is at a different level in the body, meaning that each has its own OID and will be projected onto the image as different sizes. The structures with the largest OID will be projected with a larger size than structures that have a small OID.

Another size relationship controlled by OID is seen in Figure 13.19. Structure B is a smaller object than structure C, but due to the inherent OID, structure B appears as the same size as structure C on the image. A thorough knowledge of normal radiographic anatomy is necessary when making judgments about size relationships and in determining the best position for achieving the minimum OID for the specific anatomy.

Focal Spot Size

The line focus principle controls the focal spot size by reducing the effective focal spot. The angle of the anode has been designed to increase the actual focal spot to absorb the heat produced with each exposure while decreasing the size of the effective focal spot that is projected toward the patient. The line focus principle makes use of an anode surface tilted or angled with respect to the x-ray beam. A small target angle produces an effective focal spot that is smaller than the actual focal spot. The effective focal spot is the size of the focal spot as seen by the patient. Because of the tilted anode angle, the effective focal spot is smaller on the anode side and larger on the cathode side. The result is less focal spot blur on the anode side and more blur on the cathode side of the image.

X-rays diverging from different parts of the focal spot will blur the edge of an image. This blur or unsharp shadow along the edge of the image is called penumbra. Larger focal spots produce greater amounts of penumbra or blur. The size of the focal spot is a major controller of image resolution because it controls the amount of focal spot blur. When the focal spot size is decreased, the blur decreases, thereby increasing resolution. The amount of blur is calculated by using the following formula:

$$P = \frac{\text{Focal spot size} \times \text{OID}}{\text{SOD}}$$

where P is the width of penumbra, OID is object-to-image receptor distance, and SOD is source to object distance.

CRITICAL THINKING BOX 13.8

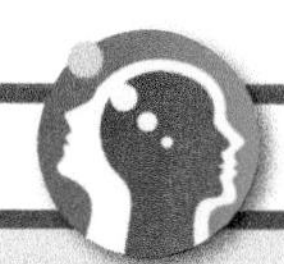

Determine the size of focal spot blur for an image taken with a 2.0-mm focal spot, at a 40-inch SID and an OID of 4 inches.

CRITICAL THINKING BOX 13.9

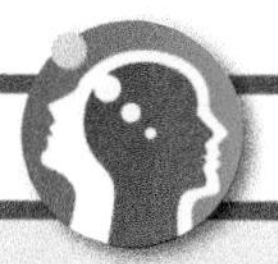

Calculate the size of focal spot blur for an image taken with a 1.0-mm focal spot size, at 40-inch SID and an OID of 4 inches.

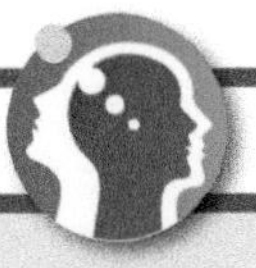

CRITICAL THINKING BOX 13.10

Calculate the size of focal spot blur for image taken with a 1.0-mm focal spot, at a 72-inch SID and an OID of 4 inches.

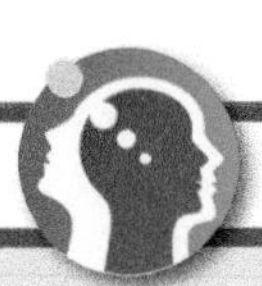

CRITICAL THINKING BOX 13.11

Determine the amount of focal spot blur for an image taken with a 1.0-mm focal spot, at a 40-inch SID and an OID of 9 inches.

These examples demonstrate how the penumbra decreases when the SID increases. The penumbra will also decrease when the focal spot size decreases and when the OID decreases. Each of these changes will result in increased resolution of the anatomy.

In Figure 13.20 A, the effect of the focal spot size on resolution is seen. When there is a large focal spot, the penumbra area is larger, whereas the small focal spot has a much smaller area of penumbra. The smaller focal spot size provides the best resolution possible because of less penumbra. Figure 13.20 B demonstrates what occurs when the SID is changed. The small SID is so close to the image receptor that it does not allow the beam to fully diverge, producing a larger penumbra. The geometry of the beam allows the longer SID to produce a smaller area of penumbra, which increases resolution of the object. Finally, Figure 13.20 C represents the effect of OID on penumbra. When there is increased OID, the area of penumbra will be larger, causing more geometric unsharpness and less resolution in the image. If possible, moving the OID closer to the image receptor will decrease the area of penumbra, which improves resolution. For all these reasons, it is clear that the best resolution can be achieved when the smallest OID and focal spot size are used with the longer SID possible for the anatomic area being imaged.

Shape Distortion

Shape distortion is dependent on the alignment of the x-ray tube, the body part, and the image receptor. Shape distortion moves the projected image of a structure away from its actual position. When the image is shorter in one direction than the object, the image is said to be foreshortened. **Foreshortening** occurs when the part is inclined in relation to the tube and image receptor. The part will appear to

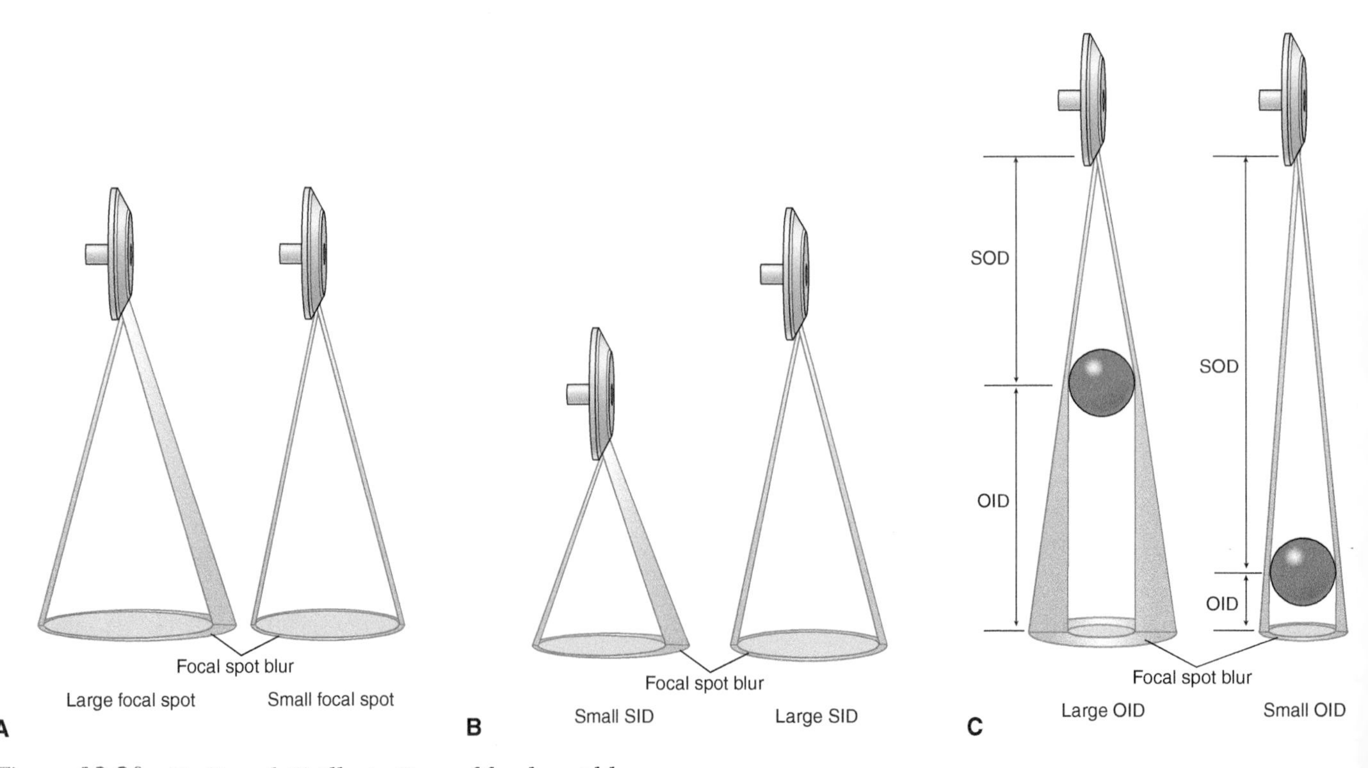

Figure 13.20. (A, B, and C) Illustrations of focal spot blur.

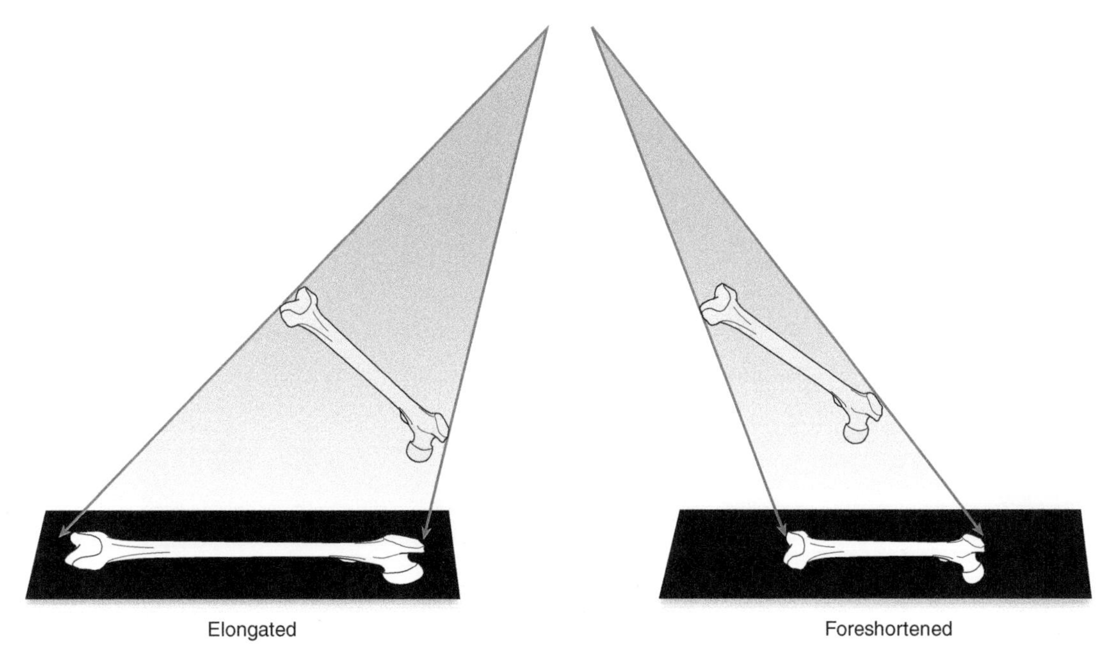

Figure 13.21. **Presents examples of foreshortening and elongation shape distortion due to changes in the alignment of the central ray.**

have a reduced size or to be foreshortened. As the incline of the part increases, the foreshortening will become greater. When the image is longer in one direction than the object, it is said to be elongated. **Elongation** occurs when the tube is angled in one direction (Fig. 13.21).

Specific imaging protocols require the use of elongation to visualize the bony anatomy such as with imaging the sacrum where the proper angle elongates the sacrum to enhance visualization (Fig. 13.22).

Three factors that must be in alignment are the tube, part, and image receptor. The central ray is the line connecting the focal spot to the center of the image receptor. The alignment of the central ray is critical in reducing or eliminating shape distortion. The central ray must be perpendicular to the image receptor and body part being examined to eliminate shape distortion. When the central ray is angled, the beam will not intersect the part correctly and will result in the part being distorted. There are specific images where the central ray is angled purposely to unsuperimpose structures or to better visualize a part. The body part and image receptor must be parallel with each other meaning the part needs to be as flat as possible. If the part is angled or inclined, shape distortion will be seen on the image.

Other alignment issues that must be corrected are off-centering of the tube, when the image receptor is off-center and when the anatomical part is incorrectly positioned in relation to the tube and image receptor. These relationships of misalignment are demonstrated in Figure 13.23. It is critical for the radiographer to properly align the tube to the image receptor to prevent alignment issues that will distort the image or result in the anatomy not being completely seen on the image.

Beam Angle

Some clinical situations use shape distortion to reduce the superimposition of overlying structures such as angling the central ray in axial images. The amount of angulation is used to create a controlled or expected amount of shape distortion. This will result in foreshortening or elongation of the structures overlying the body part of interest. Some examples include imaging the skull, clavicle, and calcaneus. The amount of angulation will cause a change in the SID; more angulation creates longer SIDs than less angulation. An angle of 5 degrees will not change the overhead display of 40-inch SID, while an angle of 25 degrees requires the overhead display to read 35-inch SID. If the SID is not changed with greater tube angles, there will be a resultant size distortion.

Tube Angle Direction

The x-ray tube is commonly directed with the longitudinal axis of the table; this avoids issues with grid cutoff. The longitudinal angles are either cephalic or caudal.

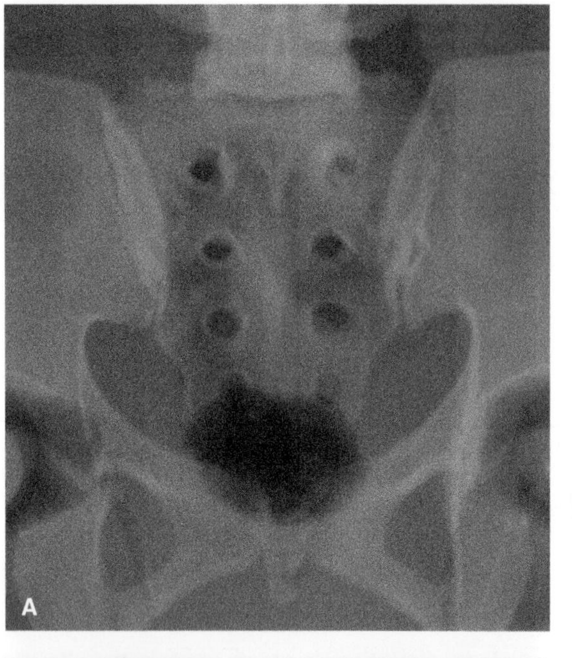

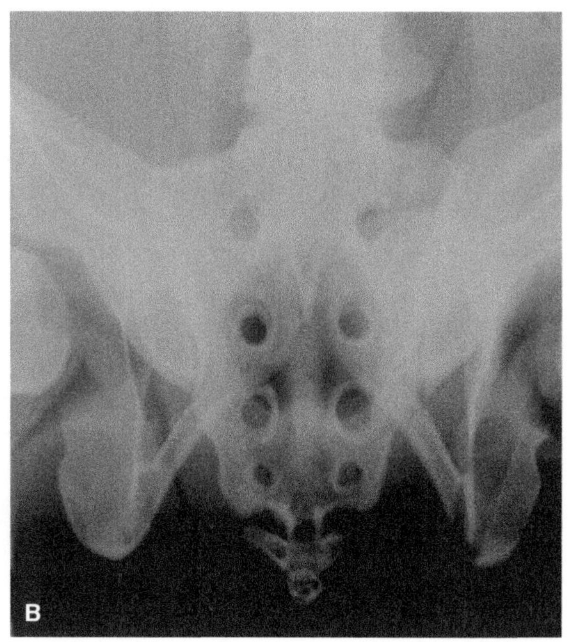

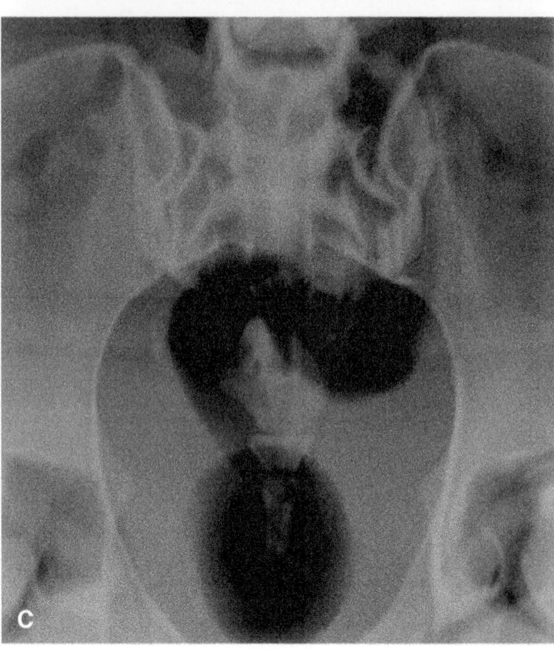

Figure 13.22. **Shape distortion. (A) Perpendicular beam. (B) 30-Degree cephalic angle. (C) 30-Degree caudal angle.**

A cephalic angle means the tube is angled toward the head of the patient, while a caudal angle is toward the patient's feet. The amount and direction of tube angle are specified by the examination and patient position. Common oblique cervical spine images are performed with the patient facing the tube and the tube angled cephalic. If the patient's position is reversed, the angle of the tube must be reversed to caudal. These principles are utilized to maintain the visualization of expected anatomy.

Motion

Motion affects the recorded detail because it appears as a blurred series of densities where no fine detail can be visualized. There are various types of motion; most are controlled by the radiographer and include

- Voluntary motion
- Involuntary motion
- Equipment motion

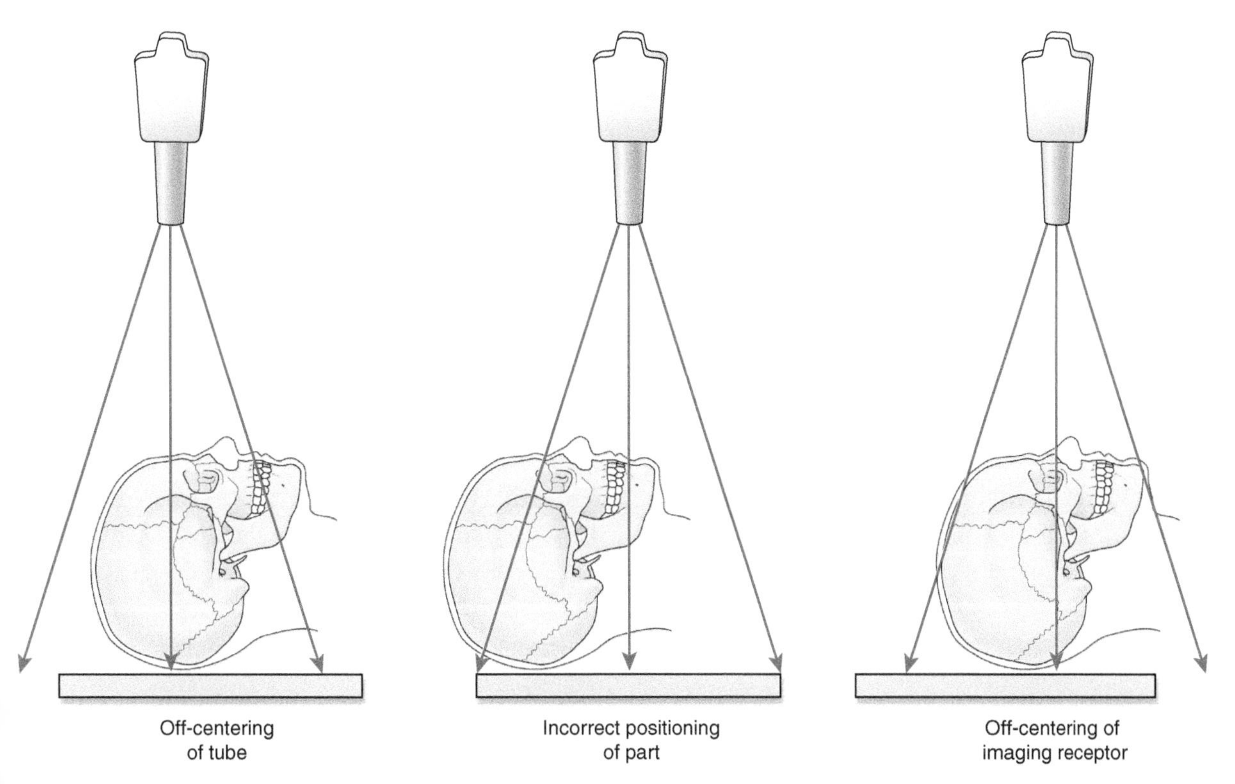

Figure 13.23. **Incorrect centering of tube, image receptor, and anatomy.**

- Communication
- Reduced exposure time
- Immobilization

Voluntary motion is motion that the patient directly controls. The radiographer must use effective communication when working with all patients to ensure that the patient understands the necessity of holding still for the exposure. For the majority of exams, the patients are able to comply with the positioning instructions as long as they understand what they are to do. The responsibility of communicating in a professional and competent manner rests with the radiographer who must determine the method of communicating with the patient. Patients of all ages will respond to a gentle touch and comforting tone. Never assume that the patient is not able to understand the instructions. Even very young children can be cooperative when they wish to be, and adults with mental impairments will be able to follow instructions when provided in a simple, clear manner.

Involuntary motion is not under the control of the patient. Examples include the heartbeat, peristalsis of the small and large intestines, and uncontrollable trembling caused by a disease process. The radiographer can reduce the motion artifact caused by involuntary motion by using the shortest exposure time possible.

Equipment motion can be caused by equipment, which is not functioning properly or is not properly maintained. Movement of a reciprocating grid that causes the grid to vibrate in the Bucky and an x-ray tube that drifts or vibrates are just a few examples of equipment motion. These types of motion artifact can be identified by reviewing multiple images that were produced with the same radiographic equipment.

Communication is the most effective method of reducing motion artifact. The radiographer must use effective communication when using positioning aids such as radiolucent pads, sponges, and sandbags so that the patient understands the purpose of the positioning aids. Clear breathing instructions and allowing the patient enough time to comply with breathing instructions will eliminate motion artifact in images of the thorax and abdomen. With patients of all ages, the radiographer must use instructions that are clear, concise, and easily understood.

Exposure time must be reduced when the patient is not able to cooperate in holding still or in holding the breath for several seconds. Reducing exposure time and increasing mA will sufficiently maintain density of the image while reducing motion artifact from involuntary motion. Other methods of decreasing exposure time while maintaining density include decreasing SID and using a higher-speed film/screen system.

Immobilization is used when communication and reduced exposure time are not sufficient to reduce motion artifact. Immobilization devices such as angled sponges, sandbags, and foam pads are routinely used to hold the patient in the necessary position. These devices can assist an ill patient or a patient in pain with holding a position because it allows the patient to rest the part of interest on the pad, thereby reducing muscle fatigue and pain. The use of positioning aids is part of providing a professional service to the patient and should be utilized as frequently as possible.

Many examinations benefit greatly from immobilization aids or devices that are specifically designed to hold the patient still. Some of these devices include pediatric boards, mummy wrapping techniques, Pigg-O-Stats, and compression bands. Many experienced radiographers believe that tape is the best immobilization aid for a vast majority of exams. A strip of tape across the forehead with the sticky side out and not touching the skin has helped avoid repeated headwork exposures. A skilled radiographer will be able to determine if an immobilization aid is warranted or if communication will suffice. As a last resort, the patient's family may be asked to hold the patient still. It is advised to have a male relative be the first choice, female relatives are second, nonradiology personnel are third, and finally nonprofessional radiology personnel.

Chapter Summary

1. The transmission of light through a radiographic film is described by the film's optical density.
2. Optical density is a measure of the degree of darkness of the film. Higher-speed films require less exposure to produce a given density.
3. High-contrast films produce large density differences for small differences in exposure.
4. Films with wide latitude produce acceptable image densities over a wide range of exposures. Higher-contrast films have narrow exposure latitude, while lower contrast films have a wider latitude.
5. Improper storage and handling can produce fog that produces unwanted densities on the film.
6. Radiographic contrast is the result of differential absorption of various tissues. This makes the recorded detail visible on the image.
7. A characteristic curve demonstrates the speed, contrast, and latitude of a film. Different films will have their own unique characteristics.
8. Speed is the sensitivity of the film to radiation exposure and has a direct relationship with optical density.
9. The slope or straight-line region on the H&D curve indicates the level of contrast in the film; the steeper the slope, the higher the contrast.
10. Distortion results from the misrepresentation of the anatomy on the radiographic image; it is seen as size (magnification) or shape of the part and should be minimized to improve radiographic quality.
11. Beam or tube angulation can be utilized for specific anatomic parts to improve visualization of the structures.
12. Spatial resolution or recorded detail is the ability to detect small, high-contrast structures on the image.
13. Recorded detail depends on focal spot size, SID, OID, and motion.
14. Sharp, high detail images are obtained using small focal spots, minimum OID, maximum SID, and short exposure times.

Case Study

Donovan performed an abdomen and a chest exam on a 57-year-old patient. When reviewing the images, he considered the density of each image and determined that the chest image demonstrated a short scale of contrast. The abdomen image also demonstrated a short scale of contrast.

Critical Thinking Questions

1. What scale of contrast is appropriate for each image?
2. What effect does the incorrect scale of contrast have on an image?
3. Does either film need to be repeated? Why?
4. How would subject contrast affect the images?

Review Questions

Multiple Choice

1. Which region of the characteristic curve represents the inherent density in the film?

a. Base plus fog
b. Toe region
c. Shoulder
d. Straight-line portion

2. On the characteristic curve, the toe region will display optical densities in which range?

a. 0.1 to 0.5
b. 0.4 to 0.8
c. 0.0 to 3.5
d. 0.1 to 0.2

3. What is the relationship between optical density and the log relative exposure on the characteristic curve?

a. Nonlinear
b. Linear
c. Curvilinear
d. Noncurvilinear

4. Which area on the characteristic curve represents high exposure levels?

a. Toe region
b. Straight-line portion
c. Shoulder
d. D_{min}

5. A high-contrast film has a ________ latitude.

a. wide
b. narrow

6. Radiographic contrast depends on:

a. tissue thickness
b. tissue density
c. kVp
d. all of the above

7. Radiographic contrast is defined as:

a. the difference in densities between adjacent areas
b. the difference in attenuation between adjacent areas
c. the difference in scattering between adjacent areas
d. the difference in bremsstrahlung between adjacent areas

8. __________ is the degree of blackening on the film.

   a. OD
   b. Radiographic density
   c. Subject contrast
   d. Tissue thickness

9. The primary controlling factor for magnification is:

   a. kVp
   b. mAs
   c. focal spot size
   d. OID

10. Changing the kVp from 60 to 70 kVp and decreasing the mAs by one-half results in:

    a. a shorter scale of contrast
    b. increased optical density
    c. a longer scale of contrast
    d. decreased optical density

11. What is the magnification factor with a 40-inch SID and a 30-inch SOD?

    a. 0.75
    b. 1.33
    c. 1.2
    d. 0.80

12. In a radiographic image, focal spot blur is decreased by increasing:

    a. the size of the x-ray field
    b. the size of the focal spot of the x-ray tube
    c. the distance from the focal spot to the patient
    d. the patient motion

13. Which of the following would improve radiographic quality if patient motion is a problem?

    a. 0.6 mm focal spot, 100 mA, 0.25 s
    b. 0.6 mm focal spot, 200 mA, 0.125 s
    c. 0.6 mm focal spot, 300 mA, 0.083 s
    d. 1.2 mm focal spot, 500 mA, 0.050 s

14. The degree of spatial resolution is determined by:

    a. line focus principle
    b. line pairs per millimeter
    c. spinning top test
    d. wire mesh test

15. When a larger focal spot size is used, how will it affect the focal spot blur?

    a. Increased
    b. Decreased
    c. No change

Short Answer

1. When the characteristic curve shows a steep slope, there is __________ contrast on the film. What type of contrast is on the film when the slope is less steep?

2. Describe a long scale of contrast and the factor that affects the scale.

3. How do variations in the anatomical part affect density?

4. How are OD and mAs related?

5. What is recorded detail?

6. Explain how SID and OID affect size distortion.

7. What is the difference between elongation and foreshortening?

8. What is the difference between voluntary and involuntary motion?

9. Explain how SID and OID affect size distortion.

14

Image Exposure

Objectives

Upon completion of this chapter, the student will be able to:

1. Define radiation quantity and its relation to x-ray beam intensity.
2. List the factors that affect the intensity of the x-ray beam.
3. Explain x-ray quality and how it is related to penetrability.
4. Explain the relationship between milliamperage and exposure time with radiation production and image receptor exposure.
5. Calculate changes in milliamperage and exposure time to change or maintain milliamperes per second.
6. Discuss how kVp affects exposure to the image receptor.
7. Calculate changes in kVp to change or maintain exposure.
8. Calculate changes in mAs for changes in source-to-image receptor distance.

Key Terms

- 15% rule
- brightness
- direct square law
- exposure time
- involuntary motion
- mAs/distance compensation formula
- kilovoltage peak (kVp)
- milliampere
- milliampere-second (mAs)
- optical density
- quantum mottle
- radiographic density
- source-to-image receptor distance (SID)
- technical factors
- voluntary motion

Introduction

Conventional radiography forms a two-dimensional image from projections through a three-dimensional patient. The appearance of the final radiographic image is affected by the technical factors of milliamperes, exposure time, kVp, distance, and focal spot size. The selections that the radiographer makes are dependent upon the anatomical area to be imaged, patient size, and known pathology. It is important for the student to have a thorough understanding of the technical factors and how each is used with regard for patient variables. We will review the proper selection of these factors as this is an essential step in the production of diagnostic quality radiographs.

Technical Factors

There are various **technical factors** that affect the appearance of the final image. It is important for the student to have a thorough understanding of each of these factors. Many of these factors are discussed throughout the textbook; however, it is appropriate to mention each here because a misstep with just one can compromise the image.

Milliampere

Milliampere, abbreviated mA, is a measure of the quantity of electrons or electrical current flowing per second through a circuit. The unit of electric current is the ampere (A). 1 ampere = 1 Coulomb of electrostatic charge flowing per second in a conductor. The mA control on the machine console is a selector that connects to one of the resistors in the filament circuit. As a higher mA setting is used, a greater flow of electricity will pass through the filament circuit to the cathode each time the rotor is depressed. When more current is forced through the thin filament wire, there is a greater amount of friction, which makes the filament burn hotter. Because of the higher temperature, more electrons are boiled off the filament wire in a process of thermionic emission. Changes in the mA setting control the number of electrons flowing from the cathode to the anode in the x-ray tube; the kinetic energy of electron flow is not affected by mA changes. The rate of electrons striking the anode per second determines the rate of x-ray photons produced. Larger mA values produce more x-ray photons. Doubling the mA setting doubles the number of x-ray photons being emitted per second. Milliampere selections on x-ray generators range from 25 to 1,000 mA (Fig. 14.1).

Exposure Time

Exposure time, abbreviated s for seconds, is the amount of time when the x-ray beam is activated when an x-ray exposure is occurring. The length of the exposure time also influences beam *quantity*. Longer time values allow for more photons to be produced if the other parameters are not changed. Exposure time can be expressed in milliseconds, or as a decimal, or a fraction of a second. Longer exposure times result in more x-ray photons striking the patient. Doubling the exposure time doubles the number of x-ray photons produced. Exposure times should be selected to allow for the shortest or fastest exposure time possible to minimize **involuntary motion** artifacts.

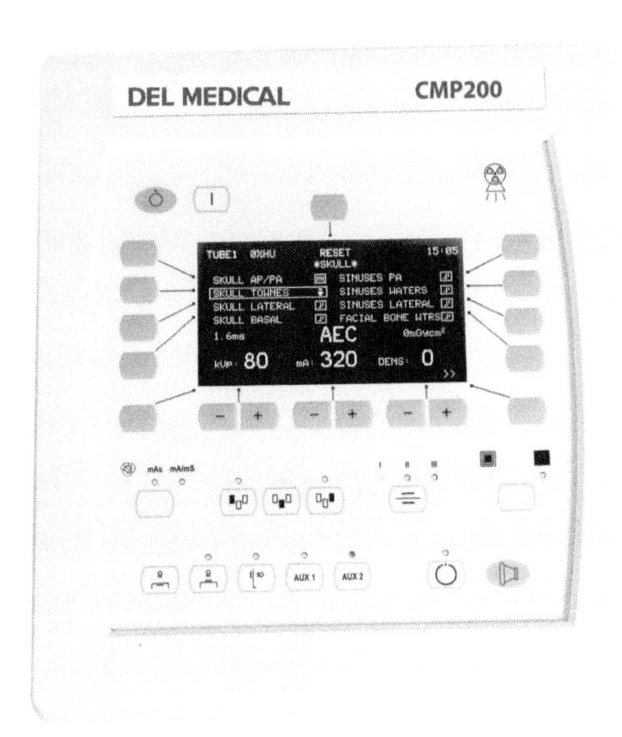

Figure 14.1. Shows a modern control panel with variable selections.

Milliampere-Second (mAs)

Milliampere-second, abbreviated as mAs, is the product of mA times exposure time in seconds and is commonly called "*mass*." mAs determines the number of x-ray photons reaching the image receptor and is the total quantity or intensity of the entire x-ray exposure that was made. The exposure can be expressed as R/s (Roentgens per second) for the exposure rate and R (Roentgens, which measures exposure in air) for total exposure. An increase in mA or time results in an increase in x-ray photon quantity or intensity, which produces an increase in the number of x-ray photons. To maintain the same exposure, the mA must be increased if the time is decreased. The effect of doubling the mA setting actually doubles both the bremsstrahlung and characteristic x-ray photons. The exposure time can be doubled instead of the mA and will result in the same amount of total exposure.

In radiography, mAs is the controlling or primary technical factor used to control the x-ray exposure because it determines the number of x-ray photons in the primary beam. Many factors can affect the x-ray exposure, but when it is stated that a variable is a "primary control," it means that it is the preferred way to control the quantity or intensity of the exposure. Changing other variables like kVp has an undesirable effect. When kVp is changed, the penetration characteristics of the beam and subject contrast in the remnant beam are affected. This is an occurrence that we may not want to tamper with as it may result in a poor quality radiographic image.

mAs is considered the key factor in controlling the optical density on the radiograph. Thicker body parts require higher mAs settings to achieve proper OD. When either mA or time is doubled, there is a doubling of exposure (OD) to the image receptor. mA and time are inversely proportional, and to maintain a given exposure if the mA is doubled, the time must be halved and vice versa. This inverse relationship is expressed in the formula:

$$mA_o \times s_o = mA_n \times s_n$$

where o is for original mA and exposure time and n is the new mA and exposure time. The product of mA times the exposure time must always yield the same total mAs to maintain a given exposure.

CRITICAL THINKING BOX 14.1

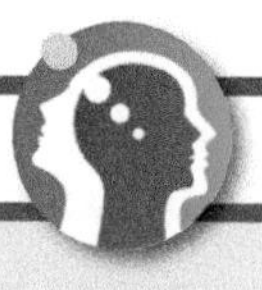

20 mA and 0.5 seconds were set and resulted in the proper exposure. If the time is decreased to 0.05 s, what is the new mA setting?

Performing the Mental Math

Working with the formula in your head can be easier when converting the mA and time into easier numbers. When calculating the total mAs, it is helpful to remember that most mA stations are in multiples of 100. Move the decimal place for the *mA to the left two places* and the *decimal two places to the right for the exposure time* so that time is multiplied by the *first* number in the mA setting. An example is:

$$200\text{ mA at }0.08\text{ seconds} = 2\text{ mA at }8\text{ seconds}$$
$$= 2 \times 8 = 16\text{ mAs}$$

Consider 200 mA at 0.04 seconds simply as $2 \times 4 = 8$mAs. An example of exposure time with only one decimal would be 300 mA at 0.8 seconds or $3 \times 80 = 240$ mAs. There are some mA stations with only two digits, but you should still "work" the mental math the same. For example, 75 mA at

CRITICAL THINKING BOX 14.2

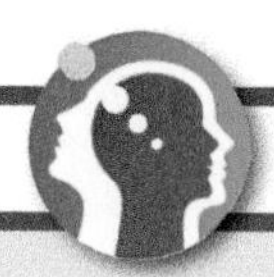

Complete the calculations for each column:

mA × decimal time = total mAs	mA × milliseconds = total mAs
1. 100 × .03 =	1. 60 × 50 ms =
2. 150 × .04 =	2. 100 × 40 ms =
3. 200 × .08 =	3. 200 × 125 ms =
4. 300 × .025 =	4. 300 × 80 ms =
5. 400 × .008 =	5. 600 × 140 ms =

0.02 seconds will become $0.75 \times 2 = 1.5$ mAs. When time has three decimal places (0.025), convert it to 2.5 seconds. Milliseconds must be converted to seconds before doing the problem (50 ms = 0.5 seconds).

Radiographic Density

Radiographic density was discussed in Chapter 13, but a further discussion is warranted here to further a student's understanding on the effect mAs has on optical density. A film that appears too light is lacking sufficient density and warrants an increase in mAs. On the other hand, a film that is too dark has excessive density and warrants a decrease in mAs. Radiographers must assess the level of density in film screen images to determine if the proper density is seen to adequately visualize the area of interest. **Optical density** that is not acceptable is seen outside of the straight-line region on the characteristic curve and may indicate that the image must be repeated. The question becomes how much of an increase is needed to make a visual difference on the radiograph? The answer is simply a 30% change is the least amount of change necessary to see a visible difference in the image density. Density errors often require the mAs to be adjusted by a factor of two, either double or half. This change will bring the ODs back into the straight-line region. When a greater adjustment in density is needed, the radiographer should multiply or divide by a factor of 4. This is simple to do and produces an acceptable level of density on a repeat radiograph. If an image was produced with 5 mAs and is too light, the image should be repeated at 10 mAs. This will produce an image with acceptable density (Fig. 14.2).

Radiographic images that have sufficient but not optimal density are usually not repeated. If there is another

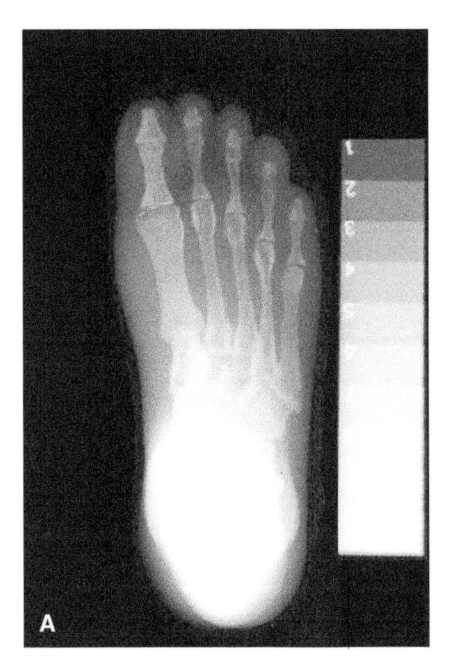
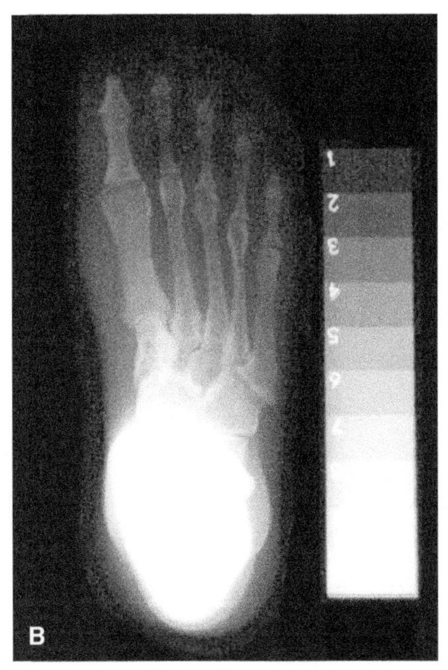
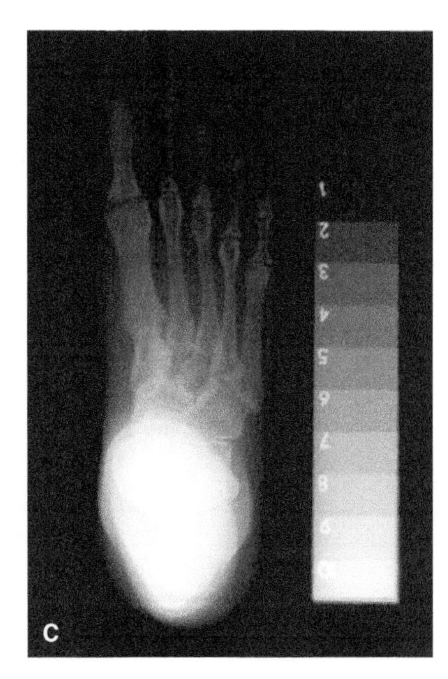

Figure 14.2. **Three-foot images demonstrating a doubling of mAs with each image. (A) 65 kVp at 3 mAs. (B) 65 kVp at 6 mAs. (C) 65 kVp at 12 mAs.**

error, such as in positioning that will require a repeat, the radiographer may use the opportunity to make an adjustment in mAs to produce an optimal quality radiograph.

On a daily basis, radiographers perform multiple mAs calculations with a desired mAs in mind. The best mA-time combination must be determined. First, decide on the size of focal spot; extremities use a small focal spot. Set the highest mA setting possible to keep the length of time short. This will minimize the chance of patient motion. This combination of settings provides a higher exposure dose to the patient but results in a sharper image. This same density can be accomplished by using smaller mA values with a longer time. However, the radiographer must determine if the patient can hold completely still for the longer exposure. If the patient cannot hold still and moves during the exposure (**voluntary motion**), motion blur will be seen on the image, which would make a repeat image necessary, effectively giving a double exposure to the patient. Longer exposure times are beneficial when imaging anatomy that requires a breathing technique; this effectively blurs anatomy, which superimposes the anatomy of interest (Table 14.1).

When patient exposure is more important than fine detail, the large focal spot is used. In chest and abdomen

TABLE 14.1 **RELATIONSHIP BETWEEN DIFFERENT METHODS OF EXPRESSING MAS, WITH TYPICAL MA VALUES AND EXPOSURE TIMES**

Time			mAs from			
Milliseconds	Decimals	Fractions	25 mA	100 mA	300 mA	400 mA
10	0.01	1/100	0.25	1	3	4
25	0.025	1/40	0.625	2.5	7.5	10
50	0.050	1/20	1.25	5.0	15	20
100	0.1	1/10	2.5	10	30	40
200	0.2	1/5	5.0	20	60	80
250	0.25	1/4	6.25	25	75	100
333	0.33	1/3	7.5	33	99	132
500	0.50	1/2	12.5	50	150	200
1,000	1.0	1	25	100	300	400

imaging, it is preferred to use 500 or 600 mA stations and short amounts of time to reduce exposure to the patient. When employing a "breathing technique," the settings are reversed—use low mA and the longest practical times (3 to 4 seconds) when long exposures are required. To calculate the length of the exposure when the mAs and mA station are known, simply divide the mA station into the desired mAs.

$$\text{mAs} = \text{mA} \times \text{time}$$
$$90 \text{ mAs} = 300 \text{ mA} \times \text{time}$$
$$90 = 300(x)$$
$$\frac{90}{300} = x$$
$$0.3 \text{ s} = x$$

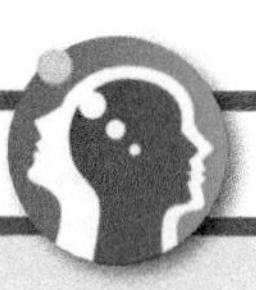

CRITICAL THINKING BOX 14.3

Calculate the length of the exposure for each combination.

1. 2.4 = 100 mA × _____
2. 45 mAs = 150 × _____
3. 1.3 mAs = 50 mA × _____
4. 80 mAs = 300 mA × _____
5. 240 mAs = 600 mA × _____
6. 150 mAs = 50 mA × _____

Density and Brightness

As previously discussed, density is the amount of exposure to the radiographic image. Density is seen as levels from white to gray to black. On a film screen image, intensity must be neither too low nor too high, but an optimum level is needed to convey the maximum amount of information about the anatomic region of interest. In a digital image, **brightness** is the term used to describe density. The digital image is composed of pixels (picture elements), which each displays its own level of brightness or density. The brightness should fall in a broad range of "gray shades" from very light gray to very dark gray within the anatomic area of interest. An image with many shades of gray or intermediate brightness indicates there was proper attenuation of the x-ray beam. As with film screen images, areas of black indicate the x-ray beam was not absorbed by the patient while areas of white show complete absorption of the x-ray photons. Under these conditions, only the outline or edges of the anatomy are seen, and we are not able to see "inside" the organ. With proper penetration and absorption of the x-ray beam, the whole organ including edges and internal structures will be seen. Partial penetration results in various gray shades along the appropriate range of image brightness. A further in-depth discussion of brightness/density occurs in Chapter 19.

Quantum Mottle

Radiographic noise or **quantum mottle** is the speckled appearance on an image. The x-ray beam contains a random pattern of photons. We cannot see the photons, but we can imagine they are snowflakes. During a light snow shower, we can see individual snowflakes landing on the sidewalk. Some are close together, while others are farther apart; this pattern is random. Now, imagine a heavy snow shower where you cannot see each snowflake but rather a blanket of snow that covers the sidewalk. When very low mAs is used, there are only a few photons striking the image receptor and it is easy to see the uneven distribution of the exposure. This is caused by the fluctuations in x-ray interactions. The radiograph has a "grainy" appearance or blotches of dark and light are seen. This "grainy" appearance is called quantum mottle. A mottled appearance on the image is caused by the decreased quanta or photons in the remnant beam. Quantum mottle indicates an insufficient amount of x-ray photons have reached the image receptor and represents a form of image or radiographic noise. A radiographer can overcome quantum mottle by selecting the proper mAs settings for the anatomical area of interest.

Kilovoltage

Kilovoltage peak (kVp) controls the energy of the x-ray photons, and when the kVp is increased, the quality of the beam is increased and the x-ray photons are able to penetrate the tissue of interest. As previously discussed in Chapter 12, radiographic contrast depends on the quality of the x-ray beam and subject contrast of the anatomical part imaged. Increasing the kVp increases the amount of exit radiation through the patient and decreases differential absorption. Higher-energy x-ray photons are more penetrating and produce more scatter radiation by way of increased Compton interactions.

When imaging the body, a sufficient amount of contrast improves visibility of tissues within the body. The kVp setting is the primary controlling factor of radiographic contrast.

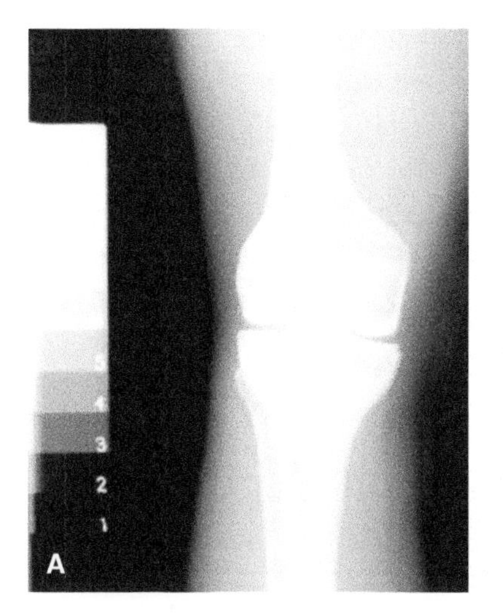

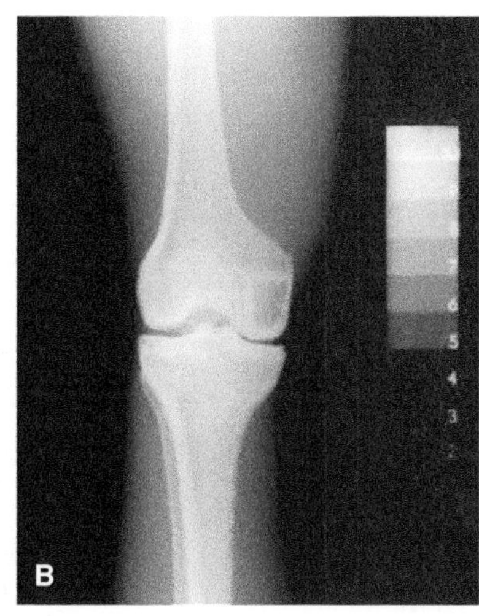

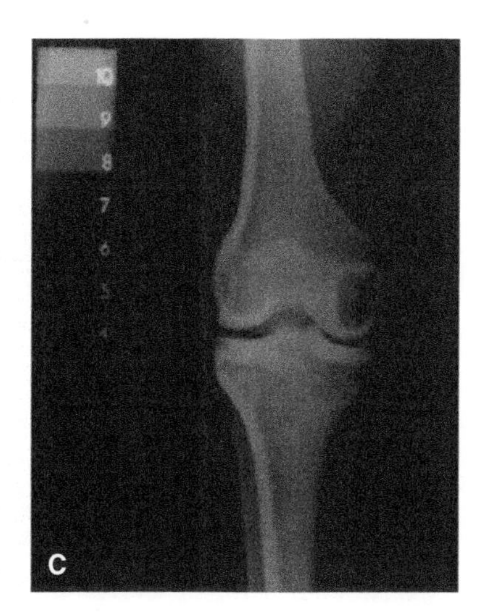

Figure 14.3. Demonstrates images of an aluminum step wedge and a knee phantom. (A) 55 kVp at 2 mAs. (B) 65 kVp at 2 mAs. (C) 75 kVp at 2 mAs.

Figure 14.3 demonstrates how high-kVp images have a long-scale contrast and smaller-density differences between black and white. The mAs was adjusted to maintain the same image density for each image. The number of density differences visible in the 55 kVp image is less than the number of density differences visible in the 75 kVp image. The 75 kVp image is a long-scale contrast, low-contrast image. The 55 kVp image is a short-scale contrast, high-contrast image.

kVp and Image Density

A change in kVp will also alter the image density because the penetration or quality of the x-ray photons changes. An increase in kVp results in an increase in exit radiation. When the x-ray quality is increased with higher kVp, less x-ray quantity is needed due to the higher penetration of the beam, so fewer x-ray photons are needed to produce the same optical density. A 15% change in kVp is equivalent to changing the mAs by a factor of 2. This is termed the 15% rule for kVp. If the kVp is decreased from 100 to 85 kVp, the mAs must be doubled to maintain the same image density. The same is true if the kVp is increased by 15%, the mAs should be decreased by a factor of 2.

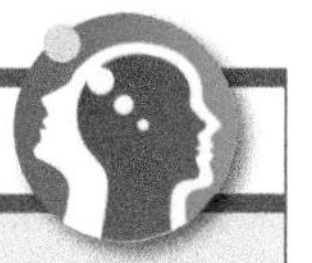

CRITICAL THINKING BOX 14.4

An IV contrast study of the urinary system, which is obtained at 100 kVp and 10 mAs, has acceptable density but demonstrates low contrast. What mAs should be chosen if the new kVp is decreased by 15%?

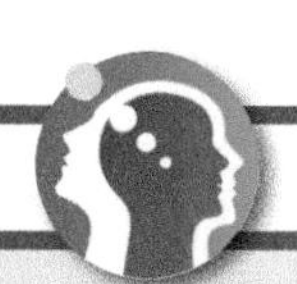

CRITICAL THINKING BOX 14.5

A radiographer reduces the mAs by one-half to reduce motion artifacts. What new kVp should be selected to maintain the same density as originally obtained from 60 kVp at 10 mAs?

Changes in kVp will change radiographic contrast when utilizing the **15% rule** with the appropriate change in mAs. These adjustments will result in changes in the image contrast by creating a long scale of contrast (Table 14.2).

TABLE 14.2 DENSITY AND CONTRAST ARE ALTERED BY ADJUSTING TECHNICAL FACTORS

Factor	Density Change	Contrast Change
mA increase	Increase	Unchanged[a]
mA decrease	Decrease	Unchanged[a]
Time increase	Increase	Unchanged[a]
Time decrease	Decrease	Unchanged[a]
kVp increase	Increase	Decrease
kVp decrease	Decrease	Increase
SID increase	Decrease	Unchanged[a]
SID decrease	Increase	Unchanged[a]
Focal spot increase	Unchanged	Unchanged
Focal spot decrease	Unchanged	Unchanged

[a]When mAs is changed and a corresponding change in SID is made to maintain density.

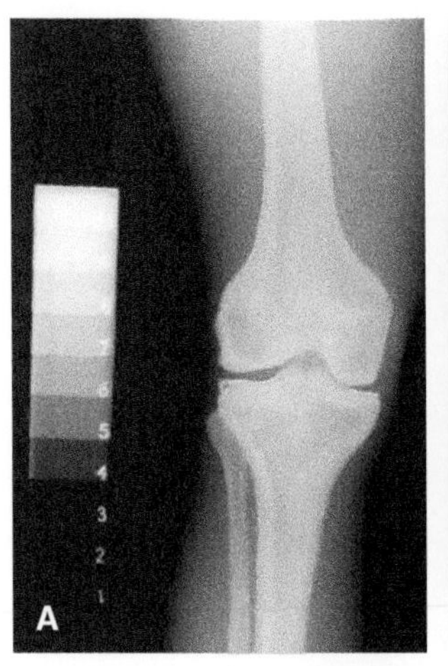

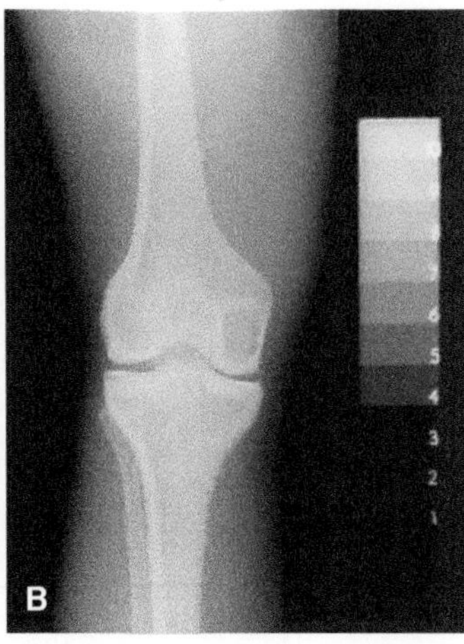

Figure 14.4. (A) AP knee using 70 kVp at 4 mAs. (B) AP knee using 80 kVp at 2 mAs. Using the 15% rule to increase kVp and using half the mAs resulted in a long scale of gray, which obscured the fine bony detail and a nondiagnostic image.

The radiographer must select different combinations of kVp or mAs to optimize image density and contrast. Higher mA settings should be chosen to minimize the exposure time and patient motion artifacts. It is often possible to obtain further reduction in exposure time by increasing the kVp by 15% and reducing the mAs by one-half. The skilled radiographer will be able to determine when this change will not affect the diagnostic quality of the image.

When using kVp to add density to the image, one must be careful because the additional kVp will add density in the form of scatter radiation. Scatter radiation will change the contrast on the image, which will increase the gray scale and may be detrimental to the image. A skilled radiographer will be able to distinguish the appropriate factor to use to make the desirable change in exposure on an image while maintaining density and gray scale. As seen in Figure 14.4, the change in gray scale on the image obscured the fine detail of the knee anatomy, thereby compromising the final interpretation of the image.

Source-to-Image Receptor Distance

The distance between the x-ray source or focal spot and the image receptor influences the image density. This distance is termed the **source-to-image receptor distance (SID)**. Changes in SID influence the quality of the beam and the radiographic contrast; therefore, a change in distance requires a change in mAs to maintain beam intensity.

The x-ray intensity (measured in mR or R) decreases with the square of the distance from the x-ray source because the x-rays are spread out over a larger area as the distance to the source increases. This is a result of the inverse square law. Doubling the distance decreases the x-ray intensity by a factor of 4 to one-fourth of the original intensity. Increasing the SID decreases the number of x-ray photons striking the film. Reducing the SID to one-half the original distance increases the intensity by a factor of 4 to four times the original intensity. The variation of x-ray intensity as a function of distance is given by the inverse square law:

$$\frac{I_1}{I_2} = \frac{(D_2)^2}{(D_1)^2}$$

where I_1 is the old intensity, I_2 is the new intensity, D_1 is the old distance, and D_2 is the new distance. This relationship is known as the inverse square law because the new intensity is inversely related to the ratio of the distances squared. An increase in distance results in a decrease in intensity.

CRITICAL THINKING BOX 14.6

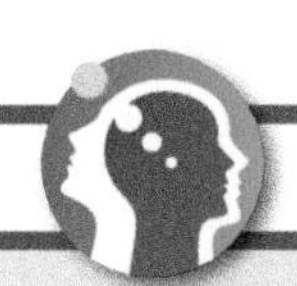

An exposure was made with 60 mR at 40-inch SID. What is the intensity of the beam if the new distance is 80 inches?

As demonstrated, the new beam intensity is one-fourth the intensity of the beam at the original distance.

Figure 14.5 illustrates how the beam intensity is changed with an increase or decrease in SID. A decrease in the SID results in an increase in the number of x-ray photons striking the image receptor because the intensity is much greater and more easily penetrates the anatomy. As seen in the Critical Thinking exercise, when the distance is decreased by one-half, the x-ray intensity will increase by four times.

CRITICAL THINKING BOX 14.7

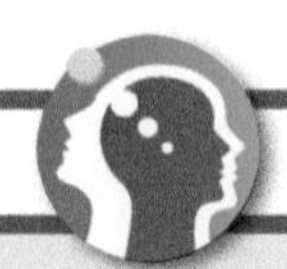

60 mR is used to make an exposure at 80 inches. Determine the new intensity when the SID is decreased to 40 inches.

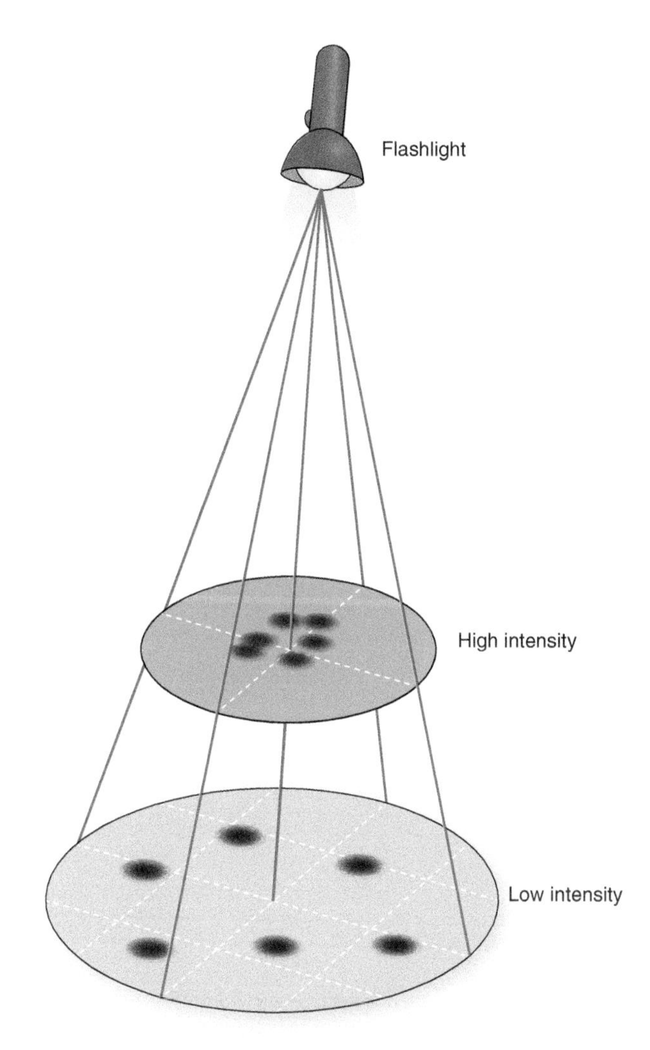

Figure 14.5. Illustrates the decrease in x-ray intensity as the distance to the source increases.

Optical Density and SID

Standard distances are used in diagnostic imaging to provide more consistency in radiographic quality. The majority of radiographic images are performed at either a 100-cm (40-inch) SID or 180-cm (72-inch) SID. Special circumstances, such as trauma or mobile radiography, do not allow for standard distances to be used. The radiographer must determine the change needed in mAs to produce a quality radiograph when the SID is not one of the standard distances. During these special circumstances, the radiographer must make quick adjustments in mAs based on commonly used SIDs. For example, when a 72-inch (180-cm) SID cannot be used, adjust the SID to 56 inches (140 cm) and decrease mAs by one-half. When a 40-inch (100-cm) SID is increased to 56 inches (140 cm), twice the mAs is needed. By using this quick method of changing mAs, the radiographer can be confident there will be sufficient exposure to the image receptor.

When other SIDs are used, the quick method will not apply and the radiographer will need to use a calculator to determine the changes in mAs. To maintain the density on the image, mAs must be changed to compensate for the change in distance; this is called the exposure maintenance formula or density maintenance formula. This formula is similar to the inverse square law but is reversed to a **direct square law** because, as already stated, the mAs must increase when the distance is increased or vice versa to maintain image density. The **mAs/distance compensation formula** is stated as:

$$\frac{\text{mAs}_1}{\text{mAs}_2} = \frac{(\text{SID}_1)^2}{(\text{SID}_2)^2}$$

where mAs_1 is the original mAs, mAs_2 is the new mAs, D_1^2 is the old distance squared, and D_2^2 is the new distance squared. The following examples will help explain the mAs/distance compensation formula.

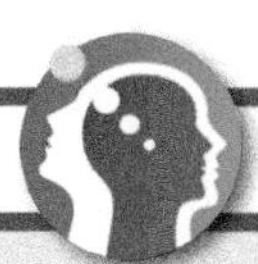

CRITICAL THINKING BOX 14.8

A lateral C-spine projection examination in the emergency room was taken at 40 inches, 70 kVp, and 10 mAs and produced an image with satisfactory density. A follow-up lateral is to be taken in a general x-ray room where a 72-inch SID is utilized. What new mAs should be selected for this new distance?

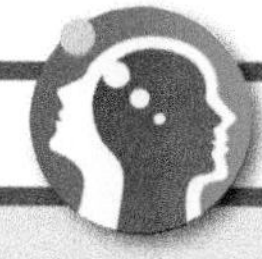

CRITICAL THINKING BOX 14.9

A radiograph is produced using 16 mAs at 72-inch SID with adequate density. What mAs will be required to maintain the density at 40-inch SID?

Even though changes in the SID change the OD of the film, the SID is usually not adjusted to change the OD. Multiple problems would arise if the distance from the x-ray tube to the image receptor was changed frequently. As seen with the mAs/distance compensation formula, a change in SID creates a change in density thus requiring an adjustment in mAs to compensate for the SID change. Figure 14.6 demonstrates the effect to the density on an image when SID is changed and all other factors remain

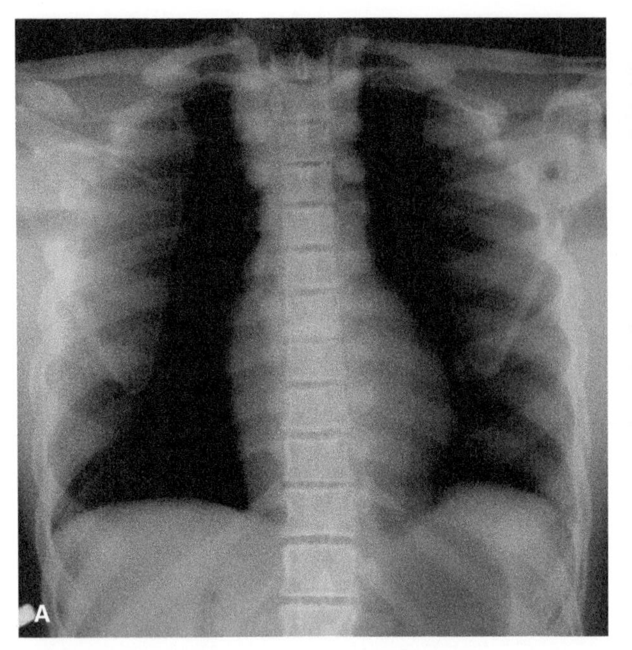

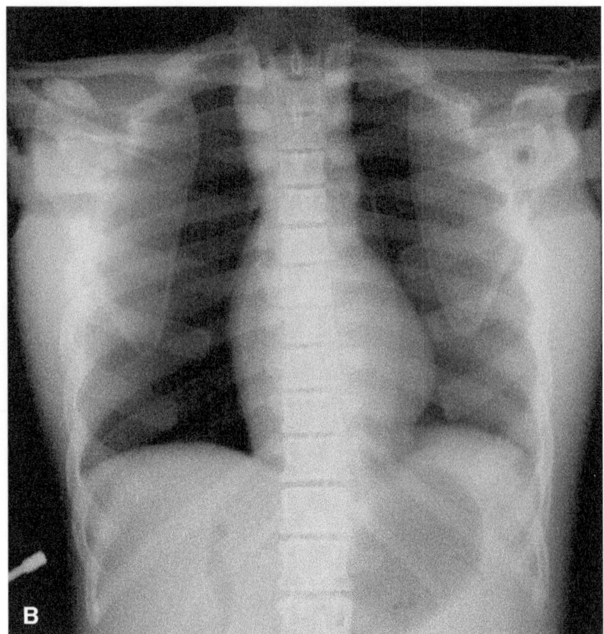

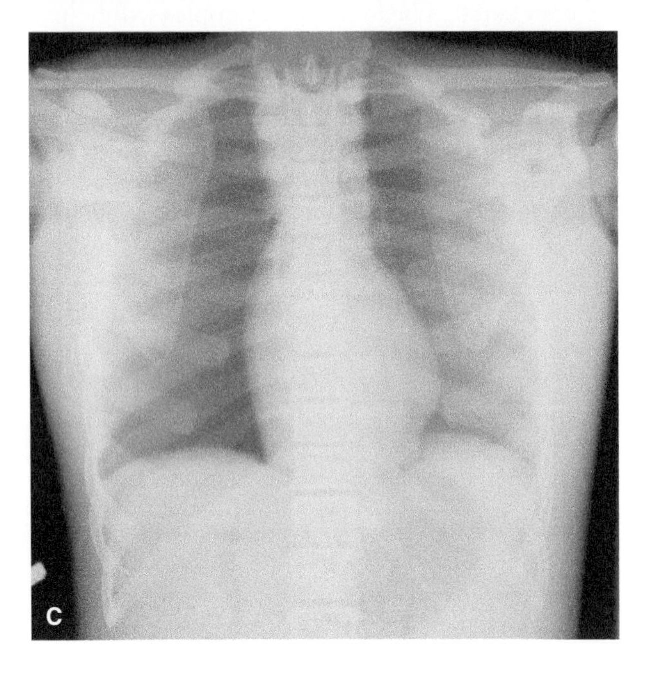

Figure 14.6. All three images were produced using the same kVp and mAs. (A) The SID was 30 inches and resulted in an overexposed image. (B) A 40-inch SID produced an image with optimum density. (C) The SID was at 60 inches, which produced an image that was underexposed.

the same. The mAs is used to change OD at one of the standard SIDs.

Digital Concepts

The fundamental principles of selecting the appropriate kVp and mAs to image a body part are just as important for digital radiography as they are for film screen radiography. There are some distinct differences between film screen and digital radiography principles. In film screen, the image receptor captures the remnant beam and ultimately displays the image. The film is a static image, which cannot be manipulated in any manner to improve the density or contrast in the image. Digital radiography uses a detector to capture the remnant beam and displays the image on a computer monitor. The computer adjusts density or brightness in the image to predetermined levels.

mAs controls the amount of density on film and is a representative of the exposure to the film as well as the patient. When the image has excessive density, it means that the mAs setting was too high; this is called an overexposed image. On the other hand, when the image lacks density, it is called an underexposed image. In the digital world, mAs no longer controls density in the image but it still represents the quantity of radiation dose. If too little radiation was used, then the image will have quantum mottle or excessive noise. The computer makes adjustments to the density or brightness to produce a quality image. When there is an overexposure, the computer will rescale the image lighter, and for underexposure, it will rescale the image darker. The computer rescales and adjusts images to provide consistent appearing diagnostic images; however, if there is excessive lack of exposure, quantum mottle will still be visible even though the brightness and contrast appear acceptable.

Digital systems have a wider dynamic range than film screen. The computer has imaging-processing software that will produce an image with a specified level of contrast even when higher kVp values are used. kVp can be increased to help reduce patient radiation dose. The 15% rule can be applied to increase the kVp, but it does not change the scale of contrast in the image. In an effort to reduce radiation dose, the radiographer can use the 15% rule to increase kVp while reducing mAs by one-half. This rule can be applied one time without affecting the final image, and in some cases, it can be used twice but more than that will cause a lack of sufficient radiation exposure (mAs) and greater amounts of scatter radiation, which will negatively affect the image.

Whether using film screen or digital imaging, the radiographer must select the appropriate kVp for optimum penetration of the part and sufficient mAs for exposure or quanta to create an image. Unfortunately, the use of excessive mAs has become a common practice in radiography. In an attempt to eliminate the possibility of quantum mottle or to make the image "look better," many radiographers use excessive mAs settings. This is not an acceptable practice because excessive radiation dose is being given to the patient. The ARRT and ASRT codes of ethics and the ALARA principle must be followed to prevent exposing patients to excessive radiation. In Part Four, there will be an in-depth discussion of digital imaging concepts, which students must learn so that they can ethically utilize radiation to create a quality diagnostic image.

Chapter Summary

1. X-ray quantity is determined by mAs, which is the product of milliamperes and time. Image noise is primarily controlled by mAs.
2. Increasing the mA or exposure time increases image density. Increasing the SID decreases image density.
3. Quantum mottle is the result of a lack of exposure to the image receptor.
4. Image contrast is primarily controlled by kVp. High-kVp techniques produce images with long-scale contrast and low contrast. Low-kVp techniques produce images with short-scale contrast and high contrast.
5. The inverse square law states that x-ray intensity varies inversely with the square of the SID. As an example, the intensity decreases by a factor of 4 when the SID is doubled.
6. Image noise increases as intensity decreases. To compensate for intensity changes produced by SID changes, the mAs must be changed.
7. A 15% change in kVp is equivalent to changing the mAs by a factor of 2.

Case Study

Amanda performed an oblique hand image on a 78-year-old patient who had fallen and was complaining of severe pain. She used 55 kVp, 50 mA, 0.06 s, and 40-inch SID and did not use a radiolucent sponge. When Amanda viewed the image, the metacarpals and phalanges demonstrated a blurring effect that partially obscured areas of the anatomy. The overall density of the image is appropriate for this patient. Amanda decided to make some modifications and repeat the radiograph.

Critical Thinking Questions

1. What modifications to the exam should Amanda make?
2. Should she use an immobilization aid?
3. Will she need to change kVp and mA or time?
4. How might communication help improve the next image?

Review Questions

Multiple Choice

1. **Radiographs are obtained utilizing 70 kVp and 10 mAs for proper density. The kVp is decreased by 15%. In order to obtain the same film density, the mAs must be:**

   a. 2.5
   b. 5
   c. 20
   d. 40

2. **If the distance from the source is increased from a 36-inch to 72-inch SID, the exposure at 36-inch SID used 70 kVp and 10 mAs, what new mAs should be chosen to maintain the same image density?**

   a. 2.5 mAs
   b. 5.0 mAs
   c. 20 mAs
   d. 40 mAs

3. **If the distance from the source is decreased by a factor of 2, the mAs must be ________ to maintain the same image density.**

   a. increased by a factor of 2
   b. decreased by a factor of 4
   c. increased by a factor of 3
   d. decreased by a factor of 3

4. **Which of the following would improve radiographic quality if patient motion is a problem?**

   a. 100 mA, 0.25 seconds
   b. 200 mA, 0.125 seconds
   c. 300 mA, 0.083 seconds
   d. 500 mA, 0.050 seconds

5. **Which rule is used to determine how much kVp should be changed to allow for mA to be halved?**

   a. 15% rule
   b. 50% rule
   c. 30%rule
   d. 25% rule

6. An image is produced with 110 kVp and 4 mAs at 72-inch SID. To maintain density, what will be the new mAs if the distance is reduced to 40-inch SID?

   a. 8 mAs
   b. 1.2 mAs
   c. 5 mAs
   d. 2.8 mAs

7. The milliampere is a measure of the quantity of electrical current flowing per second through a circuit.

   a. True
   b. False

8. What is the effect on the filament wire when a high amount of current is flowing?

   a. A greater amount of friction is produced.
   b. Filament wire will burn hotter.
   c. Increase in the number of electrons boiled off filament.
   d. A and B.
   e. A, B, and C.

9. When the exposure time is increased two times, how does this affect the number of photons in the beam?

   a. One-half the number of photons are produced.
   b. Four times as many photons are produced.
   c. There are twice as many photons produced.
   d. One-fourth the number of photons are produced.

Short Answer

1. What is the difference between voluntary and involuntary motion?

2. What formula is used to determine the intensity of the x-ray beam when the SID is changed?

3. An image of a hand is produced using 3 mAs and 50 kVp. What kVp would be required to halve the mAs to the image receptor while maintaining density?

4. The image of an abdomen was created using 10 mAs and 70 kVp. What change in kVp would be required to double the mAs while maintaining density?

5. How are OD and mA related?

6. An increase in SID will cause a __________ in mAs.

7. Write the formula for mAs/distance compensation or maintenance.

8. What is the controlling factor for density and how does it affect it?

9. How much of a change in kVp is needed to decrease mAs by one-half? To double mAs?

15

Controlling Scatter Radiation

Objectives

Upon completion of this chapter, the student will be able to:

1. Describe the effect of scatter on radiographic contrast.
2. Identify the factors that affect the amount of scatter.
3. Identify methods of scatter reduction.
4. Describe the construction of an antiscatter grid.
5. Identify the types of grids.
6. Explain the types of grid errors.

Key Terms

- air gap technique
- aperture diaphragm
- automatic collimator
- beam-restricting device
- Bucky
- Bucky factor
- collimation
- collimator
- cone
- crossed grids
- cylinder
- exit radiation
- focal range
- focused grids
- grid
- grid caps
- grid cassette
- grid conversion factor (GCF)
- grid cutoff
- grid frequency
- grid ratio
- interspace material
- oscillating grid
- parallel grids
- positive beam-limiting (PBL) device
- reciprocating grid

Introduction

Radiographic contrast is an important characteristic of image production. Contrast provides the many shades of gray that make a manifest image possible. Most of the x-ray photons entering a patient undergo Compton scattering before they exit the patient. Scattered photons contain no useful information and create fog or noise on the image, which decreases the contrast of the image making the image less visible. Two types of devices are used to control scatter radiation: beam-restricting devices and grids. A thorough understanding of the use of these devices is paramount in producing a quality radiographic image with the appropriate level of radiographic contrast.

Factors Affecting Amount of Scatter Produced

The intensity of scatter radiation reaching the image receptor depends on three primary factors: patient thickness, high kVp settings, and field size. The radiographer can change the x-ray photon energy by changing the kVp and the field size by adjusting the **collimator** to reduce the amount scatter radiation. Unfortunately, there is very little a radiographer can do to affect part thickness. Careful selection of the field size and kVp can significantly reduce the amount of scatter radiation produced thereby improving image quality.

Patient Thickness

The volume of tissue irradiated or patient thickness directly correlates to the amount of scatter radiation that is produced. When the part is sufficiently thick to warrant an increase in kVp, there will be a greater amount of scatter produced. The patient is the source of scatter radiation that is degrading the image. An increase in tissue thickness increases the amount of scatter because there are more atoms available for interactions in the thicker tissue. The greater number of these interactions produces more scatter. It is sometimes possible to reduce the patient or part thickness and reduce the amount of scatter with some examinations. Compression in mammography, for example, reduces tissue thickness and scatter radiation.

Another source of scatter radiation is the type of tissue being irradiated. Tissue with a higher atomic number will absorb more of the x-ray beam than tissue with a lower atomic number. Bone is an example of high–atomic number tissue. Bone will absorb more of the beam and produce less scatter radiation because bone absorbs more photons photoelectrically. Soft tissue has a lower atomic number and less ability to absorb the photons, which then creates more Compton scatter radiation (Fig. 15.1). It is this scatter radiation that decreases radiographic contrast in either digital or film screen imaging.

The grid is designed to absorb the unwanted scatter radiation that occurs with larger, thicker body parts and with procedures that use higher kVp techniques. Radiographers must keep in mind the following to determine if a grid is needed for a given procedure:

1. Body part thickness >10 cm
2. kVp settings higher than 60 kVp

When either of these factors applies to the patient, a grid must be used to clean up or absorb scatter radiation. Higher kVp settings will produce higher energy scatter radiation that can penetrate through the anatomic part and strike the image receptor. Photoelectric interactions are lost with higher kVp, which results in more scatter reaching the image receptor as noise.

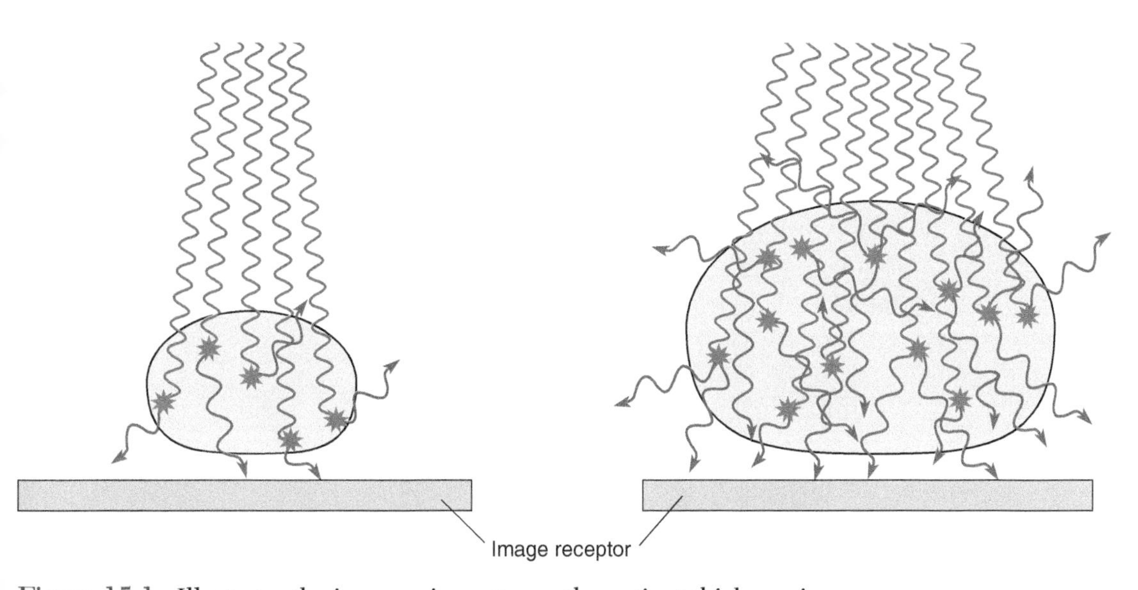

Figure 15.1. **Illustrates the increase in scatter as the patient thickness increases.**

X-Ray Beam Energy

kVp is the factor that controls x-ray photon energy or the penetrability of the beam. Increasing the kVp energy results in higher energy scatter radiation, which is emitted in a more forward direction to exit the patient and strike the image receptor. Decreasing the kVp decreases the x-ray beam energy and the amount of scatter. However, lower energy x-rays have decreased penetration and result in higher patient dose because more x-ray photons are absorbed in the patient's tissue. The kVp selected must be tailored to the body part under examination. For example, higher kVp settings are desirable to penetrate the tissue so that the remnant beam carries sufficient subject contrast. Higher kVp settings are useful for exams that use contrast media and for body parts with higher proportions of bone. An advantage of using higher kVp is the corresponding decrease in mAs that is needed to create the image. Overall, this is a reduction in the amount of radiation the patient receives. Higher kVp also produces a long scale of gray, which provides more information in the final image.

The benefits of using higher kVp outweigh the small amount of scatter that reaches the image receptor. When deciding on correct kVp settings, consider penetration of the part and subject contrast; if either of these is lacking on the radiographic image, the image will require a repeat exposure, which will effectively double the amount of radiation the patient received.

Field Size

Larger field sizes produce more scatter radiation because the larger area results in more tissue being irradiated. The light field should match the size of the image receptor. Extending the light field well beyond the image receptor results in primary beam striking the tabletop. Upon impact, scatter radiation will be produced, which may then reach the image receptor and cause noise on the radiographic image. The image receptor and light field should be correctly sized to the part being imaged. The light field should never extend past the edges of the image receptor. Often, it is acceptable to decrease the field size to reduce the area of tissue available for x-ray interactions. Smaller field sizes result in less scattered radiation and higher image contrast. Of course, this comes with the caveat that all necessary anatomy must be included in the radiographic image.

Effect of Scatter on Contrast

Exit radiation is a combination of transmitted and scattered radiation that passes through the patient. Transmitted radiation undergoes no interaction in the patient. The transmitted radiation passes through the patient with no change in direction or loss of energy (Fig. 15.2). Scattered radiation has undergone multiple Compton scattering interactions. Each Compton interaction causes the scattered radiation to change directions and lose energy before leaving the patient. Scattered radiation has lower energy and is emitted in all directions from the patient; it reduces radiographic contrast by adding a general density over the entire image. Because the photons have changed direction, they no longer relay anatomic information to the image receptor. For this reason, scattered radiation provides no diagnostic information. The presence of scatter lowers image contrast, which creates a longer scale of gray that

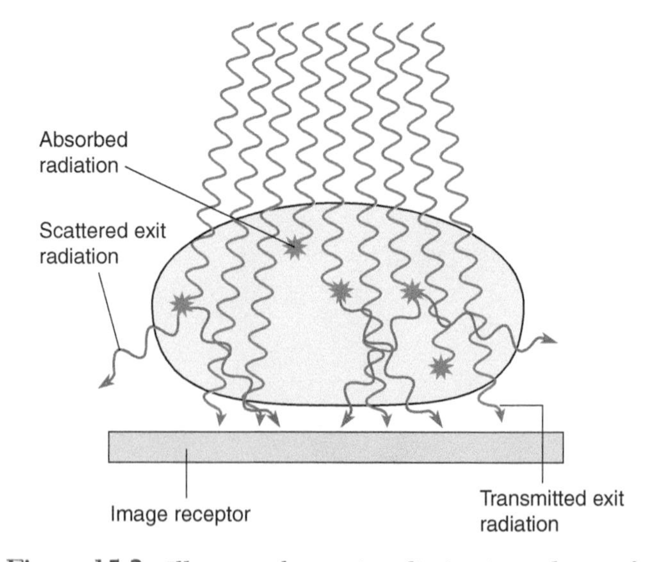

Figure 15.2. Illustrates how exit radiation is made up of transmitted and scattered radiation while some photons are absorbed in the tissue.

affects the visibility of objects in the radiographic image. The scattered radiation is the source of exposure to personnel in the room during fluoroscopy and portable examinations.

Beam Restriction

As previously discussed, one of the most important characteristics of image quality is radiographic contrast. Depending upon the anatomy to be imaged, the scale of gray will be long or short. Regardless of the intended gray scale, scatter radiation will have an effect on the final amount of optical density and the levels of gray seen in the image. A radiographer can use beam restriction to decrease the amount of scatter radiation produced, which will result in a higher-quality radiographic image. There are various methods a radiographer can use to restrict the beam. It is crucial for the radiographer to use the appropriate method for the examination.

Collimation

The most frequently used beam restriction method is **collimation**. These devices are the most advanced, useful, and accepted beam-restricting device. The purpose of collimation is to define the size and shape of the primary x-ray beam striking the patient and to provide a visible light field that outlines the x-ray field (Fig. 15.3). The old term of *coning* is used in the same way as collimation, meaning to restrict the field size. As you will learn later in this section, the phrase *coning* more accurately describes another device for restricting the field size.

A light-localizing variable-aperture collimator consists of two pairs of lead shutters that are adjusted to intercept x-ray photons outside the desired x-ray field. Located immediately below the tube window, the entrance shutters limit the size of the x-ray beam. The entrance shutters absorb off-focus radiation as it leaves the anode. The second set of shutters has one or more sets of adjustable lead leaves that are at least 3 mm thick. This set of shutters is located 3 to 7 inches below the tube. These shutters work in pairs and are independently controlled, which allows the radiographer to adjust the longitudinal and transverse edges of the field. The field shape produced by the collimator is always

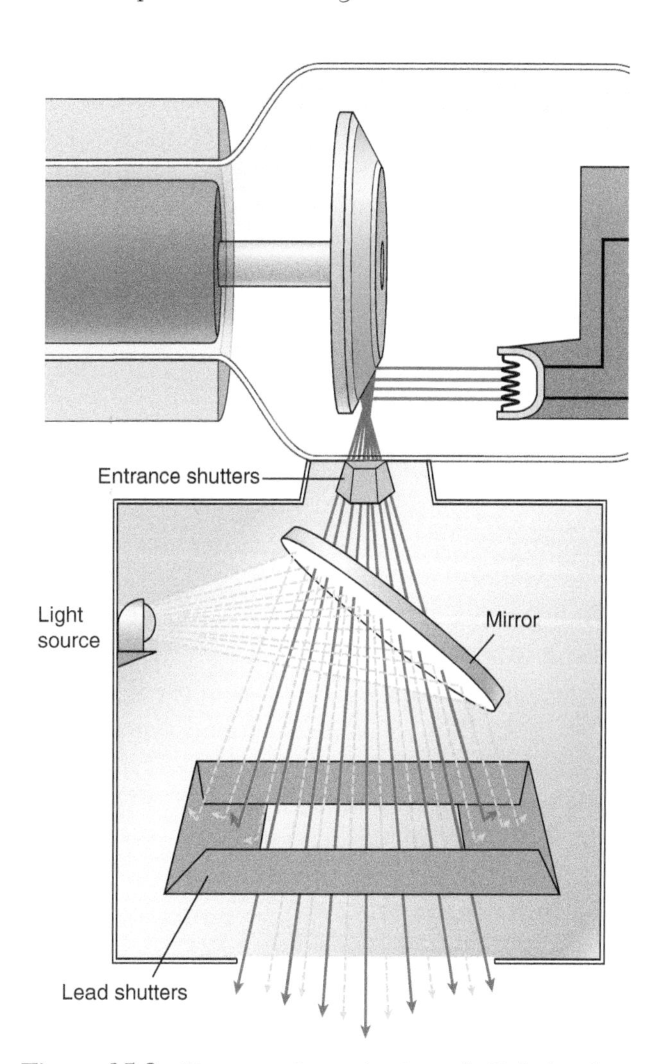

Figure 15.3. **Shows a schematic view of a light-localizing collimator.**

rectangular or square. This allows for infinite possibilities when matching the field size to the patient's anatomy.

Collimators have a light source and a mirror that projects the light through the shutters and onto the patient. The mirror is placed between the tube and light source so that a sharp light pattern can be projected through the collimator leaves or blades when the light is on. The projected light field coincides with the size of the x-ray beam and must remain accurate. Misalignment of the light field with the x-ray beam can result in anatomical parts being "cut off."

The collimator adjustment controls have indicators to show the field size in centimeters or inches at varying SIDs. IF the light source were to burn out, the x-ray field measurement guide will indicate the projected field size based on the adjusted size of the collimator opening. The x-ray field measurement guide is located on the front of the collimator box along with the button to turn on the light source. At the bottom of the collimator is a clear sheet of plastic with crosshairs affixed to the bottom, which indicates the center of the primary beam or central ray (CR). The size of the light field should never exceed the size of the image receptor since this would cause primary radiation to directly strike the table and create more scatter.

Automatic Collimators

An **automatic collimator**, also called a **positive beam-limiting (PBL) device**, automatically adjusts the size and shape of the x-ray beam to the size and shape of the image receptor. In 1974, the U.S. Food and Drug Administration mandated the use of PBLs on all new radiographic installations in an effort to protect patients from overexposure to radiation. The law has since been rescinded, but today, nearly all light-localizing collimators manufactured in the United States are automatic for fixed radiography equipment. Sensors in the **Bucky** tray detect the size of the image receptor and automatically adjust the collimator shutters to match the cassette size. The PBL makes it difficult for a radiographer to expand the light field beyond the size of the image receptor unless an override mechanism is used that will disengage the PBL feature. The field size can be reduced to limit the field to the area of interest and decrease scatter. Whether or not a PBL is used, the radiographer should collimate tightly to the area of interest to improve image quality and minimize patient dose.

Cassette-based image receptors vary in size from 8 × 10 inches to 14 × 17 inches. The PBL will automatically size to the specific image receptor that is placed in the Bucky. When using a digital flat panel detector, the x-ray field size should be restricted to the area of interest. The digital plates typically come in one size and are significantly larger than many anatomic areas. It cannot be stressed strongly enough that a radiographer must collimate appropriately for the anatomy being imaged. Practicing appropriate collimation for each image will ensure that the patient is not exposed to unnecessary radiation.

Aperture Diaphragms

A very simple **beam-restricting device** is the **aperture diaphragm**. An aperture diaphragm is a flat piece of lead (diaphragm) that has a hole in the middle (aperture). The aperture is attached to the tube head directly below the x-ray tube window. The aperture size is designed to cover an area slightly smaller than the dimensions of the image receptor. The aperture cannot be adjusted from the designed size, which means the projected field size cannot be adjusted. Figure 15.4 illustrates the relationship of the x-ray tube, diaphragm, and image receptor.

Cones and Cylinders

Radiographic extension cones and cylinders are essentially an aperture with an extension flange attached to it. The flange is a metal structure, which restricts the useful beam to a required size. The flange can be either one piece or two pieces and can vary in length. The two-part flanges are

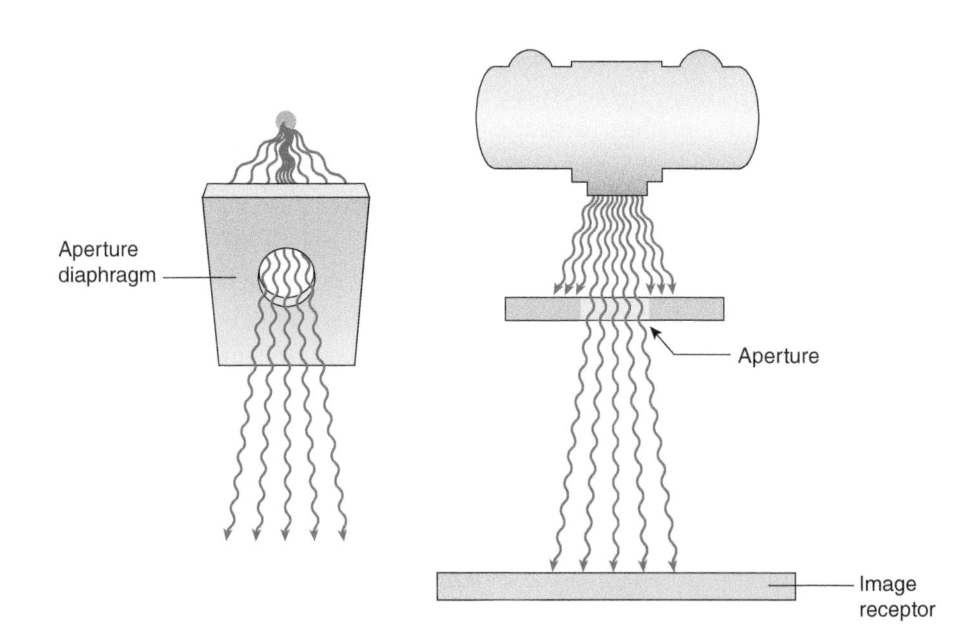

Figure 15.4. Illustration of a commercially made aperture diaphragm and its location between the tube and image receptor.

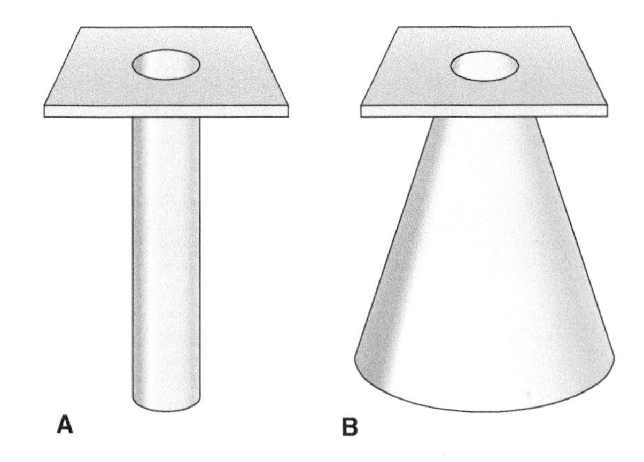

Figure 15.5. **(A) Cylinder. (B) Cone.**

made to telescope, which increases the overall length of the flange. As seen in Figure 15.5, the **cylinder** is a long tubular structure while the **cone** flares out toward the distal end. Cones and cylinders are usually circular where an aperture may be rectangular. Both the cone and cylinder are routinely called *cones* with the cylinder being the most common device used. At one point, cones were used extensively in radiographic exams, but today, the cones are more commonly used for examinations of the paranasal sinuses.

Radiographic Grids

A radiographic **grid** is a device used to absorb scatter radiation before it can reach the image receptor and fog the film. Grids are used with radiographic exams on large body parts >10 cm. These require a high-kVp setting; this high kVp creates a high-intensity x-ray beam and results in more Compton interactions. Controlling the amount of scatter radiation that reaches the image receptor controls the radiographic contrast on the image. Therefore, grids absorb or clean up scatter, which improves image contrast and produces a higher-quality image.

In 1913, Dr. Gustave Bucky, an American radiologist, designed a grid in an attempt to absorb scatter before it reached the image receptor. The first grid was a rather crude design with strips running in two directions, which left a checkerboard pattern superimposed over the patient's anatomy. Despite the checkerboard artifact, the grid removed scatter radiation and improved the contrast of the image. Although this was a step in the right direction, the thin white lines did obscure information on the image.

Grid Construction

A grid is a thin, flat, rectangular device that consists of alternating strips of radiopaque and radiolucent materials. The radiopaque material is usually lead foil due to its high atomic number and increased mass density. Lead foil is easy to shape and is relatively inexpensive; these properties along with the high atomic number make it the best material to clean up or absorb scatter. A grid absorbs scatter from the **exit radiation** before it reaches the image receptor. The grid is located between the patient and the image receptor. Scattered x-ray photons spread in various angles as they leave the patient and are preferentially attenuated by the lead foil strips, because the scattered photons are not parallel or in line to the grid interspaces.

The **interspace material**, which is the radiolucent space between the lead strips, is made of plastic fiber or aluminum. Aluminum has a high atomic number and produces less visible grid lines on the image. The use of aluminum increases the absorption of primary x-ray photons in the interspace, especially at low kVp. Higher mAs factors are required to maintain image density or receptor exposure (when referring to digital imaging) but increase patient dose by ~20%. Plastic fiber interspace materials are preferred to aluminum interspace materials because there is no need to increase patient dose with these types of grids. There are positive and negative attributes to each type of interspace material; therefore, both are manufactured.

The radiolucent interspace materials allow transmitted x-rays to reach the image receptor while intercepting or absorbing scattered x-ray photons. Only x-ray photons that are parallel with the interspaces pass through the grid. When to use a grid is a matter of professional judgment. As a general rule, grids are employed when the body part is >10 cm thick or when kVp settings are higher than 60 kVp (Fig. 15.6).

thePoint® ***An animation for this topic can be viewed at http://thepoint.lww.com/Orth2e***

Grid Ratio

The **grid ratio** has a major influence on the grid's ability to clean up scatter and improve radiographic contrast. The amount of scattered radiation removed by the grid depends on the height of, and the distance between, the

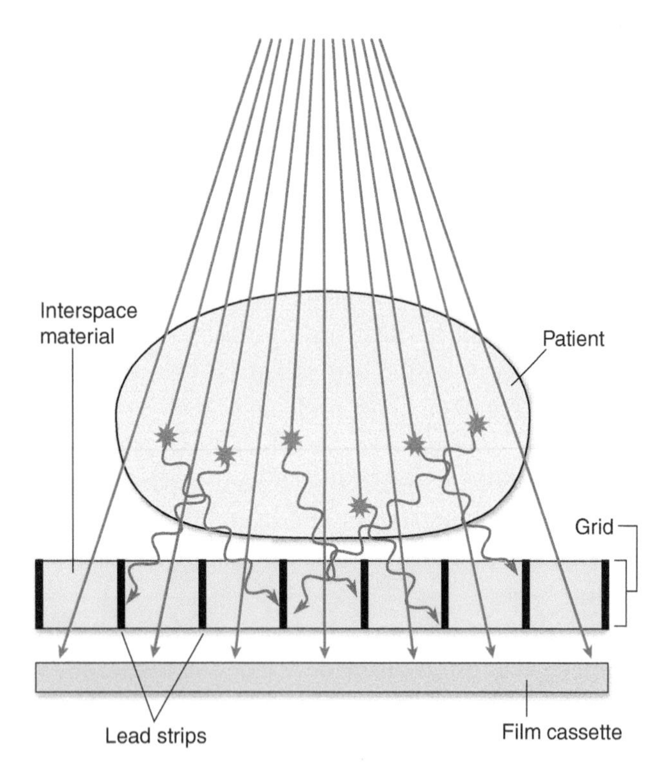

Figure 15.6. **Illustrates the construction of a typical grid and the absorption of scatter.**

lead strips, which make up the factor called a grid ratio. The amount of scatter eliminated, often called the scatter cleanup, depends on the grid ratio. The grid ratio is defined as the height of the lead strips divided by the thickness of the interspace material (Fig. 15.7). The formula to determine the grid ratio is

$$GR = h/D$$

High grid ratios are made by reducing the width of the interspace material, increasing the height of the lead strip, or using both methods. With high grid ratios, higher exposure factors are required to permit a sufficient number of x-ray photons to reach the image receptor. Grid ratios typically range from 5:1 to 16:1. Grids with higher

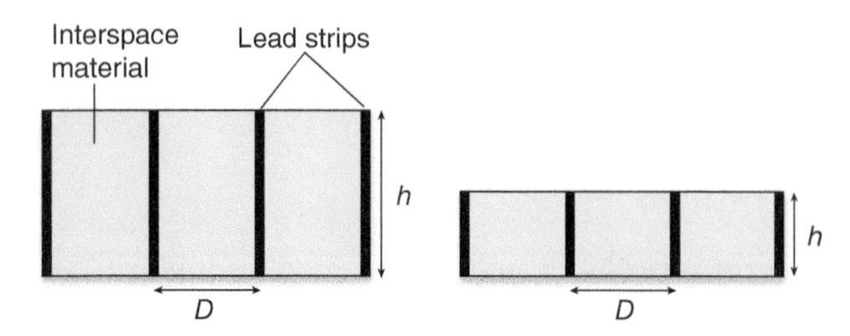

Figure 15.7. **Illustrates the grid ratio of high-ratio and low-ratio grids.**

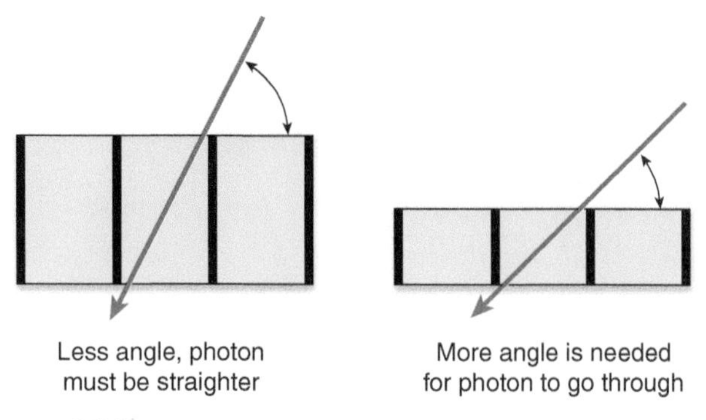

Figure 15.8. **Grid ratio. Smaller angle = less scatter reaching image receptor.**

grid ratios remove more scattered radiation but are much more difficult to align properly. Closer attention to grid placement must be used to make sure that the grid and x-ray tube are properly aligned to avoid errors in positioning. For this reason, portable examinations are usually taken using grid ratios of <12:1. General radiography examinations utilize an 8:1 or 10:1 grid ratio. Figure 15.8 demonstrates the effect of grid ratio and the angle of scatter photons. The high-ratio grid absorbs scatter that is at a small angle to the lead strip, meaning that less scatter reaches the image receptor. The height of the lead strips in high-ratio grids makes the grid more effective at absorbing scatter.

CRITICAL THINKING BOX 15.1

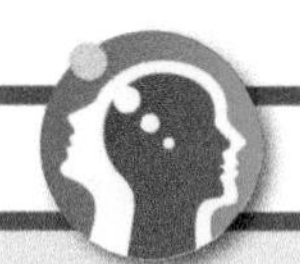

A grid is made of lead with 40 μm thick placed between aluminum interspace material 350 μm thick. The height of the grid is 3.5 mm. Determine the grid ratio. (Hint: first change the grid height to micrometers.)

Grid Frequency

Improvements in technology and manufacturing have led to a broader variety of interspace materials and lead foil strips that are incredibly thin. The **grid frequency** is the number of lead strips per centimeter. Grids with thinner strips have higher grid frequencies because the lead strips are closer together. The lead strips of a high-frequency grid are less visible on the radiographic image. The higher the grid frequency, the thinner the strips of interspace material must be and the higher the grid ratio.

Typical grid frequencies range from 25 to 45 lines per centimeter (60 to 110 lines per inch). As the grid frequency increases, higher technical factors are required to produce an image with sufficient density or receptor exposure; this results in greater patient dose. This occurs because as the grid frequency and grid ratio increase, there are more lead strips absorbing the photons, which means fewer photons are reaching the image receptor. For a given grid frequency, when the grid ratio increases, scatter cleanup improves and radiographic contrast increases; as grid ratio decreases, scatter cleanup is less effective and radiographic contrast decreases.

Types of Grids

Parallel Grids

The simplest type of grid is the parallel grid. **Parallel grids** have parallel lead and interspace strips running parallel. Parallel grids are sometimes called linear or nonfocused grids because the lead and interspace strips run in one direction. This grid is easy to manufacture, but it has some negative aspects. Parallel **grid cutoff** arises because parallel grids are constructed with the lead strips parallel to the central axis of the x-ray beam, but x-ray photons diverge from the focal spot. Grid cutoff occurs because x-rays near the edge of the field are not parallel to the lead strips and are attenuated. Parallel grid cutoff is greatest when the grid is used with short SID or with a large image receptor because the x-ray beam has a wide divergence at a shorter SID. The pronounced angle of divergence will cause more of the primary beam to be attenuated in the lead strips and grid cutoff will be seen along the outer edges of the image (Fig. 15.9).

Parallel grids should be used with smaller field sizes and longer SIDs to reduce grid cutoff. The divergence of the beam is less with a longer SID; in other words, the beam will be straighter. This works well as the beam is more parallel to the grid strips and less attenuation will take place. Parallel grid cutoff produces a radiographic image that has the correct intensity in the center but is lighter at both edges.

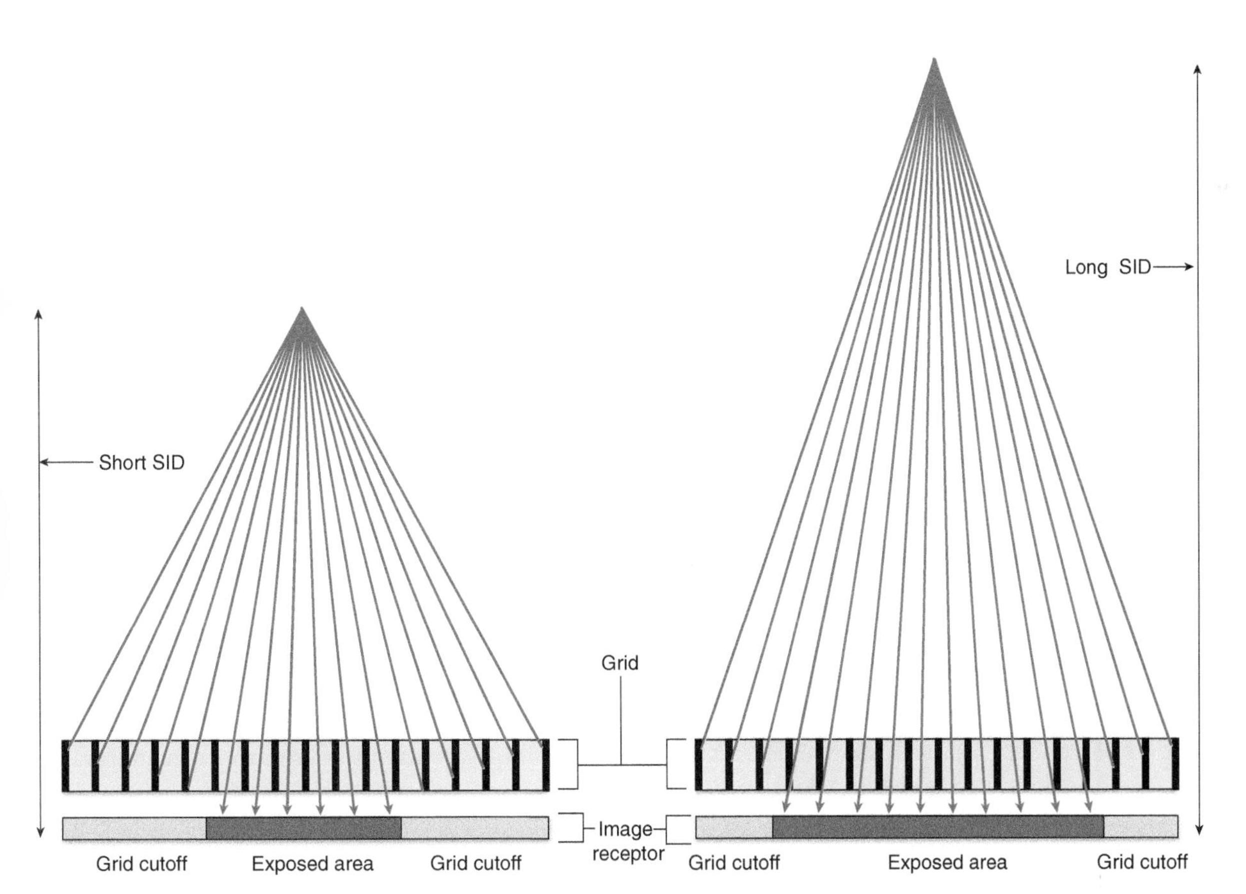

Figure 15.9. Longer SID results in less beam divergence and less parallel grid cutoff.

Focused Grids

Focused grids have the lead strips that are parallel at the center of the grid, and as the strips move away from the center of the grid, they become progressively more angled. If imaginary lines were extended from the lead strips toward a fixed focal distance, the lines would meet at a point, and this is called the convergence line. The distance from the front surface of the grid to the convergence line is called the grid radius. The focused grid is designed to match the divergence of the x-ray beam from a particular distance. The divergent rays transmitted from the x-ray source pass through the focused grid interspaces while the scattered x-ray photons are intercepted.

Focused grids eliminate grid cutoff at the edges of the field because the lead strips are angled toward the center and converge at the focal distance. When the x-ray source is in line with the center of the grid and located at the grid focal distance, there is no grid cutoff because the transmitted radiation passes through the radiolucent interspaces as seen in Figure 15.10. Focused grids are recommended for examinations that must use large fields or short SIDs. An example would be abdominal imaging that requires both the large field size and short SID to produce an acceptable image. Typical focused grid distances are 100 and 180 cm (40 and 72 inches).

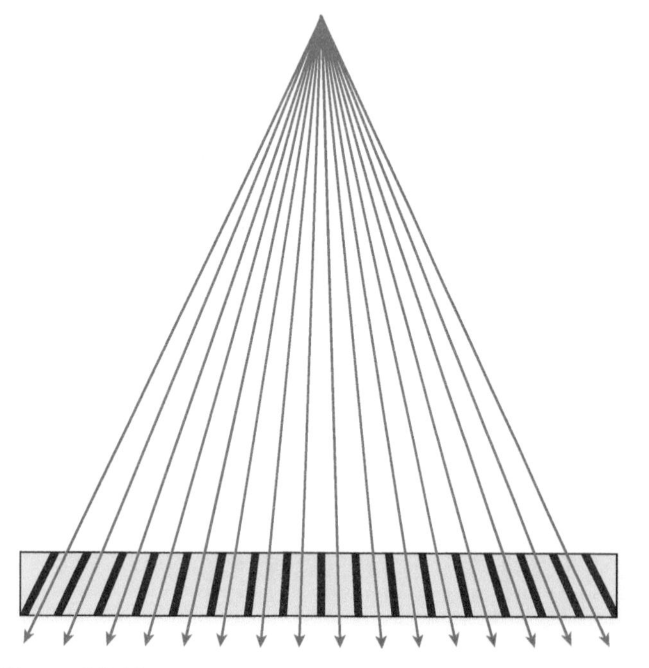

Figure 15.10. Illustrates the construction of a focused grid.

Each focused grid must be used with the appropriate **focal range** for which it was designed. The focal range includes short, medium, and long focal ranges where each is designed to be used with a specific SID. Mammography uses the short focal range grid, whereas chest radiography requires the long focal range grid. Focused grids can be used at distances within about 13 cm of the focal distance with no noticeable grid cutoff. Low grid ratio focused grids allow more latitude or leeway in the alignment of the tube to the grid before grid cutoff occurs. The higher the grid ratio, the less latitude the radiographer has with grid and tube alignment.

When using a focused grid, the x-ray tube must be located along the length of the strips. If the tube were placed so that the divergence of the beam ran perpendicular to the strips, grid cutoff would occur. Grid cutoff can affect a portion of the image or the whole image and results in reduced density or total absence of film exposure. The term defines what occurs to the primary x-ray photons, they are cut off from the image receptor. Focused grids that are not used at the proper SIDs will show grid cutoff. Focused grids used outside the focal range show a decreased intensity toward both edges. Focused grids located off-center or not perpendicular to the central ray show reduced intensity on only one side of the image.

The images in Figure 15.11 were taken with an 8:1 focused grid at 40-inch SID; image A is centered appropriately, while image B is off-center 6 cm. Although the grid cutoff is subtle, there is a noticeable blurring of bony markings. The images demonstrate the increased degree of grid cutoff when the tube is off-centered from the grid. Grid cutoff can also occur with parallel grids if the tube and grid are misaligned.

Crossed Grids

Crossed grids overcome the limitation of parallel or linear grids where the grids clean up scatter in only one direction. These grids are made by placing two linear grids on top of each other with the grid lines perpendicular to each other. Crossed grids are more efficient than linear grids at cleaning up scatter. The crossed grids will clean up at least twice the amount of scatter when compared to a linear or parallel grid. An 8:1 crossed grid will clean up more scatter than a 16:1 linear grid. The crossed grid is constructed by placing two 8:1 linear grids together (Fig. 15.12).

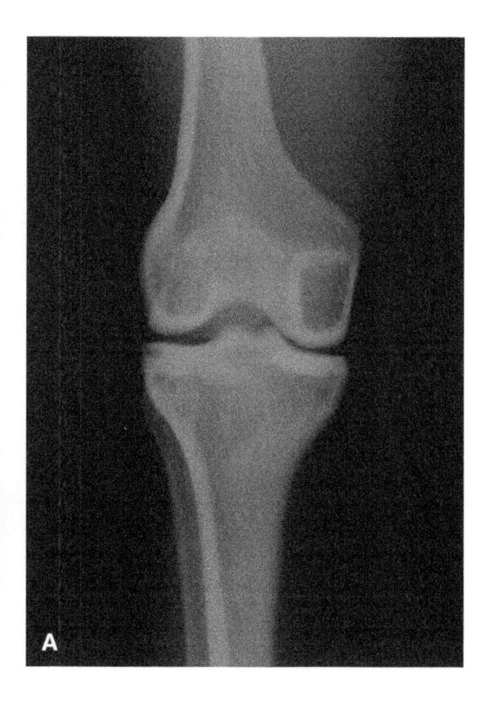

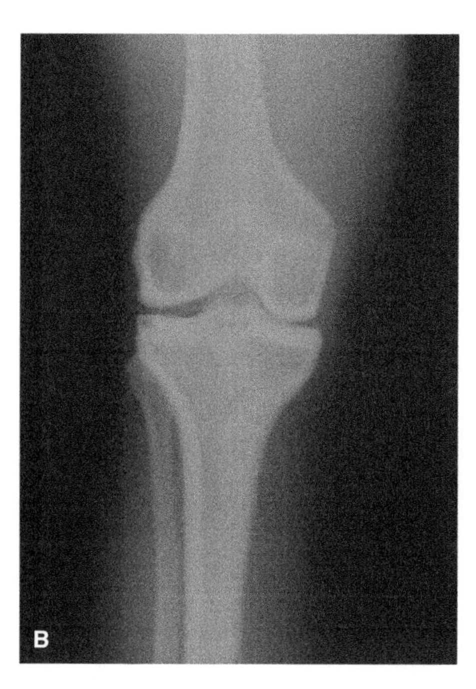

Figure 15.11. **Grid cutoff. (A) 40-inch SID on center. (B) 40-inch SID, 6 cm off laterally.**

There are three serious disadvantages associated with crossed grids. The radiographer must use precise positioning of the center of the grid to the center of the x-ray beam. Grid cutoff will occur if the crossed grid and x-ray beam are not perfectly lined up. The second disadvantage occurs when the table is tilted and the x-ray tube is not properly aligned to the table. Lastly, using a crossed grid requires much higher exposure techniques to be used, which results in higher patient dose to radiation.

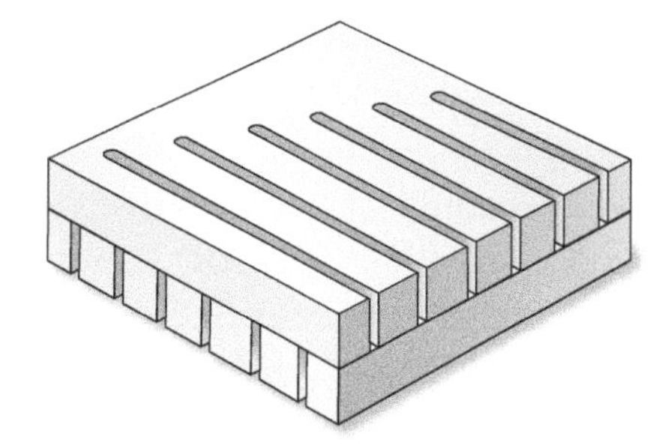

Figure 15.12. **Crossed grids constructed by placing two linear grids together with their grid strips perpendicular.**

Stationary Grids

Stationary grids are used in radiography departments for mobile examinations, upright imaging, or horizontal beam views. Most radiography departments have a supply of stationary grids; some are directly mounted to the front of a cassette and are called **grid caps**, while others are specially designed cassettes with the grid built-in called a **grid cassette**. When using stationary grids, the radiographer must be aware of the grid ratio and type of grid, whether linear or focused. The practice of aligning the x-ray tube to the grid caps or grid cassettes is also important because any misalignment can cause grid cutoff to occur.

Grid Movement

Stationary grids with low grid frequencies produce noticeable white grid lines on the final image. One way to eliminate these grid lines is to move the grid during the exposure. This motion of the grid blurs out the grid lines, so they are not noticeable. Dr. Gustave Bucky's grid design was improved upon by Dr. Hollis Potter, a Chicago radiologist, in 1920 when he placed the strips in one direction, made the strips thinner, and designed a device that allowed the grid to move during the exposure. The device is called the Potter-Bucky diaphragm or Bucky.

Reciprocating and Oscillating

Bucky grids are located directly under the table yet above the image receptor. Moving grids are typically focused grids that move when the exposure is being made. There are two types of moving grids:

- **Reciprocating grid**: The reciprocating grid is driven by a motor. During the exposure, it moves back and forth multiple times. The grid moves no more than 2 to 3 cm at a time. A selector at the control panel activates the grid motor. If the motor is not activated, the grid is stationary during exposure and grid lines will be apparent on the image.
- **Oscillating grid**: The oscillating grid is suspended in the center of a frame by four springlike devices. At the time of the exposure, an electromagnet pulls the grid to one side and then releases it. The grid will oscillate in a circular motion within the grid frame for ~20 to 30 seconds before ceasing motion.

Moving Grid Disadvantages and Advantages

The early use of grids demonstrated grid lines or the checkerboard pattern largely due to the large, thick strips and interspace material. Although cleaning up scatter and improving the contrast of the image, the grid lines were not acceptable as they distracted from the image. The moving grid was designed to remove the grid lines; however, there were some disadvantages with the design and placement of moving grids:

- Grid mechanism: Bulky, mechanical mechanism that was subject to failure.
- Increased OID: The distance between the patient and image receptor was increased due to the size of the grid mechanism. The increased OID creates magnification and blurring of the image.
- Motion: The nature of the moving grid increased the motion of the film holder; if not operating perfectly, the result would be additional image blur.

The advantages of the moving grid have greatly improved overall image quality and far outweigh the disadvantages. Advantages of the moving grid include the following:

- Motion blur: Grid mechanisms that are operating properly will completely blur out grid lines, making the overall image more diagnostic.
- Use in radiography: The moving grid is consistently used in radiography for body parts that measure >10 cm. This industry standard allows consistent imaging from one facility to the next.

Grids are very useful in radiographic exams where the tissue thickness is above 10 cm; as the tissue thickness increases, so does the amount of scatter. A skilled radiographer will be able to determine the proper grid for the examination that will be performed.

Grid Performance

Selecting the correct grid for a specific procedure requires consideration for the type of examination and the amount of kVp to be used. Examinations that require kVp settings over 95 kVp require a high-ratio grid for maximum cleanup of scatter; higher kVp results in increased amounts of scatter. High-ratio grids are more efficient at absorbing scatter, which results in less exposure to the image receptor. For some examinations, this could have a negative effect on the image, so with high-ratio grids, the exposure factors will need to be increased. mAs is typically increased to maintain image density and gray scale, but the payoff is increased patient dose. In other words, the more efficient the grid is at cleaning up scatter, the higher the dose to the patient.

Bucky Factor

The **Bucky factor** measures how much scatter is removed by the grid and how the technical factors must be adjusted to produce consistent optical density. Scattered radiation accounts for a portion of the density on the final radiographic image. When a grid removes scatter, the exposure factors must be increased to compensate for the decrease in x-ray photons reaching the image receptor. The Bucky factor or **grid conversion factor (GCF)** is used to calculate the necessary change in mAs when a grid is added, when changing to a grid with a different grid ratio or when using a nongrid. The Bucky factor depends on the grid ratio and the grid frequency but is usually in the range 3 to 5. This means that adding a grid requires an increase in mAs by a factor of 3 to 5 to obtain the same optical density compared to a nongrid technique. Table 15.1 presents specific grid ratios and grid conversion factor. When a grid is used, mAs must be increased by the indicated Bucky factor (GCF) to maintain the same number of x-ray photons reaching the image receptor. The GCF will increase with higher grid ratios and higher-kVp settings. The Bucky factor is mathematically represented as:

$$\text{GCF} = \frac{\text{mAs with the grid}}{\text{mAs without the grid}}$$

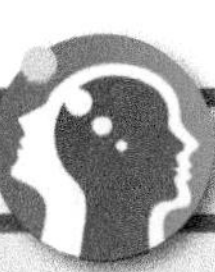

CRITICAL THINKING BOX 15.2

A satisfactory AP knee radiograph was produced using 7 mAs at 75 kVp without a grid. A second image is requested using an 8:1 grid. Using Table 15.1, what mAs is needed for the second image?

Required Change in mAs Following a Change of Grids

If a grid with a different grid ratio is used in a follow-up examination, the following formula should be used to determine the adjustment in mAs:

$$\frac{\text{mAs}_1}{\text{mAs}_2} = \frac{\text{GCF}_1}{\text{GCF}_2}$$

where mAs_1 is the original mAs, mAs_2 is the new mAs, GCF_1 is the original GCF, and GCF_2 is the new GCF.

TABLE 15.1 GRID RATIOS AND ASSOCIATED BUCKY FACTORS OR GCF

Grid Ratio	Bucky Factor or GCF
None	1
5:1	2
6:1	3
8:1	4
12:1	5
16:1	6

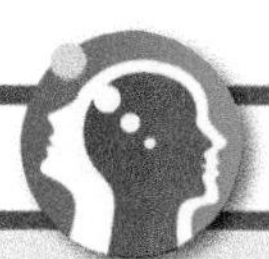

CRITICAL THINKING BOX 15.3

An abdominal examination taken in the department used 30 mAs with a 12:1 grid. What mAs should be used for the follow-up portable abdominal examination taken with an 8:1 grid?

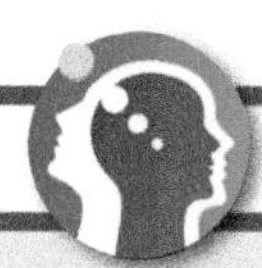

CRITICAL THINKING BOX 15.4

A satisfactory pelvis radiograph was produced using a 6:1 grid, 25 mAs, and 70 kVp. What mAs should be used with a 12:1 grid to maintain the same exposure to the IR?

As seen in the above examples, a change in mAs is required when the grid ratio changes. The major disadvantage with using a high-ratio grid is the increased patient dose (Fig. 15.13). The proper selection of the appropriate grid will increase image contrast and the diagnostic quality of the image. The radiographer must remember the following factors when selecting the correct grid for the exam:

1. High grid ratios increase patient dose.
2. High-kVp examinations typically use high-ratio grids.
3. High-kVp examinations result in decreased patient dose because the mAs can be reduced.

The utilization of grids for many examinations has required an increase in technical factors when compared to nongrid technical factor settings. The exposure time,

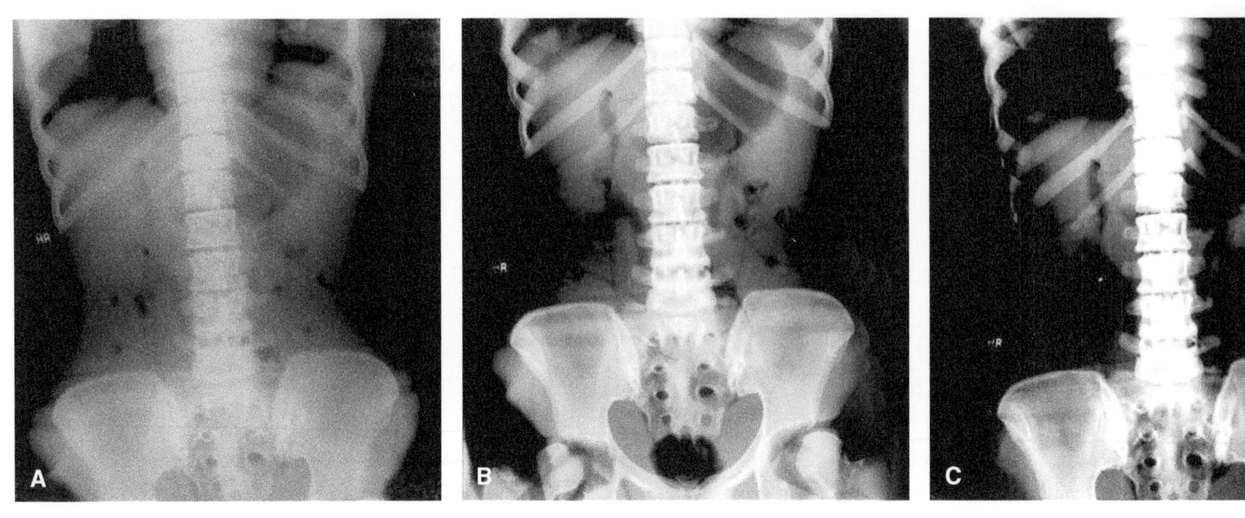

Figure 15.13. **Grid conversion. (A) The AP image of the abdomen shows low contrast due to no grid being used. This is an acceptable image for the soft tissue but does not demonstrate the bone very well. (B) The same image, except an 8:1 grid, has been used. Notice the shorter scale of gray, which demonstrates the bone. (C) A 12:1 grid has been used; the scale of contrast is too short to provide a diagnostic image of either the bone or soft tissue.**

mA, or kVp must be increased to provide adequate optical density on the image. Of these factors, kVp has been standardized in many departments and the mAs is changed to compensate for the patient's body habitus.

Grid Errors

An addition to the disadvantage of increased patient dose when a grid is used is the disadvantage of potential grid errors. Many grid errors occur because the design is a focus grid where the likelihood of an error is more common. Grid errors can be avoided if the radiographer properly centers the x-ray tube with image receptor at the correct SID and if the moving mechanism is functioning normally.

The Potter-Bucky diaphragm or Bucky is mounted underneath the tabletop directly above the image receptor. The grid in the Bucky must move side to side or in a circular pattern perpendicular to the lead strips to effectively blur out the grid lines. If the Bucky were to move in the same direction as the lead strips, the grid lines would be visible on the image.

Grid cutoff is defined as a decrease in the number of transmitted photons that reach the image receptor because of some misalignment of the grid to the tube. Improper positioning of the grid will always produce grid cutoff. The grid must be placed perpendicular to the central ray to eliminate grid cutoff. The central ray can be angled to the grid providing it is angled along the long axis of the grid strips but not across or perpendicular to the lead strips. The result of a misaligned grid is the reduction in the number of photons reaching the image receptor, resulting in a decrease in density on the image or an increase in quantum mottle.

Grid cutoff rarely occurs in the radiology department where fixed cassette holders or Bucky trays are routinely used. Grid alignment is more critical with high grid ratios and can be a serious problem with portable radiographic images. Careful positioning of grids during portable examinations is especially important because even slight misalignments will produce noticeable grid cutoff. Grid cutoff during portable examinations is a major cause of repeat imaging.

Grid errors occur most frequently because of improper positioning of the x-ray tube and grid. The grid will function correctly when the x-ray tube and grid are precisely lined up with each other. When the radiographer is not careful and misaligns the tube and grid, the following errors will occur:

- Off-level error
- Off-center error
- Off-focus error
- Upside-down error

Off-Level Error

An off-level error will occur when the x-ray tube is angled across or perpendicular to the grid strips. This can result from improper tube or grid positioning. Improper tube positioning occurs when the central ray is directed across the long axis of the table. Improper grid positioning most commonly occurs with stationary grids, which are used for mobile procedures or decubitus imaging, for example, when a patient is lying on a grid for a mobile pelvis examination and the patient's weight is not evenly distributed on the grid causing the grid to angle underneath the patient. When the vertical x-ray beam is aligned to the angled grid, off-level grid error will occur. The image will demonstrate a decrease in density over the whole image (Fig. 15.14).

Off-Center Error

The x-ray tube must be centered along with the center of a focused grid to prevent off-center error, also called lateral decentering. The center lead strips in a focused grid are perpendicular and the lead strips become more angled away from center as the strips get closer to the edges of the grid. The focused grid is designed to match the divergence of the x-ray beam. When the x-ray tube is off-centered laterally, the perpendicular portion of the x-ray beam will intersect the angled grid strips causing a decrease in exposure across the image. As demonstrated in Figure 15.15, the divergence of the beam will not line up with the angle of the lead strips. This grid error can be avoided if the radiographer correctly places the x-ray tube in the center of the grid; in some equipment, the tube will lock in place when correctly positioned to the detent in the middle of the table.

Off-Focus Error

The off-focus error results when the focused grid is used with an SID that is out of the focal range and not specified for the grid. Figure 15.16 illustrates what happens when a focused grid is not used in the proper focal range. Unlike the other grid errors, off-focus grid errors are not uniform across the entire image; rather, there is severe grid cutoff at the edges of the image. Positioning the grid at the proper focal distance is more crucial with high-ratio grids because these grids have less positioning latitude than low-ratio grids.

Upside-Down Error

This type of error is readily seen and identified immediately. When the grid is placed upside down, the lead strips are not angled toward the center of the grid. The result will be severe grid cutoff on either side of the center of the image. The x-ray beam will pass through the central axis of the grid and will be attenuated by the lead strips that are angled in the opposite direction of the beam divergence (Fig. 15.17). Focused grids are clearly marked on the tube side of the grid. The radiographer has to merely look at the grid to know which surface needs to face the tube.

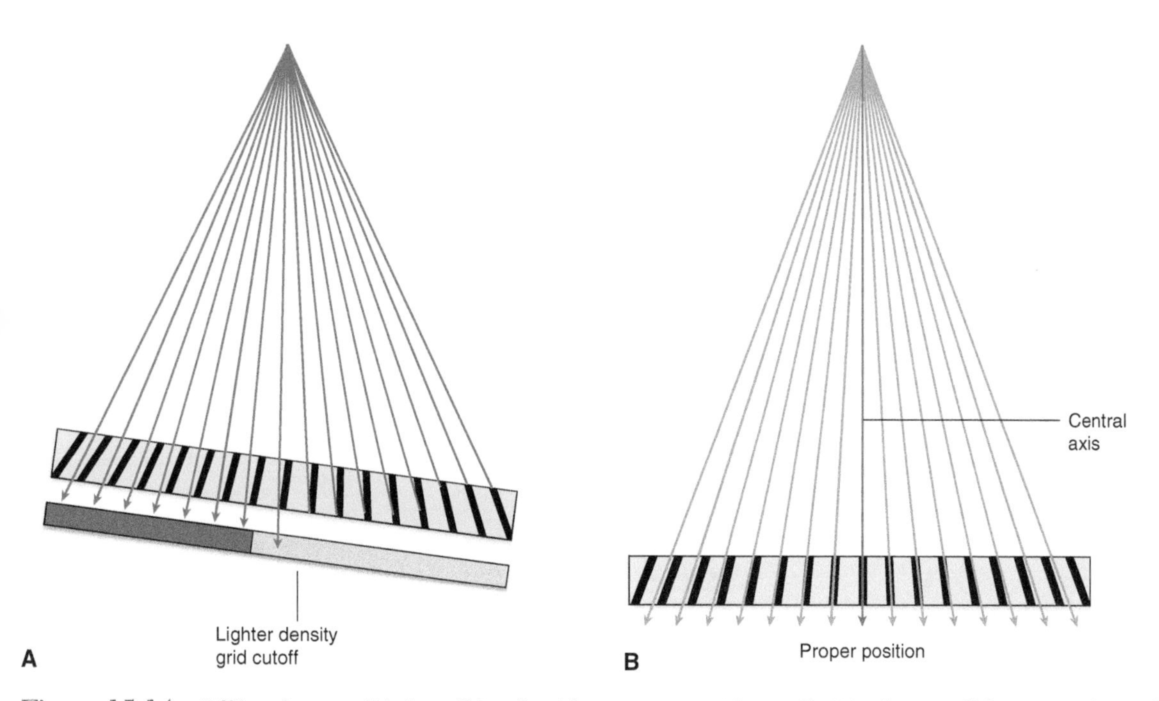

Figure 15.14. Off-level error. (A) An off-level grid can cause grid cutoff. (B) There will be no grid cutoff when the grid is perpendicular to the central axis of the beam.

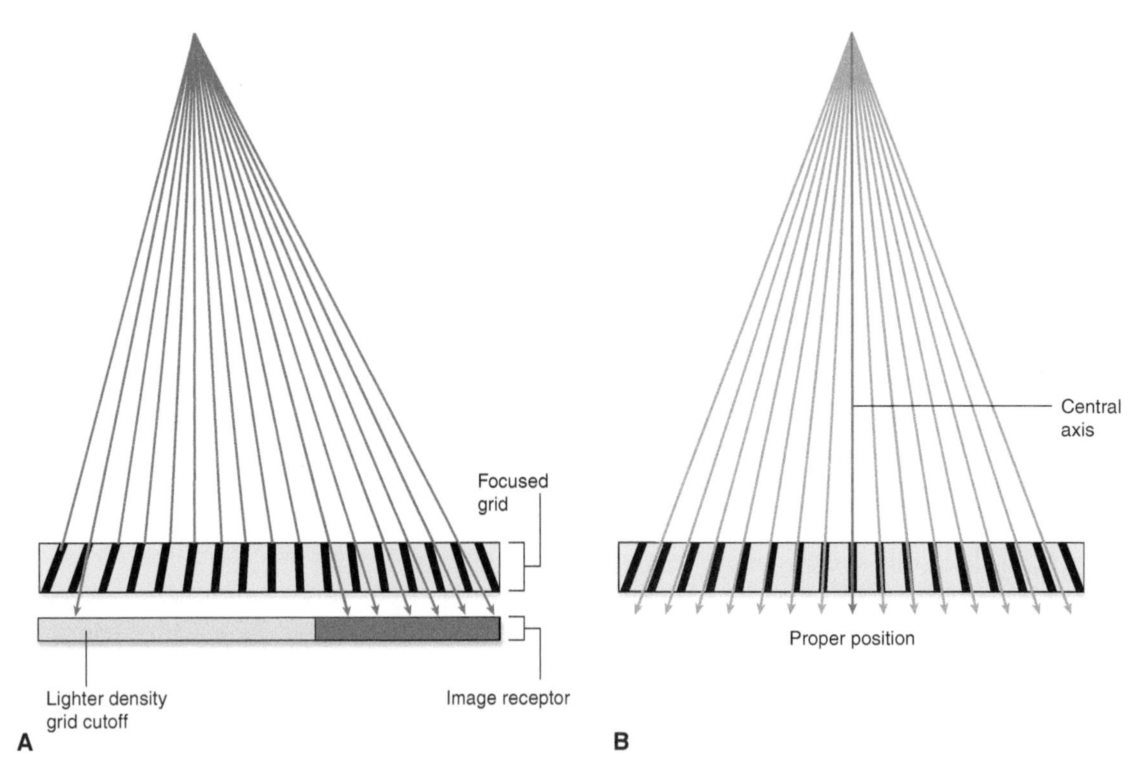

Figure 15.15. Off-center error. (A) Centering to one side of a focused grid can cause grid cutoff. (B) There will be no off-center error when the grid is perpendicular to the central axis of the beam.

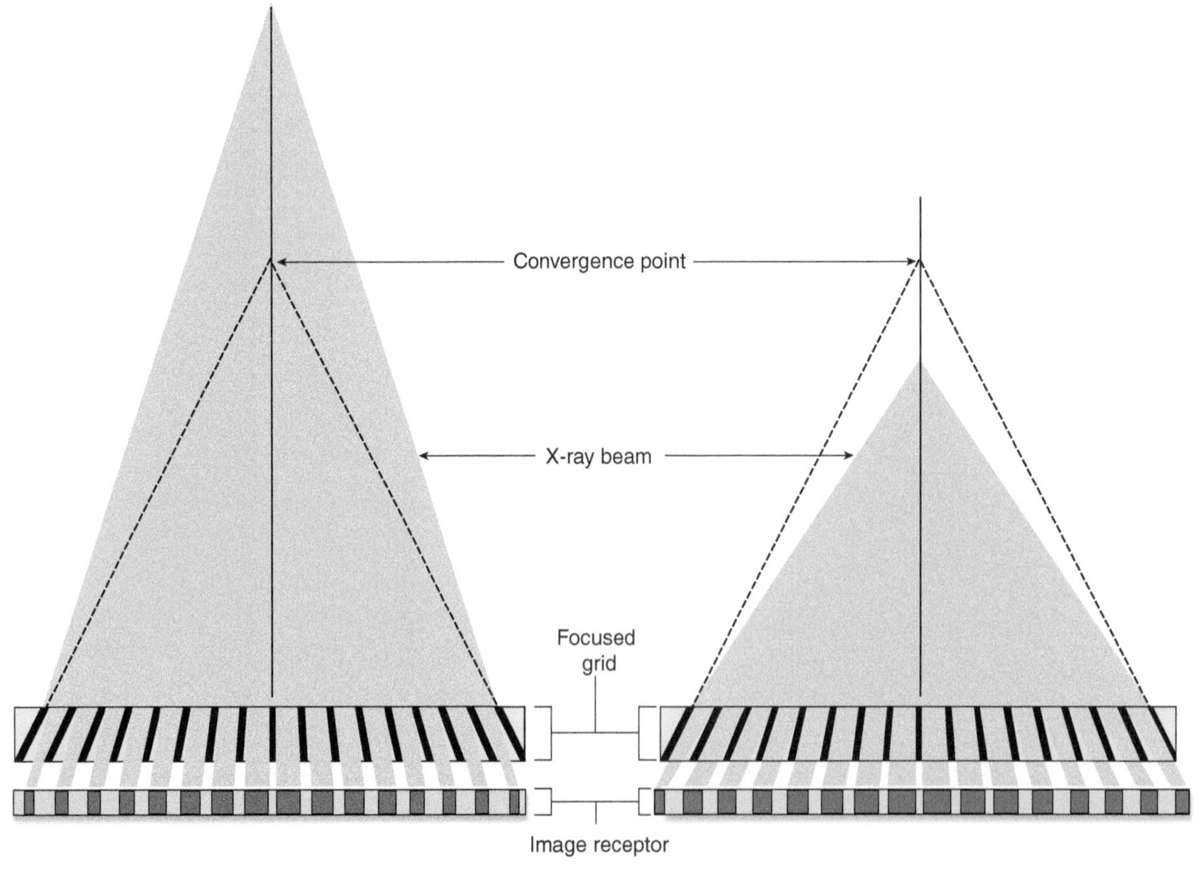

Figure 15.16. Off-focus error. (A) When the x-ray beam is outside the convergence, point grid cutoff occurs. (B) No grid cutoff will occur when the x-ray beam is within the convergence point.

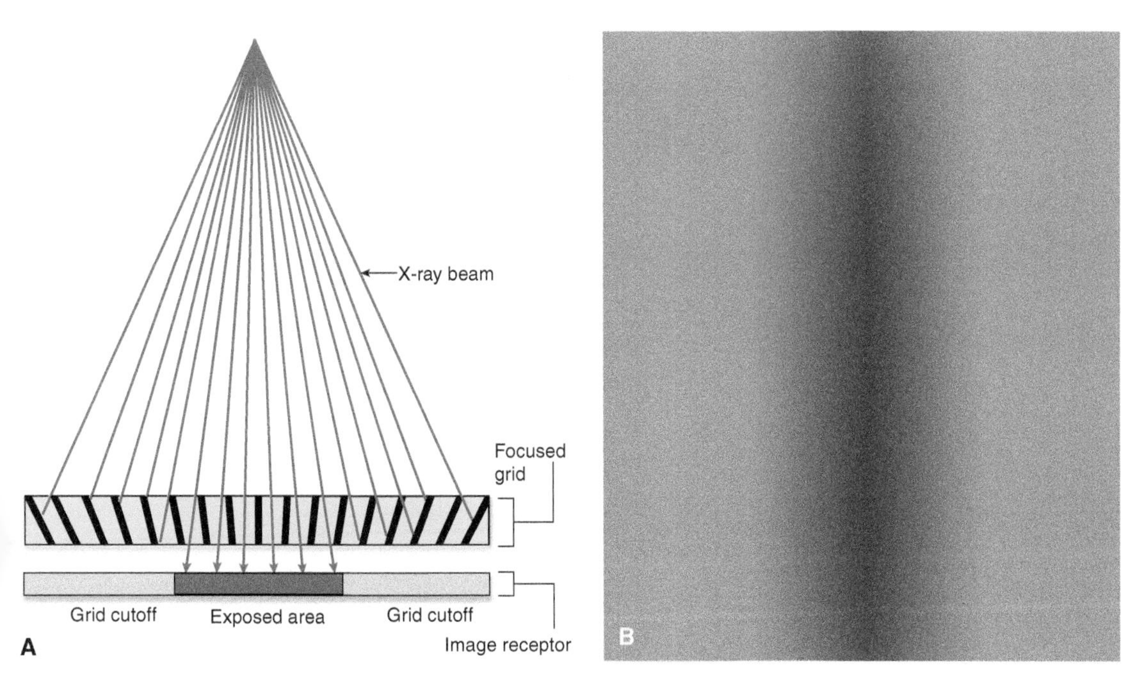

Figure 15.17. **Upside-down error. (A) Diagram of upside-down error. (B) A radiographic image demonstrating upside-down grid error.**

Table 15.2 presents the appearance of different forms of grid cutoff and the possible causes.

Alternative Method to Reduce Scatter

Air Gap Technique

The **air gap technique** is an alternate scatter reduction method and can be used instead of a grid. The air gap technique uses an increased OID to reduce scatter reaching the image receptor. This technique is used in lateral C-spine and chest radiographs. Remember that the patient is the source of scatter and the increased OID causes much of the scattered radiation to miss the image receptor. This eliminates the need for using a grid to reduce scatter and to improve the contrast of the image. A major disadvantage of the air gap technique is the loss of sharpness, which results from the increased OID. The air does NOT filter out the scattered x-rays.

An OID of at least 6 in is required for effective scatter reduction with the air gap technique (Fig. 15.18). When the

TABLE 15.2 **GRID ARTIFACT APPEARANCES AND THEIR POSSIBLE CHANGES**

Optical Density	Possible Causes
Correct density in the center, lower density on both sides of image	Parallel grid at too short SID Upside-down focused grid Focused grid outside focal distance range
Correct density in the center and on one side, low density on one side	Grid center not aligned with central axis Grid not perpendicular to central axis

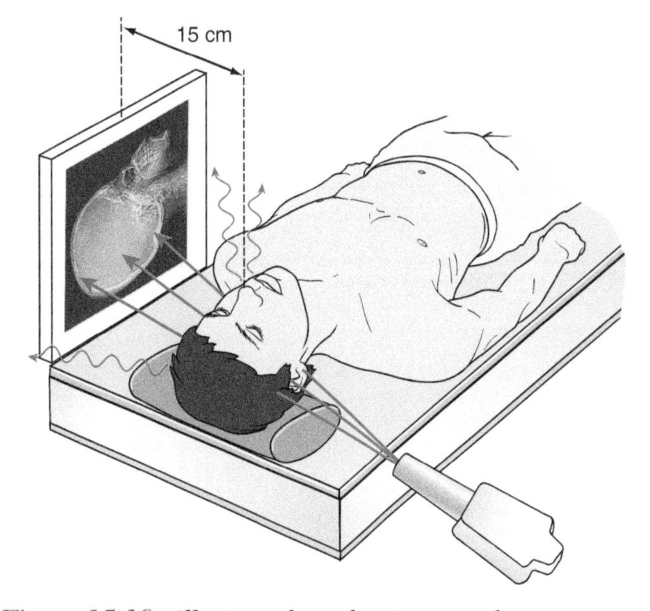

Figure 15.18. **Illustrates how the air gap technique reduces scatter.**

OID is increased, there is an increase in magnification and a reduction in detail. To compensate for this, a longer SID is utilized with a small focal spot size. Because of the longer SID, the mAs must be increased to maintain radiographic density. The patient dose does not increase because the intensity of the x-ray beam will decrease with the longer SID.

Chapter Summary

1. Radiation leaving the patient is a combination of transmitted and scatter radiation.
2. Scatter radiation decreases contrast and its production depends on field size, patient thickness, beam energy, or kVp.
3. The primary methods of scatter reduction are reduction in field size and the use of a grid.
4. In special applications, such as C-spine imaging, an air gap can be used to reduce scatter.
5. Grids are constructed of alternating strips of a radiopaque material such as lead and a radiolucent material such as aluminum or plastic.
6. Using a grid with a higher grid ratio increases the patient dose, increases the Bucky factor, increases the film contrast, and requires an increase in mAs.
7. The Bucky factor is the ratio of mAs with the grid to mAs without the grid.
8. High grid ratios are not used in portable imaging because the alignment is very critical.
9. The types of grid errors include off-center, off-level, off-focus, and placing the grid upside down. These errors can be avoided when the radiographer properly centers the tube with the Bucky and places the cassette properly with the tube side of the cassette toward the patient.

Case Study

Todd performed a portable abdominal radiograph using a 40-inch SID, 5:1 grid, 85 kVp, and 20 mAs. Upon reviewing the image, Todd noticed that the overall appearance of the anatomy was not what he expected. The image lacked sufficient contrast and had a very long scale of gray, which obscured some anatomy. There also appeared to be less density over the whole image than what he expected, and the spine was not in the middle of the image. Todd determined that the image would need to be repeated, but first he had to decide the factors that would need to be changed to produce a diagnostic image.

Critical Thinking Questions

1. Did Todd use the correct grid ratio for the technical factors he used?
2. With a higher kVp exam, should Todd have used a high-ratio grid?
3. If a change in grid ratio is determined, what will the new mAs be?
4. How will Todd address the placement of the spine in the image and how does this relate to the overall decrease in density on the image?

Review Questions

Multiple Choice

1. **Exit radiation consists of:**

   a. transmitted radiation
   b. scattered radiation
   c. transmitted plus scattered radiation
   d. transmitted minus scattered radiation

2. **Increasing the field size will __________ the amount of scatter.**

   a. increase
   b. decrease

3. **A grid is made of:**

   a. alternating strips of aluminum and plastic
   b. alternating strips of lead and plastic
   c. alternating strips of copper and plastic
   d. alternating strips of paper and plastic

4. **The number of lead strips per centimeter is called the:**

   a. Bucky factor
   b. grid ratio
   c. grid frequency
   d. grid focal factor

5. **An increase in patient thickness will increase the amount of scatter.**

   a. True
   b. False

6. **What is the grid ratio for a grid made with 20 µm of lead between 437 µm of aluminum interspace material at a height of 3.5 mm?**

   a. 12:1
   b. 8:1
   c. 5:1
   d. 16:1

7. **Which type of grid error occurs when the grid is not perpendicular to the x-ray tube?**

   a. Off-center
   b. Off-focus
   c. Upside-down
   d. Off-level

8. **Which type of tissue will attenuate more photons and create less scatter?**

   a. Soft tissue.
   b. Adipose tissue.
   c. Bone.
   d. All tissue creates the same amount of scatter.

9. **A __________ grid has lead strips and interspace material that run parallel to each other.**

   a. focused
   b. linear

10. **High-frequency grids __________ patient dose and typically have a __________ grid ratio.**

    a. increase, higher
    b. decrease, higher
    c. decrease, lower
    d. increase, lower

11. **Which material is preferred for the radiopaque grid strips?**

    a. Gold foil
    b. Platinum foil
    c. Lead foil
    d. Manganese

Short Answer

1. How does a grid improve contrast?

2. A grid should be used when which general rule is applied?

3. Gustave Bucky's original grid was a __________ grid.

4. Explain why lead is used as the grid strip material.

5. What is the advantage of a moving grid?

6. Explain how the air gap technique improves contrast.

7. As the ability of a grid to clean up scatter improves, what is the effect on patient dose?

8. How does scatter radiation affect contrast?

9. What is the difference in the Bucky factor between a nongrid and a 16:1? Refer to Table 12.1.

10. Explain the differences between a reciprocating and oscillating grid.

16

Radiographic Film and Processing

Objectives

Upon completion of this chapter, the student will be able to:

1. Discuss the components of a radiographic film.
2. Identify the stages of image formation.
3. Identify the stages in film processing.
4. List the components and describe the operation of automatic film processors.
5. Describe the purpose and construction of intensifying screens.
6. Describe the characteristics of intensifying earth screens.
7. Identify the factors that affect screen speed and spatial resolution.
8. Explain the construction of cassettes and how to care for cassettes.

Key Terms

- activator
- base
- clearing agent
- conversion efficiency
- crossover effect
- crossover network
- developing
- drive system
- emulsion layer
- film contrast
- film speed
- fixing
- fluorescence
- Gurney-Mott theory
- hardener
- hydroquinone
- intensifying screens
- latent image
- latitude
- luminescence
- orthochromatic
- panchromatic
- phenidone
- phosphor layer
- phosphorescence
- preservative
- protective coat
- rare-earth screens
- reflective layer
- restrainer
- sensitivity speck
- solvent
- spatial resolution
- transport racks
- transport system

Introduction

In this chapter, we address the composition of an x-ray film, the formation of the latent image, the image receptor, and the visible image. The exit radiation, which leaves the patient, carries the anatomic information of the part the x-ray beam has passed through. The exit radiation carries both the scattered x-rays moving away from the image receptor and the image-forming x-rays. In order to visualize the information, the exit radiation must interact with radiographic film and intensifying screens. The intensifying screens emit visible light, which exposes the radiographic film placed between the two intensifying screens. At this point, the radiographic film has been exposed and contains the latent image. The final step is to process the radiographic film so that the image can be seen. It is important for students to understand the concepts and processes involved in the creation of a radiographic image.

Film Construction

Photography and photographic film have been around since the early 19th century. The construction and characteristics of photographic film were the basis for designing and manufacturing radiographic film for medical imaging. Radiographic film is manufactured in a precise procedure unique to the manufacturer. Manufacturing facilities are kept meticulously clean to avoid contaminants on the film. These contaminants have the potential of fogging the film and degrading the image. Manufacturers designed radiographic film to image all the various body regions and in doing so found it necessary to match the size of the film to the anatomic area. Across the industry, the wide range of film sizes became standardized and the measurements were either in centimeters or inches. Table 16.1 lists the standardized film and corresponding cassette sizes. Radiographic film and cassettes are called an image receptor (IR), and the terms are used interchangeably.

Radiographic film is composed of a layer of emulsion applied to one or both sides of a transparent polyester plastic **base**. A single-emulsion film has the emulsion applied to one side where a double-emulsion film has the emulsion applied to both sides. The emulsion is attached to the polyester base by a thin layer of transparent adhesive. The adhesive layer provides uniform adhesion of the emulsion to the base. The adhesive layer maintains the contact between the emulsion and base during handling and processing. The soft emulsion layer is covered by a supercoat of hard gelatin. The supercoat layer protects the emulsion from scratching, pressure, and contamination during storage, loading, and handling (Fig. 16.1).

Base

The polyester base provides support for the emulsion. The primary purpose of the base is to provide a rigid yet flexible structure for the emulsion to be adhered to. It is

TABLE 16.1 STANDARD CASSETTE SIZES

Sizes in Centimeters (cm)	Sizes in Inches
18 × 24	8 × 10
24 × 30	10 × 12
28 × 35	11 × 14
35 × 43	14 × 17

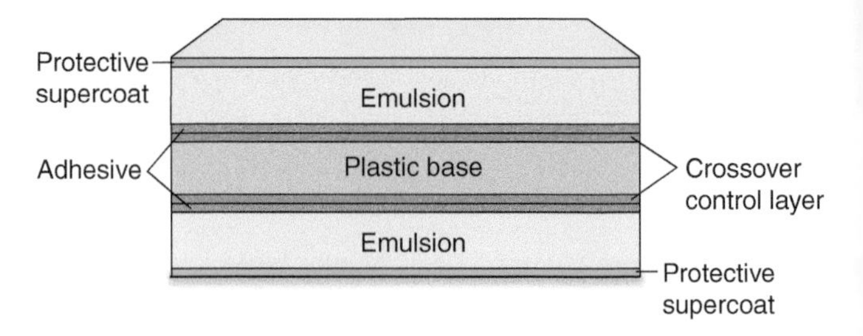

Figure 16.1. **Shows a cross section of a typical double-emulsion film.**

constructed from polyester plastic ~175 μm thick. The base layer is strong and flexible and has uniform lucency, which makes the base layer transparent, and there is no underlying pattern on the base, that would cause artifact on the image. The base is tinted blue to reduce viewer eyestrain and fatigue when the film is hung on a view box or illuminator. The film base is also coated with a substance to prevent light photons from one screen crossing over to the other screen. This reflection of light photons is called the **crossover effect**, causing blurring of the image.

Emulsion Layer

The **emulsion layer** is the material that x-ray or light photons interact with. The emulsion layer is made up of silver halide crystals uniformly distributed in a clear gelatin. The emulsion layer thickness ranges from 3 to 5 μm. The gelatin is clear and transmits light while being porous for the processing chemicals to penetrate to the silver halide crystals. The gelatin holds the silver halide crystals in place and acts as a neutral lucent suspension medium that separates the silver halide crystals. Gelatin distributes the silver halide crystals uniformly over the base, preventing the crystals from clumping and causing excessive photosensitivity in one area. Other necessary properties of the gelatin include it being clear to permit light to travel through it without interference, and it must be flexible enough to bend without causing distortion to the recorded image.

Each silver halide crystal is made up of silver, bromine, and iodide atoms in a crystal lattice. Although each manufacturer has an exact formula, the typical emulsion consists of 98% silver bromide, with the remainder consisting of silver iodide. The gelatin and base have a low atomic number ($Z = 7$), while silver halide crystals have high atomic numbers ($Z_{BR} = 35$, $Z_{AG} = 47$, $Z_{I} = 53$). The interaction between the x-ray or light photons and the high Z atoms results in the formation of the latent image on the radiographic film.

The silver halide crystals may have tabular, cubic, octahedral, polyhedral, or irregular shapes; the exact shape used is determined by the imaging application. Most radiographic film uses tabular grains, which are arranged in the crystal in a cubic pattern.

The silver halide crystals are made by dissolving metallic silver in nitric acid to form silver nitrate, which is then combined with light-sensitive silver bromide. This process takes place in the gelatin and is precisely controlled for temperature, pressure, and the rate of mixture.

The silver ion is positive because it has one electron missing from its outer shell. The bromine and iodine ions are negative because they have an extra electron in their outer shells. The presence of bromine and iodine ions in the crystal results in a negative charge on the crystal surface.

Impurities are added to the silver halide crystals to form a **sensitivity speck**. The sensitivity speck provides film sensitivity, and during processing of the radiographic image, the silver atoms are attracted to and concentrate at the location of the sensitivity speck. Changing the size and mixture of the silver halide crystals changes the response characteristics of the film. Films with larger crystals generally are faster—that is, they are more sensitive to radiation and light—than films with smaller crystals. As seen in Table 16.2, the relationships between crystal size and emulsion layer thickness directly affect the contrast, **spatial resolution**, and speed of the imaging system.

Latent Image Formation

When the remnant radiation exits the patient, it strikes the radiographic film and deposits energy into the silver halide crystals. The energy is deposited in a pattern that represents the part of the anatomy being radiographed; at this point, the image is not visible and is called a **latent image**. The **Gurney-Mott theory** indicates that x-rays and light photons from the intensifying screens cause ionization of the atoms in the crystal. The free electrons resulting from the ionization are attracted to the sensitivity speck. The collection of negative electrons at the sensitivity speck attracts positive silver ions (Ag^+), where they are neutralized to form silver atoms. When silver atoms collect at the sensitivity speck, the charge structure outside the crystal is altered and the exposed crystal becomes part of the latent image. Figure 16.2 illustrates the migration of silver ions to the sensitivity speck where they form silver atoms, altering the charge pattern of the silver halide crystal. The latent image is the distribution of exposed and unexposed crystals in the undeveloped emulsion, caused by differential absorption in the patient. The radiographic film containing the latent image must be processed to make the image visible. Processing converts the silver ions in the exposed crystals to black metallic silver, and the unexposed crystals remain crystalline and inactive, thereby making the radiographic image visible or manifest.

Types of Film

In medical imaging, there are various types of film, each used for a specific purpose. Screen film is the most commonly used film in radiography. There are several characteristics that must be considered when choosing the combination of screen film and intensifying screens. These characteristics include speed, crossover, contrast, spectral matching, and requirements for a safelight.

Screen film can be either single emulsion or double emulsion. A single-emulsion film has emulsion on only one side of the polyester film base. Single-emulsion film is processed in the same manner as double-emulsion

TABLE 16.2 **RELATIONSHIP OF CRYSTAL SIZE AND EMULSION TO FILM FACTORS**

	Crystal Size		Emulsion Layer	
	Small	Large	Thin	Thick
Speed	Slow	Fast	Slow	Fast
Resolution	High	Low	High	Low

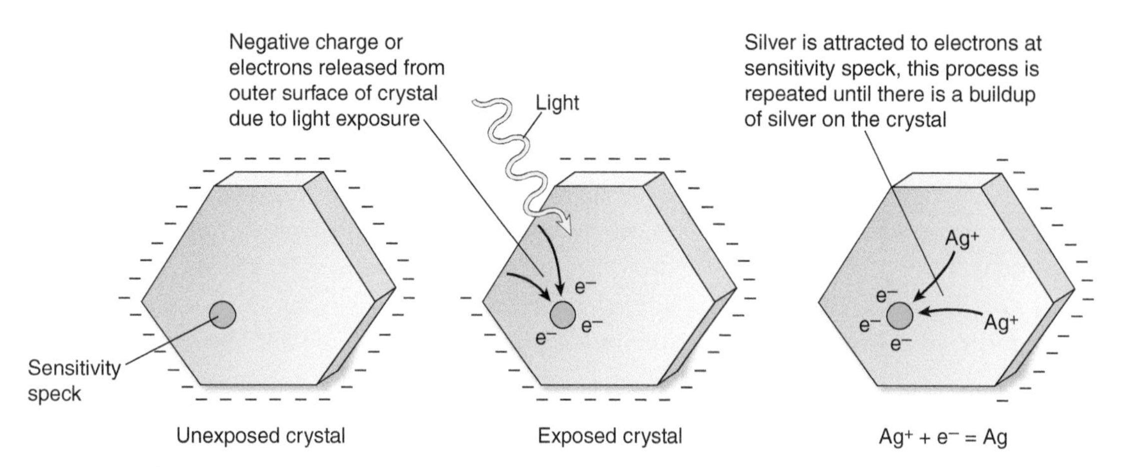

Figure 16.2. **The charge patterns surrounding silver halide crystals in the emulsion are changed after exposure.**

film. It provides better resolution than does double-emulsion film because with double-emulsion film, the images from the two sides are not exactly superimposed unless they are viewed directly head on, whereas with single-emulsion film, the image is on only one side of the base, and therefore, small objects and sharp edges are not blurred as much.

Double-emulsion screen films are designed to optimize speed. The double-emulsion films are placed between two screens, which effectively exposes both sides of the film at the same time, which increases the efficiency of the interactions in the silver halide crystals. This produces twice the speed of the screen film. The speed of the film also depends upon the different film emulsions and intensifying screen phosphors. The speed is directly related to the degree of sensitivity of the screen film combination to x-rays and light. To accurately image the areas of the body, manufacturers provide a variety of IRs with different configurations of film emulsion and different types of phosphors in the intensifying screens. To optimize the speed, the speed of the film and intensifying screens must match. When there is a mismatch in speed of the film with the intensifying screens, a significant exposure error can occur.

During the exposure, there is a possibility that light from one intensifying screen will pass through the emulsion and film base to expose the opposite emulsion. Such "crossover" light is spread out and reduces the sharpness of the image. Current emulsions have tabular silver halide crystals, which are flat and provide a larger surface area. The tabular shape reduces crossover because the shape improves the efficiency of the silver in the emulsion. Light absorption from the screen is increased but the light transmitted through the emulsion is reduced. To further reduce crossover, a crossover control layer is placed between the emulsion and base. The crossover control layer consists of a light-absorbing additive that reduces the crossover effect to near zero. The crossover layer accomplishes three critical tasks: it absorbs most of the crossover light; it is a separate layer, which does not combine with the emulsion layer; and it is completely removed during processing.

Screen film is offered with multiple levels of contrast. The contrast in the IR is inversely proportional to the exposure **latitude**. As discussed earlier, latitude is the range of exposure techniques that result in a diagnostic image. The contrast of a screen film is considered medium, high, or higher. The difference in contrast depends on the size and distribution of the silver halide crystals. The high-contrast film has smaller silver halide crystals, while the low-contrast films have larger crystals.

Spectral matching is an important consideration when selecting film with the absorption characteristics. The silver halide crystals are designed to be sensitive to different wavelengths or colors of light emitted from the screen. Calcium tungstate screens emit blue and blue-violet light and are matched to film that is sensitive to blue wavelengths or light. In the early 1970s, **rare-earth screens** were introduced; many rare-earth phosphors emit ultraviolet, blue, green, and red. Silver halide films respond to violet and blue light but not to green, yellow, or red unless spectral dyes are added to the emulsion. Green-sensitive, or **orthochromatic**, film is sensitive to green and blue light. These films are matched to the spectrum of light emitted from the intensifying screens. The construction and application of intensifying screens are covered later in the chapter.

Radiographic film is designed to be sensitive to light from the intensifying screens. It is also sensitive to visible light and will fog if it is exposed to room lights. Because of this, radiographic film is manufactured to total darkness from the beginning where the emulsion components are brought together until the film is packaged. At the imaging facility, the radiographer must take special precautions to handle the film and load it into the cassette in the darkroom. Darkrooms are designed to keep all white light out so the film does not become fogged prior to use. In order for the radiographer to "see" in the darkroom, it is equipped with safelights. Safelights are designed to filter out light that is energetic enough to expose the film. Blue-sensitive film is not sensitive to amber light, so an amber safelight filter is used with blue-sensitive film. Green-sensitive, or orthochromatic, film is sensitive to an amber safelight and therefore requires a special deep red safelight filter such as a GBX filter (Fig. 16.3).

It is possible to identify the emulsion side, even in the darkroom under safelights, because light reflection makes the emulsion side appear dull and the base side appear shiny. The manufacturers place notches on one edge of single-emulsion film to aid in identification of the emulsion side in the dark. When the film is positioned with the notches at the upper right corner of the film, the emulsion is facing up. It is important to have the emulsion side of single-emulsion film facing the intensifying screen, which is the light source. If the film is facing backward, the image will be blurred because the light must pass through the base before reaching the emulsion.

Hard Copy, Laser Printer, or Multiformat Film

Hard copy film is used to provide a permanent record of an electronically displayed image. Digital images from computed tomography, ultrasound, nuclear medicine, or magnetic resonance imaging units are initially presented on monitors or on electronic "soft" displays, and only certain images are selected for the permanent hard copy record. Hard copies can be produced by a laser printer or a multiformat camera. In a laser printer, the intensity of the laser beam depends upon the strength of the electronic image signal in a process called laser beam modulation. While the beam is modulated, the laser beam writes in a raster fashion over the entire film. The spatial resolution of the laser printer is superior to that of the multiformat camera. The number of images on one film, known as the image format, can be selected by the technologist. Typical image formats are 4, 6, or 12 images on one film.

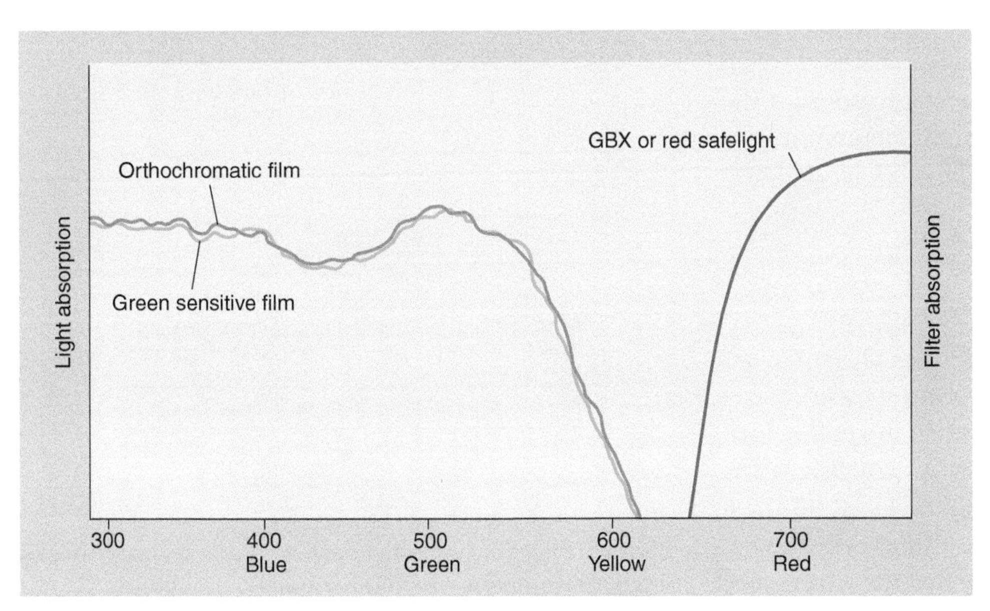

Figure 16.3. Safelight curves for different types of film.

Film Storage and Handling

Film is very sensitive to storage and handling conditions. Improper storage or handling can produce fog or artifacts. Fog is an increase in density on areas of the film. Artifacts are unwanted local densities on the final image. Radiographic film is sensitive to light, temperature, humidity, radiation, and improper handling. Exposed but undeveloped film is much more sensitive to radiation than unexposed film.

Temperature, Humidity, and Storage

Film should be stored in a cool, dry place with a temperature <68°F and with <60% relative humidity. Storage under heat conditions above 75°F will increase the fog and decrease the image contrast. Storage under conditions of low humidity, less than about 40%, will increase static artifacts.

Storage of film should not be longer than the expiration date on the box of film. Forty-five days should be the average storage time. Film must be stored in a climate-controlled environment. Film boxes must be carefully opened, and the film and cardboard insert should be removed carefully to avoid abrasion artifacts.

Radiation

Film must be shielded from radiation exposure. Even a few milliroentgens will produce a noticeable increase in fog on the film. Exposure to scattered radiation in fluoroscopy rooms is a possible source of radiation fog. To decrease the chance of unwanted radiation exposure, the film bin is lined with lead, and the darkroom must have lead shielding in the walls if the darkroom is located next to a radiographic room.

Improper Handling of Film

Unexposed film is sensitive to shock, pressure, and improper handling. Dropping a box of unexposed film can cause artifacts on the edge or corner that strikes the floor. The sensitivity of film to pressure can be demonstrated by placing a piece of paper over an undeveloped film and writing on the paper. The pressure of the pen through the paper will alter the emulsion so that the writing will show after the film is developed. Hands need to be clean and free from lotions or creams prior to handling film. Creams and oils from the hands cause fingerprint artifacts on the film emulsion. Film boxes should always be stored on end to avoid abrasion and pressure artifacts. Rough handling can cause crease densities to appear on the developed film. Rapid removal of unexposed film from the storage box can produce static artifacts.

Intensifying Screens

The purpose of an **intensifying screen** is to increase the efficiency of x-ray absorption and decrease the dose to the patient. An intensifying screen converts a single x-ray photon into thousands of lower energy light photons that interact more efficiently with the image receptor. The conversion of x-ray energy into light energy reduces the amount of radiation required to produce an acceptable image. Most x-ray photons that pass through a 30-cm-thick patient have no trouble passing through the image receptor a few millimeters thick. Only about 1% of the interactions in the image receptor are produced directly by x-ray photons; the other 99% result from intensifying screen light. This light is produced when an x-ray photon interacts with the phosphor crystals in the screen (Fig. 16.4).

The intensifying screens are typically used in pairs and are mounted inside the top and bottom of a lightproof cassette. In a standard x-ray cassette, the film is held in a lightproof cassette, while in a direct imaging or CR system, a detector plate is in close contact with the intensifying screens (Fig. 16.5).

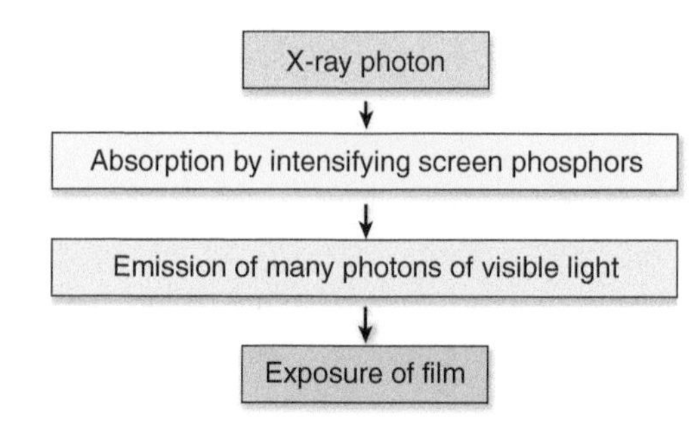

Figure 16.4. Illustrates the steps involved in converting a single x-ray photon into many visible-light photons.

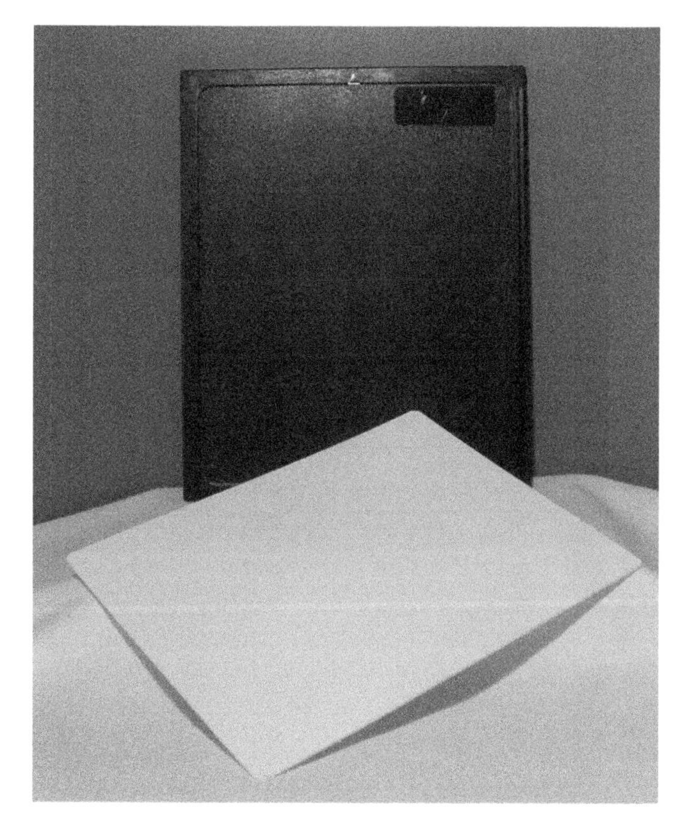

Figure 16.5. **Shows a CR cassette with the detector located next to its intensifying screens.**

Intensifying Screen Construction

thePoint® *An animation for this topic can be viewed at http://thepoint.lww.com/Orth2e*

An intensifying screen consists of a plastic base supporting a reflective layer, a phosphor layer, and a protective coat (Fig. 16.6).

- Base
- Reflective layer
- Phosphor layer
- Protective coat

Base

A 1-mm-thick polyester plastic screen base provides support for the other components of the screen. It is flexible yet tough, rigid, and chemically inert and is uniformly

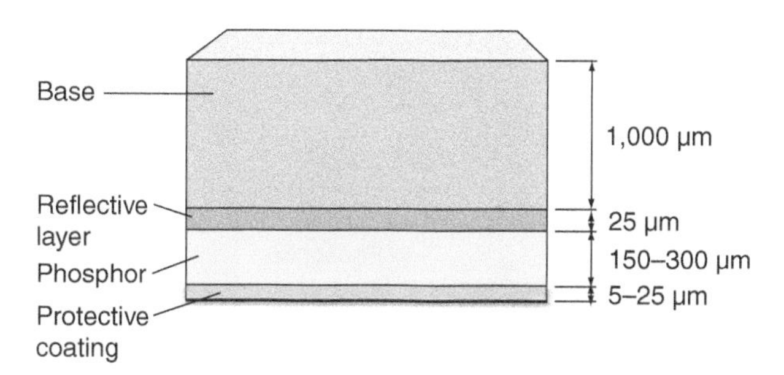

Figure 16.6. **Illustrates the construction of a typical intensifying screen.**

radiolucent. The base must be flexible enough to fit snugly when sandwiched between the top and bottom of the cassette. It is necessary for the base to be chemically inert so that it will not react with the **phosphor layer** or interfere with the conversion of x-ray photons to light photons. The base material must also be uniformly radiolucent to allow the transmission of x-ray photons without causing artifacts to the image.

Reflective Layer

The **reflective layer** is made up of a special reflective material such as magnesium oxide or titanium dioxide that is ~25 µm thick. The screen phosphor crystals emit light with equal intensity in all directions upon interaction with an x-ray photon. Less than half the light produced by the screen phosphor crystals is directed toward the film. The reflective layer redirects the light from the phosphor toward the film, thereby increasing the efficiency of the intensifying screen (Fig. 16.7). Some intensifying screens use dyes to selectively absorb the diverging light photons that have a longer wavelength, which reduces image sharpness.

Phosphor Layer

The active layer of the intensifying screen is the phosphor layer, which is made up of crystals embedded in a clear plastic support layer. The phosphor crystals convert incident x-ray photons into visible-light photons. The phosphor layer varies from 50 to 300 µm, depending on the speed and resolving power of the screen. Prior to 1980 calcium, tungstate was embedded in a polymer matrix in the screen. The rare-earth screens use the elements of gadolinium, lanthanum, and yttrium. The phosphor action can be seen by placing an open cassette on a radiographic table and exposing the intensifying screen to x-rays. As long as the x-ray beam is on, the phosphors will glow and emit light.

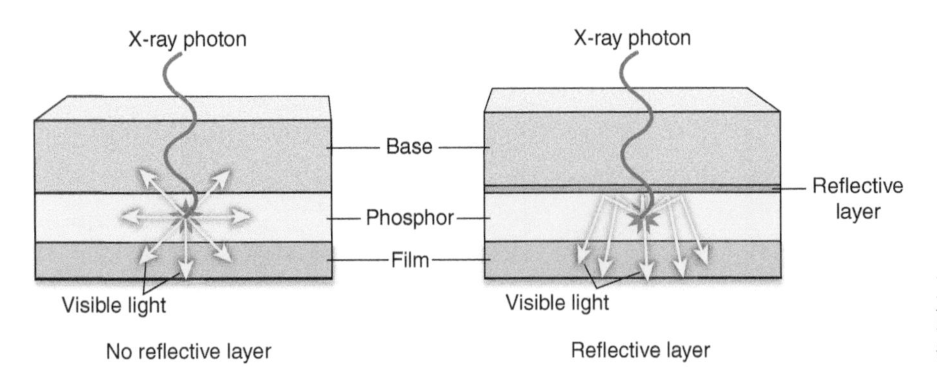

Figure 16.7. Shows how the reflective layer redirects screen light back toward the film.

At the time Roentgen made his discovery of the invisible rays, he noticed that barium platinocyanide glowed when the x-rays were being emitted. American inventor Thomas A. Edison developed calcium tungstate to use during his experiments with x-rays. He also is the first to use intensifying screens, but the common practice of using the screens didn't occur until much later. As manufacturers improved their techniques and processes, calcium tungstate proved to be a superior phosphor and was used in nearly all screens. As with screen film, the 1970s brought a change to screens with the use of rare-earth phosphors. Using spectral matching with the film and screens resulted in lower patient dose.

The material, size, and distribution of the phosphor crystals and the thickness of the phosphor layer determine the speed and resolution of the intensifying screen. There is a trade-off between speed, patient dose, and resolution. Thicker screens have higher speed and require lower patient dose but have poorer spatial resolution. Different film screen combinations are chosen for different clinical applications.

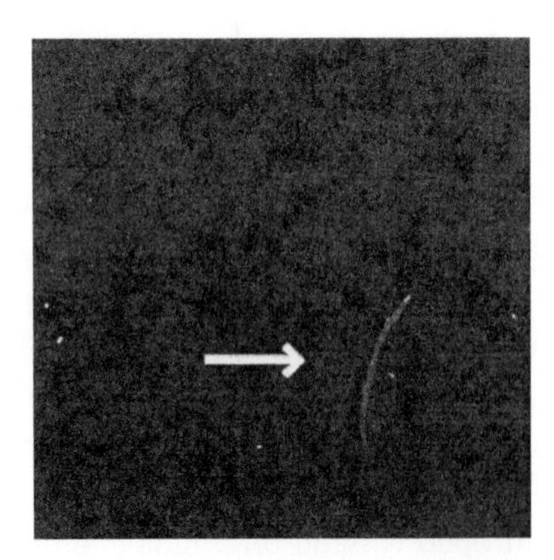

Figure 16.8. The arrow is pointing to an artifact produced by a scratch on the intensifying screen.

Protective Coat

The **protective coat** is the layer that is closest to the screen film. The protective coat is a thin plastic layer 10 to 20 μm thick that protects the phosphor layer from abrasion. It also helps to eliminate the buildup of static electricity. The protective layer cannot withstand scratches from fingernails, rings, or hard objects. As seen in Figure 16.8, scratches that remove the protective layer also remove the phosphor layer producing white, negative density artifacts. The protective layer provides a surface for routine cleaning and protects the active phosphor from the cleaning chemicals. The protective coat is transparent to light.

Phosphor Materials

The primary characteristics of phosphor materials that are important to radiography are

- Atomic number
- Conversion efficiency
- Luminescence

Atomic Number

Intensifying screens are made of higher atomic number (higher Z) phosphors to increase x-ray interaction. Historically, several different phosphors have been used: calcium tungstate, zinc sulfide, and barium lead sulfate in addition to the rare-earth phosphors of gadolinium, lanthanum, and yttrium. Approximately 5,000 light photons are produced by each x-ray photon absorbed by the phosphor crystal. To permit photoelectric and Compton interactions, the phosphor must have a high atomic number.

Conversion Efficiency

The number of light photons produced by one x-ray photon is described by the **conversion efficiency**. It is a measure of the screen's efficiency in converting x-ray energy into light energy. As the conversion efficiency increases, the radiation dose to the patient decreases.

Luminescence

Luminescence is the ability of a material to emit light in response to excitation. Luminescent materials will emit light with a wavelength that is specific to that particular luminescent material. The result is light emission of a specific characteristic color. There are two mechanisms that produce light, **fluorescence** and **phosphorescence**. Fluorescence is the production of light during the stimulation of the phosphor by the x-ray photons. Fluorescence is an instantaneous emission of light. Phosphorescence is the continuation of light emission after the stimulation ceases. Most of the light output from intensifying screens is due to fluorescence. Delayed phosphorescence creates screen lag or afterglow and becomes increasingly more pronounced as the phosphor ages.

Screen Speed

Screen speed or sensitivity is a term used to describe how much light is obtained from a given x-ray exposure. Screen speeds range from 50, which are slow and used for detail, to 1,200, which are very fast. Standard speed is set as a speed of 100 for historical reasons. The speed is controlled by phosphor size, layer thickness, kVp, and temperature. An increase in phosphor size and layer thickness will also increase the screen speed. When kVp is increased, the screen speed will also be increased. Intensifying screen phosphors have a high atomic number, so increasing kVp will increase the likelihood of light producing interactions within the phosphors. Increases in temperature can cause a significant decrease in screen speed, especially in hot climates.

Types of Screens

Film/screen systems range in speeds from 50 to 1,200. There are three types of screens: detail, medium or par speed, and high speed. Detailed screens, valued at 50 to 80, are used for higher-resolution imaging, such as extremity examinations. Medium- or par-speed screens, valued at 100, are used for routine imaging. High-speed screens, valued at 200 to 1,200, are used for examinations that require short exposure times. A chest x-ray exam is an excellent example of the need for short exposure time because of the difficulty of holding breath for more than a few seconds. Table 16.3 illustrates the screen types and speeds associated with each of the three types of screens. The mAs must be changed to compensate for a change in screen speed. The amount of change is given by the ratio of the screen speed:

$$mAs_2 = mAs_1 \left(\frac{\text{old screen speed}}{\text{new screen speed}} \right)$$

where mAs_2 is the new mAs and the mAs_1 is the old or original mAs used.

CRITICAL THINKING BOX 16.1

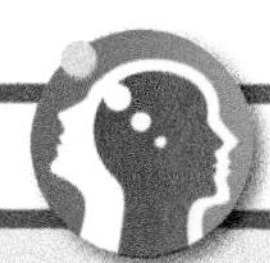

Changing from high-speed to detail screens requires an increase in mAs to maintain the same optical density. As an example, if a 400-speed screen is replaced by a 50-speed screen, if the original mAs was 5 mAs with the 400-speed screen, what is the new mAs for the 50-speed screen?

K-Shell Absorption Edge

Calcium tungstate ($CaWO_4$) screens will absorb ~30% of the incident beam, while rare-earth screens will absorb ~50% to 60%. The percentage varies depending on the keV of the incident beam. Practically all of the absorption takes place during photoelectric absorption. Photoelectric absorption in the screen depends on the x-ray photon energy and the K-shell–binding energy of the specific phosphor material. The K-shell absorption energy refers to the x-ray photon energy just high enough to remove a K-shell electron

TABLE 16.3 SCREEN TYPES AND SPEEDS

Screen Type	Speed
Detail	50
Medium speed	100
High speed	200–1,200

from its orbit. In a $CaWO_4$ screen, the tungsten has an atomic number of 74 and a K-shell–binding energy of 70 keV; therefore, the incident x-ray photon must have energy of at least 70 keV to remove the K-shell electron. When the incident x-ray photon matches the K-shell binding energy, there is a dramatic increase in characteristic photon production, which is called K-shell absorption edge.

The sharp rise in x-ray absorption occurs at the K-edge–binding energy. X-ray energies above the K-shell–binding energy have enough energy to interact with and remove a K-shell electron. X-ray energies below the K-shell–binding energy can only remove L-, M-, or N-shell electrons. If the x-ray energy is above the K-edge, energy absorption is much higher. Rare-earth phosphor materials are chosen because their K-edge energies occur in the diagnostic energy range of 35 to 70 keV. Additionally, rare-earth screens absorb approximately five times more x-ray photons than do the calcium tungstate screens, which correlates to more light being emitted by the rare-earth screens.

Radiographic Noise and Quantum Mottle

Radiographic noise or quantum mottle is the random speckled appearance of an image. It is similar to the "salt and pepper" or "snow" seen with poor TV reception. It is caused by the statistical fluctuations in x-ray interactions. Quantum mottle is noticeable when the number of x-ray photons forming the image is too low. Screens with greater conversion efficiency convert more x-ray photons into light so they require fewer photons and produce images with more noise. Radiographic noise or quantum mottle depends on the number of x-ray photons interacting with the phosphor crystals in the screen. Faster screen images have more image noise because they require fewer x-ray photons to produce the image. The technical factor that influences the amount of image noise or quantum mottle is mAs. The radiographer controls the quantity of the photons with the mAs setting. Increasing the mAs setting will effectively eliminate quantum mottle. Quantum mottle is commonly seen in fluoroscopy due to the low mA settings. The image appears to be very grainy on the monitor. The radiographer can increase kVp, but this often results in lower subject contrast; however, increasing the mA setting and exposure rate will improve the fluoroscopic image.

Spatial Resolution

Spatial resolution is the minimum distance between two objects at which they can be recognized as two separate objects. Spatial resolution is measured using a line pair test pattern and has units of line pairs per millimeter (lp/mm). Spatial resolution of the intensifying screen depends on the thickness of the layer, the phosphor size, and the concentration of the crystals. Intensifying screens with smaller crystals and a thinner layer increase resolution but cause a decrease in screen speed. Thicker layers with larger crystals have poorer spatial resolution because the light spreads sideways and blurs out the edges of an image but increase screen speed (Fig. 16.9). As described, the phosphor crystal size and layer thickness are both inversely related to resolution and directly

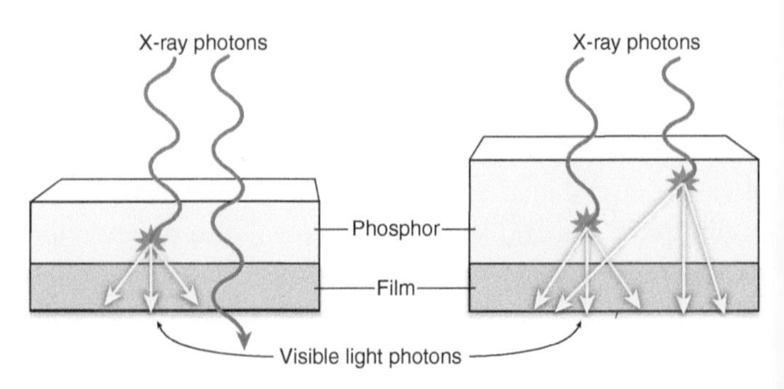

Figure 16.9. Illustrates how thicker screens have poorer spatial resolution.

related to screen speed. Thicker high-speed screens have poorer spatial resolution than do slower-speed screens. A screen with a larger concentration of crystals will have an increase in both spatial resolution and screen speed; therefore, phosphor concentration is directly related to spatial resolution and screen speed.

Spectral Matching

Spectral matching refers to matching the wavelength or color of the light from the screen to the film sensitivity. Figure 16.10 compares the light output from calcium tungstate ($CaWO_4$) and rare-earth screens.

Different screen phosphors emit light of different colors or wavelengths. The response of the film must be matched to the light wavelength of the intensifying screen. There are two classes of intensifying screens, those that emit blue light and those that emit green light. $CaWO_4$ and some rare-earth materials emit blue light. Other rare-earth materials emit green light. There are two general groups of film whose sensitivities are designed to match the light from the different types of intensifying screens. Blue-sensitive, or **panchromatic**, film is used with calcium tungstate and other blue-light–emitting screens. Green-sensitive, or orthochromatic, film is used with green-light–emitting rare-earth–intensifying screens. A mismatch between intensifying screens and film results in reduced efficiency and increased patient dose. Table 16.4 presents representative screen materials, their K-shell absorption edge energy, and the color of light emitted.

TABLE 16.4 SCREEN MATERIALS AND THEIR CHARACTERISTICS

Phosphor Material	K-Edge Energy	Emitted Light Color
Calcium tungstate	70	Blue
Gadolinium	50	Green
Lanthanum	39	Blue
Yttrium	17	Blue

Rare-Earth Screens

The intensifying screens developed by Thomas Edison in the early 1900s used $CaWO_4$ crystals as the phosphor. $CaWO_4$ crystals give off blue light and are 3% to 5% efficient in converting x-ray energy into light (Fig. 16.10). They were in common use until the mid-1970s when rare-earth screens were introduced. Rare-earth screens use elements from the rare-earth section ($Z = 57$ to 70) of the periodic table. Rare-earth elements used in intensifying screens include gadolinium, lanthanum, and yttrium. They are 15% to 20% efficient in converting x-ray energy into light as compared to the calcium tungstate ($CaWO_4$) because their K absorption edges are closer to the average energy of diagnostic x-ray beams.

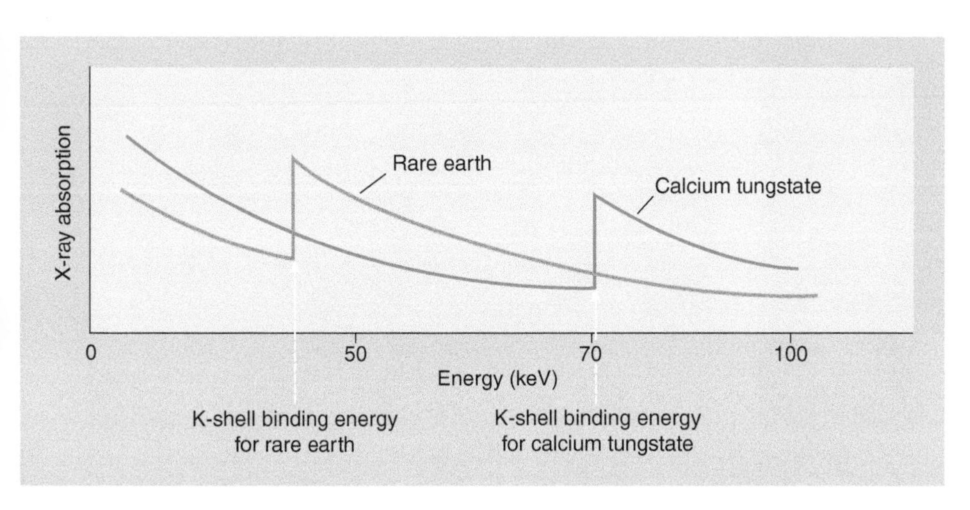

Figure 16.10. Absorption of x-ray photons by calcium tungstate and typical rare-earth screen materials.

Film/Screen Cassettes

Diagnostic films are held inside of film cassettes. A cassette has a pair of intensifying screens glued to the interior front and back. The purpose of the cassette is to provide a lightproof holder for the film. The front side of the cassette is constructed of carbon fiber, which is a low atomic number material that attenuates approximately one-half of the x-rays entering the cassette compared to aluminum cassettes. The cassette also contains a thin layer of lead foil in the back to attenuate exit radiation. For this reason, the tube side is always indicated on the cassette. Film cassettes come in a variety of sizes.

Film/Screen Contact

Poor film/screen contact destroys detail and spatial resolution because the light from the screen diffuses before it reaches the film. Many cassettes have a slight curve on the door side of the cassette so that pressure is applied when the cassette is closed. This extra pressure ensures good film/screen contact. Film/screen contact can be evaluated using the wire mesh test. A screenlike wire mesh embedded in plastic is placed over the film cassette to be tested. After exposure, the film is developed. Any areas of poor film/screen contact will appear as blurred or unsharp areas on the image. Figure 16.11 shows an image of a wire mesh test pattern showing good and poor film/screen contact.

Cassette Care

Every screen cassette has an identification number that appears on every exposed film and can be used to trace artifacts or poor film/screen contact to a particular cassette. For example, a series of fogged films caused by a light leak due to a dropped cassette, or a white area on the film caused by removal of the intensifying phosphor by a scratch on the screen, can be readily traced to the damaged cassette. Screens should be cleaned according to manufacture specifications regularly and whenever artifacts appear on the images. Dirt on the screens will result in white or negative density spots on the image. Areas of darker density are caused by fingernail impressions or scratch marks on the screen.

Automatic Film Processing

thePoint® *An animation for this topic can be viewed at http://thepoint.lww.com/Orth2e*

Processing a film transforms the invisible latent image into a permanent visible image. The visible image is produced by reducing silver ions in the exposed crystals to black metallic silver. The metallic silver on the film appears black instead of the familiar shiny silver color because the silver crystals are so small that they scatter

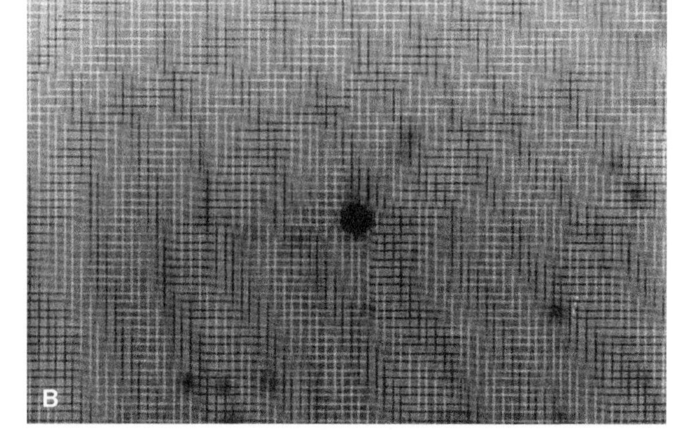

Figure 16.11. Examples of good (A) and poor (B) film/screen contact.

light instead of reflecting it. Film processing consists of four stages: developing, fixing, washing, and drying. Each stage of processing is essential in the production of a diagnostic quality radiograph.

Developing

Developing is the first step in processing a film. The developer is a water-based solution containing chemicals that will reduce the exposed silver halide crystals to metallic silver without changing the unexposed silver halide crystals. The reducing agents used in automatic processors are **phenidone** and **hydroquinone**. Phenidone rapidly reduces silver and enhances fine detail and subtle shades of gray. It is not able to reduce heavily exposed areas of an image. Hydroquinone slowly reduces silver and produces areas of heavy density or the darkest shades. Combining these two chemicals creates a solution with exceptional reducing abilities that controls the optical density of the processed radiograph. Other chemicals are used during the developing stage, which assist in producing a radiographic image.

- **Activator**: Enhances developer solution by maintaining an alkaline state
- **Restrainer**: Added to developer solution to restrict the reducing agent
- **Preservative**: Helps reduce oxidation when reducing agents are combined with air
- **Hardener**: Controls swelling of gelatin, maintains uniform thickness, and hardens emulsion; insufficient hardener causes films to have moist, soft surfaces
- **Solvent**: Filtered water that dissolves chemicals prior to use

Fixing

The action of the developer must be stopped before the film can be exposed to light; this is done by a process called **fixing**. The fixer stops the reducing action of the developer and removes the unexposed silver halide crystals. The fixer solution is also called the **clearing agent** because it removes unexposed and undeveloped silver halide crystals from the emulsion. The clearing agent in the fixer solution is ammonium thiosulfate. The action of the clearing agent prepares the film for archiving. If the fixer does not completely remove the unexposed silver halide crystals, the film will have a milky appearance and will not stand up to the archival conditions. Although the clearing agent is the primary agent in the fixer, other chemicals are also used to complete the fixation process (Table 16.5).

- **Activator:** Acetic acid maintains the pH to enhance the clearing agent
- **Preservative:** Dissolves silver from the ammonium thiosulfate
- **Hardener:** Prevents scratches and abrasions during processing; insufficient hardener causes films to have moist, soft surfaces
- **Solvent:** Dissolves other chemicals

TABLE 16.5 **CHEMICALS CONTAINED IN THE DEVELOPER AND FIXER SOLUTION AND THEIR FUNCTIONS**

Chemical	Function
Developer	
Hydroquinone	Reducing agent, slowly produces dark areas
Phenidone	Reducing agent, rapidly produces fine detail shades of gray
Sodium carbonate	Activator, swells gelatin, maintain alkaline pH
Potassium bromide	Restrainer, decreases reducing agent activity, antifogging
Sodium sulfite	Preservative, controls oxidation
Glutaraldehyde	Hardener, hardens emulsion, controls emulsion swelling
Water	Solvent, dissolves chemicals for use
Fixer	
Ammonium thiosulfate	Clearing agent, removes undeveloped silver halide crystals from emulsion
Acetic acid	Activator, provides acidic pH
Potassium alum	Hardener, hardens and shrinks emulsion
Sodium sulfite	Preservative, maintains acidic pH
Water	Solvent, dissolves chemicals

Washing

Developer or fixer chemicals that are left in the emulsion will slowly be oxidized by the air and will turn the film brown. The washing stage removes all chemicals remaining in the emulsion. The incoming wash water is filtered before it enters the wash tank. The water is constantly circulated and drained to ensure that it is clean. Unremoved fixer can combine with metallic silver crystals to form silver sulfide or dichroic stains. Incomplete removal of the fixer solution is known as hyporetention. Degradation of the image quality of stored films as a result of incomplete washing will appear only after several years.

Drying

Most of the wash water is removed by the processor rollers as the film is transported into the drying chamber. The final drying of the film is done by blowing hot air over both sides of the film as it begins to exit the processor. Drying removes the remnants of the water on the film. It also shrinks and hardens the emulsion and seals the supercoat to protect the film during handling and storage. In order to sufficiently dry the film, the hot air must be between 120°F and 150°F (43°C to 65°C).

Contamination

Contamination of the basic developer by the acid fixer lowers the pH, reducing the effectiveness of the developer and producing lower-contrast, "washed-out" images. Contamination can occur when new chemicals are added or during the cleaning of film transport components. Drops of warm fixer can condense and contaminate the developer solution when the processor is turned off. For this reason, the lid of the processor should always be lifted and propped partially open when the processor is turned off. This will allow vapors to escape and reduce cross-contamination and corrosion of processor parts.

Contamination of the fixer by the developer is not a problem. Some developer is inevitably carried along when the film is transferred into the fixer tank. The processor system is designed to compensate for this contamination.

Recirculation and Replenishment

The developer and fixer solutions must be constantly mixed to ensure that their chemical strength is uniform. Mixing also ensures that fresh chemicals come in contact with the emulsion. This mixing or agitation is produced by circulation pumps. A microswitch on the first set of transport rollers senses each film as it enters the processor and turns on the transport system and the pumps to replenish the developer and fixer solutions. The microswitch remains on for the length of time that it takes the film to travel through the microswitch.

The processing of each film uses up small amounts of the developer and fixer chemicals. The replenishment system automatically maintains the correct chemical concentration. Each time a film is processed, the microswitch activates the replenishment pumps to add developer and fixer solutions. The replenishment solutions are contained in large replenishment tanks located near the processor.

Copy films are different from conventional films. Replenishment rates adjusted for conventional double-emulsion films will not maintain the proper chemical concentrations after a large number of copy films have been processed because copy film has only a single-emulsion layer. This is especially important if the processor is also used to develop mammography films, which require critical control of processor chemistry.

Automatic processors have a standby switch that turns the transport roller drive motor off after a few minutes of inactivity. This motor must be restarted before another film can be processed.

Film Transport System

The film **transport system** carries the film through the developer, fixer, and wash tanks and through the dryer chamber. The film transport system regulates the amount of time the film is immersed in each solution and agitates the chemicals to ensure maximum reaction. The feed tray at the entrance to the automatic processor guides the film into the processor. Entrance rollers grip the film as it begins the trip through the processor. At this point, there is also a microswitch that is activated by the film. When feeding films in the processor, it is necessary to place the film on the tray so that the short axis enters the processor. This allows for the least amount of chemicals to be used to adequately process the film. When feeding multiple films into the processor, it is also necessary to alternate sides from film to film. This allows for even wear of the transport system components. The transport system consists of three distinct subsystems: transport racks, **crossover network**, and drive system.

Transport Racks

There are three types of rollers used in the **transport racks**: transport rollers, master rollers, and planetary rollers. Transport rollers, 1 inch in diameter, grip the film at the feed tray and guide the film into the processor.

As seen in Figure 16.12, the rollers are positioned opposite each other in pairs or are offset from one another; this provides constant tension to move the film down into and up out of the processing tanks. When the film reaches the end of a series of rollers, it must be bent and turned to travel in the reverse direction. At the bottom of each vertical rack, there is a turnaround assembly containing a large master roller, smaller planetary rollers, and guide shoes that hold the film against the master roller while the film reverses direction. The guide shoes have ribs to reduce friction and keep the film in alignment. Guide-shoe misalignment can remove some of the soft emulsion, causing processor artifacts, which appear as white scratch lines in the direction of film travel (Fig. 16.13).

After the film has cleared the master roller, it will then be pointing upward and will be pulled along by the next set of offset rollers. When the film reaches the top of the transport rack, it is guided into the next set of racks by a crossover network.

Crossover Networks

As seen in Figure 16.14, at the top of each tank, the film is carried across to the next tank by a crossover network. The crossover network also contains rollers and guide shoes. The rollers squeeze out the chemicals in the emulsion prior to the film entering the next tank. The assembly is similar to that in the transport racks. If the guide shoes become misaligned, the film emulsion will be scratched. The primary cause of guide-shoe misalignment is the improper seating of the transport racks and crossover networks.

Drive System

The **drive system** is a series of mechanical devices designed to turn the rollers in the processor. The speed of the drive system is usually set to move the film from the entrance rollers to the output bin. The transport system drive motor and gears are usually set for 90-second

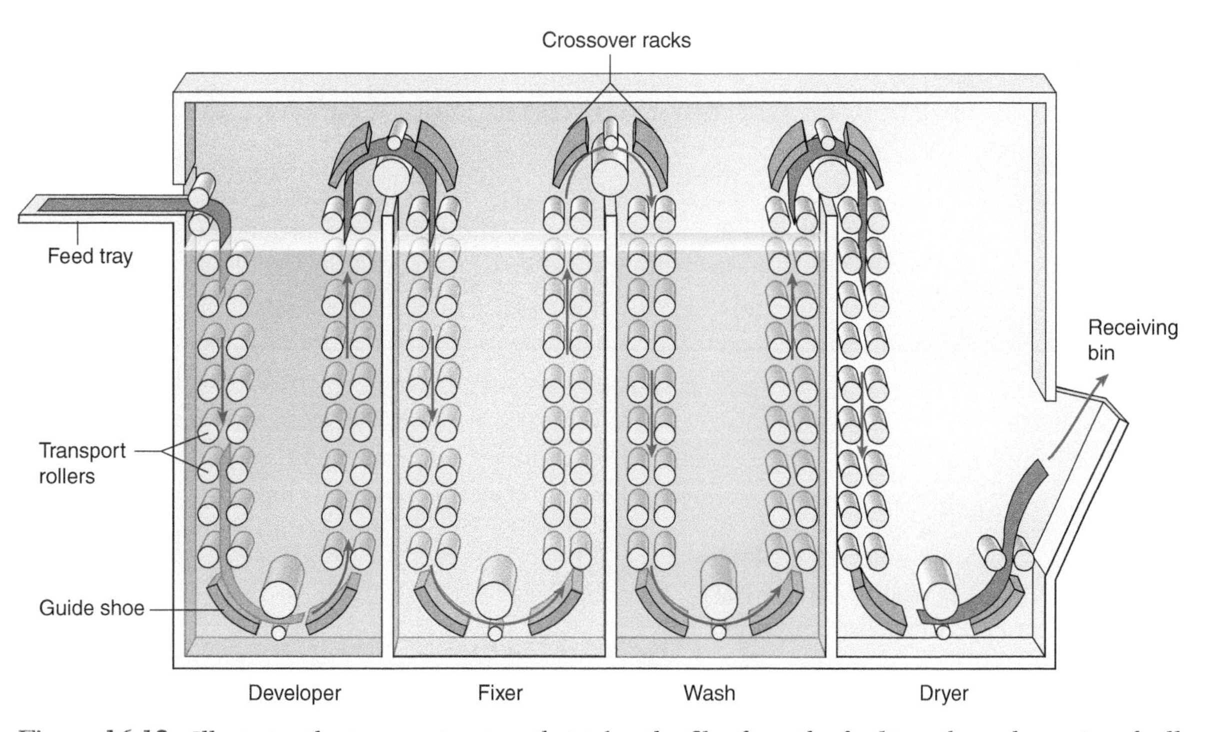

Figure 16.12. **Illustrates the transport system that takes the film from the feed tray through a series of rollers into the development tank, the fixer tank, the wash tank, and finally the drying chamber.**

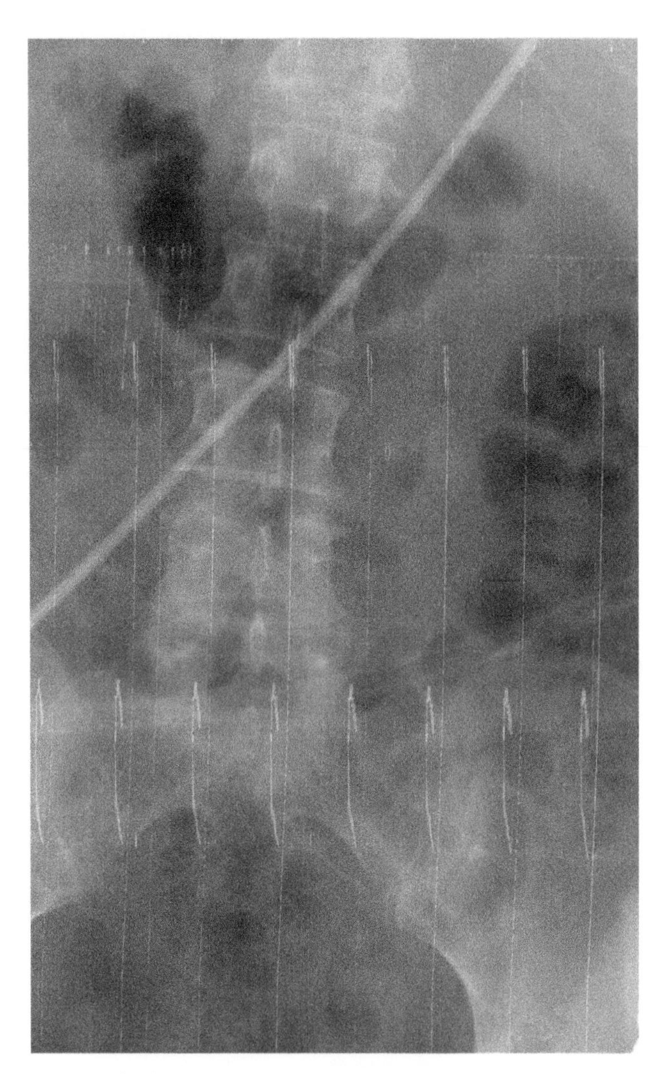

Figure 16.13. **Image shows artifacts produced by misaligned guide shoes.**

processing. The speed controls the length of time the film spends in each solution. After washing, the film passes through the dryer and is deposited in the output bin. The film transport rollers, crossover racks, and guide shoes must be periodically cleaned to maintain good quality images.

Effect of Concentration, Time, and Temperature

Any change in developer concentration, developing time, or developing temperature will change the speed, contrast, and base fog of the image. An increase in time, temperature, or concentration will increase the **film speed** and base plus fog. An increase in the time, temperature, or concentration will also increase the contrast of the film.

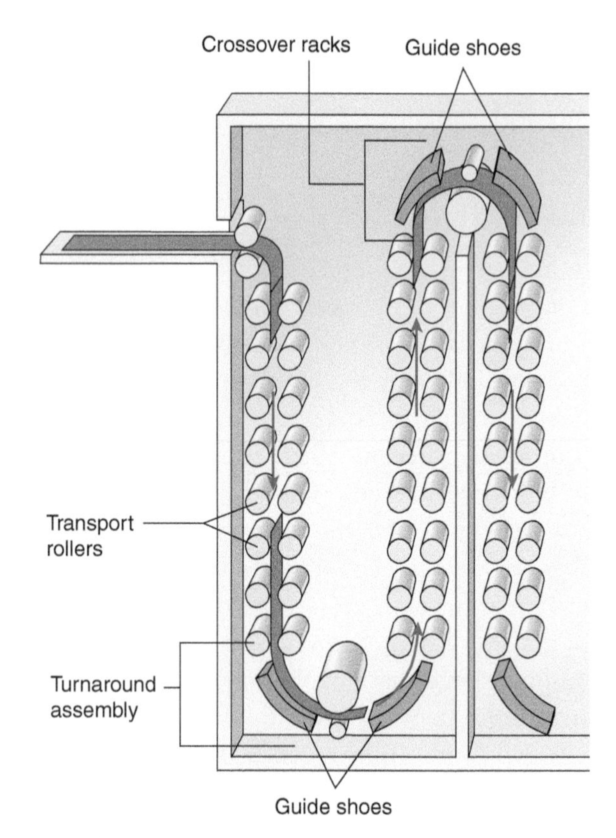

Figure 16.14. **An expanded view of the transport system guide shoes and crossover rack.**

The speed of the transport motor controls the amount of time the film is immersed in the developer, fixer, and wash tanks. Time and temperature are inversely proportional; as one is increased, the other must be decreased to maintain the same optical density for the same exposure.

A thermostat controls heating elements to maintain the developer and fixer at the proper temperature. The thermostat is set to maintain the developer temperature in the range between 92°F and 95°F in 90-second automatic processors. Developer temperatures below this range result in slower chemical reactions and an underdeveloped film with decreased density and low contrast. Temperatures above this range result in rapid chemical reactions, overdeveloped film, increased image density, and a high-contrast, narrow-latitude image.

Rapid Processing

By increasing the temperature and chemical concentrations, the total processing time can be reduced to 45 seconds. The sensitometric characteristics of rapid processing films are designed to be identical to conventional 90-second processed film.

Extended Processing

Extended processing is used in mammography to increase the **film contrast** and speed and reduce the patient dose. Standard chemicals and temperatures are used, but the processing time is extended to 3 minutes by slowing the film transport speed.

Processor Quality Assurance

Processing is the last in a long series of careful steps designed to produce a diagnostic quality image. Any error in processing will prevent the production of high-quality radiographs. Processor cleanliness, temperature, and chemical effectiveness must be maintained within strict limits. The rollers and gears must be periodically inspected for wear and replaced before their degradation affects image quality.

The Darkroom

The darkroom is an essential part of a radiology department. The darkroom entrance should be designed so that entry does not inadvertently expose films. Lightproof mazes, rotating doors, interlocks, and double-entry doors are used to eliminate the possibility of exposure of an undeveloped film to light. The darkroom temperature and humidity must be controlled to avoid artifacts.

Darkroom Safelights

An exposed film is much more sensitive than an unexposed film because some silver halide crystals may have been partially exposed. Darkrooms do not have to be totally dark, but the light level must be very low. Safelights provide low-level illumination without exposing the film. A safelight contains a low-wattage (7 to 15 W) light bulb with a special filter to maintain low light intensity. An amber filter is used with a blue-sensitive film. The GBX filters produce a deep red light. Red light from the GBX filter has low energy and is safe for green-sensitive orthochromatic films. The safelight must be 4 feet from the work area to prevent safelight fogging of the film.

Figure 16.15. **Result from a darkroom safelight test.**

A test can be performed to determine the amount of safelight fogging. Half of a uniformly exposed but undeveloped film is covered with a piece of cardboard, and the film is left on the darkroom table under the safelight for 2 minutes. The film is then developed in the usual way. After processing, the difference in the optical density between the covered and uncovered sides should be <0.05 OD (Fig. 16.15).

Silver Recovery

The final processed film contains only about half the silver contained in the original emulsion. Silver is classified as a toxic heavy metal by the Environmental Protection Agency. Environmental laws restrict the amount of silver discharged in waste liquid to <5 parts per million. Therefore, the silver must be removed from the fixer solution before that solution is discarded as waste. The most common method of silver removal is the electrolytic recovery system. This system is attached to the drain or waste line of the fixer tank; the used fixer solution circulates through the recovery system where an electric current removes the silver ions from the fixer solution and converts them into metallic silver. The recovered silver can be sold to commercial companies.

Daylight Processing Systems

With daylight processing systems, a darkroom is not required in order to load and unload the film cassettes. All film handling is done automatically inside the daylight processor. An exposed cassette is placed in the entrance slot, and the cassette is drawn into the daylight processor and opened. The film is removed from the cassette and started through the processing cycle. The cassette is then reloaded with an unexposed film, which is stored in a bulk magazine inside the daylight processor, and returned ready for another exposure (Fig. 16.16). The daylight processor has a storage magazine for each size film used by the department. Of course, a darkroom is still needed to load the daylight processor's magazines. The development, fixing, washing, and drying cycles are the same as in a conventional automatic processor.

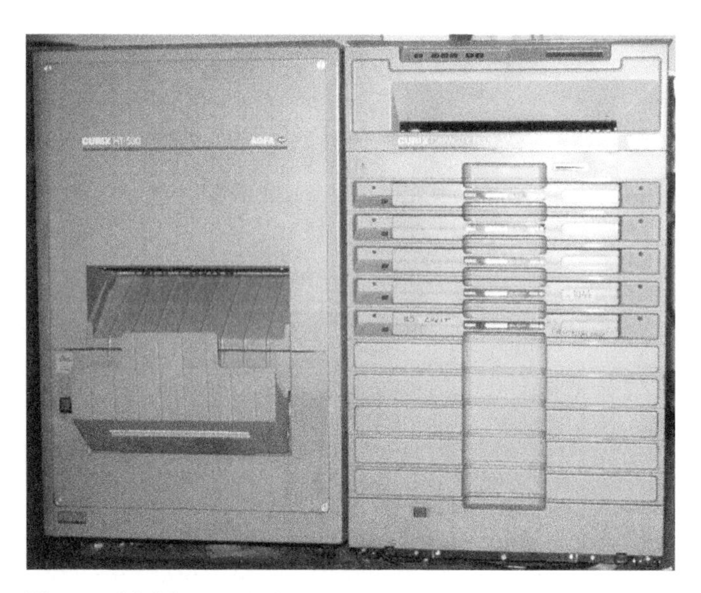

Figure 16.16. **Daylight processing system.**

Dry Processing Film

Dry processing film (Fig. 16.17) is used to permanently record digital images from computed tomography, magnetic resonance imaging, ultrasound, and digital radiographic systems. The digital image data are transferred with a laser beam onto a special film, which is then processed using heat to fix the image on the film. There are no chemicals used for dry processing and there is no need for silver reclamation.

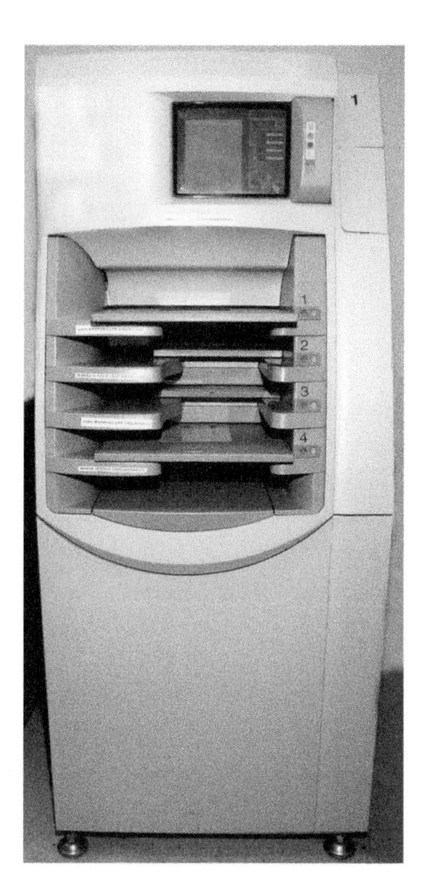

Figure 16.17. **Dry film processing system.**

Chapter Summary

1. Radiographic films consist of an emulsion containing silver halide crystals coated on a polyester base. Exposure to x-rays and visible light produces changes in the silver halide crystals to form a latent image.
2. The latent image is the distribution of exposed and unexposed silver halide crystals on the film.
3. Developing the film changes the latent image into a permanent visible image. Film development converts exposed silver halide crystals to black metallic silver and removes the unexposed crystals.
4. The transmission of light through a radiographic film is described by the film's optical density. Optical density is a measure of the degree of darkness of the film.
5. Higher-speed films require less exposure to produce a given density.
6. High-contrast films produce large density differences for small differences in exposure. Films with wide latitude produce acceptable image densities over a wide range of exposures.
7. Orthochromatic film is sensitive to green light and requires a special deep red safelight filter.
8. Radiographic film is sensitive to light, temperature, humidity, radiation, and pressure during storage and handling.
9. Improper storage and handling can produce artifacts and fog that produces unwanted densities on the film.
10. Intensifying screens convert x-ray photon energy into light energy.
11. Upon stimulation by x-ray photons, these phosphors emit green or blue light, which is matched to the spectral sensitivity of the film.
12. There are three classes of screen speeds: high, medium, and detail. High-speed screens require fewer x-rays resulting in lower patient doses but have greater quantum noise. Detail screens produce superior spatial resolution but require increased patient dose.
13. Cassettes, which provide a light-tight container for the film, must be cleaned and checked regularly for good film/screen contact. Cassettes utilize intensifying screens to improve the image quality through increasing the number of conversions from x-ray photons to light photons.
14. Film processing consists of developing, fixing, washing, and drying. Film processing converts the latent image in the emulsion into a permanent visible image by reducing the exposed silver halide grains to black metallic silver.
15. Chemical agents in the basic developer solution include two reducing agents, hydroquinone and phenidone. The fixer is an acidic solution that stops the developer action. It contains ammonium thiosulfate, which dissolves away the unexposed silver halide crystals. Changing the developer chemical concentrations, the time, or the temperature will change the speed, contrast, and base fog of the final image.
16. Film must be processed in the dark, either in a darkroom or in a daylight film processor. The darkroom safelight and filter must match the characteristics of the film used.
17. Daylight processors permit the development of exposed film without the need to open the exposed cassette in a darkroom.
18. Dry film systems do not require developing solutions; instead, they use heat to fix the image on the film.

Case Study

Janet has just arrived at 6:00 AM for her shift and turned on the processor. There is an emergency room patient who must have a single-view chest exam STAT. She performed the exam and has run the film through the automatic processor. When the film drops into the output bin, Janet notices that the film has scratch lines in the direction the film traveled through the processor. The film also has a decreased amount of density and lower contrast than Janet expected. Using your knowledge of automatic processing, determine answers to the following questions.

Critical Thinking Questions

1. How did scratch lines get on the film?
2. Is this an adjustment Janet can make?
3. What has changed the appearance of the image?
4. Did Janet use enough kVp and mAs?
5. Or is it another problem?

Review Questions

Multiple Choice

1. **A high-contrast film has a __________ latitude.**
   a. wide
   b. narrow

2. **The developer solution:**
   a. softens the emulsion
   b. reduces the exposed silver halide crystals to black metallic silver
   c. produces an alkaline pH
   d. does all of the above

3. **Replenishment systems in an automatic processor replenish:**
   a. unexposed film emulsion
   b. developer and fixer solutions
   c. used wash water
   d. drying racks

4. **Which of the following is a reducing agent?**
   a. Glutaraldehyde
   b. Hydroquinone
   c. Acetic acid
   d. Alum

5. **The hardening agent in the fixer is:**
   a. glutaraldehyde
   b. sodium sulfite
   c. potassium alum
   d. ammonium thiosulfate

6. **The purpose of the guide shoes in the transport racks is to:**
   a. allow the film to move up or down
   b. force the edge of the film around the master roller
   c. bend the film in the crossover network
   d. pull the film from the film tray into the transport rack

7. **The GBX filter is safe for use with which type of film?**
   a. Films that are sensitive to blue light
   b. Films that are sensitive to green light

8. **What effect does increased developer solution temperature have on the film?**
   a. The speed of the film will decrease.
   b. The amount of fog on the film will be decreased.
   c. The amount of contrast will be unchanged.
   d. The amount of contrast will be increased.

9. **The emulsion layer must have a thickness of:**
   a. 3 to 5 µm
   b. 10 to 20 µm
   c. 25 to 30 µm
   d. 150 to 300 µm

10. **In order to increase the spatial resolution of a film/screen system, the most important factor would be to change:**
    a. to a faster film
    b. to a faster-speed film
    c. to a slower-speed film
    d. to extended processing

11. **Film/screen contact is evaluated by a:**
    a. line pair test
    b. densitometer
    c. wire mesh test
    d. sensitometer

12. **Which of the following are rare-earth phosphor materials?**
    1. Calcium tungstate
    2. Gadolinium
    3. Lanthanum
    4. Yttrium
    a. 1, 2, and 3
    b. 2, 3, and 4
    c. 1, 3, and 4
    d. 1, 2, 3, and 4

13. **When changing from a detail screen to a high-speed screen, the mAs should be:**
    a. increased
    b. decreased
    c. not changed
    d. none of the above

14. **Radiographic noise or quantum mottle can be reduced by using:**
    a. high kVp and a small focal spot
    b. low kVp and high mAs
    c. high kVp and low mAs
    d. low mAs and large focal spot

15. **What is the purpose of the phosphor layer in the intensifying screen?**
    a. To decrease the conversion from x-ray photons to light photons
    b. To aid in increasing mAs
    c. To protect the screen base from harm
    d. To increase the number of conversions from x-ray photons to light photons

16. **Which part of the intensifying screen intercepts light photons going in various directions and redirects them to the film?**
    a. Reflective layer
    b. Base
    c. Phosphor layer
    d. All of the above redirect light

17. **The reflective layer utilizes which of the following materials?**
    1. Magnesium oxide
    2. Calcium tungstate
    3. Titanium dioxide
    a. 1 and 2
    b. 2 and 3
    c. 1 and 3
    d. 1, 2, and 3

18. **Dirt trapped inside a cassette will have a ________ or ________ appearance on the film.**
    a. white, positive
    b. black, negative
    c. black, positive
    d. white, negative

Short Answer

1. **List the four primary steps in automatic processing.**

2. What is the problem with the developer solution if the film drops into the output bin damp or wet?

3. What is the purpose of the fixer tank?

4. Explain the relationship between film resolution and the size of the silver halide crystals.

5. Radiographic film that has emulsion on both sides is ___________.

6. Explain the difference between panchromatic and orthochromatic films.

7. Which type of image archival requires a laser beam and high heat?

8. The intensifying screens serve what purpose in the radiographic cassette?

9. Describe the difference between fluorescence and phosphorescence.

10. List the four layers that make up the intensifying screen.

11. Why is afterglow not desirable for a radiographic image?

12. Name the properties of an intensifying screen base.

13. Describe the relationship between resolution and phosphor crystal size, layer thickness, and phosphor concentration.

14. Describe the difference between panchromatic and orthochromatic.

15. Discuss the process of luminescence.

16. Why is it necessary to have the film and intensifying screen spectrally matched? List the rare-earth phosphors and their colors.

17. How do intensifying screens reduce patient dose?

17

Radiographic Technique

Objectives

Upon completion of this chapter, the student will be able to:

1. Identify patient factors that may affect image receptor exposure.
2. Describe the exposure factors that can affect patient radiation exposure.
3. State the differences between the types of technique charts.
4. Differentiate technical factor modifications for additive versus destructive pathologies.
5. State technical factor considerations for body habitus, pediatric patients, soft tissue, and casts.
6. Describe the advantages and disadvantages of fixed and variable kVp systems.
7. Discuss why measurement of part thickness is critical to the accurate use of technique charts.
8. State the steps used to develop a technique chart.

Key Terms

- additive disease processes
- asthenic
- body habitus
- calipers
- contrast medium
- destructive disease processes
- fixed kVp-variable mAs technique chart
- high-kVp technique chart
- hypersthenic
- hyposthenic
- optimal kVp
- radiolucent
- radiopaque
- sthenic
- variable kVp-fixed mAs technique chart

Introduction

The world of radiography revolves around radiographers who determine the optimal kVp and mAs for each image that is produced. It is quite easy for radiographers to become accustomed to selecting factors based off their experience in working with patients of similar age, size, and pathologic processes. Radiographers evaluate each image to discern whether the correct technical factors were used; if there is a need for a repeat image because of incorrect technical factors, the radiographer again relies on his or her experience. This is an imperfect method for determining optimal kVp and mAs for an image; this method cannot be reproduced by other radiographers with consistency. The knowledge of how these factors affect the image individually and when combined assists radiographers in producing consistently high-quality radiographic images.

Regardless of the type of equipment utilized in producing an image, the patient should be exposed to the least amount of radiation necessary to produce an image with adequate optical density. This chapter will build upon the information of the primary factors in Chapter 14 to provide additional knowledge in specific patient factors that will affect the kVp and mAs that is used for the image. The methods that are used to formulate a technical factor chart will assist the student and radiographer in building a chart for each radiographic unit in the department. The information in this chapter is for film screen radiography; special considerations for CR and DR will be discussed in Chapter 21.

Patient Factors

There are several patient-related factors that must be discussed to provide a basis for selecting exposure factors. A thorough knowledge of each will assist the radiographer in determining the best combination of factors to use for each patient.

Body Habitus

Body habitus refers to the size of build of the body. It is important for the radiographer to consider the body habitus when establishing technical factors. There are four types of body habitus: **sthenic**, **hyposthenic**, **hypersthenic**, and **asthenic**.

The sthenic body habitus refers to the average-sized adult and accounts for ~ 50% of adult patients. Hyposthenic patients are taller and have a more slender build. Hypersthenic patients are larger individuals who have a stocky build.

The hypersthenic build is becoming more prevalent in the patient population. These patients have thicker body part sizes compared to sthenic and asthenic patients; the technical factors must be increased for adequate penetration of the body part. On the opposite end of the spectrum is the asthenic patient who has a very slender build. Their body parts are thinner than are those of sthenic body types; therefore, technical factors must be decreased for asthenic body types. Figure 17.1 represents the four types of body habitus.

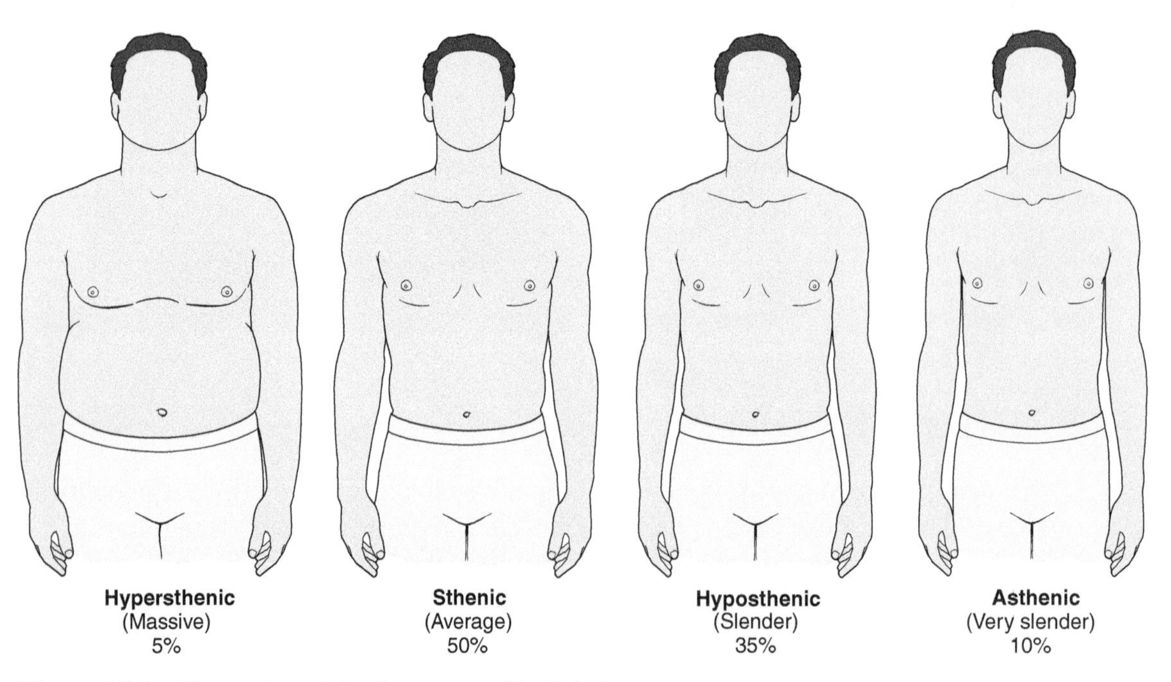

Figure 17.1. Illustration of the four types of body habitus.

Part Thickness

The thickness of the anatomic part being imaged will affect the amount of attenuation of the x-ray beam as well as how much remnant radiation reaches the image receptor. Thinner body parts will have less attenuation with more remnant radiation reaching the image receptor, while thicker body parts will have more attenuation (Table 17.1). To maintain adequate exposure to the

TABLE 17.1 **AVERAGE ADULT PART THICKNESS**

Region		Average Thickness Adult—CMS			Percent Frequency
		AP	PA	Lat	
Thumb, fingers		1.5–4 (AP, PA, Lat)			99
Hand		3–5 (AP, PA)			99
				7–10	93
Wrist		3–6 (AP, PA)			99
				5–8	98
Forearm		6–8 (AP, PA)			94
				7–9	92
Elbow		6–8			96
				7–9	87
Arm		7–10			95
				7–10	94
Shoulder		12–16			79
Clavicle			13–17		82
Foot		6–8 (AP, PA)			92
				7–9	91
Ankle		8–10			86
				6–9	96
Leg		10–12			85
				9–11	89
Knee		10–13 (AP, PA)			92
				9–12	92
Thigh		14–17			77
				13–16	76
Hip		17–21			76
Cervical	C1–3	12–14			77
Vertebrae	C4–7	11–14			98
	C1–7			10–13	90
Thoracic vertebrae		20–24			76
				28–32	81
Lumbar vertebrae		18–22			69
				27–32	77
Pelvis		19–23			78
Skull			18–21		96
				14–17	88
Sinuses	Frontal		18–21		97
	Max.		18–22		88
				13–17	96
Mandible				10–12	82
Chest			20–25		82
				27–32	84

 Average Adult Part Thickness by Region from Arthur W. Fuch's Relationship of tissue thickness to kilovoltage. Published in *The X-ray Technician*, 19:6, 287–293, 1948.

image receptor, the mAs will need to be either increased or decreased for hyposthenic or asthenic patients, respectively.

For the radiographer to determine how much of a change in mAs is needed, an accurate measurement of the body part is in order. A **caliper** is the measuring tool that is used and provides an accurate measurement when used correctly (Fig. 17.2). Each radiography room should have a caliper. When producing and using a technique chart, it is necessary to measure through the central ray location for the body part to be imaged. It is critical that all radiographers using a particular technique chart measure in exactly the same manner. A common mistake is

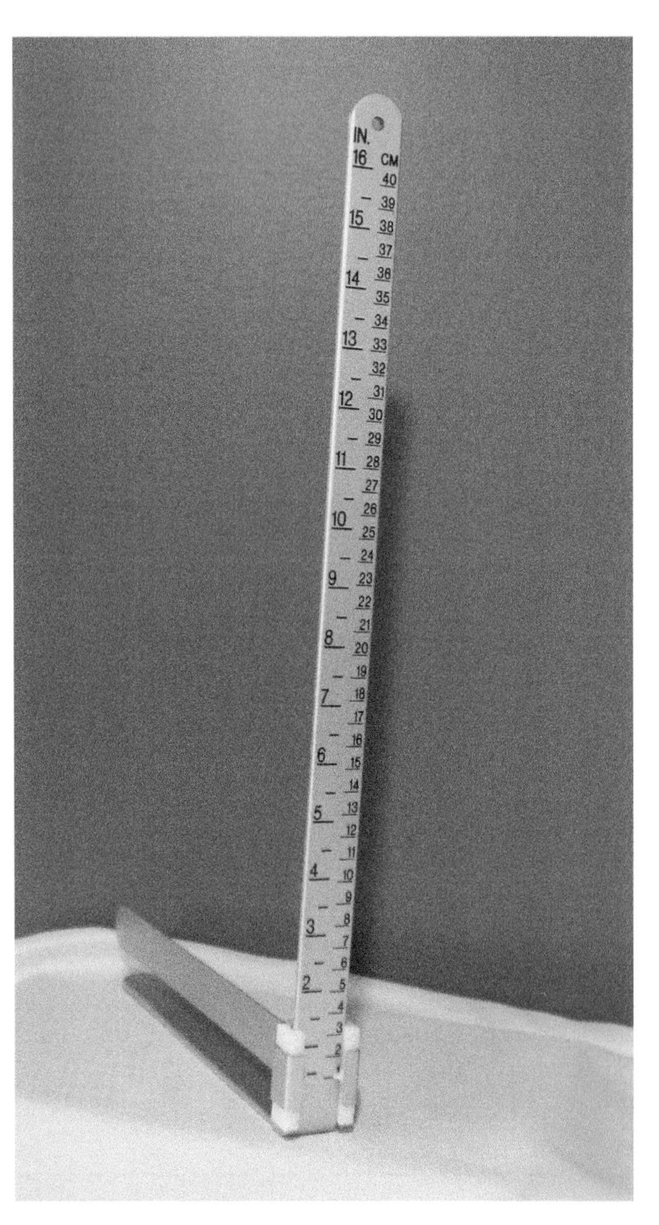

Figure 17.2. **Caliper to measure part thickness.**

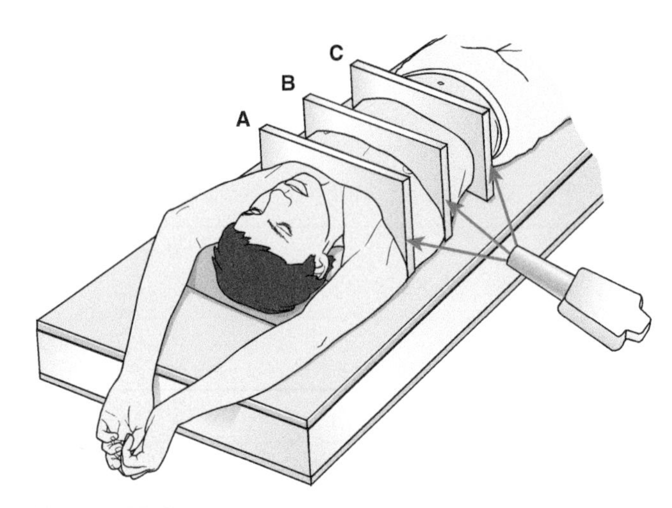

Figure 17.3. **Illustration of accurate caliper measurement of the thorax.**

not measuring accurately and using the incorrect technical factor settings from the chart.

Central ray measurements should be made at the point where the central ray will enter and then exit the body. For example, in Figure 17.3, the measurement at the thickest part of the region should be used to determine the technical factors to be selected. The thickest part is at B, which corresponds to the thickest portion of the thorax. Points A and C do not correspond to the thickest part of the region, and using either measurement to determine technical factors will compromise radiographic quality.

Four-to-Five-Centimeter Rule

Because x-rays are attenuated exponentially, a general rule to follow is that for every change in part thickness of 4 to 5 cm, the radiographer should change the mAs setting by a factor of 2. For example, patient A anatomical part measured 8 cm, and 10 mAs was used for an adequate image. The same body part measured 12 cm for patient B. What is the new mAs? Because the size of the part is 4 cm thicker, the original mAs is multiplied by 2 or doubled; the new mAs will be 20. This method can be used when a body part measures 4 to 5 cm less than the listed part thickness on the technical factor chart. For patient C, the body part measured 4 cm; the original mAs will be divided by 2 or halved for 5 mAs.

This rule is applied to mAs settings; however, if a change in kVp is needed for penetration of the beam, the 15% rule must be used. Remember that when kVp is increased by 15%, the mAs can be halved to maintain exposure to the image receptor. A decrease in kVp of 15% requires mAs to be doubled to keep adequate radiation exposure.

CRITICAL THINKING BOX 17.1

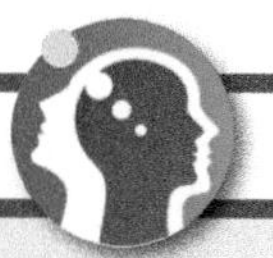

For the technique chart, determine the adjustments in mAs needed for changes in part thickness.

Technique Chart

Part	mAs	Thickness	Actual Thickness	New mAs
Ankle	5	7 cm	11 cm	______
Knee	8	10 cm	14 cm	______
Thoracic spine	20	24 cm	20 cm	______
Chest	6	27 cm	29 cm	______

CRITICAL THINKING BOX 17.2

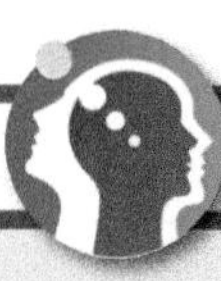

For the technique chart, determine the adjustments in kVp needed for changes in part thickness.

Technique Chart

Part	kVp	Thickness	Actual Thickness	New kVp
Ankle	64	7 cm	11 cm	______
Knee	70	10 cm	14 cm	______
Thoracic spine	80	24 cm	20 cm	______
Chest	110	27 cm	29 cm	______

Minimum Change Rule

When a radiograph is evaluated for optical density and it is determined that there needs to be a change in mAs to improve the OD, the radiographer has two options to consider. The first option: Is the optical density too low or too high, requiring mAs to be either halved or doubled? The second option: If the mAs does not need to be doubled or halved, how much of a change is needed to affect optical density? These are important questions to answer because this means that the radiographer has determined that a repeat exposure is needed. To make sure the adjustment is adequate and will result in a diagnostic image, it takes more than a guess to determine the new mAs.

When the optical density is too light, a 100% increase in mAs is the same as doubling mAs, but the image may not need this much of a change. The opposite is true if less mAs is needed. Changes in mAs must be fine-tuned more than just doubling or halving mAs as this change may not lead to the intended result.

To see a visible difference in the optical density in a radiographic image, the mAs must be changed by at least 30% (Table 17.2). Images with excessive density will have the mAs decreased by at least 30%, while images with less than adequate density will require at least a 30% increase in mAs. When making an equivalent change using the 15% rule for kVp, consider that a change of one-third or 5% is needed. Keep in mind that if penetration of the x-ray beam through the anatomical part is the problem with optical density on the image, the kVp must be adjusted.

Tissue Composition

The type of tissue to be imaged must be considered when determining the appropriate technical factor selection. Chest and abdomen anatomy may have the same

TABLE 17.2 COMMON OPTIMUM KVP RANGES FOR BODY REGIONS

Region	Optimal kVp Range
Small extremities (hand, foot, etc.)	50–60
Iodine-based contrast media exams	68
Large extremities (shoulder, knee, etc.)	70
Skull	80
Abdomen and ribs	80
AP vertebral column	80
Lateral vertebral column	90
Barium exams (double contrast)	90–110
Chest	120
Barium exams (single contrast)	120

thickness, but each requires a different mAs and kVp to properly image the structures. Soft tissue structures in the abdomen use low kVp and higher mAs compared to chest techniques. Extremities are a combination of soft tissue and bone; low kVp is used because the extremities are thinner parts compared to the chest and abdomen.

The chest has a variety of tissue types; the lungs have low mass density, while the ribs and sternum have high mass density. The mediastinal structures are intermediate mass density. To properly image all these structures, high kVp is needed for sufficient penetration, and low mAs is used. This combination provides the proper radiographic contrast to accurately image the various types of tissues. An added benefit is that the radiation dose to the patient is low.

Subject Contrast

In any radiographic image, the subject contrast is needed to visualize structures adjacent to one another. Each structure will absorb the radiation differently based on the composition of the tissue. Tissue thickness and atomic number affect absorption characteristics. High atomic number tissues have higher absorption of the radiation (bone), while low atomic number tissues have lower absorption (soft tissue).

Pediatric Patients

Pediatric patients pose a challenge when choosing the appropriate kVp and mAs for the image. Pediatric patients have a smaller size compared to adults, so it makes sense that lower kVp and mAs would be used. When imaging, the chest radiographers must use a fast exposure time, which helps to stop the motion of the diaphragms when the patient cannot or will not hold the breath. The fast exposure time may eliminate the use of an automatic exposure control (AEC) for pediatric chest x-ray images.

As pediatric patients age, their bones increase in mass density. At the age of 6, a pediatric skull has approximately the same mass density as does an adult skull. If the radiographers do not have a technical factor chart for pediatric patients, they can use the same kVp and mAs for a skull x-ray as they would for an adult. When the patient is under the age of 6, it is appropriate to decrease kVp by 15% or more to adjust for the lack of bone density.

The use of calipers to accurately measure the anatomy of interest in pediatric patients will assist the radiographer in determining the proper technical factors to select. A technical factor chart should be developed for pediatric patients to include the anatomical part, part thickness, kVp, and mAs used for each projection. The chart should be referred to prior to each exposure to make sure the correct technical factors are being used. This practice will increase consistency when producing radiographs and should result in a decrease in the number of repeat images because of the use of incorrect technical factors.

Pathologic Conditions

The greatest variable in producing a diagnostic radiograph is the condition of the patient. In addition to the normal types of tissues, the radiographer must also consider the abnormal changes caused by disease, trauma, or medical procedure. The radiographer must review the exam orders carefully to determine the reason for the exam and any prior images to gain knowledge about the patient's condition. Gathering a medical history from the patient will also provide knowledge that will be used to ascertain the technical factors to be used. All this information is considered in the final selection of kVp and mAs.

Pathologic conditions that can affect the absorption characteristics of the anatomical part are considered to be either additive or destructive pathologies. Many disease processes do not require an adjustment in technical factors. A pathologic condition that substantially alters the tissue composition will require an adjustment in kVp and/or mAs. Radiographically demonstrated pathologies or materials include air, fluid, fat, bone, and metals from surgical procedures.

Additive Disease Processes

Abnormal conditions that lead to an increase in fluid, bone, or metal are additive pathologies. **Additive disease processes** or conditions increase absorption of the beam and require an increase in kVp because the part is more difficult to penetrate. The presence of excessive bone tissue, calcification of joints, or metal prosthesis increases the atomic number of the tissue. Fluid accumulation in the lungs substantially increases the tissue density compared to the normal air-filled lung tissue.

TABLE 17.3 ADDITIVE DISEASE PROCESSES

Abdomen	Chest
Aortic aneurysm	Atelectasis
Ascites	Cardiomegaly
Cirrhosis	Congestive heart failure
Hypertrophy (e.g., splenomegaly)	Hydropneumothorax
	Pleural effusion
Skeleton	Pneumonia
	Tuberculosis
Hydrocephalus	**General Sites**
Metastases	
Osteoarthritis (degenerative joint disease)	Abscess
	Edema
Osteochondroma	Sclerosis
Osteopetrosis	
Paget's disease (late stage)	

TABLE 17.4 DESTRUCTIVE DISEASE PROCESSES

Abdomen	Chest
Bowel obstruction	Emphysema
Free air	Pneumothorax
Skeleton	**General Sites**
Gout	Atrophy
Metastases (osteolytic)	Emaciation
Multiple myeloma	Malnutrition
Osteomyelitis	
Osteoporosis	
Paget's disease (early stage)	
Rheumatoid arthritis	

Fluid in the abdomen distends the part and increases overall part thickness. The abdomen is quite rigid and hard to the touch.

To image additive diseases, it may be necessary to increase techniques from 30% to 100% or more when the disease is in advanced stages. A general rule to follow is to measure the part thickness and determine the techniques to use based on that measurement and then increase technique by an additional 50%. This method will produce an acceptable optical density on the image. Table 17.3 lists common additive disease processes.

Destructive Disease Processes

Abnormal disease processes that lead to an increase in air or fat, or to a decrease to normal body fluid, are considered destructive conditions. **Destructive disease processes** or conditions decrease the absorption of the x-ray beam and require a reduction in technical factors to produce the acceptable optical density in the image. Air and fat have low atomic numbers, which makes them significantly less dense than other tissues. Because of their composition, air and fat are easier to penetrate and absorb fewer x-ray photons.

The kVp can be changed because it affects the penetration of the primary beam, and destructive conditions affect how the x-ray beam penetrates the tissue. It can be difficult to estimate exactly how much of a change to make, but a general rule is to start with the 15% rule. Areas with large amounts of gas also require a decrease in mAs, for example, a bowel obstruction where the bowel has large amounts of gas. If the mAs is not decreased, there will be too much density on the image and the bowel pattern will be obscured. Common destructive disease processes are listed in Table 17.4.

Special Considerations

Selecting the correct technical factors is a challenging aspect of radiography. The radiographer must be able to recognize a wide variety of patient and procedure variables that will affect the decision for the amount of kVp and mAs to be used for the image. A radiographer must gain a thorough understanding of each of these variables and how each affects the resultant radiographic image.

Soft Tissue Imaging

Soft tissue imaging is most frequently used to image the hands and neck. When small objects like wood or glass become embedded in the soft tissue of the hand, it becomes necessary to adjust technical factors to adequately visualize the embedded foreign object. When the physician suspects a patient has croup, a soft tissue image of the neck is needed to demonstrate the larynx. Soft tissue techniques also demonstrate a foreign object that has been swallowed, for example, when a child swallows a quarter. In these types of images, the normal subject contrast of an anatomical part is not of interest and can be sacrificed to adequately image the soft tissue. When using film screen image, the mAs will be reduced for better visualization of the soft tissue.

Casts

Casts are used in postreduction of fractures in the extremities. Orthopedic surgeons will manipulate the fracture to align the bone fragments and thereby stabilize the bone for healing. The extremity then has a cast applied to provide a means of support to prevent the bone from moving during the healing process. The traditional casts were made of plaster, which is a dense material that attenuated the x-ray beam. When a plaster cast is used, the mAs will need to be doubled or kVp increased by 15%. Because of the weight of a plaster cast, they were quite uncomfortable; this led to the development of fiberglass casts. Fiberglass is a much lighter, less dense material that is **radiolucent**. Because of this, there is no need to adjust technical factors.

Contrast Medium

Imaging low-contrast soft tissue structures requires the use of **contrast medium** or agents to better visualize the structures. Arteries, veins, and soft tissue organs are virtually invisible on a radiographic image because the tissue lacks sufficient density to be seen. Contrast media can be injected or ingested into the body; it changes the absorption characteristics of soft tissue structures by increasing or decreasing attenuation of the x-ray beam.

Positive contrast medium contains iodine or barium sulfate; both have high atomic numbers and efficiently absorb x-ray photons. Positive contrast media is called **radiopaque** because it is easily seen on x-ray images. When the barium sulfate is ingested, it fills the esophagus and allows the outline of the esophagus to be seen. Because of the high atomic number of the positive contrast media, an increase in kVp will be needed for penetration. Iodinated contrast media is injected into arteries, veins, or organs and is an effective method of increasing the radiographic contrast of the structure. The utilization of iodinated contrast media makes it possible to visualize pathologies within a vessel or organ. The iodine absorbs the x-ray photons; reducing the number of photons to reach the image receptor provides an image of the structure.

Negative contrast media is composed of air or special gas such as carbon dioxide. Negative contrast media is called radiolucent because the x-ray photons are not absorbed and pass through the tissue quite easily. Negative contrast media typically does not require a change in technical factor settings. Often positive and negative contrast media are combined to coat and expand structures like the esophagus; this would require an increase in kVp to penetrate the barium.

The use of contrast media is an effective method to increase radiographic contrast when imaging low-subject contrast structures. Pathologies are better demonstrated when the radiographic contrast is sufficient enough to highlight the tumors, cysts, etc.

Technique Charts

Technique charts have been a standard tool in radiography departments for quite some time. Every radiography department should develop technique charts for each unit including mobile units. The purpose of developing and using technique charts is to standardize protocols and techniques. A standardized approach provides consistency in producing diagnostic images from one image to the next and from one radiographer to the next radiographer. In the process of developing a technique chart, it is necessary for all radiographers to write down what works; in this way others will benefit from the knowledge. This sharing of information is a starting point and will be a reference in selecting the technique for subsequent images. The best approach is one that is simplified and easy to use. A standardized approach reduces the number of errors and also reduces the number of repeat images, which ultimately reduces patient radiation exposure.

In addition to developing a technique chart, the administration in the facility must encourage the use of the chart and support continuous review of the charts to make improvements. All staff radiographers should be allowed to provide input and feedback on the accuracy of the charts. The process of gathering information helps to assure the feeling of "ownership" and increases the likelihood the radiographers will use this important tool that they helped to develop.

There are different types of technique charts: **variable kVp-fixed mAs**, **fixed kVp-variable mAs**, and **high-kVp**. It is necessary to understand that regardless of which technique chart is used, the minimum kVp required for adequate penetration of the anatomical part should always be used. The type of technique chart that is used in a department will depend upon many considerations; regardless of the type of chart used, the best results will be obtained when the chart is actually used.

Variable kVp-Fixed mAs

The variable kVp-fixed mAs approach has the primary argument that mAs can be kept low to reduce patient radiation exposure. kVp will change to accommodate part thickness. kVp has less impact on patient radiation exposure compared to increasing mAs. It is a valid consideration to keep radiation exposure as low as reasonably achievable. Typically, the variable kVp systems require an adjustment in both kVp and mAs for each projection, making for a very complicated approach. When considering body habitus, the mAs has to be lowered for asthenic patients rather than kVp to prevent inadequate penetration from using a kVp setting that is too low to penetrate the bony anatomy.

As the part thickness increases, kVp must also be increased; however, a 15% increase is not always applicable. A general rule is that when kVp will be increased by 2 for every 1-cm increase in part thickness, mAs will be maintained. Accurate measurement of the part is critical to ensure the 2 kVp adjustment is applied consistently. All radiographers must become skilled with using the calipers properly and measuring through the central ray location to obtain the most accurate measurement possible.

A baseline or original kVp for a specific part must be established. Historically, the specific baseline kVp has been 30, 40, or 50; the one that is used will depend upon which one is the best number for the equipment in the facility. Using a base kVp of 50 and then adding two times the part thickness is a valid method. For example, an AP knee measures 11 cm, 11 × 2 = 22 + 50 = 72 kVp for the AP projection. Phantom exposures are then taken to test the kVp to ascertain the optical density in the image. Once the optimal OD has been found for the given projection, that kVp is listed on the technique chart as the average kVp (Table 17.5).

TABLE 17.5 **VARIABLE KVP-FIXED MAS PELVIS**

Part Thickness	Optimal kVp	mAs
15 cm	80	20
19 cm	88	20
23 cm	96	20

The variable kVp-fixed mAs chart may be most effective for pediatric patients or when imaging small extremities such as hands, fingers, toes, and feet. These exams use low kVp because the part is thin and does not require higher kVp like abdomen or chest images. At low kVp settings, small changes may be more effective at changing OD on the image compared to changing mAs, which is already low. As a general practice, changing kVp may be ineffective for elderly patients, pathologic conditions, or extremes in part thickness.

The main advantage of the chart is that it is easy to formulate variable kVp because making changes to compensate for part thickness is relatively simple. By adjusting the baseline kVp according to the part thickness, a radiographer can be fairly certain the image will have adequate penetration. One consideration that must always be considered is the effect variable kVp changes have on the radiographic contrast. For thick body parts only increasing the kVp can cause a very long scale of contrast which may obscure essential anatomy. The variable kVp-fixed mAs charts tend to be less accurate for part size extremes.

The fixed mAs must still be established for each general body area. The body areas can be listed as:

1. Upper extremities, nongrid
2. Lower extremities, nongrid
3. Pelvis and femurs
4. Head procedures
5. Abdomen and urinary procedures
6. Gastrointestinal barium procedures
7. Shoulder and thorax procedures

Grid and nongrid procedures must be grouped together as the part thickness will determine the amount of mAs to be used. The 10-cm rule of part thickness is applied to extremities to determine if the part will use a grid or nongrid. When the knee is imaged with a grid, it will be grouped with the femur, which requires a grid.

Shoulders require gridded techniques because of their thickness and should not be grouped with nongrid upper extremities.

Grouping similar part thicknesses together further simplifies the technique chart and makes it easier for radiographers to use the chart. For example, if an AP foot and AP elbow have equivalent technical factor combinations, the kVp and mAs will be the same for both. This also works for the lateral ankle and AP humerus, AP pelvis and AP lumbar spine, AP cervical spine and lateral skull, etc. Using this approach of comparative anatomy, grouping similar parts will make it easier to memorize the chart.

CRITICAL THINKING BOX 17.3

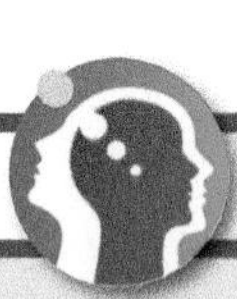

Using the base 50 method for variable kVp, a base mAs of 5.5 is used for all nongrid upper extremities. Using the formula, find the solutions for the kVp for each projection.

AP wrist: 3.5 cm
AP forearm: 5 cm
AP humerus: 8 cm

The one exception to the above rule is thorax radiography. The thorax is a complex area where the structures range from bone to soft tissue. By using the above method, a PA chest measuring 24 cm would use 98 kVp, and the lateral chest measuring 32 cm would use 114 kVp—these are both lower than the typical kVp used by radiographers. The optimum kVp for chest imaging is 110 to 120 kVp for both the PA and lateral projections with a 72″ SID. The mAs is typically 3 mAs for the PA and 6 mAs for the lateral. Using the higher kVp ensures adequate penetration of the thorax while using lower mAs for acceptable radiographic contrast to visualize lung tissue, ribs, and mediastinum structures.

Fixed kVp-Variable mAs

The fixed kVp-variable mAs technique chart is the most commonly used chart. This chart uses the method of selecting the **optimal kVp** required for the procedure and adjusting mAs for part thickness. Optimal kVp is described as the kVp that is high enough to ensure penetration but not too high to compromise radiographic contrast. Radiographers tend to develop their own optimal kVp based off their knowledge of imaging a variety of body habitus and pathological conditions.

TABLE 17.6 **FIXED KVP-VARIABLE MAS PELVIS**

Part Thickness	Optimal kVp	mAs
15 cm	80	20
19 cm	80	40
23 cm	80	60

Once optimal kVp has been established for each type of procedure, it will not vary according to part thickness (Table 17.6). The mAs will be changed for variations in part thickness.

As discussed earlier, x-ray photons are attenuated exponentially and the general guideline is to adjust mAs by a factor of 2 for every 4- to 5-cm change in thickness. For example, an AP knee measuring 10 cm is imaged with 70 kVp and 8 mAs. A patient with a knee that measures 14 cm would require mAs to be increased by a factor of 2; $8 \times 2 = 16$ mAs. The new technical factors would be 70 kVp and 16 mAs.

Accurately measuring the part thickness is still important but not as crucial as it is for the variable kVp-fixed mAs system. The fixed kVp-variable mAs technique chart is relatively easy to use, and similar anatomic areas can be listed together to aid memorization. For most x-ray procedures of the extremities where nongrid is used ~60 kVp is considered optimal. Optimal kVp for the abdomen is ~80 kVp, while lateral spine procedures require ~90 kVp. Using this fixed kVp-variable mAs, there is more consistency in producing quality radiographs, greater assurance of adequate penetration of the part, and improved accuracy with extreme variations in thickness of anatomical parts.

Sufficient kVp

The importance of using sufficient kVp to adequately penetrate the tissue cannot be overstated. This is especially important when imaging extremely large anatomical parts on obese patients. As previously learned, kVp is the driving force for the x-ray photons. For example, if the pelvis is imaged using 50 kVp, the bone will absorb the x-ray photons, and none will reach the image receptor.

The outline of the pelvis will appear as a blank area on the radiographic image. ***IF*** mAs is doubled, twice the number of photons are present in the beam and will be incident on the bone. Again, the bone will absorb the photons, but because of lack of penetration, the resultant image will not demonstrate the pelvis. The patient has just received two exposures and will require a third exposure to attempt to image the pelvis. This is a tremendous amount of radiation exposure to the patient!!! The problem is the photons lack sufficient energy (kVp) to penetrate the part.

The average abdomen is 22 cm thick and 80 kVp is optimal. If an abdomen measures 28 cm, the kVp should be increased by 2 for every 1 cm of tissue thickness to ensure adequate penetration. Because the abdomen is 6 cm thicker, an additional 12 kVp must be used for a new setting of 92 kVp. Each anatomical area has a minimum optimal kVp and adjusting that number based on part thickness will help the radiographer in formulating the most accurate combination of kVp and mAs for the procedure. Remember…**NO** amount of mAs will compensate for kVp that is too low.

High kVp

The kVp selected for a high-kVp chart is typically >100 kVp. Certain radiographic procedures require kVp above 100 to adequately penetrate the tissue. Routine chest radiography is performed with a 72″ SID; 110 to 120 kVp is needed to penetrate all bony structures and to enhance soft tissue mass densities. Procedures that use barium sulfate need to use 110 to 120 kVp; barium has a high atomic number of 56, which means the barium is very dense and requires higher kVp for sufficient penetration.

Preparing a high-kVp chart uses the same steps as preparing a fixed-kVp chart. Because all the exposures for an anatomical region use the same kVp, the mAs will have to vary based on part thickness. Because the kVp is so high, the mAs will be much less; the advantage is decreased patient radiation dose.

Experimental exposures are performed using a phantom to determine the appropriate mAs and optical density for all projections. For chest radiographic images, correct mAs settings will enhance visualization of anatomical parts like the bronchial tree, pulmonary markings, and mediastinal structures.

Developing a Technique Chart

Radiographers can develop effective technique charts for each unit that will assist in selecting technical factors for the various procedures that are performed. Many radiographers have their "go-to" technical factors that they use because experience has shown that the factors work. It is important to write these down and use these factors as the starting point for developing a technique chart. The tools needed to develop a chart include radiographic phantoms, calipers, and a calculator.

Initial Phantom Images

Using radiographic phantoms, an initial set of images will be produced. It is preferred to use an AEC to control the exposure, or if one is not available, an exposure reference control point is determined and the optical density is measured with a densitometer. When using an abdomen phantom, the exact center of L2 (exposure reference control point) could be measured for each image. 80 kVp will be used and several images will be taken with various mAs settings. The images must be shown to all radiologists and supervisory radiographers for their review of image quality. It is important for the individuals to select the images that are outside the acceptable parameters of image quality. In this way, the resulting images will be acceptable to all. Once the optimal radiographs are produced of each phantom exposure, techniques can be generalized for imaging similar body parts.

Comparative Anatomy

Comparative anatomy of similar size can be imaged using the same technical factors as long as the minimum kVp needed to penetrate the part is used. It is critical to find the minimum kVp needed to adequately penetrate the anatomical part so the scale of radiographic contrast will be acceptable. An example is when imaging an elbow measuring 7 cm in the AP projection with known technical factors that produce a high-quality image, the radiographer needs to image an ankle in the AP projection but has no specific technique for the radiographic unit. The ankle measures 7 cm in the AP projection. Using comparative anatomy approach, the ankle can be imaged using the same techniques as were used for the elbow as long as minimum kVp is used to penetrate the part. This method allows the radiographers to extrapolate technical factors for similar anatomical areas.

Stages for Development

Regardless of the type of chart being developed, the stages of development are the same. The construction and use of technique charts must include the following:

1. Establish a quality control program for each machine and standardized processing.
2. Produce phantom images with various mAs settings and a minimum kVp setting.
3. Review and select the optimal phantom image.
4. Extrapolate technique chart: fixed kVp, variable kVp, or other chart.
5. Perform further phantom images to assess effectiveness for small, medium, and large part thickness.
6. Perform limited clinical trial using the new chart. Each procedure should be recorded and all repeat images analyzed. Make any adjustments to the chart based on the clinical trial.
7. All radiographers should periodically review each chart to determine the need for updates.

Once established, the chart should not be altered but used as developed. Often when individual radiographers make alterations to the technical factors, their decision to alter is based off of using incorrect SID, image receptors, or positioning errors. The urge to rewrite the techniques must be strongly discouraged.

Evaluating Quality Images

Poor-quality images may result when the chart is not properly used. It is crucial to critically review variables that may have caused the poor result. When a radiographer consistently produces a poor quality image, steps must be taken to determine why this is happening. The radiographers may choose to follow their own technique chart because it has always worked for them; this approach does not take into consideration changes in equipment or patient variables. Administrators must be involved in periodically reviewing images to ascertain that quality images are being produced by all radiographers.

Chapter Summary

1. Patient variables of body habitus and part thickness determine the technical factor selection.
2. Technical factors (kVp, mAs) are manipulated by radiographers to produce high-quality radiographs.
3. A 4- to 5-cm change in part thickness requires mAs to be changed by a factor of 2.
4. The tissues and materials demonstrated radiographically are air, fluid, fat, bone, and metals from surgical procedures.
5. Minimum change in mAs is 30% to demonstrate a visible difference between structures in the image.
6. Additive and destructive pathologies must be considered when selecting the kVp and mAs for a given procedure.
7. Procedures where contrast media (iodine or barium) is used to enhance visualization of soft tissue structures require a change in kVp.
8. The two most common technical factor charts are variable kVp-fixed mAs and fixed kVp-variable mAs.
9. Technical factor charts standardize the selection of kVp and mAs for the average patient so that consistently high-quality radiographs can be produced.
10. Technical factors may need to be modified for pediatric patients, casts, body habitus, pathologic conditions, and contrast media procedures.

Case Study

Judy is a chief radiographer in an imaging department that recently installed a new radiography room. She must develop a technique chart for this new unit to ensure quality images are consistently produced by all the radiographers who use the room.

Critical Thinking Questions

1. Which tools will Judy need to assist her in formulating the new chart?
2. When making exposures of the phantoms, should Judy use the AEC or common technical factors that other units use? Why?
3. After obtaining the optimal radiographs of the phantoms, which method will Judy use to build the remainder of the chart?
4. Once the chart is developed, is it ready to be used on the entire patient population?

Review Questions

Multiple Choice

1. Using a base kVp of 50, how much kVp is needed for a cervical spine that measures 13 m in the AP projection?

a. 60
b. 58
c. 76
d. 80

2. Which is considered a destructive pathology?

a. Ascites
b. Pneumonia
c. Tuberculosis
d. Gout

3. 5 mAs is used for an elbow measuring 6 cm thick. What is the new mAs for a 10-cm-thick elbow?

a. 10
b. 7
c. 4
d. 6

4. The average ankle thickness for an adult is:

a. 10 to 13 cm
b. 8 to 10 cm
c. 10 to 12 cm
d. 6 to 8 cm

5. When using a variable kVp chart, how much is kVp changed for each 1 cm change in part thickness?

a. 4
b. 5
c. 3
d. 2

6. An AP lumbar spine is imaged, and the resultant image demonstrates the outline of the vertebral bodies but no bony markings. Which factor must be changed first?

a. kVp
b. mAs

7. **High-kVp charts are developed for which procedures?**
   a. Barium procedures
   b. Routine chest exams
   c. Lower extremity
   d. a and b
   e. b and c

8. **The stocky, larger body type is termed:**
   a. Sthenic
   b. Hypersthenic
   c. Asthenic
   d. Hyposthenic

9. **What is the primary purpose of using a fast exposure time when performing a chest exam on a pediatric patient?**
   a. Improves visualization of lung tissue
   b. Creates a blurred image of the ribs
   c. Helps to stop the motion of diaphragms
   d. Mediastinal structures are better demonstrated

10. **How will kVp be changed when imaging the skull of a 4-year-old patient compared to the technique for an adult?**
    a. kVp will be decreased by 15%.
    b. kVp will not be changed.
    c. kVp will be increased by 15%.
    d. kVp will be increased by 50%.

Short Answer

1. **How does the asthenic body habitus differ from the hyposthenic body habitus?**

2. **Measurement of body parts should generally be taken:**

3. **Will a fiberglass cast on a forearm require a change in technical factors?**

4. **What percentage of change in kVp is equivalent to a 100% change in mAs?**

5. **An abdomen radiograph was obtained using 80 kVp and 15 mAs. The image demonstrates adequate penetration but has a very long scale of contrast. What change is needed and why?**

6. **__________ kVp is recommended for small extremities.**

7. **An AP knee measures 15 cm, selecting 70 kVp and 16 mAs produces a quality image. What is the change in mAs for an AP knee that measures 11 cm?**

18

Automatic Exposure Control

Objectives

Upon completion of this chapter, the student will be able to:

1. State the purpose of using automatic exposure control (AEC) in radiography.
2. Distinguish between the various types of radiation detectors.
3. Describe how the detector size and configuration affect the AEC response to radiation.
4. Explain the positioning errors, which affect how the AEC responds to radiation.
5. Discuss patient and exposure technical factors and their effect on the AEC detector.
6. Describe anatomically programmed radiography (APR).
7. Explain the purpose of the mAs readout and how it can be used to learn manual technique.
8. Discuss the effect the backup timer/mAs has on the length of the exposure when the AEC malfunctions.
9. List the various types of operator errors that are seen when using the AEC device.
10. State the purpose of the density controls.

Key Terms

- anatomically programmed radiography (APR)
- automatic exposure control (AEC)
- backup timer
- density controls
- detectors
- ionization chamber
- mAs readout
- minimum response time (MRT)
- photomultiplier (PM) tube
- phototimers

Introduction

The automatic exposure control (AEC) is a device available on modern radiographic equipment and is designed to compensate for differences in patient size by adjusting the exposure time. The AEC measures the exit radiation and adjusts the exposure time to produce a proper density in the image. The general purpose of the AEC is to assist the radiographer in producing more consistent exposures resulting in fewer repeat images and ultimately reducing radiation exposure to the patient.

The radiographer is responsible for selecting the techniques and detector configuration to produce the quality image. There are thousands of potential combinations of kVp, mA, SID, exposure time, image receptor, and grid ratios. The radiographer must be knowledgeable about each of these factors in addition to patient variables and pathologic conditions; this makes for a challenging task. The radiographer's judgment is crucial to determine how to manually set the technical factors or to use the AEC or combining both practices. In this chapter, you will learn about the evolution of detectors, the proper use of these detectors, positioning considerations, limitations of using AEC, and the use of automatically programmed radiography (APR) to produce a quality image.

Detectors

All **automatic exposure control** devices work on the same principle: As the radiation exits the patient, it strikes the **detectors** that convert the radiant energy into electrical current, which terminates the exposure time. The exposure time is terminated when the preset amount of radiation has been detected; the electrical current exiting the detector indicates the level of radiation received by the chamber.

There are two basic types of AEC devices used to convert radiation into electrical current. Automatic exposure devices called phototimers were the first generation for use, and this is the origin for the term phototiming that is still used today. The current generation in use is the ionization chamber. Regardless of the type of detector used, most systems use three radiation measuring devices in a triangle configuration. Each detector can be used independently or in combination with other detectors to measure the radiation exposure reaching the image receptor. The radiation monitoring devices are called by various names such as sensors, chambers, cells, or detectors. In this text, they will be referred to as detectors.

Phototimers

Phototimers are AEC devices that use **photomultiplier (PM) tubes** or photodiodes; there have been other AEC devices developed, but an understanding of the photomultiplier tube is in order. The photomultiplier tube is an electronic device that converts light energy into electrical energy. The photodiode is a solid-state device that performs the same function as the PM tube. Phototimer devices are considered exit-type devices because the detectors are located after the image receptor. The exit radiation passes through the image receptor and is then measured by the detectors (Fig. 18.1). The detectors are light paddles that are coated with fluorescent material,

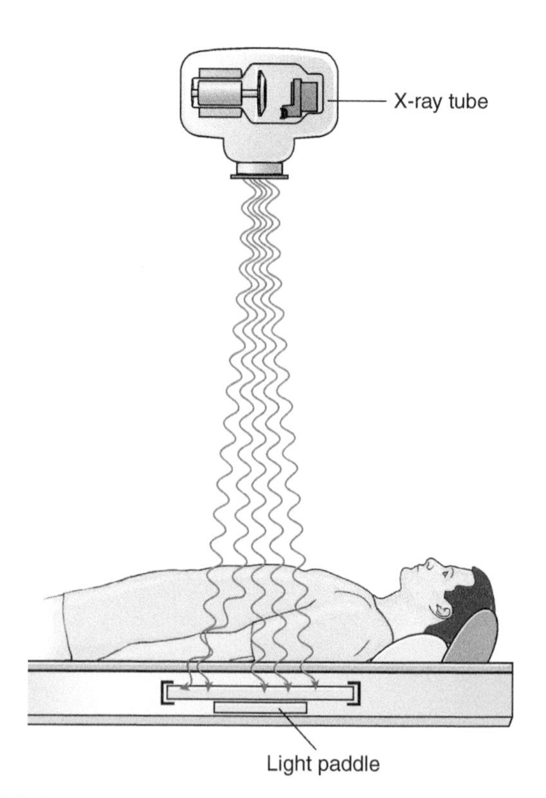

Figure 18.1. **Phototimer automatic exposure control: The detectors are located directly behind or below the image receptor. This is called an exit-type device because the x-ray photons must exit the image receptor before they can be measured by the detectors.**

the exit radiation strikes the paddle, and visible light energy is produced. The light is transmitted to the photomultiplier tubes or photodiodes, which convert the light to electricity. When the preset amount of exposure is reached, the timer is tripped and the exposure terminated. Although the phototimers have been mostly replaced by ionization chambers, the term *phototiming* is still used by radiographers.

Ionization Chamber

An **ionization chamber** (Ion chamber) is a flat, rectangular, double-plate of very thin aluminum or plexiglass with a layer of gas encased in the middle. This chamber is connected to the timer circuit by an electrical wire. Ionization chambers are entrance-type devices because they are positioned before the image receptor (Fig. 18.2). The radiation will leave the patient and interact with the chamber before reaching the image receptor; therefore, the radiation enters the ionization chamber first. The gas atoms are ionized by the radiation-freeing electrons. The electrons are attracted to and strike the positively charged anode plate at one end of the chamber. The electrons then flow out of the anode plate and down a very thin wire, becoming an electric charge. The electric charge is proportional to the radiation to which the ionization chamber has been exposed. The ion chamber is the most commonly used AEC device.

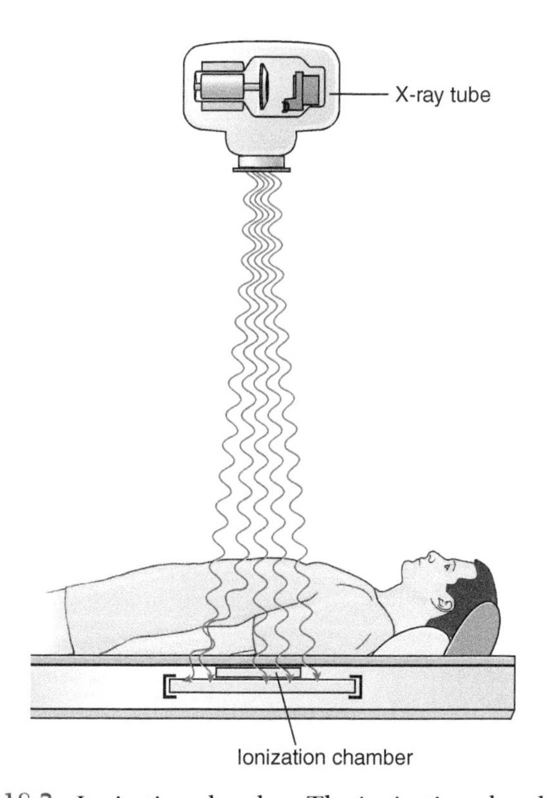

Figure 18.2. **Ionization chamber: The ionization chamber automatic exposure control device has the detectors that are between the patient and image receptor. This is called an entrance-type device because the x-ray photons are measured in the chamber before reaching the image receptor.**

kVp and mA/s Selection

The AEC controls the quantity of radiation reaching the image receptor and has no effect on image contrast. The radiographer must always select the correct kVp for the exam regardless of using an AEC or manually setting a technique. As discussed in Chapter 17, the minimum kVp necessary to sufficiently penetrate the part must always be set. To produce the correct scale of contrast in the image, the proper kVp must be selected; using very high kVp will create excessive scatter radiation, which will negatively affect the contrast of the image. Changing the kVp will change the image contrast but not the image density when an AEC circuit is operating. When the image contrast is degraded, a repeat image will be required; this in turn increases the radiation dose to the patient, which is the very thing we wanted to avoid by using higher kVp.

Digital imaging measures the exposure to the AEC, and using higher kVp results in a shorter exposure time needed to provide a sufficient amount of radiation to the AEC. Higher kVp is more penetrating, and detectors measure the quantity of radiation; the preset amount of radiation is reached faster with higher kVp because more x-ray photons are exiting the patient. This results in decreased exposure time and overall mAs needed to produce the image. The main advantage is a decreased radiation dose to the patient.

The radiographer will also select the milliamperage (mA) station that is appropriate for the part being imaged whether or not an AEC is being used. When using AEC, the mA station is set independently from the exposure time, which the AEC controls. mA directly effects the exposure time needed to produce the correct quantity or mAs for the image. Increasing the mA station will result in a lower exposure time and vice versa. When radiographers want to use a very short exposure time, they simply select a higher mA station on the control panel.

mAs Readout

The **mAs readout** displays the total amount of radiation (mAs) required to produce an appropriate exposure to the image receptor. The AEC system determines the length of time the exposure will last. Radiographic units have a mAs readout display that shows the actual amount of mAs used for the image. The mAs readout will be displayed for a few seconds immediately after the exposure. Advantages to reviewing the mAs readout include the following:

1. When a radiographer is not comfortable setting manual exposure factors, he or she can make note of the mAs readout, which aids in learning manual exposure technical factors.
2. When a suboptimal image is produced, the mAs readout provides a basis for making an adjustment and using manual exposure technique.

Many exams have different positions where the AEC is difficult to use. For these select exams, the radiographer should use both the AEC and manual techniques. An example: An AP lumbar spine can be easily imaged with the AEC; the radiographer must make note of the mAs readout. The oblique lumbar spine is difficult to position directly over a detector. To assure a proper image, the radiographer should manually set the kVp and mAs for the oblique image. A skilled radiographer will utilize all the tools in the imaging department to produce quality images and reduce the number of repeat images that are needed because of poor use of an AEC. With an AEC circuit in operation, changing the mA setting will not change the image density, because the AEC circuit will adjust the exposure time to obtain the same image density.

Minimum Response Time

Minimum response time (MRT) is the shortest exposure time the system can produce. The MRT for modern AEC systems is 1 millisecond (ms) for the chamber to detect and react to the radiation exposure. MRT is state-of-the-art equipment that can produce exposure times as low as 0.002 s. High-power generators combined with higher digital processing speeds make it possible for the actual exposure time to be so reduced that the AEC circuit will not respond correctly. The machine will not shut off until the MRT is reached, which results in overexposure to the patient. An alternative solution is to reduce the mA station to produce sufficient exposure. For example, a 300 mA station × 0.005 s exposure = 1.5 mAs. The ideal technique for a pediatric AP chest image is 65 kVp @ 0.8 mAs. AEC set with the 300 mA will result in overexposure to the patient by twice the radiation. The solution is to lower the mA station to 100 or 150, which will result in 0.5 or 0.75 mAs, respectively.

Ion chambers, scintillation detectors, or solid-state detectors are used as AEC detectors. Regardless of the type of detector used, there are three detectors located in a triangular configuration. The two outer detectors are located on either side and slightly above the central detector.

The radiographer is responsible for properly selecting the appropriate detectors and positioning the patient or the body part over the active detectors. Positioning the patient over the photocell must be accurate to ensure proper exposure. When the patient's anatomy does not completely cover the photocell, the primary beam will expose the detector and the exposure will terminate prematurely. The result will be a lack of density in the image, likely resulting in a repeat exposure. The type of examination determines which detectors should be selected. For example, the posteroanterior chest examination employs the two outer detectors to ensure proper density of the lung field rather than the spine, whereas the lateral chest examination uses only the central detector.

Backup Timer

The **backup timer** is the maximum length of time the exposure continues when using an AEC. The backup timer or backup mAs can be set either by the radiographer or automatically by the unit. The AEC circuit rarely fails, but if it does, the backup timer is a safety mechanism that terminates the exposure after a maximum time, which prevents excessive duration of exposure. The backup timer or backup mAs is designed to protect the patient from excessive and unnecessary exposure and to prevent the tube from reaching or exceeding heat-loading capacity. A backup timer is always set in case the AEC circuit fails.

Historically, a typical backup timer setting of 5,000 ms was used. This means that the backup timer shuts off the x-ray beam after a 5-second exposure, which would deliver an incredible amount of radiation to the patient. A general rule to follow is to set the timer or mAs for two times the expected exposure time or mAs for the projection. For example, an AP abdomen manual technique of 20 mAs was obtained using 300 mA station and 0.066 s. Multiplying the time by two for a backup time of 0.13 s, the maximum exposure delivered would be 40 mAs. If the backup time had been set for 5 seconds, the patient would have been exposed to 1,500 mAs!

Operator error plays a major role in the importance of the backup timer. A common error is when the wall Bucky is selected and the x-ray tube is directed toward the table Bucky or vice versa. Selecting the incorrect image receptor activates the wrong AEC. Example is when the table Bucky is selected but the vertical Bucky is being used for a thoracic spine exam. The exposure will continue indefinitely because the table detectors are forced to wait an extremely long time to measure enough radiation to terminate the exposure. The backup time is reached and exposure is terminated, which limits patient exposure and prevents tube overload. Without the backup timer, the exposure would continue until the tube failed. Modern units are designed with a sensor in the Bucky tray and will not allow an exposure to activate if the table Bucky detectors are selected when the x-ray tube is centered to the vertical Bucky.

In units where the radiographer is able to set the backup timer, he or she must be sure to set the backup time high enough to be greater than the desired exposure needed for an optimal image but low enough to protect the patient from excessive exposure if the x-ray tube fails to function properly. Another general rule to follow is setting the backup timer 1.5 times longer than the expected time. If the backup time is too short, it will result in the exposure terminating prematurely, which will result in a poor quality image. A backup time that is too long would result in unnecessary radiation exposure to the patient if a problem occurs and the exposure does not end until backup time is reached. This would cause too much radiographic density on this image, and it may have to be repeated because of poor quality.

It cannot be stated too frequently that any time an image is repeated, the dose to the patient is doubled! Producing diagnostic quality images on the first attempt requires a skilled radiographer who understands the functions of the equipment, patient anatomy, and pathologic processes. Combining all this knowledge is essential to producing a quality image with the first exposure.

Density Controls

Density controls or adjustments allow the radiographer to adjust the amount of preset radiation detection sensitivity. The control console has knobs or buttons labeled density, and these are applied to the AEC circuit. The unit may display the change using a bar display that becomes wider with increased density and narrower for decreased density. Other manufacturers use body habitus illustrations for small, medium, and large figures that are selected to change density. The preset sensitivity of the detectors is increased or decreased by specific percentages. Because the mA is set, it is the exposure time that is automatically extended or shortened by these percentages.

In digital imaging, the controls are called intensity controls because the detector actually determines the intensity of exposure at the plate.

There are various formats for the density button or knobs. One method is to use small, average, or large settings. The small setting uses one-half the exposure time than the average setting, while the large setting is twice the exposure time. A second type of configuration is to have ½, ¾, N, 1½, 2 where N is normal or average. 1½ is 50% more than average.

A seven-station configuration has AEC density controls of −3, −2, −1, N, +1, +2, and +3, which permit adjustment of the image density. N is the normal or average setting. Each incremental step changes the image density by 25%. The +3 setting is three steps of 25% for an increase of 75% above normal.

In Chapter 17, the minimum change rule of 30% increase or decrease in mAs is needed to visually demonstrate a difference in image density. The +1 setting would not be enough for substantial improvement in exposure to the image receptor because it would only be a 25% change; therefore, the +2 setting is recommended selection.

When it is desirable to decrease the density, the −1 selection does provide sufficient change because it is a 25% reduction of the normal exposure. This equates to ¾ of the original exposure. For example, 15 mAs for AP abdomen is normal, −1 = 75% of 15 for 11.25 mAs. Using the 30% rule is a great method to check the math for the −1 setting. For example: 15 mAs × 30 % = 4.5, 15 − 4.5 = 10.5 mAs; as you can see either the 11.25 or 10.5 mAs setting would be appropriate.

A properly calibrated AEC unit should not require adjustment of the density controls to produce an acceptable radiograph. Changing the mA or kVp selectors on an x-ray unit with a properly functioning AEC will not change the image density. The AEC circuit changes the exposure time to maintain the same density following changes in mA, kVp, or distance.

When radiographers find that they need to make constant adjustments by using the density buttons, this means there is a calibration problem or poor positioning of the part. Poor centering of an AP hip may have a significant portion of the detector beneath the soft tissue rather than the bone tissue. The radiation penetrates more easily through the soft tissue resulting in the AEC terminating the exposure early, which underexposes the anatomy of interest, which is the femoral head, femoral neck, and acetabulum.

In digital imaging, the computer can compensate for an overexposure to display an acceptable image, but if it cannot compensate for underexposure; the information is simply not present on the plate! With film screen imaging, an overexposed image can be viewed with a hot light to view the anatomy; however, this is not optimal as an overly dark image may obscure the information. An underexposed image is missing information on the x-ray film, which prevents the anatomy from being visible.

In radiography, the frog-leg lateral hip image can be quite challenging because of the tissue thickness. Properly centering the femoral neck over the detector will demonstrate proper exposure of the femoral neck but the femoral head and acetabulum will be underexposed. This occurs because the thickest part of the anatomy is not over the detector but is in the corner of the image (Fig. 18.3). Using the +2 density control is indicated for routine frog-leg lateral hip to add sufficient mAs to demonstrate the femoral head and acetabulum.

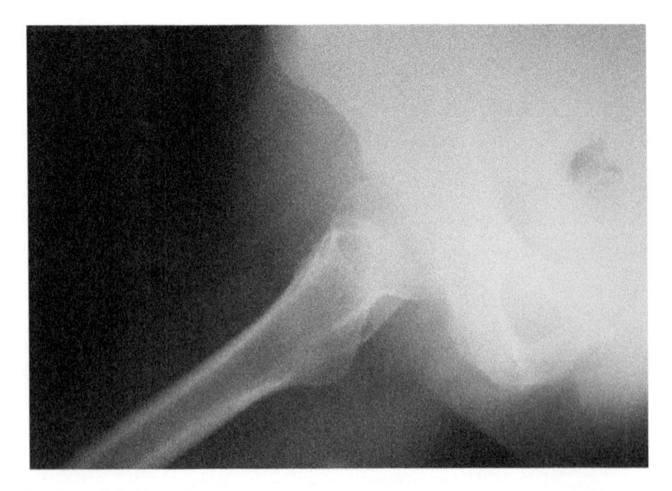

Figure 18.3. **Illustrates a detector that is only partially covered by the anatomy of interest. Underexposure of the acetabulum and femoral head will result in the AEC shutting off too early.**

AEC Limitations

The AEC detectors were never intended to replace the radiographer's knowledge and critical thinking abilities. Rather, it was meant to be used as a tool to produce a quality radiographic image in concert with setting manual techniques. Unfortunately, too many radiographers use the AEC as a "crutch" so they don't have to remember the various combinations of kVp and mAs required for specific anatomical imaging. The AEC is a wonderful tool, but it does have its limitations, and if not used properly, it may cause the need for repeat images.

Each radiographic procedure has specific central ray locations, image sizes, and collimation, which must be carefully used to provide a quality image. The goal is to properly align the anatomical part of interest to the image receptor and to use either the AEC or manual technique.

The AEC limitations that all students and radiographers must consider include the following:

1. Never use the AEC for anatomy that is too small or narrow to completely cover at least one detector. Distal extremities and extremities in general on small children fit into this category. The detector measures the average amount of radiation striking the area. Uncovered sections receive too much radiation, which prematurely terminates the exposure; this results in an underexposed image.
2. Anatomy that is close to the edge of the body like the clavicle or lateral sternum will not be correctly imaged with the AEC. Portions of the detector may not be covered with anatomy. The exposure terminates too early and results in an underexposed image as seen in Figure 18.4.
3. The proper positioning and centering of the anatomy of interest must be perfected! Tissue of interest must cover the detector that was selected for use. Near-perfect centering can be very difficult to obtain especially for spine imaging. Correct positioning and centering is quite easy to do on an AP projection of the lumbar spine, but on the oblique and lateral projections, it can be very challenging especially on larger patients. The lateral lumbar spine is nearly the same width of a detector, and near-perfect centering is a must for the detector to receive sufficient radiation to image the spine (Fig. 18.5).

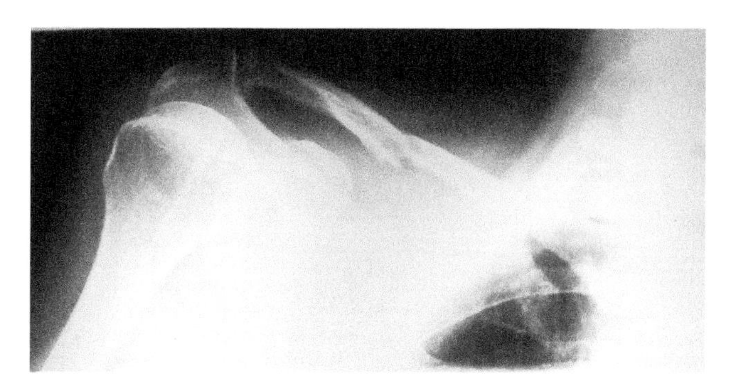

Figure 18.4. **Clavicle image illustrating incorrect placement of the anatomy in relation to the AEC detector. A portion of the detector is not covered by tissue and will receive primary x-ray beam exposure. This will result in early termination of the exposure and an underexposed image.**

4. The field must be properly collimated to the anatomy of interest. When the field is too large, there is excessive scatter radiation from the patient's body and table. Detectors cannot distinguish between scatter and transmitted radiation. The scatter radiation will be absorbed by the detector and will cause the detector to prematurely stop the exposure. When the field is collimated too tightly, the detector does not receive sufficient exposure initially, and a longer exposure time is needed, which results in overexposure. In digital imaging, the plates are very sensitive, and when the exposure is terminated too early, the image will appear "washed out," which is an overall light appearance. The image may also begin to show quantum mottle because of the insufficient amount of radiation. The art of closely collimating side to side is quickly becoming a lost art as many radiographers leave the field open to the size of the image receptor or plate. Cervical spine projections, Swimmer's lateral spine images, and cross-table lateral hip images all require a tightly collimated field. The previous three anatomical examples are imaged with a 10 × 12 in.-sized light field. In digital imaging, DR plates come in the standard size of 14 × 17 inches. It would be irresponsible to image a hip using a 14 × 17 inch field size. It is essential that the radiographer use the correct field size or smaller to decrease the amount of tissue, which is exposed to radiation.

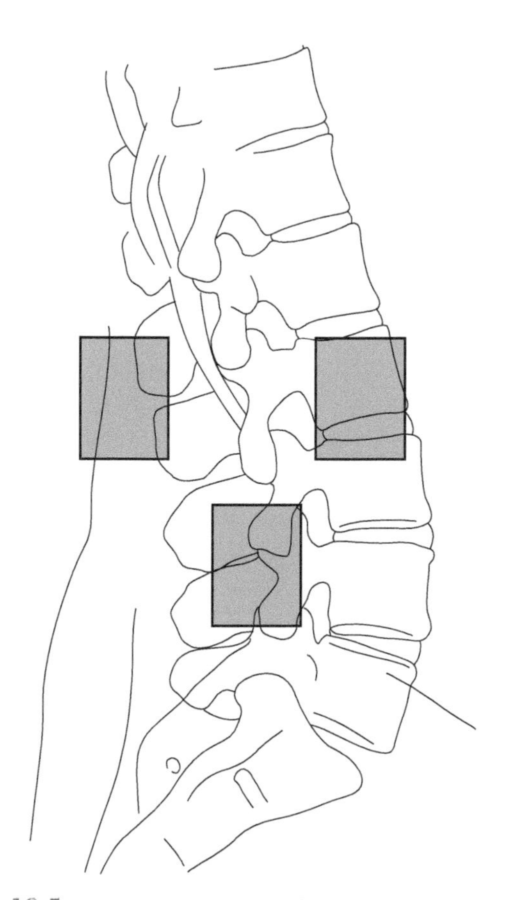

Figure 18.5. **Positioning error. The centering for the lateral lumbar spine is posterior to the lumbar vertebral column. The resulting image demonstrates vertebral bodies that are underpenetrated; it is determined that the image is underexposed.**

5. The AEC should never be used when the patient has an additive pathology, surgical prosthesis, orthopedic corrective device, or other large metal artifacts that cannot be removed, or in the presence of positive contrast media. The effect of the metal is that it lowers the measured intensity of the beam at the detector, and the AEC will stay on much longer to reach the preset value. The result is excessive exposure to radiation when the AEC overextends the exposure time. For example, a patient has a prosthesis in the hip, and a frog-leg lateral hip is positioned (Fig. 18.6). Upon exposure, the metal will effectively block the radiation from reaching the detector, and the exposure time can run all the way up to the backup time or mAs. The radiation dose may be up to 20 times higher than if manual technique had been used!!! The unacceptability of such levels of radiation dose goes without saying.

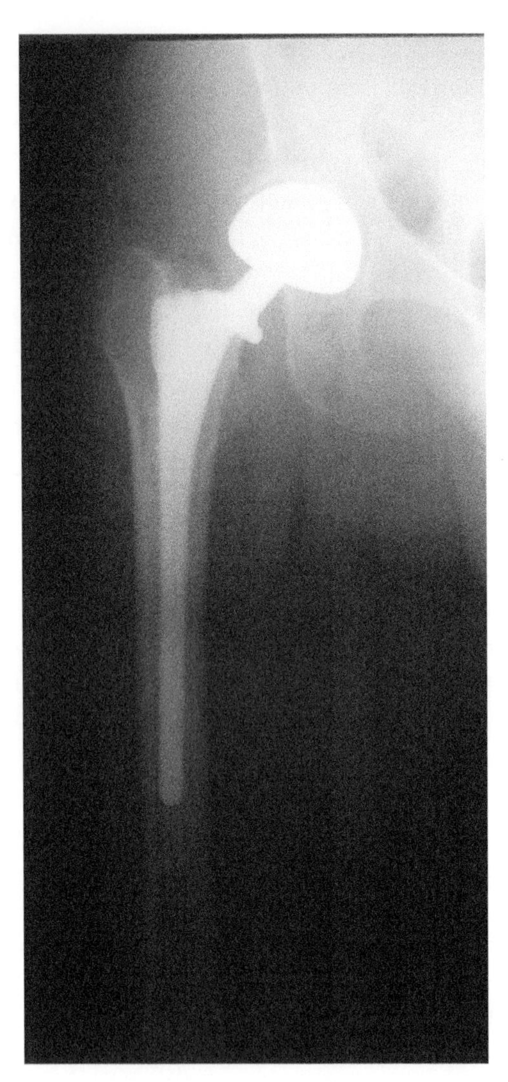

Figure 18.6. **Large metal orthopedic prosthesis such as seen in this hip image leave large areas where the x-rays are not able to penetrate through the metal. The detector cells will average the measured exposure across the entire area, the exposure time will be extended, and overexposure will occur at the image receptor. The patient will also receive a higher dose of radiation than is necessary for the exam.**

Detector Configuration

The standard configuration of detectors is a triad of rectangular-shaped demarcated lines on the tabletop or vertical Bucky (Fig. 18.7). The radiographer can select 1, 2, or 3 detectors for the image. Careful positioning and selection of the proper combination of detectors are essential in producing a satisfactory radiograph with the AEC unit. The thickest anatomy needs to be positioned over the energized detector to assure adequate exposure to the image receptor. Determining which of the three detectors to energize is part of the positioning consideration for each image. Experienced radiographers develop a sense of tissue densities and anatomy to be visualized; they use this knowledge to their advantage and become creative in selection of detectors.

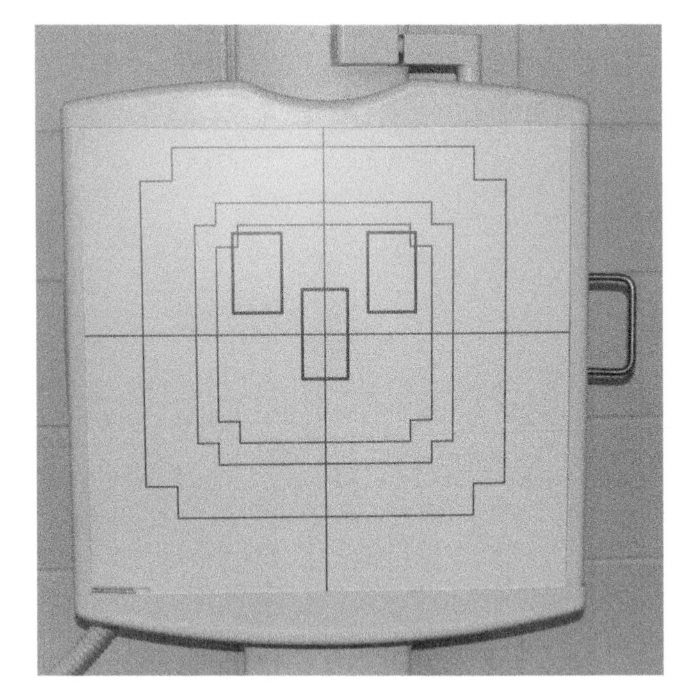

Figure 18.7. **AEC detector configuration. Triad configuration of three automatic exposure control detectors on an upright Bucky.**

As previously discussed, improper selection of detectors can result in either underexposure or overexposure of the image receptor. Figure 18.8 illustrates a frog-leg lateral hip. When imaging the hip, there must be sufficient penetration of the acetabulum and head of the femur. As seen in the illustration, the three detector locations do not all cover the anatomy of interest. The upper cell that is closest to the acetabulum can be selected because this is the thickest part of the anatomy. It would be acceptable to *also* select the center detector, which lies under the proximal femur. The selection of either or both detectors will ensure adequate exposure to the image receptor. Selecting the detector that is partially covered by anatomy would result in the exposure terminating prematurely and therefore would not be chosen.

Imaging the thorax presents a challenging mixture of tissue types. The anatomy includes the lungs, whichare air-filled radiolucent structures, and the heart, which is a muscular structure filled with blood that has a radiopaque appearance. This presents a unique situation in selecting the best configuration of detectors, especially when using digital imaging. For film screen imaging, the outside detectors are selected because the lungs are the critical

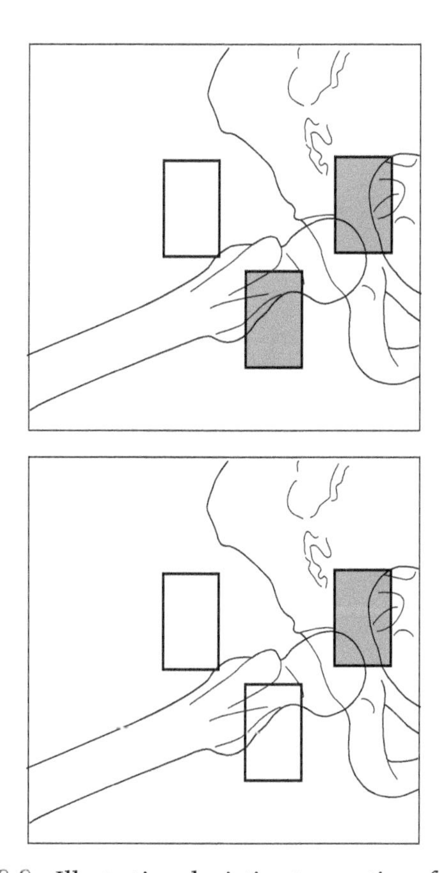

Figure 18.8. **Illustration depicting two options for proper configuration of AEC detectors for a frog-leg lateral hip. The medial cell and center cell are placed under the thickest anatomy.**

area of interest. The detectors will quickly receive adequate amounts of radiation to reach the preset exposure amount. This will produce an image with the best scale of contrast to adequately visualize the lung structures. However, the heart and mediastinum area are underexposed and show up as very light areas. The thoracic spine is over the center detector, and if the center cell is chosen, the exposure would last longer until there was adequate penetration of the spine. This would result in better visualization of the heart and mediastinum but would produce overexposure to the lung tissue. One major advantage of digital imaging is the ability of the system to make corrections in exposure. It is better to have adequate exposure through the heart and mediastinum and let the digital system lighten the lung fields; therefore, the center cell would be used in digital imaging (Fig. 18.9).

For the lateral lumbar spine, the center detector is selected. If the lumbar spine is positioned too posterior and the spine is not placed directly over the center detector, the spine will not be properly penetrated and will be underexposed, requiring a repeat image. With digital imaging, the computer can adjust for exposure error and provide an acceptable image; however, image quality and patient exposure are compromised. Underexposure is seen as quantum mottle that degrades the image.

Abdominal imaging is commonly performed for patients who are experiencing excessive amounts of bowel gas. This pathologic condition extends the abdomen, which makes the patient's abdomen thicker than normal. An experienced radiographer will recognize the special imaging considerations caused by the excessive bowel gas. The detectors will be covered by areas of excess bowel gas, which permits the x-ray beam to pass through the tissue with little attenuation. The timer will stop prematurely and result in underexposure of the abdomen tissue. When imaging destructive pathologies, there is a higher chance of the image being underexposed. For these reasons, a manual technique would best image the anatomy.

Precaution Checklist

Digital imaging systems do a terrific job of covering up errors, which makes it very difficult to determine if the AEC is working properly. Film screen imaging is much easier to see errors because the image will appear too light when underexposed or too dark when overexposed. Digital systems have exposure indicator (index) numbers that indicate exposure to the patient. It is critical that the radiographer monitor the exposure index for each exposure. This is an ethical and professional practice that radiographers must develop the habit to always check the index number. It is becoming more common to overexpose a patient when using digital systems because as long as the image "looks good," that is all that matters. Our mission as radiographers is to use the least amount of radiation necessary to produce a diagnostic image. Manufacturers use different exposure indicator ranges that indicate if the exposure was within range and acceptable. When the number is higher than the indicator range, it indicates an overexposure for the projection, and when the number is lower, it indicates underexposure because of insufficient penetration of the beam. As already stated, this leads to quantum mottle, which requires a repeat exposure that effectively doubles the amount of radiation dose or exposure to the patient.

Tables 18.1 and 18.2 provide a checklist of common errors that would explain high- or low-exposure indicator numbers. Whenever the exposure indicator number is curiously high or low, the radiographer must investigate the reasons why this occurred. Through

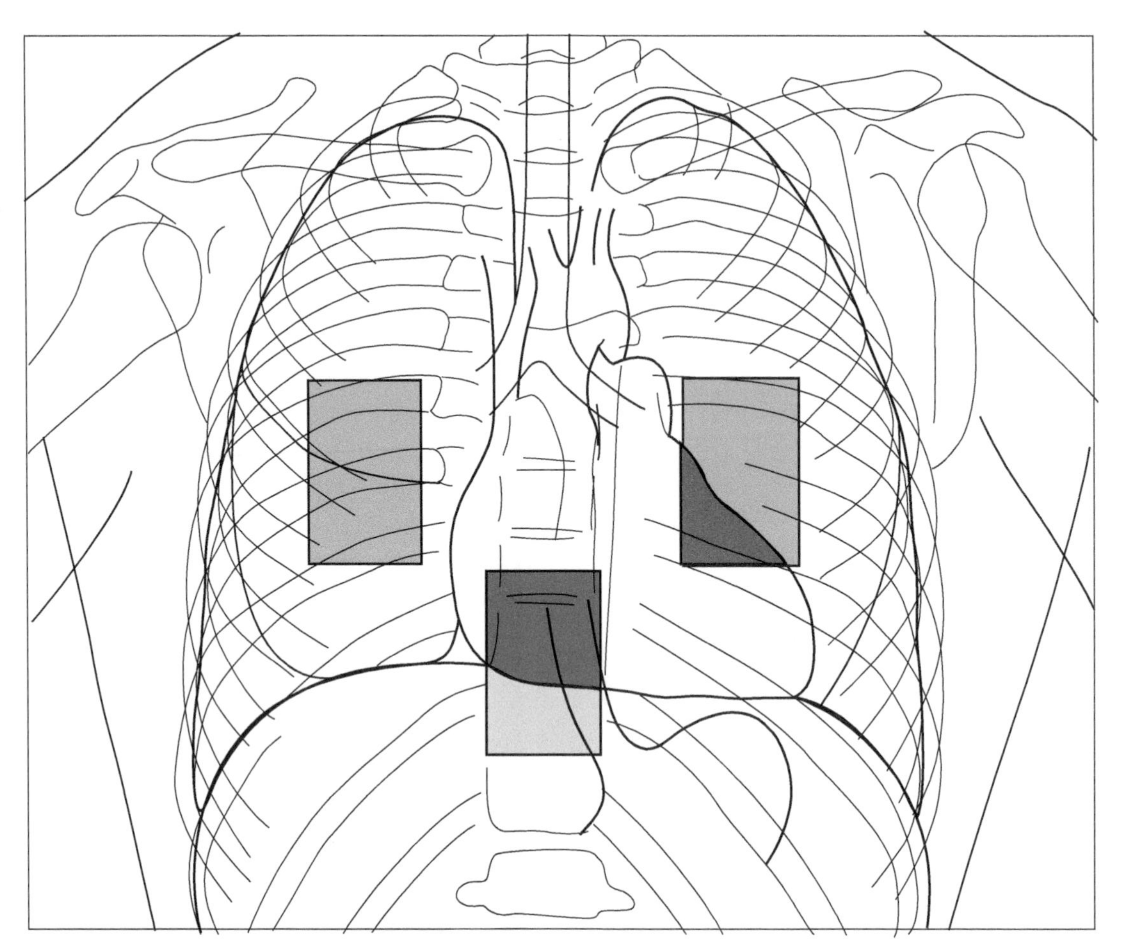

Figure 18.9. **Illustration of use of AEC detectors for a digital chest image. Using the two outer detectors will result in underexposure of the heart and mediastinum because the majority of the detector is under lung tissue. Adding the center detector will ensure adequate exposure through the mediastinum.**

a process of elimination, the checklist will help the radiographer narrow down the cause of the incorrect exposure.

TABLE 18.1 CAUSES OF OVEREXPOSURE USING AEC

Incorrect Bucky activated
Exposure time less than minimum response time
Density control left on +1, +2, etc. from previous patient
AEC malfunctioned
Incorrect detector cell configuration selected, energized detector(s) are under anatomy that is more dense or thicker than the anatomy of interest.
Presence of orthopedic metal prosthesis, which cause radiopaque artifacts
Presence of any external artifact like a sandbag or lead strip over the detector

TABLE 18.2 CAUSES OF UNDEREXPOSURE USING AEC

Backup timer set shorter than the necessary exposure time
Density control left on −1, −2, etc. from previous patient
Lack of adequate collimation resulting in excessive scatter radiation to the detector
Incorrect detector cell configuration, energized detector(s) are under tissue that is less dense or thinner than the tissue of interest.
Detector(s) not completely covered by tissue of interest:
• Anatomy peripheral to detector
• Anatomical part too small to effectively cover detector
• Specific tissue area too small to effectively cover detector
• Anatomical area of interest not centered over energized detector(s)

AEC Technique Charts

Chapter 17 covered information for developing a technique chart for setting manual technique. The use of AEC does not mean a technique chart should not be used. The only thing the AEC controls is the exposure time; the radiographer still selects the optimum kVp and optimum mA station for the anatomy to be imaged. The correct detector configuration must also be made, and backup time should be set.

To provide a consistent method of obtaining images, an AEC technique chart should be developed for each unit. The imaging department needs to standardize the AEC technique chart so that regardless of which radiographer is performing the exam, a consistent, quality image can be obtained. Table 18.3 provides an example of a technique chart for the use of an AEC. The use of

TABLE 18.3 **AEC TECHNIQUE CHART**

Procedure	Projection	kVp	mA	Detector(s)	Density Control	SID and Notes
Chest	PA/AP	110–125	200	■ ■ □	N	72″
	Lateral	110–125	200	□ □ ■	N	72″
Ribs above diaphragm	AP/Obl	70	300	□ □ ■	N	40″
Ribs below diaphragm	AP	70–80	400	□ □ ■	N	40″
KUB	AP	80	400	□ ■ ■	N	40″
Pelvis	AP	80–85	400	■ ■ □	N	40″
Hip	AP/Lat	80–85	400	■ □ ■	+2	40″ Medial and/or center
Lumbar spine	AP/Obl	75–85	400	□ □ ■	N	40″
	Lat	80–90	400	□ □ ■	N	40″
	L1/S1	85–95	400	□ □ ■	N	40″
Thoracic spine	AP	75–85	300	□ □ ■	N	40″
	Lat	80–90	400	□ □ ■	N	40″ Breathing
Swimmers C/T	Lat	80–95	400	□ □ ■	N	40″
Cervical spine	AP/Odontoid	75–85	150	□ □ ■	N	40″
	Obl/Lat	75–85	150	□ □ ■	N	72″
Skull (sinus) (facial bones)	PA/Caldwell	70–80	150	□ □ ■	N	40″
	Waters	70–80	150	□ □ ■	N	40″
	Townes	70–80	150	□ □ ■	N	40″
	Lateral	70–80	150	□ □ ■	N	40″
Shoulder	AP	70–85	200	□ □ ■	N	40″
Knee	AP/Obl/Lat	70–85	200	□ □ ■	N	40″

any technique chart makes it easier for students and new radiographers to produce quality images.

Radiographers must learn to use both the AEC and manual technique settings and maintain clinical proficiency with both. To exclusively rely on the AEC is a practice that compromises image quality and that has led to increasingly higher radiation doses to patients. Imaging the distal extremities, cross-table projections, mobile trauma imaging, and the presence of metallic artifacts are all situations where the use of manual techniques is a best practice. As advancements in digital systems continue to progress, there will always be situations where manual techniques will still need to be used instead of the AEC. A great radiographer will know how to use both!

Anatomically Programmed Radiography

Anatomically programmed radiography (APR) has been designed to simplify the selection of technical exposure factors by incorporating preprogrammed technical factors for each type of procedure. The design and appearance of the control panels may vary, but each provides an easy selection of the main anatomical area of interest (thorax) and more refined exam (ribs). The radiographer simply selects the button on the control panel that represents the area of interest, and the preprogrammed set of technical factors (kVp and mAs) is displayed. Additional settings for large, average, and small patients may be available. The appropriate AEC detectors are also indicated. The control panel has a computer chip or circuit that is programmed for various exams and projections as well as positions of the part. The APR can be used to view kVp, mA, and time when learning how to set manual technique. The APR and AEC together display the factors and cell configuration for specific exams. For example, PA chest, 120 kVp, 200 mA station, large focal spot, vertical or wall Bucky, and two outer cells.

The APR settings do not take into account variations in body habitus, pathology, and conditions that occur from patient to patient. The patient size indicators of large, average, and small are limited and do not cover all possibilities. APR settings should never be considered the "final word"; they can and should be overridden when appropriate. Preprogrammed settings simplify and expedite the setting of techniques. All the advancements in technology do not and should never replace the independent judgment and discretion of the radiographer in determining the final set of exposure factors to obtain the best possible exposure results for each projection.

Chapter Summary

1. AECs improve the consistency of radiographic exposures; however, there are limitations to the effectiveness of using AECs.
2. The selected detectors must be completely covered by anatomy for an adequate exposure to occur.
3. It is crucial that proper positioning of the part not be compromised to allow for the use of an AEC.
4. It is acceptable to use the density controls for specific projections and situations. The +2 density setting should be used to make a significant difference when increasing exposure.
5. The x-ray field must be well collimated when using AEC. It is especially critical when using digital imaging.
6. The correct configuration of AEC detectors is necessary for a proper exposure to be made.
7. Optimum kVp and mA must still be set by the radiographer. The AEC controls the amount of time it will take for the preset exposure to be reached.
8. MRT is the minimum amount of time and signal needed to operate the AEC.
9. Backup timer or mAs settings terminate the exposure when the AEC circuit fails to end the exposure when the preset limit has occurred. The backup timer prevents excessive exposure to the patient and excessive heat overload to the tube.
10. The detectors are in a triad configuration and can be selected individually or in a combination.

11. The ionization chamber is the common type of detector currently in use. The ionization chamber contains air that becomes ionized by radiation, which creates an electric charge.

12. APR is another system that allows selection of a specific body part and position, which results in a display of preprogrammed exposure factors. The APR can also include AEC configuration.

Case Study

Joanie is preparing to perform a routine two-view chest x-ray on a patient. The x-ray unit has AEC capabilities, and Joanie decides to use AEC for the exam. She uses the preprogrammed settings for chest anatomy and one outer cell for the PA and lateral projections. Upon review of the images, Joanie notices the lateral image has a lack of contrast and density resulting in an underexposed image.

Critical Thinking Questions

1. What is the primary error that produced the underexposed image?
2. Which detector should Joanie use for the repeat lateral projection?
3. Should Joanie use manual technique for the repeat image or the preprogrammed setting?

Review Questions

Multiple Choice

1. What is the resulting exposure when the incorrect Bucky is activated during an AEC exposure?

a. The exposure will terminate prematurely.
b. The exposure will remain on for a longer time because the detectors are not sensing radiation.
c. The backup timer will be activated because of the long exposure time.
d. a and b.
e. b and c.

2. The backup time should be set at __________ the expected exposure.

a. Three times
b. Six times
c. Two times
d. Four times

3. The most critical factor in obtaining diagnostic quality images using an AEC circuit is the use of correct:

a. positioning
b. focal spot size
c. SID
d. backup time

4. When utilizing the AEC, changing the mA from 100 to 300 will result in:

a. more density
b. less contrast
c. less distortion
d. a shorter exposure time

5. Phototimers are electronic devices that use a(n) __________ to convert light energy into electrical energy.

a. ionization chamber
b. photodiode
c. p–n junction
d. rectifier

6. **The mAs readout display will show:**

   a. only the mA used for the exposure
   b. only the length of time for the exposure
   c. the mAs required to produce an appropriate exposure
   d. the backup mAs

7. **Which of the following is an operator error?**

   a. Selecting the incorrect image receptor.
   b. Using the wrong detector configuration for the exam.
   c. Positioning the anatomy in such a way that the detector is not completely covered.
   d. Each of these is an operator error.

8. **Each incremental step change in the density control will change the density by:**

   a. 25%
   b. 55%
   c. 75%
   d. 60%

9. **It is acceptable to use the AEC for distal extremity imaging.**

   a. True
   b. False

10. **A 14 × 17 detector plate is used to image a cervical spine projection. There was minimal collimation evident on the image. How will the excessive scatter radiation affect the AEC?**

    a. Detector will absorb radiation and terminate the exposure too quickly.
    b. Image will appear "washed out."
    c. Quantum mottle will be present because the exposure terminated too soon.
    d. Each will affect the AEC.

Short Answer

1. **Explain the two reasons why backup timers are still very important.**

2. **When an image is produced and the exposure indicator is high, what does this indicate?**

3. **Explain why it takes longer for the AEC to terminate the exposure on thicker body parts.**

4. **Which detectors are used for a hip image? Explain why.**

5. **Describe the exit-type detector.**

6. **List three causes of overexposure when using an AEC.**

7. **The APR serves what purpose in selecting exposure technical factors?**

PART IV

Digital Imaging and Processing

19

Basic Principles of Digital Imaging

Objectives

Upon completion of this chapter, the student will be able to:

1. Describe how a matrix of pixels is used to form a digital image.
2. Identify the relation between matrix size, pixel size, and field of view.
3. Identify the differences between spatial resolution and contrast resolution.
4. Describe how postprocessing manipulation allows for improved visualization of the image on the monitor.
5. Compare the dynamic range between digital imaging and film screen.
6. Discuss how digital image characteristics of brightness, contrast, and resolution compare to film screen imaging.
7. Recognize the effect of quantum noise, scatter, and artifacts on the quality of a digital image.

Key Terms

- artifact
- bit depth
- brightness
- contrast resolution
- dynamic range
- gray scale
- matrix
- pixel
- pixel density
- pixel pitch
- quantum noise
- spatial frequency
- spatial resolution
- window level
- window width

Introduction

Digital images are used throughout medical imaging. They appear as computed tomographic (CT), magnetic resonance (MR), ultrasound, mammography, computed radiography (CR), direct radiography (DR), fluoroscopy, and diagnostic images. Unlike film screen images, whose contrast, speed, and latitude are fixed during processing, the appearance of digital images can be altered after they have been recorded and stored. Changes in the processing and display of the digital data can enhance visualization of information and suppress quantum noise in the final image. The advantages of digital imaging include the ability to adjust the contrast after the image has been recorded, to process the image to emphasize important features, and to view the image on a high-resolution monitor immediately after the exposure has terminated. In this chapter, the material will focus on the characteristics of digital images with comparison to film screen images.

Creating the Digital Image

Digital image receptors respond to a wider range (dynamic range) of x-ray exposures than do film screen images. Traditionally, the film screen images are static images that cannot be manipulated if they are underexposed or overexposed. Like the old saying, "What you see is what you get!" The computer systems utilized in digital imaging are capable of taking a moderately underexposed or overexposed image and displaying it as an acceptable diagnostic image. In digital imaging, the response of the image receptor is linear as compared to the curvilinear response of film screen (Fig. 19.1). The linear response displays a greater range of radiographic densities, which makes all anatomic tissues easier to visualize.

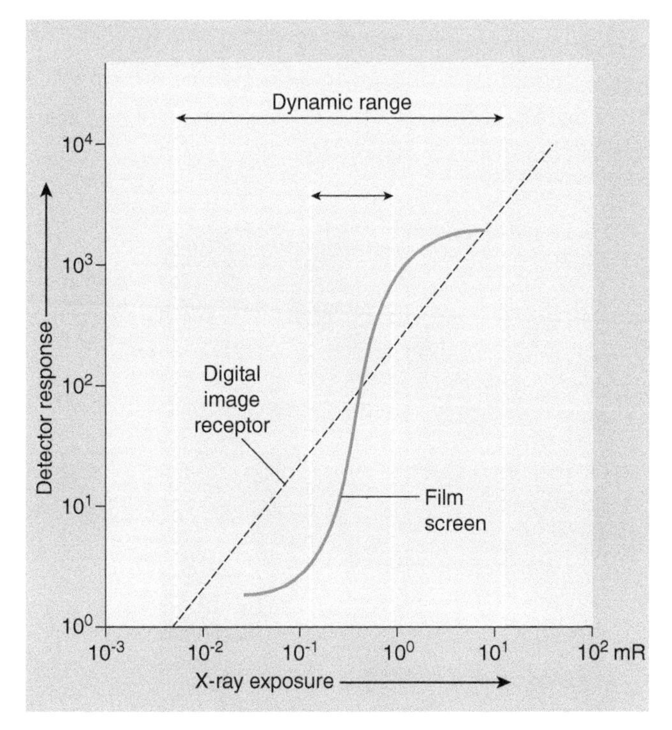

Figure 19.1. **The digital image receptor has a wider dynamic range compared to film screen.**

The images are constituted of numerical data, which are easily manipulated by a computer. When the image is displayed on a monitor, there is flexibility in altering the brightness and contrast of the digital image. One advantage is that any anatomic structure can be independently and optimally visualized. Another advantage is that the computer can perform postprocessing manipulations that will further improve the visibility of the digital image.

A digital image is made up of a matrix of picture elements or **pixels**. A **matrix** is an array of cells, which is arranged in rows and columns that is stored in computer memory. The designation of each cell corresponds to a row and column that identifies the specific location of the pixel in the image (Fig. 19.2). The numeric or pixel value of each cell represents the level of **brightness** or density assigned to that location in the image. Pixels with a higher number have greater density than do pixels with a lower number. The pixel value represents the area within the patient or volume of tissue that is being imaged.

The size of the matrix is described by the number of pixels in the rows and columns (Fig. 19.3). A small matrix has fewer pixels compared to a large matrix, which has many pixels. For example, a matrix with 256 pixels in each row and column is called a 256 × 256 matrix (written 256 × 256); one with 512 pixels in each row and column is called a 512 × 512 matrix. Some systems have a 1,024 × 1,024 matrix size, which provides a very small size of pixels in the matrix. A 1,024 × 1,024 has 1,048,576 pixels while a 2,048 × 2,048 matrix has 4,194,304 pixels. Think of the matrix as a box in which you want to put in smaller boxes or pixels. In order to increase the number of boxes in the matrix, the size of each box must decrease to fit more boxes in the matrix. The higher number of small boxes or pixels there are in the matrix, the better the resolution of the image.

		COLUMNS				
		1	2	3	4	5
ROWS	1	1-1	2-1	3-1	4-1	5-1
	2	1-2	2-2	3-2	4-2	5-2
	3	1-3	2-3	3-3	4-3	5-3
	4	1-4	2-4	3-4	4-4	5-4
	5	1-5	2-5	3-5	4-5	5-5

Figure 19.2. **A matrix is made up of rows and columns of individual picture elements, each designated by its row and column number.**

7	20	23	37	21
21	80	85	92	7
26	10	88	40	11
17	75	93	100	35
4	15	23	19	42

A

7	6	2	19	8	12	43	58	46	38
11	13	6	9	13	15	23	65	50	27
15	18	9	8	10	9	16	40	37	21
12	12	21	77	78	60	65	23	12	6
20	22	11	2	8	10	80	9	3	7
20	23	30	9	6	85	22	17	6	9
26	30	15	16	95	30	34	20	19	12
17	14	26	94	6	3	4	8	1	2
8	5	7	93	88	91	85	2	3	8
6	4	3	7	2	1	6	5	2	6

B

Figure 19.3. **Two sizes of matrices each covering the same physical area. Image A is a 5 × 5 matrix and B is a 10 × 10 matrix. Image A has 25 pixels while image B has 100 pixels. Notice that the pixels in image B are much smaller. Because the smaller pixels produce sharper resolution, it is easier to distinguish the pattern of larger numbers in B.**

Larger size matrix = Smaller pixels
= Improved image sharpness

Picture Elements or Pixels

Each pixel in the matrix is capable of representing a wide range of shades of gray from white to black. The maximum range of pixel values is determined by the amount of exit radiation that is detected and recorded. Each pixel contains bits of information, and the number of bits per pixel that determines the shade of gray is called the **bit depth**. Bit depth is the exponent of a base of 2 that produces the equivalent binary number for the range of gray shades in the image. The number of shades of gray for various ranges includes the following: a pixel with a bit depth of 6 has a range of 2^6 or 64 shades, 7 bits deep for a range of 2^7 or 128 shades, 8 bits deep for a range of 2^8 or 256 shades, and 10 bits deep for a range of 2^{10}, which is 1,024 shades of gray. Most digital radiography systems use an 8, 10, or 12 bit depth. The human eye can only distinguish 32 shades of gray or 2^5; however, the computer with sufficient capacity can distinguish up to 4,096 bit depth (Fig. 19.4). A higher bit depth will provide better contrast resolution. The level of gray will be a determining factor in the overall quality of the image.

Spatial Resolution

Spatial resolution is described as the minimum separation between two objects at which each can be distinguished as two separate objects in the image. Specific to digital imaging, spatial resolution describes the ability of an imaging system to accurately display objects in two dimensions. Digital images with smaller pixel sizes have better spatial resolution. In film screen imaging, the crystal size and thickness of the phosphor layer determine resolution; in digital imaging, pixel size is a limiting factor of resolution. Spatial resolution can be measured in terms of the **spatial frequency** that is measured in line pairs per millimeter (lp/mm). At least two pixels are required in order to image one line pair because a line pair consists of one brighter shade and one darker shade of density. A pixel which is 0.4 mm in size will only measure 2 lp/mm while a 0.1-mm pixel can measure 6 to 8 lp/mm. By comparison high-speed film screen measures 8 to 10 lp/mm while slow-speed film screen measures 10 to 12 lp/mm. Spatial frequency in lp/mm is derived from the minimum object size that can be imaged (a single pixel). The formula for this relationship is written as:

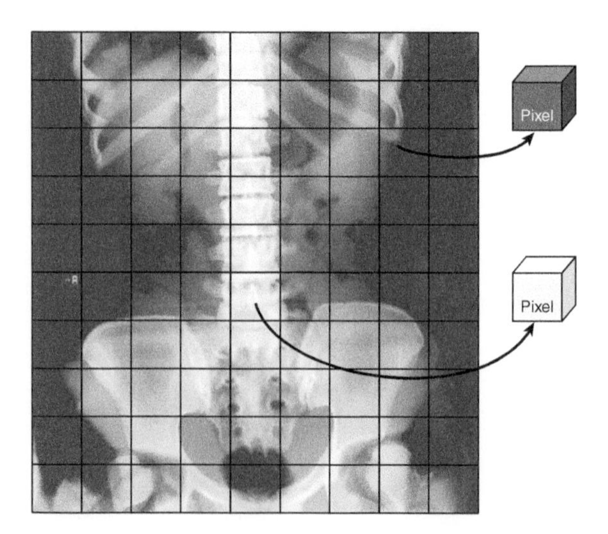

Figure 19.4. **Zero represents white or no intensity while higher numbers show darker shades of gray or more intensity.**

$$SF = \frac{1}{2}(PS)$$

where *SF* is the spatial frequency in lp/mm and *PS* is the pixel size in millimeters. This formula demonstrates that spatial frequency is a measure of image resolution.

CRITICAL THINKING BOX 19.1

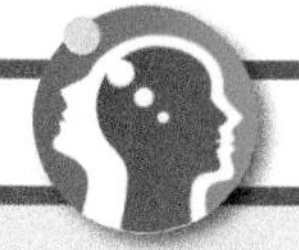

For a pixel size of 0.4 mm, what is the resolution in line pairs per millimeter?

Specifically, it can be stated that the size of the matrix is inversely proportional to pixel size and directly proportional to spatial resolution.

$$\text{Large matrix} = \text{Small pixel size} = \text{Improved spatial resolution}$$

As digital systems have evolved to use smaller pixels, the spatial resolution has improved and comes close to that of film screen but is not quite as good. Digital systems may have poorer spatial resolution, but this is offset by the vast improvement in contrast resolution. As illustrated in Figure 19.5, a small matrix contains fewer pixels

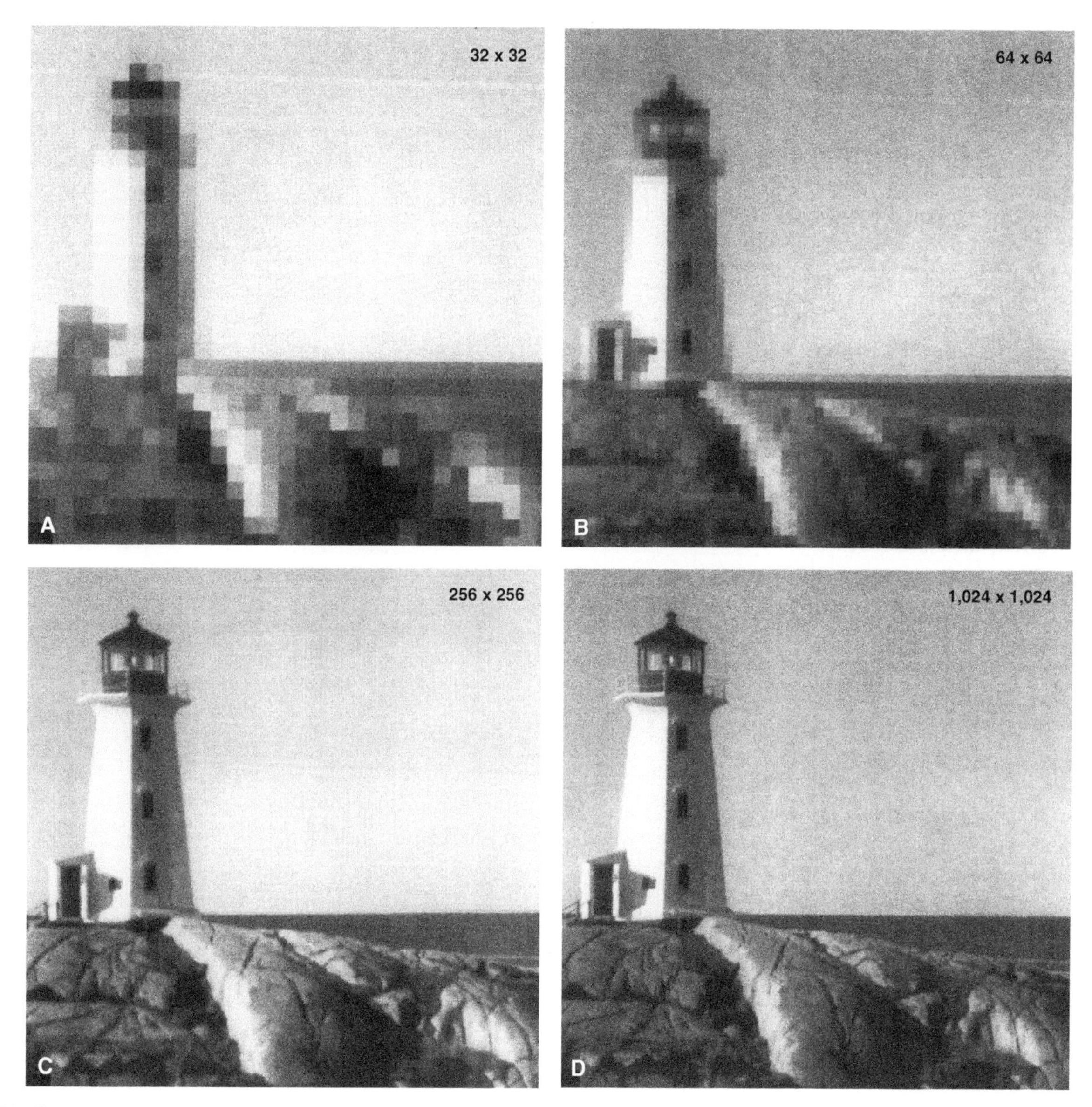

Figure 19.5. Demonstrates the improvement in spatial resolution and appearance of a digital image as the matrix size and pixel size change. (A) Large pixels are easy to distinguish. (B) The pixels are twice as small, but it is still easy to determine individual pixels. (C) The pixels are even smaller and more difficult to see, but the image has a blurred appearance. (D) Notice how the structures in the image are sharp and clear; the individual pixels cannot be distinguished.

to adequately demonstrate the many details in an image. As the matrix size increases, the details in the image become more and more distinct. When the matrix has reached maximum size, the image details are sharp and crisp making it easy to see the many parts of the lighthouse and rocks.

Field of View and Pixel Size

The size of the pixel is related to the size of the matrix, but it is also related to the field of view (FOV) seen on the display monitor. In conventional radiography, the FOV included the anatomic structures, which were in the collimated x-ray beam that was projected onto the radiographic film. In digital radiography, the FOV is the portion of the imaging plate that contains the relevant anatomical information (latent image), which is displayed on the monitor. For example, the FOV for an infant chest x-ray would be considerably smaller than that for an adult chest x-ray. Each image is displayed on the monitor using the same image matrix, and the smaller FOV will contain more pixels in a given display area than will the larger FOV for the adult chest.

The size of pixels in an image is directly proportional to the size of the displayed FOV and inversely proportional to the size of the matrix. The relationship of the pixel size to the size of the matrix and FOV is explained in the formula:

$$\text{Pixel Size} = \frac{\text{FOV}}{\text{Matrix}}$$

CRITICAL THINKING BOX 19.2

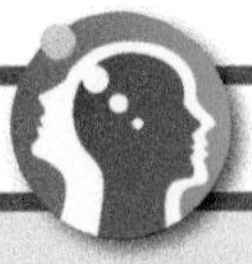

What is the pixel size in millimeters (mm) of a 256 × 256 matrix for an image with a 20-centimeter (cm) FOV?

When the FOV increases and the matrix size remains the same, the pixel size must increase. On the other hand, when the FOV decreases and the matrix size remains the same, the pixel size decreases. It is easy to see there is a direct relationship between FOV and pixel size.

If the FOV remains the same and the matrix size changes, the pixel size changes. An increase in the matrix size results in a decreased pixel size (Table 19.1).

TABLE 19.1 SHOWS THE RELATIONSHIP BETWEEN FOV, MATRIX SIZE, PIXEL SIZE, AND SPATIAL RESOLUTION

FOV	Matrix Size	Pixel Size	Spatial Resolution
Increases	Remains constant	Remains constant	Decreases
Decreases	Remains constant	Remains constant	Increases
Remains constant	Increases	Decreases	Increases
Remains constant	Decreases	Increases	Decreases

CRITICAL THINKING BOX 19.3

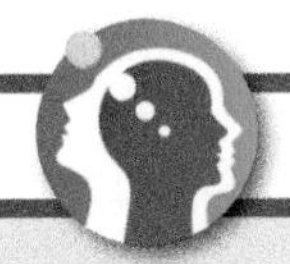

What is the pixel size for a 10 × 10 in. digital image that is reconstructed at the display screen on a 512 × 512 matrix?

CRITICAL THINKING BOX 19.4

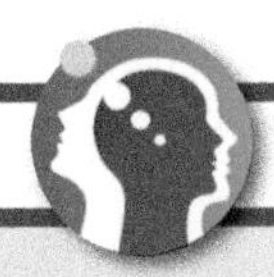

An 82 × 82 cm FOV is projected onto a monitor screen with 0.8 mm pixels. What is the size of the matrix on the monitor screen?

Displayed Image Characteristics

The visibility and accuracy of the anatomical structures on the display monitors is just as important as viewing the anatomical structures on film. The characteristics include brightness, contrast, spatial resolution, and image noise. Each of these will be further explored in this section.

Brightness

When viewing an image on the monitor, densities seen in the image are described as levels of **brightness**. Brightness is described as the amount of luminance or light emission of the display monitor. In the radiographic image, areas of decreased density are seen as increased areas of brightness on the monitor. Bone is a great example of an anatomical area in an image that has decreased density. Because bone has a higher atomic number, it will attenuate more of the beam, and fewer photons will reach the image receptor. On the image, the appearance of the bone is white or a light shade of gray; this correlates to more luminance seen on the monitor in this area. Therefore, bony structures display more brightness than do other anatomical structures. Conversely, areas of increased density on the image are seen as areas of decreased brightness, for example, abdomen tissue.

In digital imaging, the brightness level is easily manipulated on the monitor to improve the visualization of the range of anatomic tissues. The manipulation is possible because the intensity of a digital image is controlled by the numerical value of each pixel. Manipulating the level of brightness displayed on the monitor assists in creating a quality diagnostic image.

The human eye can distinguish 32 shades of gray; however, the x-ray beam that exits the patient contains over 1,000 intensities. The image receptor must be able to capture this broad range of intensities to adequately image all the structures in the FOV. To accomplish this, the image receptor needs to have a wide dynamic range. Because digital imaging has a wide dynamic range combined with computing ability to adjust for exposure errors, there is a greater margin of error to produce acceptable densities. This means that if the exposure technique used is not perfect for the anatomical area, the radiographer can manipulate the image to compensate and still produce a diagnostic image. The vast range of densities can be manipulated by radiographers, and it is their responsibility to choose the appropriate density ranges to be displayed. When processing the digital image, the radiographers must use discretion in manipulating the image so they do not inadvertently obscure diagnostic information.

Although it is wonderful to have such a wide dynamic range, it is only useful when it can be seen by the human eye. The displayed image brightness can be altered to optimize viewing. The adjustment is made by using a windowing function of the system. The **window level** control sets the density value displayed at the center of the density range because it sets the center point of the entire gray scale at a selected gray level. The center point of the gray scale also sets the average gray level in the image. As seen in Figure 19.6, the window level can be adjusted up or down the density scale from white to black. As the level is adjusted up or down, the entire window of displayed gray shades adjusts with it. The window level must be set to the diagnostic range for the anatomy being visualized so the proper level of diagnostically relevant information will be displayed.

Imagine a scale of eleven gray shades that are arranged from white on the bottom to black on top. Over the scale is a sliding window of a fixed size with a red circle at the center point. In **A**, the center point is level with the third step on the gray scale, a light-to-medium shade of gray. Within the borders of the window, you can see five steps of the gray scale; the average brightness of the entire image being visualized is 3.0 (the third step which is the center point). Now, move the red circle up four steps. In **B**, the range of visualized steps remains at five but the overall appearance is darker. The average brightness is now a 7.0 or the seventh step. The window level has been increased, resulting in a darker average brightness that makes the overall appearance darker.

There is a direct relationship between displayed image density and window level; as the window level is increased, the displayed image brightness (density) will increase. An example is a dark area that is hard to see (high pixel value). To compensate, turn up the brightness on the monitor to make it easier to see the area. In film screen, an image was held up to a hot light to improve visualization! Areas on an image that appear very bright (low pixel value) or glaring on the monitor can make it difficult to visualize the anatomy. To compensate, the window level will need to be adjusted to make the image appear darker, which will decrease the brightness seen on the monitor. Turning down the brightness on the monitor will reduce the glare and make it easier to visualize that area of the anatomy.

Recall that pixel values can range from 0 to 1,024, depending on the size of the matrix, and are used to signify the range of image densities or brightness levels in the image. A low pixel value could signify an area of tissue where the x-ray beam was highly attenuated; this would be displayed as an area of increased brightness (or decreased density) on the monitor. A high pixel value would signify a volume of tissue where the x-ray beam had minimal attenuation and would be displayed as an area of decreased brightness (or increased density) on the monitor.

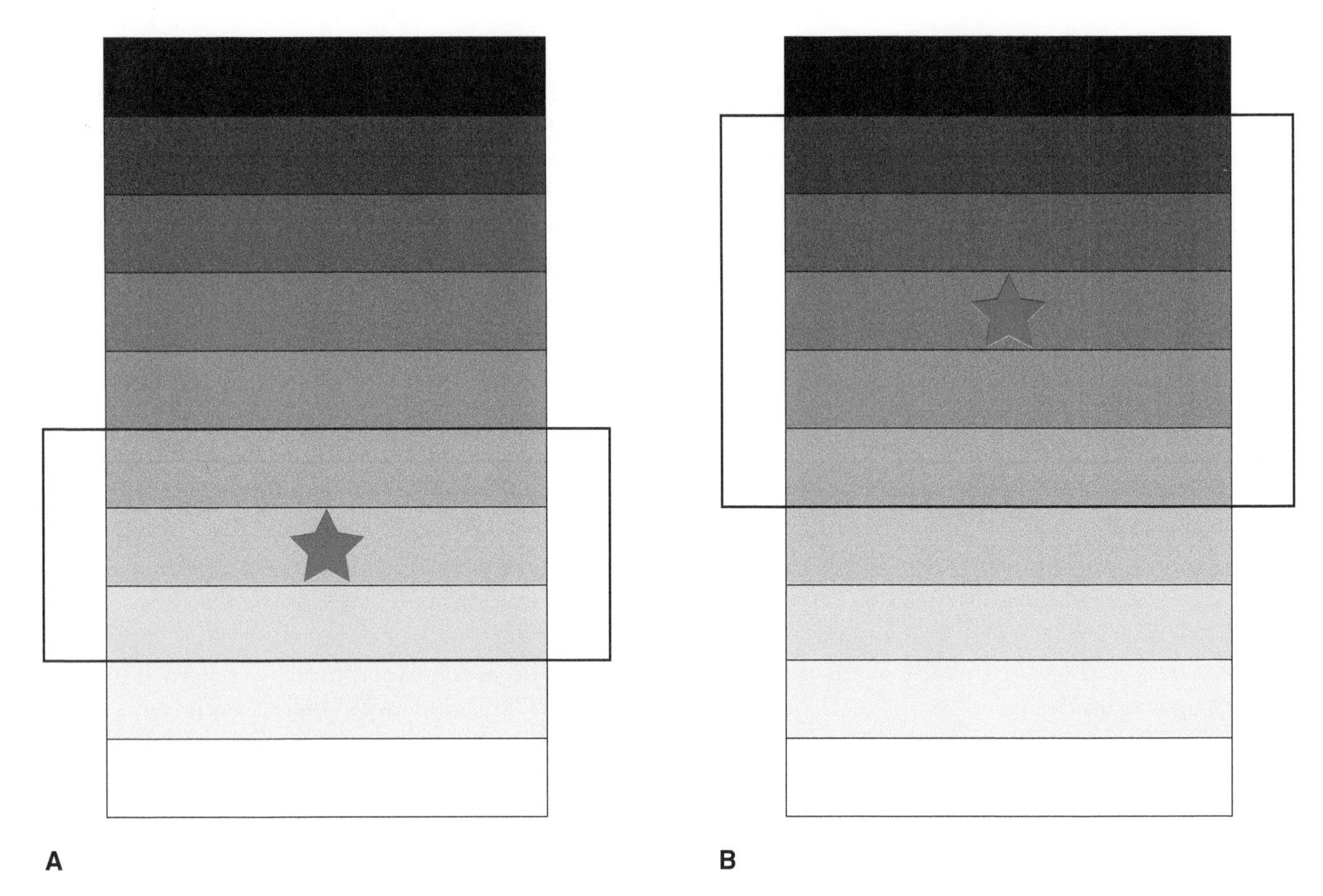

Figure 19.6. **Image A, the window level is at the lower end of the range of gray shades while image B is at the upper end of the range. Both images include the same number of shades, but image B appearance is an overall darker image.**

- Low pixel value = high attenuation = increased brightness = decreased density
  - Example: bony structures
- High pixel value = low attenuation = decreased brightness = increased density
  - Example: lungs or soft tissue

Contrast

As previously discussed in this text, contrast is a term used to describe the shades of gray seen in an image. In digital imaging, it is called **gray scale** and represents the number of different shades that can be stored and displayed on the monitor. In digital imaging, **contrast resolution** describes the ability of the imaging system to distinguish between small objects that attenuate the x-ray beam in a similar manner. In comparison to film screen, contrast resolution is much improved in digital imaging. The contrast resolution improves the visibility of the minimum density differences or shades of gray between two tissues that can be detected in an image. Contrast resolution depends on the depth of the pixels (8, 10, 12, etc.) because the bit depth directly affects the number of shades of gray available on the display monitor. Increasing the bit depth produces more shades of gray, which increases contrast resolution and the visibility of the recorded detail along with the ability to distinguish between small anatomic areas of interest. As seen in Figure 19.7, **A** is an image with only two shades, black and white, which displays a high contrast image, yet the small details are obscured. The bit depth is higher in **B** and **C** where more gray shades are seen; however, the subtle details in the image are still not visible. **D** has the highest bit depth of 256, which allows the visualization of small areas of interest.

After processing, the radiographic contrast can be adjusted to vary the visualization of the anatomy of interest. The human eye is limited in the number of shades of gray that can be visualized and having the ability to adjust the contrast in the image improves visualization. The **window width** is the adjustment that is used to

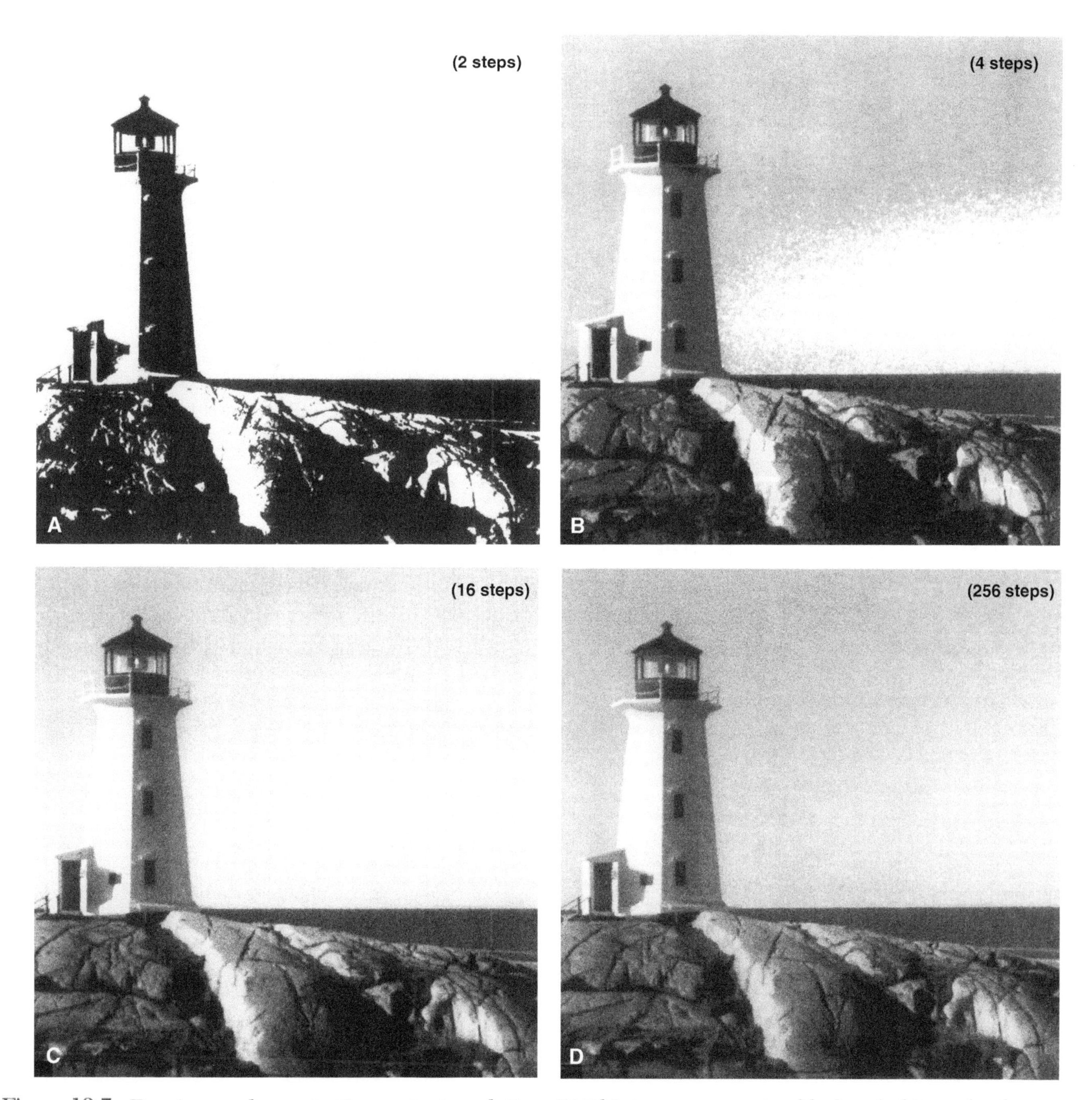

Figure 19.7. **Four images demonstrating contrast resolution. (A) This image represents a black and white scale of contrast. Much of the detail of the image is obscured because there is not enough information to form a complete image. (B) With four steps of gray scale, we can now begin to distinguish more areas of the picture. (C) The sky, rocks, and lighthouse are beginning to demonstrate more detail because there are more shades of gray. (D) An image with the maximum number of data values has pixels with densities covering a vast range; this provides the most comprehensive set of data for the image.**

change the radiographic contrast. Because the gray scale ranges from black to white, the display monitor can vary the range of densities visible on the image to show all of the anatomy of interest. Adjusting the range of densities varies the image contrast. Displaying the entire range of densities, wide window width, results in an image with lots of shades of gray and lower contrast in the image. In abdominal imaging, a wide window width allows the visualization of the various tissue structures located in the abdomen. When a smaller range of densities is displayed, narrow window width, the image has fewer shades of gray and higher contrast. Extremity imaging benefits from a narrow window width to improve visualization of fine trabecular markings in the bone.

Similar to film screen, radiographic contrast is inversely related to the range of visible densities.

Smaller range = few shades of gray
= high contrast resolution

Greater range = many shades of gray
= low contrast resolution

The center or midpoint of the window width determines the contrast of the displayed image. Using the sliding window and eleven-step gray scale, we can visualize the length of gray scale present in an image (Fig. 19.8). The slide window in both **A** and **B** is centered on the scale at step six. Window **B** is vertically wider and you can see nine steps on the gray scale compared to five steps in window **A**. By focusing on the gray scale seen within the slide window, the gray scale in image **B** has been increased although the average gray level is the same. This is an example of changing window width without changing window level.

Dynamic Range

The **dynamic range** is the range of gray levels available to construct the image. Images are represented by binary numbers in 2, 4, 8, 16, 32, 64, 128, 256, 512, 1,024, etc. gray levels. The binary number correlates directly to the shade of gray, which is represented in each pixel. When the dynamic range is too low, the gray scale will be too short resulting in a loss of image detail. A greater dynamic range combined with a longer gray scale produces more details represented in the image.

When "selecting" the bit depth, a consideration must be to determine the ideal dynamic range. A narrow dynamic range will improve computing power while maintaining enough correct levels of gray and brightness. However, the range chosen must allow postprocessing manipulation of the image to adjust the brightness or contrast. A range of 256 (2^8) is eight times the capability of the human eye and would allow for overall brightness to be doubled or halved without running out of available gray levels. For most images, the range that is eight bits deep would be sufficient while maintaining the ability

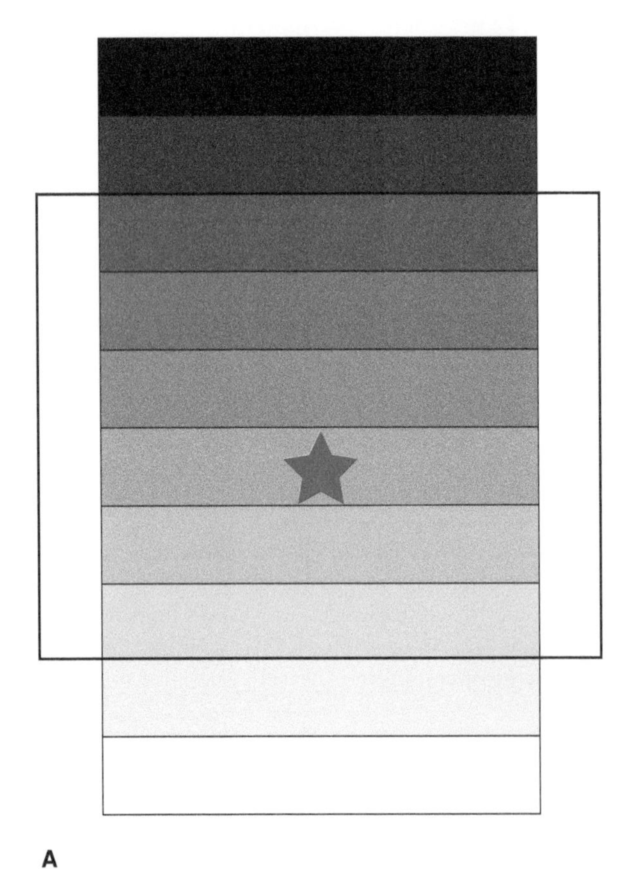

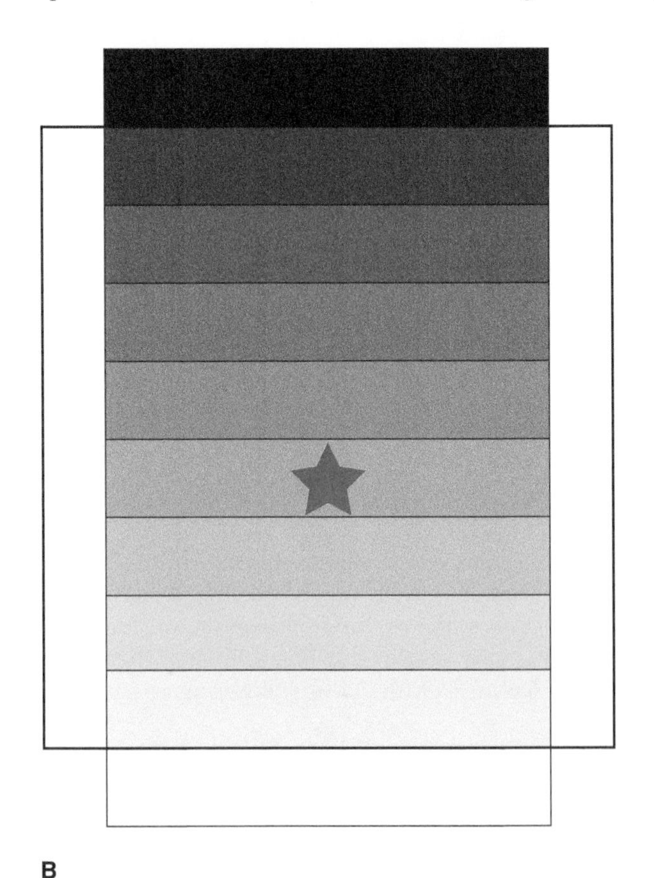

Figure 19.8. Window B is wider including nine steps on the gray scale compared to five steps in window A. The gray scale in image B is wider although the average gray level has not changed.

to use postprocessing manipulation of the image. When compared to film screen imaging, the main advantage of digital imaging is the enhanced contrast resolution, which depends upon an extended dynamic range and the processing latitude it provides.

Spatial Resolution of the Display

Spatial resolution is a characteristic of digital imaging that is comparable to recorded detail in film screen imaging. Over time, the monitor and image receptors have evolved in design elements that have improved the spatial resolution, but it is still low compared to film screen. The displayed digital image is composed of discrete information in the form of pixels that display shades of gray in the image. As mentioned earlier, the greater number of pixels in the matrix, the smaller their size. In digital imaging, an image with a greater number of pixels in a given area or **pixel density** has improved spatial resolution. In addition to the size of the pixel, the distance or spacing from the middle of one pixel to the middle of an adjacent pixel determines the **pixel pitch** and affects the spatial resolution (Fig. 19.9).

Various methods are used to alter the continuous exit radiation intensities into the array of discrete pixels for image display. Digital image receptors can use sampling techniques or fixed detector elements to capture the exit radiation intensities. No matter what the method used, the major determining factor of spatial resolution is the pixel size and pixel pitch. The display device also affects the ability to view anatomical area of interest. High-resolution monitors are required to maximize the visibility of the spatial resolution in the image to further improve the ability to visualize the smallest details in the image.

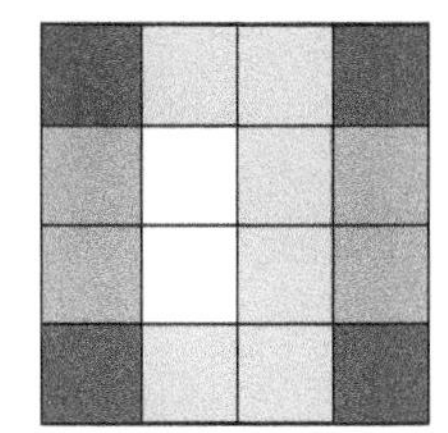

Figure 19.9. **The pixel pitch is measured by the distance from the center of one pixel to the center of an adjacent pixel. This affects the spatial resolution of the digital image.**

Image Noise

Image noise is made up of random background information, due to the constant flow of current in the circuit that is detected but does not contribute to the diagnostic information and detracts from image quality. On a digital image, noise looks like quantum mottle but it is really more like the effect of base plus fog on a standard radiographic image.

Quantum noise, which is seen in the digital image, is dependent upon the photons in the x-ray beam. With fewer photons reaching the image receptor to form the image, a greater amount of quantum noise will be visible on the digital image. Quantum noise is seen as density fluctuations in the image, much like quantum mottle in film screen where the image has a grainy appearance.

The computer system can adjust for low or high exposures during acquisition. When the exposure is low, there is a decreased number of photons striking the image receptor. The computer will compensate for the lack of density as long as there is sufficient contrast in the image for the computer to distinguish acquired data from noise. The appearance of the image will be altered to make brightness more acceptable but the image will display increased quantum noise. Utilizing postprocessing options can make quantum noise more noticeable or less noticeable. Increased noise decreases image contrast; however, increased image contrast tends to decrease noise. In digital systems, there will not be added density to the image because of noise.

The radiographer is responsible for selecting the appropriate exposure technique for the exam. The principles of using the maximum kVp and minimum mAs to produce a quality image are valid for either film screen or digital imaging. The goal is to produce an image with acceptable quality while keeping dose as low as possible to the patient (ALARA). With the development of digital imaging, the unacceptable practice of increasing mAs for the exposure has become much too common. A recommendation to follow is for the radiographers to continue to select techniques that will produce diagnostic quality images, regardless of whether film screen or digital systems are used. In addition, the foundation principles of correctly positioning the patient and using correct beam-limiting devices (collimators) should be used for every image where necessary.

Scatter Radiation

As previously learned, scatter radiation produces unwanted density on the image as a result of Compton interactions. The unwanted density degrades or decreases the visibility of the anatomic structures seen in the image. The increased density changes the ratio of density differences. Just like film screen, scatter radiation is a concern in digital imaging. Although the computer is able to change contrast or gray levels in the image, the additional density from the scatter does not provide any information of the area of interest. Digital image receptors are extremely sensitive and can detect low levels of radiation intensities, and they are more sensitive than film screen. Measures must be used control the amount of scatter radiation and to prevent the degradation of the image. These include the proper use of collimators, lead strips to absorb scatter radiation, etc.

Image Artifact

An **artifact** is an unwanted item visualized on an image. Artifacts are detrimental to images because they can affect the visualization of anatomy, pathologic processes, or patient identifying information. Artifacts are classified as either plus density or minus density. Plus-density artifacts are greater in density than the surrounding tissue. Minus-density artifacts have a lower density than does the surrounding tissue.

Common causes of image artifacts include double exposing the image receptor, improper use of equipment, clothing, or other items like IV lines or telemetry monitors. These errors are seen in both film screen and digital imaging. The radiographers must identify potential artifacts like clothing or items and remove them from the area of interest prior to the exposure.

Scatter radiation or fog and quantum noise can be classified as artifacts because they add unwanted information to the image. In regard to film screen, the artifacts are typically the result of handling the film as well as film storage and chemical processing.

Errors that are specific to digital imaging include errors that occur during the extraction of the latent image from the image receptor or the performance of electronic detectors. More discussion regarding errors in digital imaging will be discussed in Chapter 20 Capturing the Digital Image.

Chapter Summary

1. A digital image is formed by a matrix, which is made of rows and columns that are made up of numbers called pixels.
2. Each pixel specifies a unique location and contains information about the image intensity at that location.
3. The FOV describes area of tissue of the patient imaged.
4. The spatial resolution of the digital image is limited by the pixel size. Smaller pixels provide better spatial resolution and improved image quality.
5. The contrast resolution of a digital image is established by the number of discrete values stored in the pixels.
6. The window width control determines the number of density differences between black and white in the display.
7. The window level control sets the center brightness (density) by allowing manipulation of the midpoint of the range of densities visible in the display.

8. The digital IR detects a wider range of x-ray intensities, which provide a greater range of visible densities on the monitor.
9. Window width adjusts the gray scale to display the level on contrast in the image.
10. Bit depth is the number of shades of gray the digital image can display. A larger bit depth will have a greater number of gray shades displayed to improve the image quality.
11. Digital imaging systems can adjust for errors in selecting an incorrect set of technical factors.
12. Quantum noise occurs when there is a lack of sufficient photons reaching the image receptor.
13. Scatter radiation provides unwanted density on the image, which does not add useful information to the image.
14. Image artifacts decrease the quality of the image and must be avoided.

Case Study

Tony, a first year radiologic technology student, is giving a presentation about digital radiography to her classmates. His assignment is to explain the benefits of using a 1,024 × 1,024 size matrix compared to a 512 × 512 size matrix.

Critical Thinking Questions

How many pixels are in each matrix?

1. What effect does a larger matrix have on image resolution?
2. What is the bit depth of each pixel?
3. Which matrix has the greater range of gray shades?

Review Questions

Multiple Choice

1. If the FOV increases and the matrix size remains unchanged, the contrast resolution will be:

a. improved
b. degraded

2. Spatial resolution describes:

a. the maximum separation of two objects that can be distinguished as separate objects on the image
b. the minimum density difference between two tissues that can be distinguished as separate tissues
c. the maximum density difference between two tissues that can be distinguished as separate tissues.
d. the minimum separation of two objects that can be distinguished as separate objects on the image

3. The window control sets the:

a. number of density differences in the display
b. number of pixels in the matrix
c. number of matrices in the pixel
d. density value in the middle of the display

4. What is the pixel size in millimeters of a 512 matrix with a 15-cm FOV?

a. 0.03
b. 0.3
c. 3.0
d. 30

5. How many pixels are necessary to image one line pair?

a. 1
b. 2
c. 3
d. 4

6. The contrast in a digital image is best described as:

a. the maximum separation of two objects that can be distinguished as separate objects on an image
b. the minimum separation of two objects that can be distinguished as separate objects on the image
c. the maximum density difference between two tissues that can be distinguished as separate tissues
d. the minimum density difference between two tissues that can be distinguished as separate tissues

7. The range of the image gray scale is called:

a. window
b. window width
c. center
d. window level

8. __________ is the average brightness level of the image.

a. Window width
b. Window
c. Density
d. Window level

9. A matrix size with a smaller number of pixels will result in an image that is:

a. higher contrast
b. lower in image detail resulting in an unclear image
c. resolved with more sharpness
d. darker

10. A digital image containing a discrete number of rows and columns of picture elements is called:

a. detection array
b. display table
c. matrix
d. pixel

11. __________ would result in a displayed digital image that is brighter.

a. Increased window level
b. Decreased window width
c. Decreased window level
d. Increased window width

12. Digital imaging exhibits __________ compared to film screen imaging.

a. Greater luminance
b. Wider exposure latitude
c. Lower contrast resolution
d. Superior detail

Short Answer

1. What are the principal advantages of digital radiography over conventional radiography?

2. For the same FOV, spatial resolution will be __________ with a __________ image matrix.

3. Explain how window level and window width can change a digital image.

4. What is image noise and how does it affect the digital image?

5. The human eye is capable of seeing approximately __________ shades of gray.

6. A digital image with a 12-bit depth will contain how many gray values?

7. Change FOV from 20 to 30 cm: What is the pixel size in millimeters of a 256 × 256 matrix for an image with a FOV of 30 cm?

8. Change matrix size from 256 × 256 to 512 × 512: What is the pixel size in millimeters of a 512 × 512 matrix for an image with a FOV of 20 cm?

20

Capturing the Digital Image

Objectives

Upon completion of this chapter, the student will be able to:

1. Explain the function of an analog-to-digital converter.
2. Describe the design of the cassette-based detectors.
3. Identify the components of a digital imaging system.
4. Describe the operation of a computed radiography system.
5. Explain elements used in the digital radiography system.
6. Explain the process of image extraction for CR and DR.
7. Discuss the features of a storage phosphor plate.
8. Describe the process used by the CR reader to scan the imaging plate and produce an image.
9. Define the difference between indirect capture and direct capture radiography.
10. Describe the use of silicon, selenium, and cesium iodide in digital radiography.

Key Terms

- active matrix array
- analog-to-digital converter (ADC)
- antihalo layer
- computed radiography (CR)
- charge-coupled device (CCD)
- detector array
- dexel
- direct radiography (DR)
- digital-to-analog converter
- dynamic range
- exposure latitude
- fill factor
- flat-field correction
- flat panel detector
- imaging plate
- latent image
- manifest image
- phosphor layer
- photoconductor
- photodetector
- photostimulable luminescence
- photostimulable phosphor plate (PSP)
- quantization
- reflective layer
- sampling
- scanning
- storage phosphor
- thin-film transistor (TFT)

Introduction

Digital images are used throughout radiology. They appear in computed tomography (CT), magnetic resonance (MR), ultrasound, mammography, computed radiography (CR), direct radiography (DR), fluoroscopy, nuclear medicine (NM), and cardiovascular procedures. Unlike film images, whose contrast, speed, and latitude are fixed during processing, the appearance of digital images can be altered after they have been recorded and stored. Changes in the processing and display of the digital data can enhance information and suppress noise in the final image. An understanding of digital imaging systems will aid in producing diagnostic-quality digital images. The advantages of digital imaging include the ability to adjust the contrast after the image has been recorded, to process the image to emphasize important features, and to transfer the images to a remote site.

Digital Imaging Systems

thePoint® *An animation for this topic can be viewed at http://thepoint.lww.com/Orth2e*

Radiographic film screen imaging uses x-ray–sensitive film in a cassette, any x-ray unit can use the cassette, and the **latent image** is produced by processing the film. Computed radiography (CR) is similar to film screen in that an x-ray–sensitive plate is placed inside a cassette, any x-ray system accommodates the CR cassette, and the latent image is produced by processing the plate. These similarities are very general in understanding how an existing x-ray unit can use either system. There are distinct differences in the two systems, which demonstrate the advancements in computer technology. Screen film uses an intensifying screen, which emits light when struck by x-ray photons that interact with scintillator crystals. In the CR system, electrons become trapped in response to x-ray interaction with the plate.

Digital imaging systems replace the traditional film screen systems with special detectors. There are two basic groups of digital imaging systems, either "cassette based" or "cassetteless." Regardless of the system that is used, the process of obtaining an image is basically the same. After the primary x-ray beam passes through the patient, the exit radiation is detected, and the signal data are processed, displayed, and stored. Figure 20.1 illustrates the basic components of a digital imaging system. Later in the chapter, computed radiography and digital radiography will be discussed separately for a better understanding of the principles of each system.

Image Acquisition

Image acquisition begins with performing an x-ray exposure. The rules for positioning the part and correctly placing the central ray hold true for traditional and digital radiography. Digital systems cannot compensate for

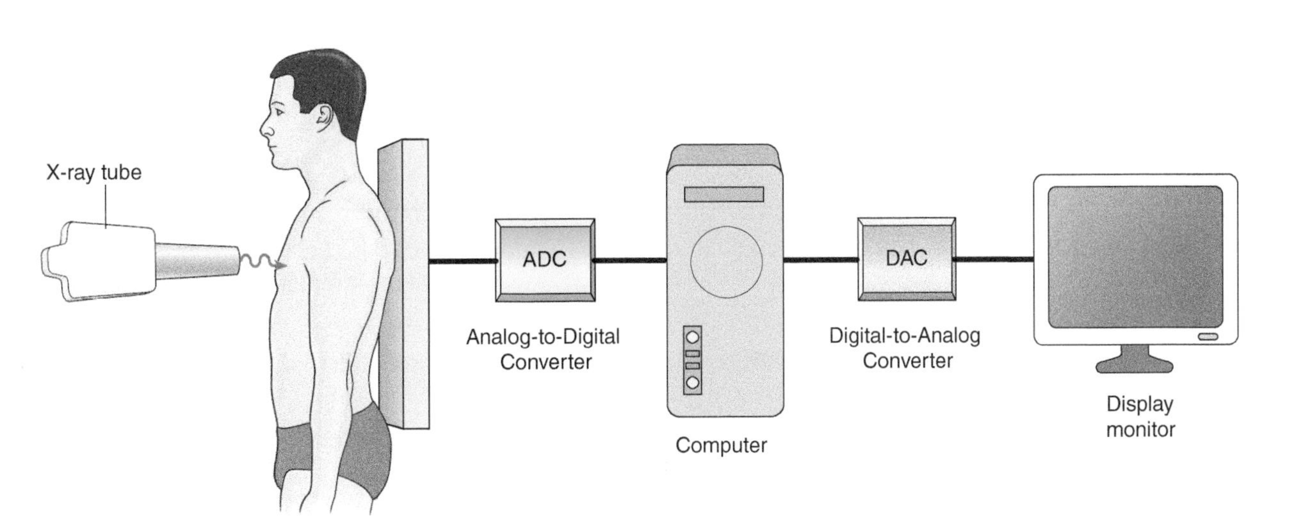

Figure 20.1. **Shows the basic components of a digital imaging system.**

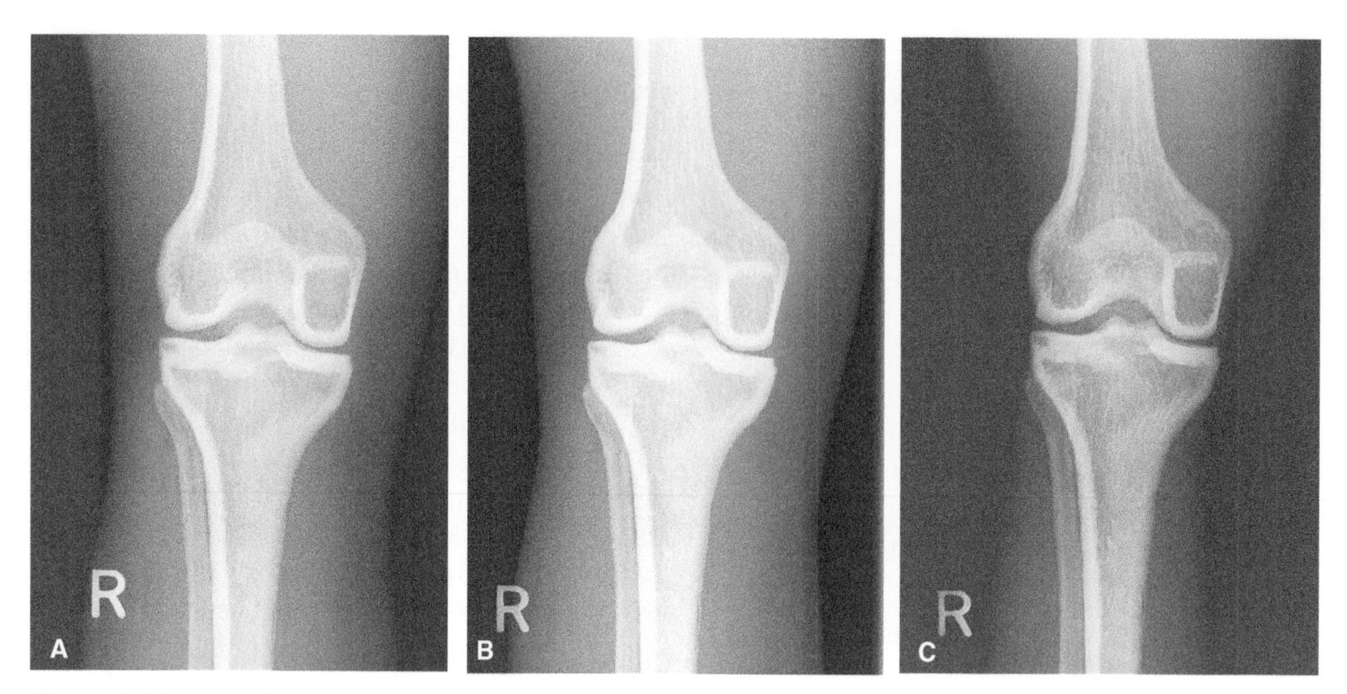

Figure 20.2. **Knee phantoms using CR system. (A) Underexposed. (B) Adequate exposure. (C) Overexposed.**

anatomy that is clipped or poorly positioned or for the lack of collimation. It is the responsibility of the radiographer to properly position the part of interest, to select the correct technical factors for the exposure, and to correctly collimate to the area of interest.

Figure 20.2 illustrates the importance of selecting the optimum kVp and mAs for every exposure. Upon viewing each of the three images, it is difficult to distinguish if the image is underexposed, overexposed, or adequately exposed. Each phantom image appears to be of diagnostic quality for the bony trabecular markings. Regardless of the exposure to the imaging plate, the computer will process the information and produce an image with acceptable levels of contrast. Image **C** has been overexposed, which resulted in higher radiation dose to the patient. With film screen, it is very easy to distinguish an overexposed image as there is increased radiographic density, which may obscure the anatomic information. In digital imaging, this is no longer the case unless an incredibly high set of exposure factors is used. As mentioned previously in this text, many technologists have been using higher mAs settings than are necessary. The danger in this practice is chronic overexposure of patients to radiation. Chronic overexposure must be avoided at all times. This only increases the dose of radiation to the patient and does not result in a better image. A skilled radiographer will be aware of the range of exposures for the specific digital equipment in his or her department and will use the equipment with respect for patient safety.

Analog-to-Digital Converter

An analog signal is a continuously varying quantity while a digital system can have either one value or the next value, but no value in between because each value is discretely assigned through computer coding. Common examples of analog and digital are clocks. An analog clock is mechanical and has hands that are continuously moving around the face of the clock. A digital clock uses a computer chip to demonstrate numbers. Digital clocks are easier to read and can be more precise.

In digital imaging, detectors produce continuously varying signals (analog signals), which make up the latent image. All digital systems initially convert the analog signal from the detector to a digital signal using an **analog-to-digital converter** (**ADC**). Digital systems represent the signal by a series of discrete values, which make up the intensity of the pixels. The digital data are then available for processing, display, and storage.

Digital-to-analog converters convert digital signals to analog signals. Digital signals with more discrete values will more closely represent the analog signal. Conventional cable TV is an analog signal because the voltage signal is continuously changing. Digital satellite

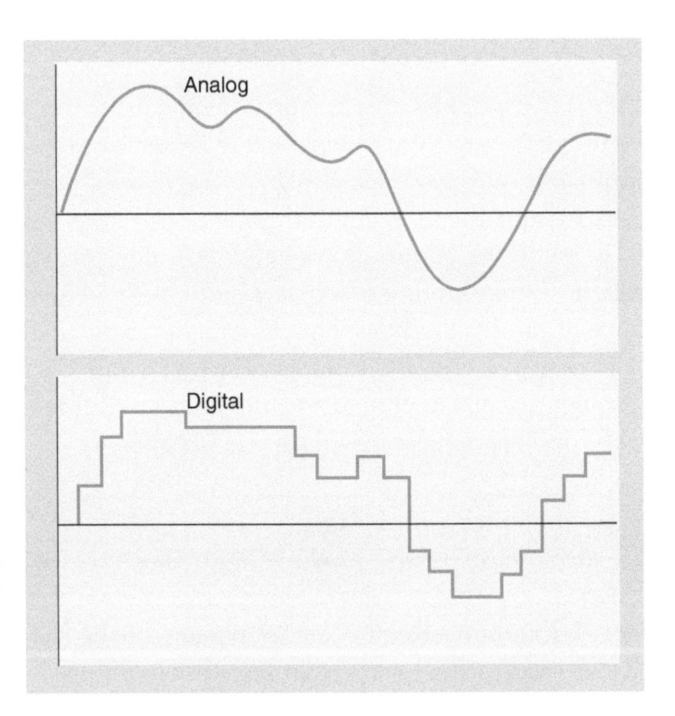

Figure 20.3. **Illustrates an analog signal and the corresponding digital signal.**

TV is sent from the satellite to the home as a digital signal and then converted into an analog signal at the input to the home TV set (Fig. 20.3).

Now that we have discussed the conversion of analog signals to digital signals and vice versa, we will move on to more exciting information regarding computed and digital radiography!

Computed Radiography

Computed radiography (CR) is a cassette-based system, which can be used with existing radiographic equipment without the need to modify the equipment. An existing radiographic unit will readily accept the CR cassette, which makes the conversion from film screen to CR very cost effective. Units with an AEC may need to be recalibrated prior to use as the speed of the CR system may be different from the film screen system. Preprogrammed anatomy settings may need to be adjusted as well to ensure the correct kVp and mAs settings are used for each anatomical area.

The primary components of a CR system include a photostimulable phosphor plate (PSP) housed in a cassette, plate reader, and computer workstation. CR uses a special detector plate instead of a film inside a cassette. As an image receptor, it is called an **imaging plate (IP)**. The exterior dimensions and appearance of the CR cassette are the same as those of a conventional film cassette. The CR cassette is comprised of a lightweight plastic with a low-absorbing carbon fiber front (Fig. 20.4). It is lined with felt to prevent static buildup and dust collection while protecting the plate from minor jolts. The back of the cassette has a sheet of lead foil to absorb x-rays that penetrate through the plate reducing backscatter radiation from reaching the plate thereby improving contrast resolution. The CR cassette is placed in the Bucky tray or used for portable examinations and exposed in the same manner as a conventional film cassette.

The CR cassette contains a **photostimulable phosphor plate (PSP)** that responds to radiation by trapping electron energy in the locations where the x-ray photons strike. The CR detector plate is made of a thin, plastic material and is extremely fragile. Radiographers must be aware that the PSP plate is a single emulsion plate and must be placed facing

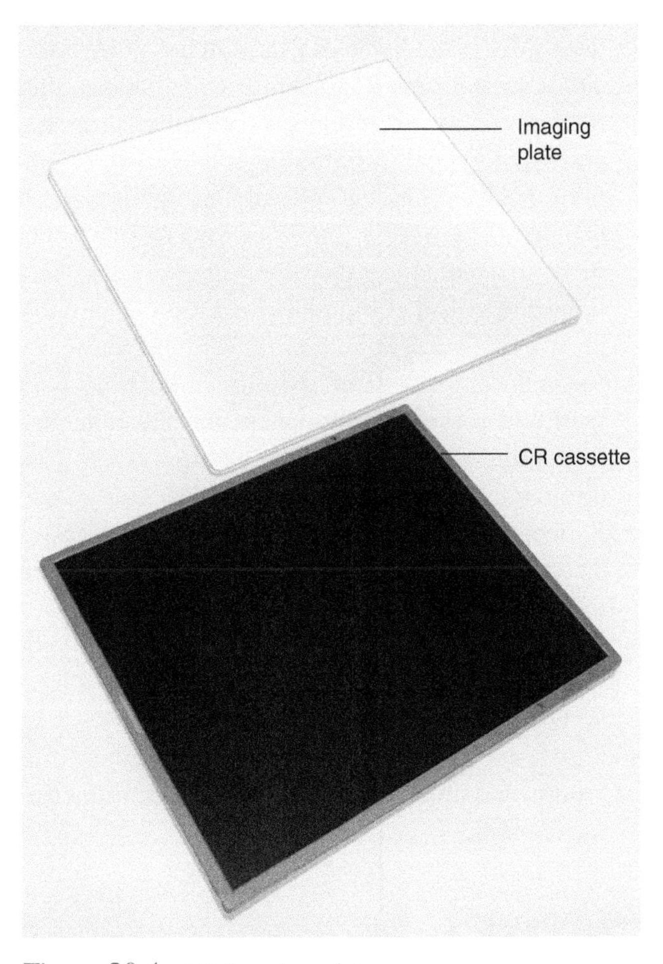

Figure 20.4. **CR imaging plate.**

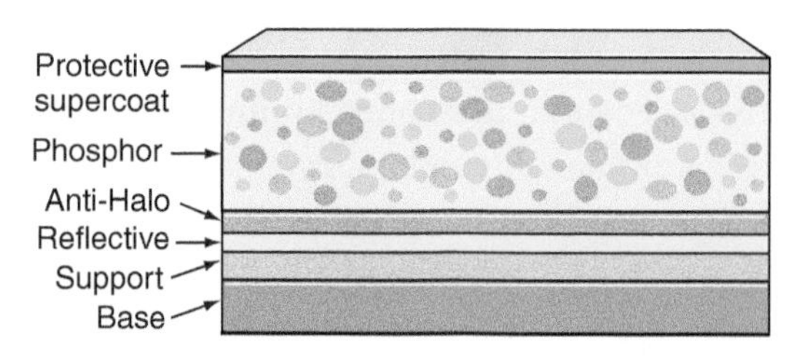

Figure 20.5. **CR photostimulable phosphor imaging plate demonstrating layers.**

forward in the cassette. CR plates and cassettes can be reused thousands of times but will be damaged when dropped.

The PSP plate is constructed with several layers (Fig. 20.5):

- Protective layer: This is a very thin, tough, clear plastic that protects the phosphor layer from handling trauma.
- **Phosphor layer**: This is the layer of photostimulable phosphor that traps electrons during exposure. It is typically made of barium fluorohalide and europium phosphors held in place by a binding material. The phosphor design is either turbid or structured. A turbid phosphor layer has randomly distributed phosphor crystals within the active layer. These crystals are 3 to 10 μm in size and scatter light excessively. A structured phosphor layer has columnar crystals within the active layer resembling needles standing on end and tightly packed together. The needle PSP is grown as a linear filament that enhances the absorption of x-rays and limits the spread of stimulated emission. The phosphor crystals emit light toward the reflective layer.
- **Antihalo** or color **layer**: Absorbs stimulating laser light and prevents it from reaching the reflective layer. Allows light emitted by the phosphor to pass through to the reflective layer.
- **Reflective layer**: This layer sends light in a forward direction to the photodetector when released in the reader.
- Support layer: This is a semirigid material that provides the imaging sheet with strength and is a base for coating the other layers.
- Base layer: This is a firm layer usually made of aluminum and protected from scratches by a thin coating of plastic.

thePoint® ***An animation for this topic can be viewed at http://thepoint.lww.com/Orth2e***

Photostimulable Luminescence

The PSP plate is coated with barium fluorohalide "doped" with europium, which has the desirable property of **photostimulable luminescence (PSL)**. At the time of making an exposure, the remnant x-ray photons will strike the PSP plate and the barium fluorohalide will fluoresce or emit light. Europium is a silvery rare earth metal, which is the activator for the phosphor. The europium is used in very small amounts and is responsible for storing some x-ray energy as the latent image on the PSL. For this reason, PSP screens are also called **storage phosphors**.

Process of Creating an Image

There are four steps that produce light stimulation or emission.

Step 1 Exposure: Remnant x-ray photon strikes PSP plate and causes an energy transfer, which results in excitation of the electrons into a metastable state (Fig. 20.6). Approximately 50% of these electrons immediately return to their ground state, which results in emission of light. The remaining electrons are liberated and become trapped in the conduction band. The conduction band is that energy level just beyond the outermost energy band (valence band) of the atom. The quantity and distribution of liberated electrons are proportional to the x-ray exposure to each area of the plate; these electrons make up the latent image. These metastable electrons will return to their ground state over a period of time resulting in fading of the latent image. The PSP plate should be read within 8 hours or the resultant image will be greatly compromised.

Step 2 Stimulation: Figure 20.7 illustrates a precisely focused laser beam of infrared light with a diameter of 50 to 100 μm directed at the PSP plate. The red laser light will scan the plate in a raster pattern and gives energy to the trapped electrons. The red laser light is emitted using 2 eV, which is needed to energize the trapped electrons. The trapped electrons are now able to leave the active layer where they emit blue light photons as they return to a lower energy state. As the laser beam intensity increases, the intensity of the emitted signal also increases. The laser beam will spread out as it penetrates the phosphor layer. A thicker phosphor layer will increase the laser beam spread.

Step 3 Read: The next step in the process is detecting or reading the stimulated light emission. The laser beam causes the metastable electrons to emit a shorter wavelength blue-green light, which is from the visible portion of the spectrum (Fig. 20.8). This process makes

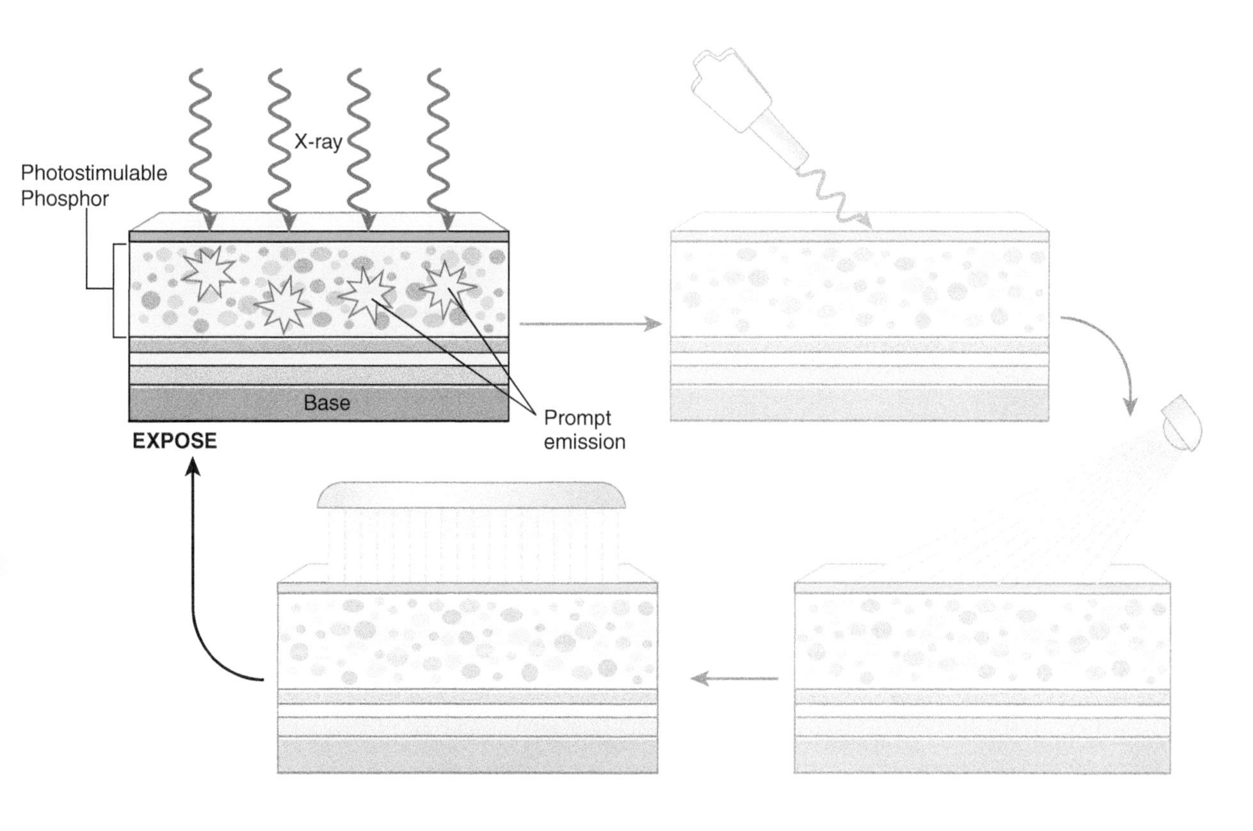

Figure 20.6. Expose. X-ray photon interaction with photostimulable phosphor.

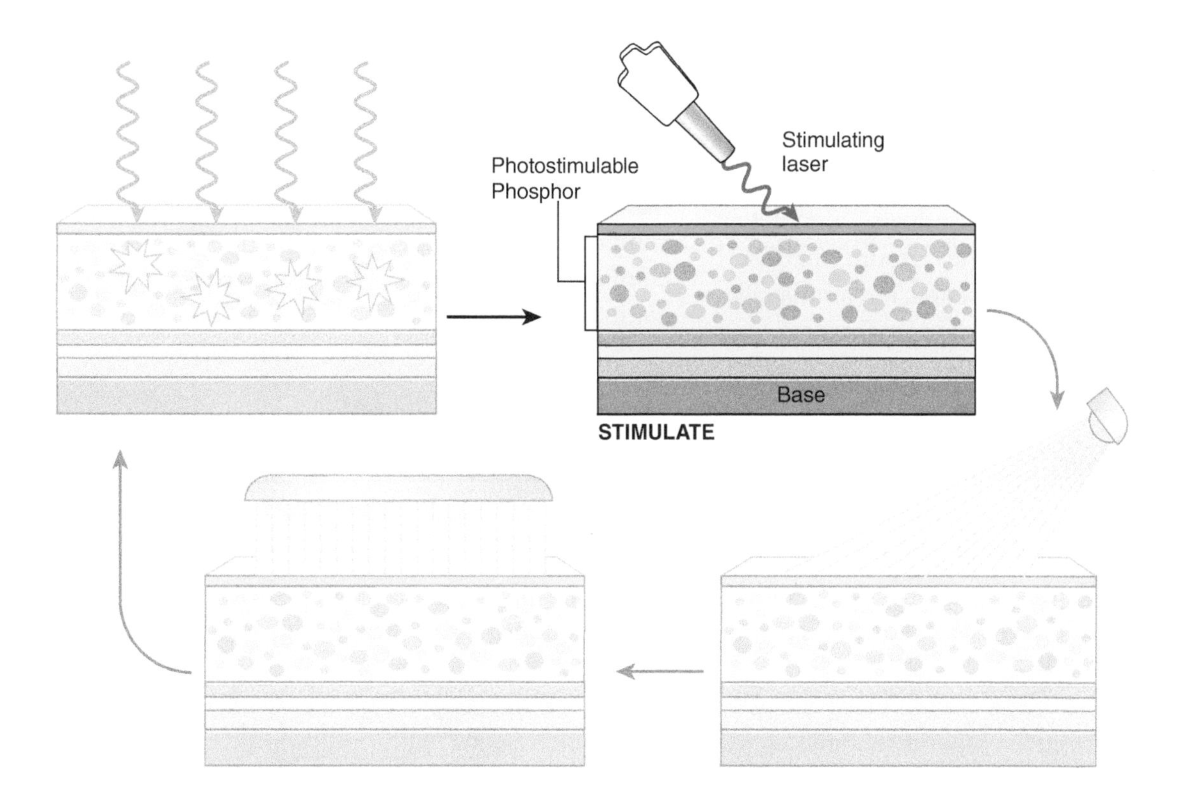

Figure 20.7. Stimulate. Stimulation of the latent image results from the infrared laser beam striking the phosphor.

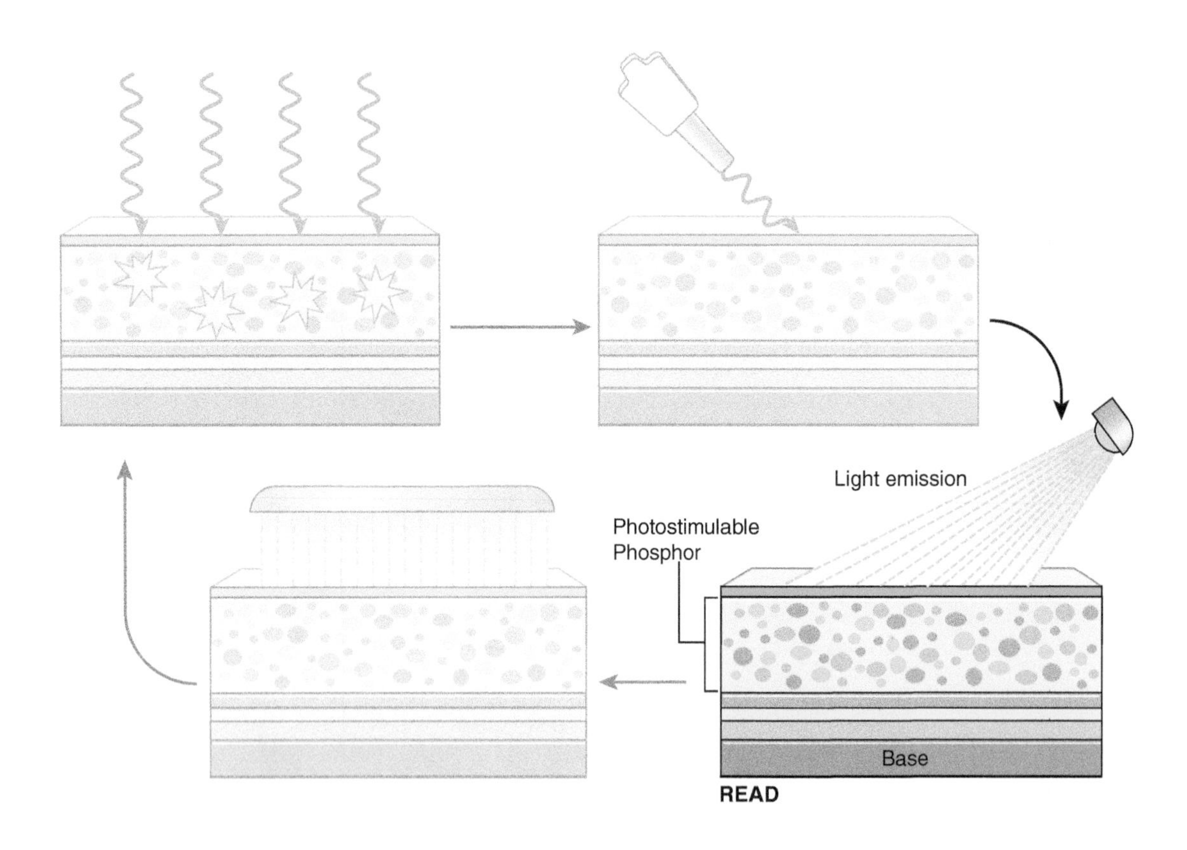

Figure 20.8. **Read. The light signal emitted after stimulation is detected and measured (read).**

the latent image visible. Some signal is lost because of the scattering of emitted light and the efficiency of the photodetector to collect the emitted light. Photodiodes are the preferred light detectors for CR.

Step 4 Erase: The stimulation phase doesn't completely move all metastable electrons to their ground state, and some stimulated electrons remain. These remaining electrons can cause an artifact called *ghosting* the next time the IP is used. After the entire plate has been scanned, the erasure process floods the IP with very intense white light from specially designed fluorescent lamps, the light source releases any remaining trapped energy, and the IP is wiped clean of any residual latent image (Fig. 20.9).

The cassette is then closed and returned to the ready bin for reuse. The entire processing cycle requires ~60 seconds (s). It is never necessary to open the CR cassette or to handle the detector plate.

IPs must be used soon after erasure. The PSP plate is sensitive to background radiation and become fogged easily. If the IP has not been used recently, it is advised to put the plate through the erasure process to clean the plate of any potential artifact on subsequent exposures.

CR Reader

A CR reader as seen in Figure 20.10 can be located in the core work area for easy use. The design of the CR reader varies between manufacturers; however, the basic components are found in each reader. There are three components to the CR reader: mechanical, optical, and computer.

Mechanical Components

After the exposure, the CR cassette is inserted into the processing reader. The processing reader opens the CR cassette and removes the IP, which is fitted to a precise drive mechanism (Fig. 20.11). The drive mechanism moves the IP at a controlled and precise speed slowly along the long axis of the IP. This is called "slow scan." Any fluctuations in drive speed can result in banding artifacts in the image. While the IP is moving a deflection device such as a rotating polygon or oscillating mirror deflects the laser back and forth in a raster pattern across the detector plate, this is called the "fast scan." The error tolerance is fractions of a pixel; a drive mechanism that is

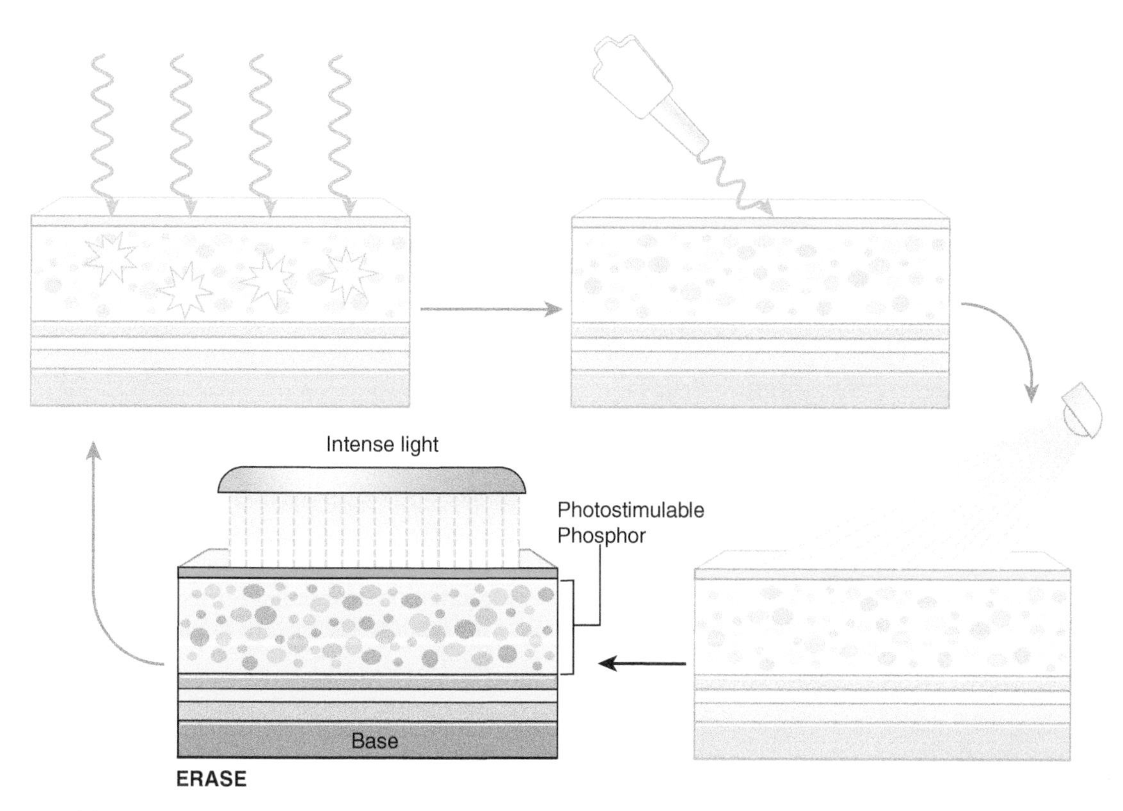

Figure 20.9. **Erase. Imaging plate is exposed to intense white light to move residual metastable electrons to ground.**

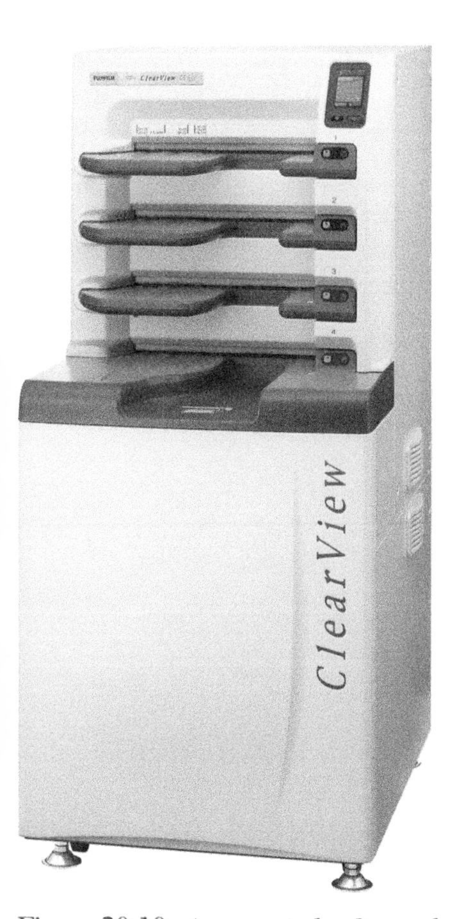

Figure 20.10. **A computed radiography reader.**

not moving the plate smoothly can result in the edges of the image having a wavy appearance.

Optical Components

The CR reader must be able to precisely "read" the intensity of each metastable electron of the latent image. The reader has specially designed optical components, which keeps the laser beam size, shape, speed, and intensity at a constant level. These components include the laser, beam-shaping optics, light-collecting optics, and optical filters (Fig. 20.12). The optical components project and guide the precisely controlled laser beam back and forth across the plate as the plate moves through the scan area. In some systems, the plate is stationary while the laser and optical system move.

The optical components can be explained by performing a simple exercise with a flashlight. Aim the flashlight toward a wall in a perpendicular manner, and note how the circle has a sharp outline. Now, slowly move the flashlight side to side and watch as the beam becomes distorted and less intense. Beam-shaping optics corrects these types of changes.

The emitted light from the PSP plate is channeled into a fiberoptic bundle or a solid, light-conducting

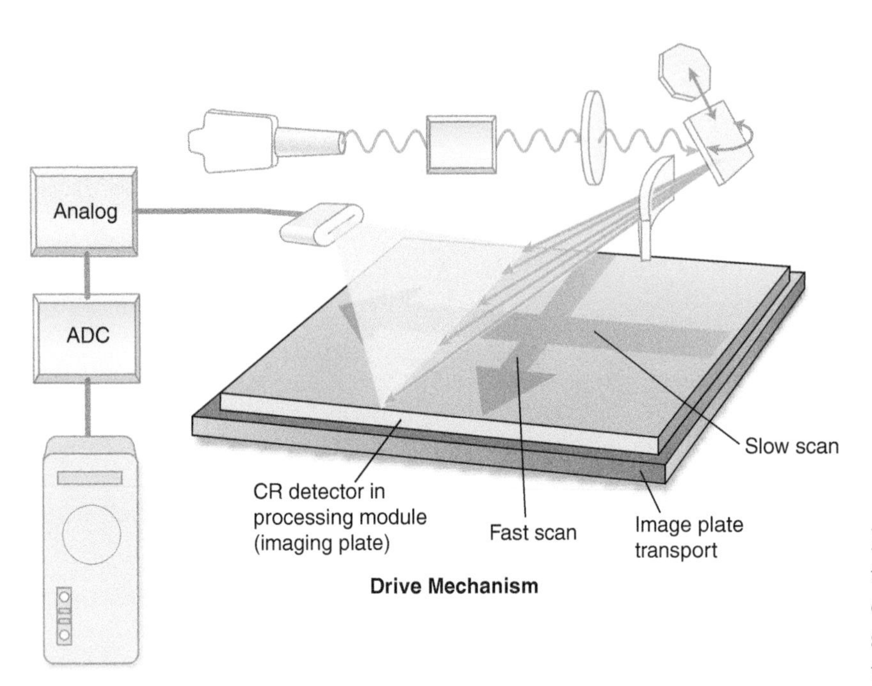

Figure 20.11. **CR drive mechanism. Moves the IP slowly along its long axis while an oscillating or rotating mirror causes the stimulating laser beam to move rapidly across the IP.**

material where it is narrowed and sent through an optical filter that removes any long-wavelength stimulation light from reaching the photodetector, photomultiplier tube (PMT), or charge-coupled device (CCD). Stimulation light is considered "noise," which drowns the emitted light or "signal" and distorts the image. The optical filter cleans up the "noise" and improves the signal-to-noise ratio in the system.

Computer Control

As the laser beam scans the imaging plate, light intensity information will be detected by a **photodetector**,

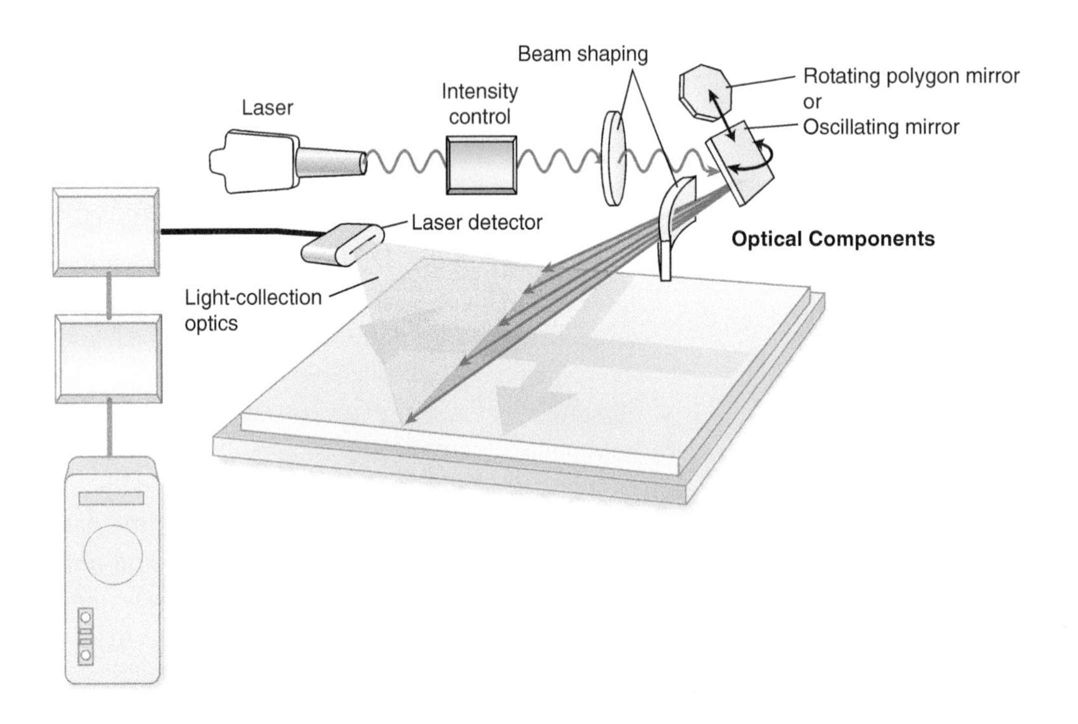

Figure 20.12. **CR optical components. Light collection optics narrow light and guide it toward the optical filter.**

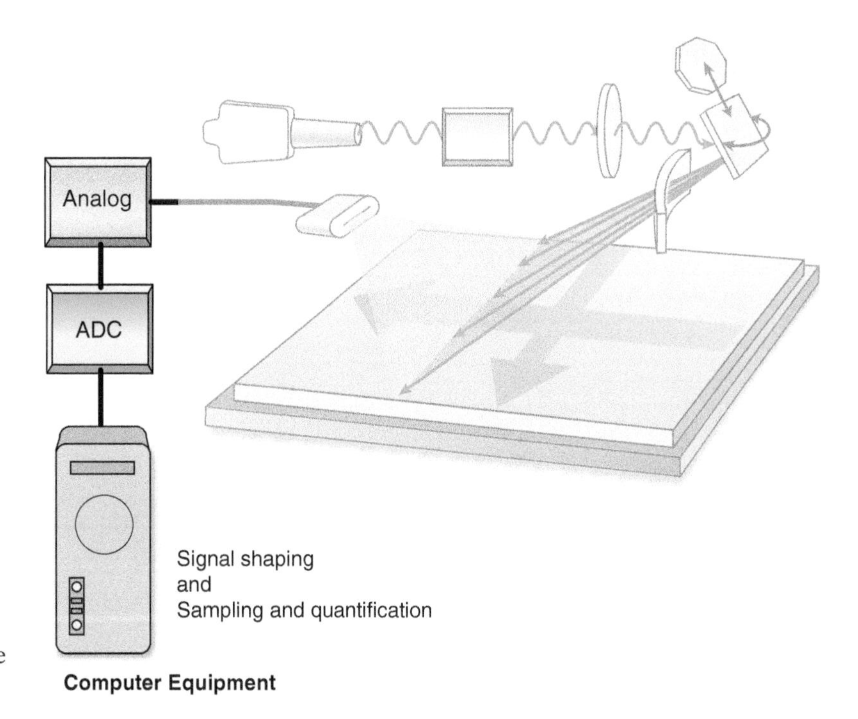

Figure 20.13. **Computer control. The computer component of the CR reader processes signal amplification, compression, scanning control, ADC conversion, and image buffering.**

PMT, or CCD. The photodetector converts the visible light into an electronic signal, which is in analog form. The analog signal is processed for amplitude, scale, and compression data, which must be converted to a digital signal for the computer to apply algorithmic formulas to the information (Fig. 20.13). Data compression reduces the number of pixels that are stored or processed in an image. Compression algorithms can reduce the size of the data in an image matrix by a factor of 30 or more while maintaining the diagnostic content of the image. Compressed images require less storage space and can be transmitted more rapidly.

At this point, the analog signal is digitized with attention to sampling (time between samples) and quantization (value of each sample). Sampling and quantization are the process of analog-to-digital conversion and will be discussed at the end of the chapter. When the laser beam scans the plate, each line of the imaging plate correlates to one pixel dimension. The analog signal emitted for each pixel has an infinite range of values, which the ADC must convert into discrete values, which can be stored as digital code. This digital code will determine the gray scale for each individual pixel. All the pixel densities will be combined to represent the many density values in the image, which affects the density and contrast of the image. Once the conversion is complete, the light intensity and the position of the laser beam are stored as digital data for each pixel. At this point, the **manifest image** is now visible on the computer monitor. Another variable related to pixels is spatial resolution; the smaller the pixel, the higher the spatial resolution. As previously discussed, matrices with more and smaller pixels have higher spatial resolution.

The benefit of using CR in radiography is utilizing your existing equipment. The other benefit is storage. Films take up a lot of room to store. They also can be misplaced or lost. With a CR system, the completed images are temporarily stored on a hard disc in the computer. The images are then transferred to a workstation for interpretation by the radiologist or archived on a backup computer. For CR radiography, you are able to transmit images to remote sites. The radiologist has quick access to previous CR images for comparison. This makes diagnosis of any abnormalities more accurate.

Image Receptor/Image Plate Response

Film screen radiography uses the characteristic curve to illustrate the response of the image receptor. In digital radiographer, the response is illustrated as a linear image receptor response function.

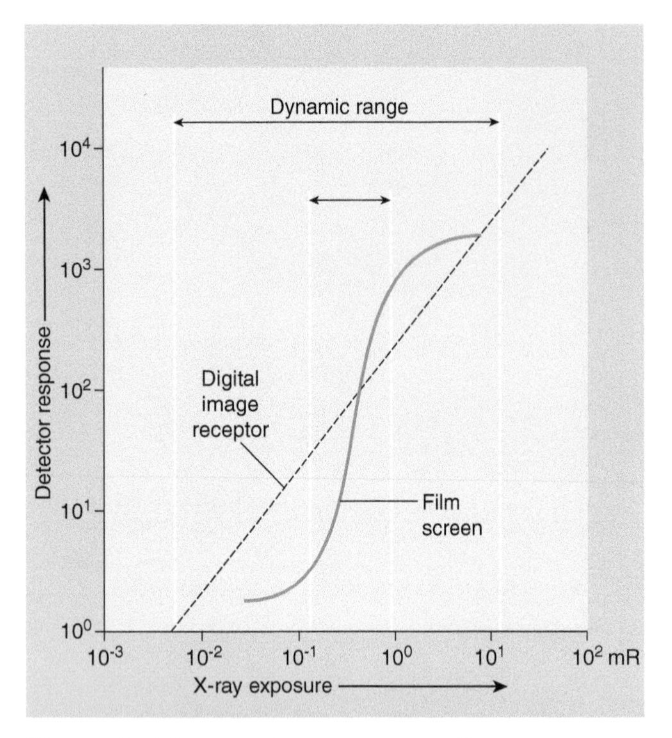

Figure 20.14. **Digital receptor versus film screen response. The image receptor response for computed radiography is linear, while the film screen response is curvilinear as seen in the characteristic curve.**

Figure 20.14 demonstrates several differences between the CR and film screen receptors. The IR response is seen as a range of optical densities between 0 and 3. OD is a logarithmic function that represents three orders of magnitude or 1,000 gray shades. Recall that film screen can only display ~30 shades of gray when the film is viewed at a view box. Because of the limited number of gray shades seen in film, it is critical to use the proper radiographic technique. Any overexposure or underexposure will result in an unacceptable film.

TABLE 20.1 SOURCES OF IMAGE NOISE IN FILM SCREEN IMAGING

- Quantum noise
- X-ray photon absorbed
- X-ray photon scattered
- Latent image fading
- Image receptor noise
- Phosphor structure
- Phosphor crystal size
- Phosphor crystal distribution
- Overcoat, reflection, or base layers

TABLE 20.2 SOURCES OF IMAGE NOISE IN COMPUTED RADIOGRAPHY IMAGING

Mechanical Component Defects	Optical Component Defects	Computer Control Defects
• Slow scan driver • Fast scan driver	• Laser intensity control • Scatter of stimulating beam • Light emitted by screen • Light collection	• Electronic noise • Inadequate sampling • Inadequate quantization

In comparison, CR has a wide **exposure latitude** of four orders of magnitude that results in 10,000 gray shades. Computerization makes it possible to visually evaluate each shade of gray through postprocessing. With CR, radiographic technique is not as critical because the contrast doesn't change over the four orders of magnitude. If a technique results in an underexposure or overexposure, the computer will adjust the contrast to produce an acceptable image. This does not imply that the radiographer can become lazy when setting technical factors; it is always preferred to select the proper kVp and mAs for an image regardless of the imaging method used whether film screen, CR, or DR.

Image Noise

The primary cause of noise in any radiographic image is scatter radiation. This is true for film screen or digital radiography. Table 20.1 lists the sources of image noise in film screen radiography. Each of these items is also considered for digital imaging in addition to those listed in Table 20.2. Luckily, CR noise sources are only an issue at very low exposures to the IP. Newer systems are more sensitive to lower exposures, which means there are lower noise levels. This can result in lower patient radiation dose.

Direct Radiography

Direct radiography (DR) is yet another way to record the x-ray exposure after it has passed through the patient. DR uses an array of small detectors to capture exit x-ray radiation and transfer it to a computer for processing into a digital image; the whole process occurs almost instantaneously. The **detector array** replaces the Bucky and generally requires a complete x-ray unit replacement. The major advantage of the DR system is that no handling of a cassette is required as this is a "cassetteless" system. The two general categories of a cassetteless systems are indirect and direct capture. Before we discuss these types of cassetteless systems, it is important to learn what a CCD is as it is a major component of DR.

Charge-Coupled Device

The **charge-coupled device (CCD)** was first developed by the military in the 1970s. CCDs are light-sensitive devices, which are used in digital cameras and other applications. Because the CCD is very light sensitive, it can respond to very low light intensities. There are three principle imaging characteristics of the CCD: sensitivity, dynamic range, and size. CCDs are silicon-based semiconductors and one is shown in Figure 20.15.

Sensitivity is the ability of the CCD to detect and respond to very low levels of visible light. This is important in radiography because it aids the radiographer in using lower technical factor settings, which correlate to low patient radiation dose.

Dynamic range is the ability to respond to a wide range of light intensities from very dim to very bright light. As seen with CR (Fig. 20.14), the radiation response of a CCD is linear while film screen is curved. Film screen has three orders of magnitude for radiation response, OD from 0 to 3, with ~30 shades of gray, which are discernable by the human eye. With the CCD image contrast is not related to IP x-ray exposure. Each of the four orders of magnitude, 10,000 shades of gray, can be visualized with postprocessing. At very low exposures, the CCD response is greater than film screen, which should result in lower patient dose when using DR.

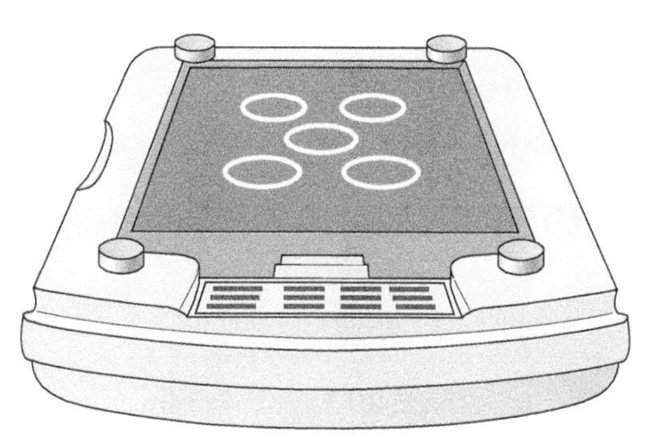

Figure 20.15. **DR detector assembly. The detector assembly replaces the Bucky tray and cassettes. Serves as the image receptor.**

The CCD is incredibly small and measures ~1 to 2 cm in size. The pixel size is an astounding 100 × 100 μm! Because of the small size, a CCD is highly adaptable to various forms of direct radiography.

There are two general categories for cassetteless or DR systems: indirect and direct capture.

Indirect Capture

There are two forms of indirect capture: one uses a CCD, x-ray scintillator, and optics while the other uses a scintillator, photodetectors, and a thin-film transistor (TFT) array. Indirect capture is a two-step process: x-ray photons are converted to light and then, the light photons are converted into an electrical signal.

Cesium Iodide CCD

The cesium iodide (CsI) CCD uses a scintillator comprised of a cesium iodide phosphor plate, which absorbs x-ray energy and emits visible light. CsI is a hygroscopic material that easily absorbs moisture. CsI must be hermetically sealed to avoid water absorption and prevent rapid degradation but is otherwise a highly efficient scintillation material.

The CsI plate is coupled to the CCD by a fiberoptic bundle or optical lens system. X-rays are absorbed by the CsI phosphor, which gives off scintillation light. The light energy is transmitted through the fiberoptic bundle to the CCD where it is converted into an electronic signal. The electronic signal is then sent to the computer workstation for processing and display. The result is a high x-ray capture efficiency and good spatial resolution up to 5 lp/mm.

CCDs are limited in size and the image receptor may have an array of several closely spaced CCDs. One major challenge to this design is the CCDs are joined at seams, which is called tiling or tiled. Tiling occurs when several CCD detectors are arranged against one another to create one large detector. Figure 20.16 demonstrates a tiled CCD where the seams are clearly visible. The seams have an unequal response to the radiation compared to each

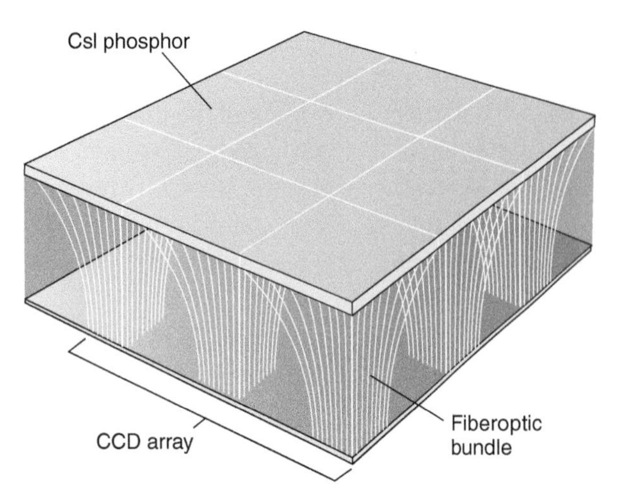

Figure 20.16. **Charge-coupled device. Basic components of the CCD detector array include a network of CsI phosphor plates that are connected to the CCD array using fiberoptic bundles.**

individual detector. The goal is to have a seamless image at the edge of each CCD. This is accomplished by computer software, which interpolates or averages the pixel values at each seam or tile interface and makes the seams disappear. This interpolation is called **flat-field correction**.

Cesium Iodide/Amorphous Silicon

The other type of indirect capture uses a scintillator with CsI as the phosphor to capture x-rays and transmit scintillation light to a collection element. The collection element consists of silicon sandwiches between TFTs. Silicon is a semiconductor, which has a crystalline form. When identified as amorphous silicon (a-Si), it is a fluid that is painted onto a glass substrate or foundation, which makes the **flat panel detectors** possible. These specially designed detectors are called photodetectors.

CsI has high photoelectric capture because the atomic number of Cs is 55 and iodide is 53; this creates a larger amount of x-ray interactions with the CsI. The technical factors can be set lower to use less radiation to produce a quality image and that results in lower patient dose.

The flat panel detector is configured into a large network of detector elements called **dexels**, which are arranged in rows and columns (Fig. 20.17). Each dexel consists of electronic components including a **thin-film transistor (TFT)**, a charge collection electrode, storage capacitor, and a photodetector. The TFT is an electronic switch that is closed during the x-ray exposure, allowing the charge in each dexel to be collected and stored. The charge collection electrode captures the electric charge that is proportional to the x-ray exposure received over the area of the dexel and the storage capacitor stores the electric charge. After the exposure is completed, the switch opens, which allows the stored electric charge to flow from the TFT to the charge amplifier. The amplifier is outside the active area of the panel. They amplify and convert the electric charge into digital code by built-in electronics; the digital code results in a gray scale value

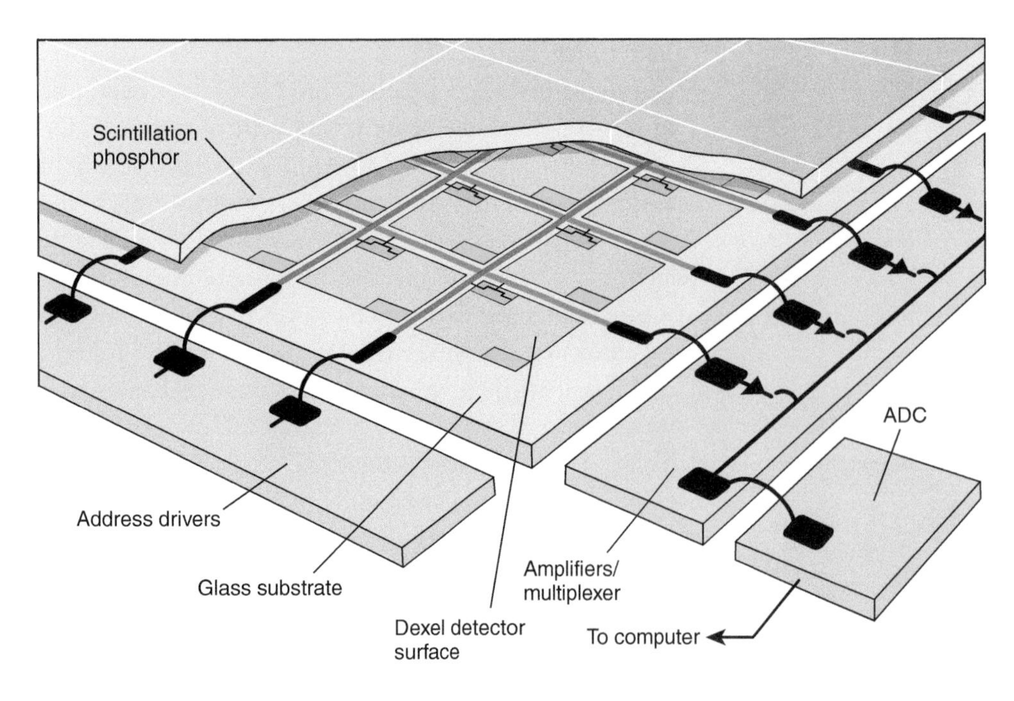

Figure 20.17. **Thin-film transistor array. Array detector elements consist of a scintillation phosphor, storage capacitor, and TFT layered on a glass substrate.**

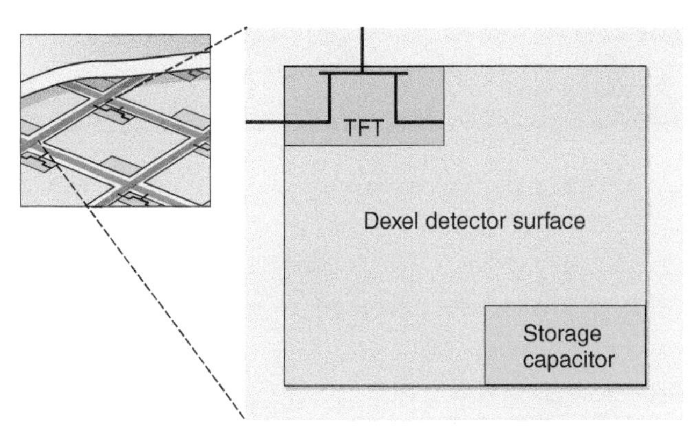

Figure 20.18. **Dexel. A hardware pixel (dexel) has three components: semiconductor detector surface area, capacitor, and thin-film transistor.**

for each dexel. The process is completed row by row until the entire array has been read.

The dexel face is occupied by the electronic components and photodetector. The percentage of the square devoted to semiconductor detection area is called **fill factor**. Eighty percent of the dexel face is sensitive to x-rays (Fig. 20.18). This reduces the efficiency of the charge collection to 80%. The remaining 20% of the area of the dexel does not contribute to formation of the image. This represents one of the challenges to digital radiography. The TFT and capacitor do not get smaller when the dexel is smaller, only the semiconductor area gets smaller. For a dexel with dimensions of 200 × 200 μm, the fill factor is 80% and it is much less (~40% to 50%) for smaller dexel dimensions. Dexels with an 80% fill factor have higher contrast resolution or signal-to-noise resolution and better spatial resolution. As smaller dexels have been designed, the spatial resolution has improved but it requires an increase in x-ray technique to offset the lower fill factor. This correlates into higher patient dose. Research in nanotechnology is showing promise in increasing fill factor for smaller dexels, improving spatial resolution while lowering patient dose.

Direct Capture

Direct capture radiography (DR) systems are the next generation in digital radiography. Direct radiography flat panel detectors or imaging plates use a TFT array and a **photoconductor** made of amorphous selenium (a-Se), which is a semiconductor with excellent x-ray photon detection ability. a-Se is ~200 μm in size and is sandwiched between charged electrodes. The array uses the same design as the CsI/a-Si indirect system. This design is called an **active matrix array (AMA)** of TFTs.

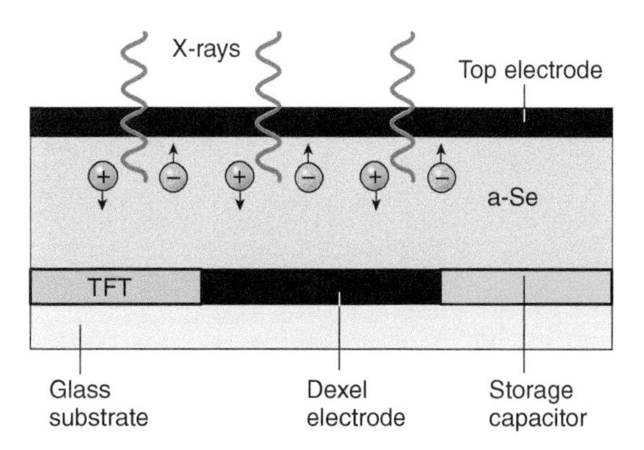

Figure 20.19. **Direct capture array. Cross-section showing the layers of a dexel.**

Figure 20.19 is a diagram of a dexel showing a thin semiconductive layer of amorphous selenium, which converts x-ray energy into electrical charge. The ionization created by the x-ray photons interaction with the selenium results in ionization of the selenium molecules freeing electrons from orbital shells. Each ionization event creates an electron-hole pair consisting of the negatively charged free electron and the positively charged "hole." The top electrode has a positive charge, which attracts the free electrons. At the same time, a negative charge is placed on the dexel electrode causing the "holes" to drift downward to build up at the bottom of the selenium layer. The positive charge is stored in the capacitor where it is amplified and converted into digital code by the built-in electronics.

An AMA of TFTs is shown in Figure 20.20. The AMA is a network of gate lines and data lines, which crisscrosses between the dexels. The address drivers control the gate lines, which permit the dexels to be read in a sequential order. When the bias voltage along the lines is changed from −5 to +10 V, it causes the TFT gates to open sequentially and dump the stored-up charge from each dexel in succession. A change in voltage causes a channel of conductivity to be opened up in the semiconductor material, which allows electrical charge to flow out and down the data lines to an amplifier, which boosts the signal before sending the signal to the ADC and finally to the computer. This process is extremely fast where more

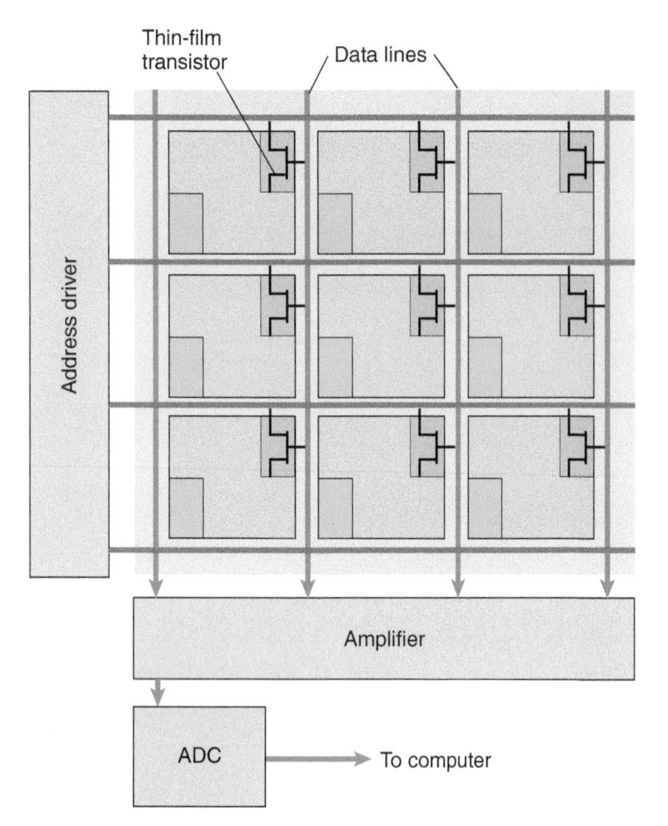

Figure 20.20. **Active matrix array. Gate lines control the sequence with which dexels release their charge into the data lines leading to the computer. The gate lines apply a charge to the TFT creating a channel of conductivity through which the stored charges can flow.**

than 1 million dexels can be read and converted into a digital image in <1 second. All this information is read with dedicated electronics that facilitate fast image acquisition and processing.

Digital radiography is similar to CR because it is filmless and the image is stored on the computer. It has the same benefit as CR. The image is displayed for the technologist to check prior to the next exposure. The images are then sent to a storage system. This storage system allows for long-term storage or the image can be printed out on a laser printer to film. There are no cassettes with digital radiography. The image is transferred directly from the detector array to the ADC and then into the computer.

When using CR or digital radiography imaging, both images are placed on computer. Once transferred, the images can be transferred electronically to "Picture Archiving and Communication System" (PACS). The images can then be sent to the radiologist and ordering physician. The images are then archived.

Digitizing an Analog Image

There are three steps to digitizing an analog image, which are relevant to all forms of digital imaging: scanning, sampling, and quantization. In the first step, the field of the image is divided up into an array of small cells by a process called **scanning**. Each cell becomes a pixel, which is assigned a designator, which is based on the column and row placement of the pixel (Fig. 20.21). The CR reader scans the imaging plate in designated number of lines, which are divided into individual sectional measurements corresponding to the pixels. In DR systems, the number of available pixels is in the number of TFTs embedded in the imaging plate. Collimation of the beam effectively selects which pixels will make up the image and is equivalent to the scanning function. Digital fluoroscopy uses a CCD, which detects the light image; it is composed of a number of electrodes that comprise pixels. Regardless of the method used, all forms require formatting of the matrix with a designated pixel size. Scanning is a term broadly applied to all approaches.

The second step in digitizing an analog image is **sampling**. In sampling, the intensity of the radiation from each pixel is measured by a detector. Sampling is the function of detecting and measuring radiation, which occurs at the imaging plate or array of detectors. The instruments used to sample the pixels have different sizes and shapes for the sampling aperture, the opening through which the pixel value is measured. In DR, the aperture is square and samplings are adjacent to each other, since the detector is a square

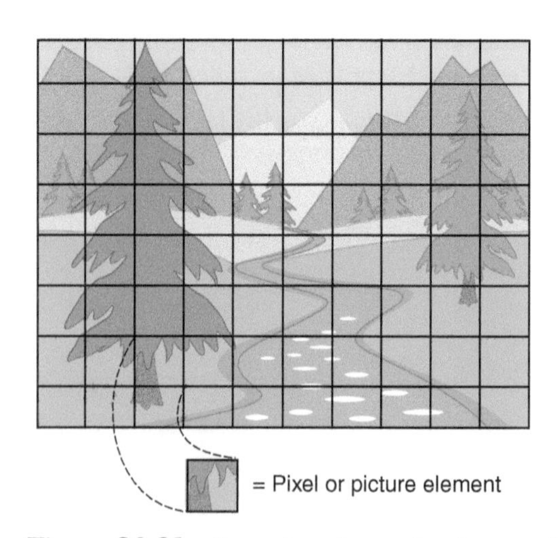

Figure 20.21. **Scanning the analog image where the matrix is formatted.**

hardware pixel. One disadvantage of the square aperture is that some of the information between the actual detection surfaces is missed. An interesting fact is the CR aperture is round because the laser beam that strikes the phosphor is round. The CR must overlap adjacent samplings in order to fill square pixels in the constructed digital image (Fig. 20.22).

The final step in digitizing the analog image is **quantization**. The result of the quantization process is to assign a value to each pixel to represent a discrete gray level; this is a number the computer can read and manipulate. Remember the gray scale is the predetermined range of gray levels seen in the image. The values of brightness (density) fall between the shades of gray and must be rounded up or down to the nearest available gray level. Recall that computers only use discrete numbers to "read" information. Analog numbers coming into the system that fall between values must be rounded up to the nearest digital number. The ADC rounds out all incoming data into digits the computer system allows.

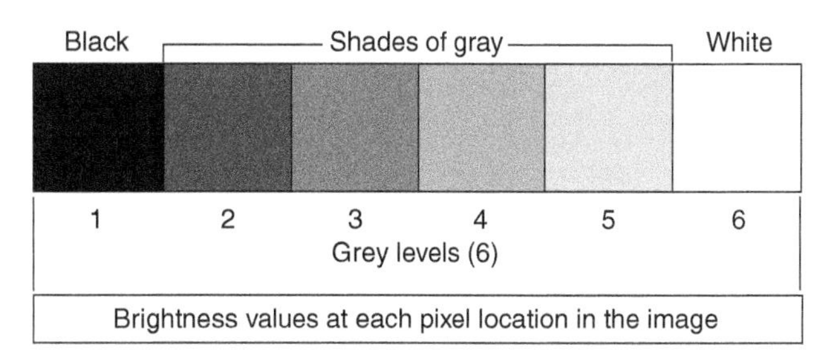

Figure 20.22. **Quantization where digital values are assigned for each pixel measurement.**

Chapter Summary

1. Digital imaging systems include CR, DR, MR, CT, NM, and fluoroscopic units.
2. Detectors used in digital imaging include fluoroscopic image intensifiers and scintillation crystals.
3. Images on film can be digitized, processed, and transmitted in PACS.
4. An ADC changes analog signals into digital signals.
5. CR employs a thin solid-state detector plate inside a special CR cassette that is the same size and shape as a conventional film screen cassette and can be used in the same Bucky holders.
6. Data compression reduces the size of the image matrix and reduces the time required to transmit, process, and retrieve the images and the memory space required to store the images.
7. Digital data can be displayed for interpretation on display monitors.
8. The PSP plate contains a phosphor that is ionized when exposed to x-ray photons.
9. Approximately one-half of the liberated electrons are trapped in the conduction band. When the plate is read, the energy from the electrons is released and converted into an electronic signal, which the computer uses to create the manifest image.
10. Cassetteless systems use a detector array that converts the exit x-ray beam into a signal that immediately displays an image on the monitor.
11. The digital image has a linear response to the x-ray exposure where the film screen has a curved response. The digital image also has a wider dynamic range and can respond to exposure levels much lower and much higher resulting in many more shades of gray.
12. The kVp still influences contrast in the digital systems. Because the systems can display a wider dynamic range, a higher kVp (adjusted using the 15% rule) can be used to produce a quality image. The benefit of this will be lowering the amount of mAs for the exposure.
13. The digitization processes for CR and DR include scanning of the image and sampling the intensity of radiation on the pixel and quantization to assign a value to the pixel.

Case Study

Jenny, a first year radiologic technology student, is giving a presentation about digital radiography to her classmates. She has decided to explain the cassette-based system. During the presentation, she will answer the following questions.

Critical Thinking Questions

1. What are the components of the cassette-based system?
2. How does the imaging plate acquire an image?
3. How is the imaging plate read?
4. What must occur for the latent image to become visible on the computer screen?
5. Where is the final image stored?

Review Questions

Multiple Choice

1. **Computed radiographic systems use:**
   a. detector plates that are read by a scanning laser beam
   b. detector plates of dry chemicals
   c. detector plates that are read by a thermal head
   d. conventional screen cassettes

2. **For the computer to process an image, the analog image must be modified into digital form by a device called a(n):**
   a. ADC
   b. SNR
   c. CRT
   d. CPU

3. **The principal limiting factor for the perception of contrast in an analog imaging system is:**
   a. the inability of the components to detect large differences in tissue density
   b. the inability of the components to provide high spatial resolution
   c. the inherent poor contrast enhancement of analog systems
   d. the limited range of gray shades that can be perceived

4. **The greatest advantage of digital imaging systems is the ability to:**
   a. improve sharpness in the image
   b. reduce radiation exposure to the patient
   c. eliminate chemical processing
   d. perform postprocessing operations on the image

5. **The __________ is the individual hardware elements of a DR receptor plate that detect radiation in the exit x-ray beam.**
   a. pixel
   b. dexel
   c. rexel
   d. diode

6. **The size of the individual dexel is closest to:**
   a. 1 cm
   b. 100 μm
   c. 1 mm
   d. 1 nm

7. **In a DR image receptor, most of the surface area of each dexel is made up of which portion of the detector element?**
   a. Thin-film transistor
   b. Capacitor
   c. Semiconductor layer
   d. Gate lines

8. **With indirect conversion DR systems, the dispersion of light emitted from the cesium iodide molecules is reduced by using:**
   a. light guides
   b. turbid phosphor structure
   c. crystalline phosphor structure
   d. scintillation optics

9. **The CR cassette is constructed to protect the phosphor plate from:**
   a. light
   b. primary x-ray photons
   c. heat
   d. static electricity

10. **The purpose of the antihalo layer of a photostimulable phosphor plate is to prevent:**
    a. laser light from penetrating through to the reflective layer
    b. emitted light from excessive diffusion
    c. back-scattered x-rays from reaching the phosphor layer
    d. external light from creating artifacts within the phosphor layer

Short Answer

1. **Explain the function of two of the layers of a photostimulable phosphor imaging plate.**

2. **Which material is used in a flat panel detector to convert x-ray photons into electrons?**

3. **Explain how the imaging plate is read in a CR system.**

4. **What is the reason that all electronic devices are inherently noise?**

5. **Identify the two principle phosphors used in DR image plates.**

6. **Why is the optical filter positioned before the photodetector?**

7. **List the three subsystems of a CR reader.**

8. **What causes "ghosting" in a digital image?**

9. **What is the purpose of europium in a photostimulable phosphor?**

10. **What is the color of stimulating laser light and emitted light?**

21

Digital Imaging Exposure Techniques

Objectives

Upon completion of this chapter, the student will be able to:

1. Identify the effects of off-centering anatomy on an image using AEC.
2. List methods for minimizing patient exposure to radiation.
3. Understand the concept behind using higher kVp levels for CR and DR.
4. Explain the foundational principles and how each applies to CR and DR.
5. Describe what "dose creep" is and how it has become common in digital imaging.
6. Differentiate between sufficient penetration, over-penetration, and underpenetration of the beam.
7. List dose reduction techniques.
8. Describe the process for aligning multiple fields on one CR image receptor.
9. Recognize and explain technique myths of CR and DR.

Key Terms

- 15% rule
- automatic exposure control (AEC)
- dose creep
- histogram analysis
- histogram errors
- off-centering
- quantum mottle

Introduction

Radiography has gone through many changes, which have expanded the field and created faster methods for capturing a quality radiographic image. Many of the foundational theories and concepts used in film-screen radiography are still valid in digital imaging. Chapter 17 discussed central concepts in selecting appropriate technical factors based on patient considerations, pathologies, and developing technique charts. In this chapter, the student will learn the rationale for adjusting film-screen techniques to digital imaging.

Procedural Considerations

Each procedure that is performed is centered on the patient and on the method used to capture a diagnostic image of the anatomy. In Chapter 17, the student learned the importance of identifying the patient's body habitus and measuring part thickness to correctly formulate adjustments in kVp and mAs. As a reminder, more hypersthenic patients are being imaged than ever before. These patients are in all age groups and genders so it is critical to use the correct combination of technical factors to reduce their radiation dose. It is important to keep the radiation dose to a minimum for ALL patients!

Tissue composition and pathologic processes must also be considered. Bone has a higher atomic number than soft tissue structures, which means the kVp and mAs settings will be based upon the anatomical structures of interest. Additive and destructive pathological processes are also considered when the technologist is selecting the technical factors for the procedure. There are many tools in the radiology toolbox, which technologists must be proficient in using. With a thorough understanding of all aspects of creating a quality image, the patient will be exposed to the appropriate amount of radiation to acquire the image. This has been a challenge in recent times with the advent of digital imaging. This chapter will dispel some myths and recent practices surrounding digital radiography.

Centering Anatomy

Centering anatomy correctly in the image receptor is a practice that must still be performed. Many technologists believe that digital radiography will compensate for their poor positioning skills; it will not. On a DR system, manual techniques can be used; however, the system is most frequently operated with the **automatic exposure control (AEC)** engaged for all procedures including extremities. Remember when the anatomy is not properly centered over the AEC detector cells, there is a portion of the detector that receives the primary beam, and the AEC will shut off prematurely, which results in underexposure of the anatomy. The digital image will display anatomy with some degree of **quantum mottle**.

CR systems are more forgiving of off-centering of anatomy in the field but are subject to **histogram errors**. It can be very difficult to perfectly center some anatomy directly in the middle of the field especially when the anatomy of interest is on the edge of the body. For example, the sternum is on the anterior surface of the body, and when the patient is positioned for a lateral view, part of the collimated field will include sternum and thorax anatomy, while the rest of the field is not over any anatomy. The resultant image will be dark because excessive background radiation caused the histogram error.

To avoid either of these problems with CR or DR, the technologists must take the time to properly center the anatomy within the image receptor and collimate to the part of interest.

Aligning Fields on IPs/IRs

In film-screen imaging, it is a common practice to put two or three images on a single image receptor. With proper use of lead strips to protect each portion of the IR, the images that were produced were of diagnostic quality. The development of digital imaging has created challenges to producing multiple images on one IR.

In CR, the computer uses the exposure field recognition program to distinguish the edges of the anatomical part against the background from the edges of the collimated field. Yes, it is still important to collimate! When multiple exposures are made on the CR plate, it makes it very difficult for the computer to distinguish between very light areas between the exposure fields and similar light areas (bone) within the image.

Multiple Fields

The area between the images must be "blank white." If the area is fogged, the computer has a difficult time distinguishing those densities from bone. In Figure 21.1A, a single knee image was taken on a 14 × 17 CR plate with proper four-sided collimation. The image demonstrates the proper radiographic contrast of an AP knee when performing only one image on the IR. In Figure 21.1B, two images were taken on the same IR with 1 inch of space between the collimated fields. There is fog present between the two fields; **histogram analysis** included this fog density, which resulted in a lengthened gray scale. When having two fields on one IR, the anatomy should be centered well within each field, and all collimation

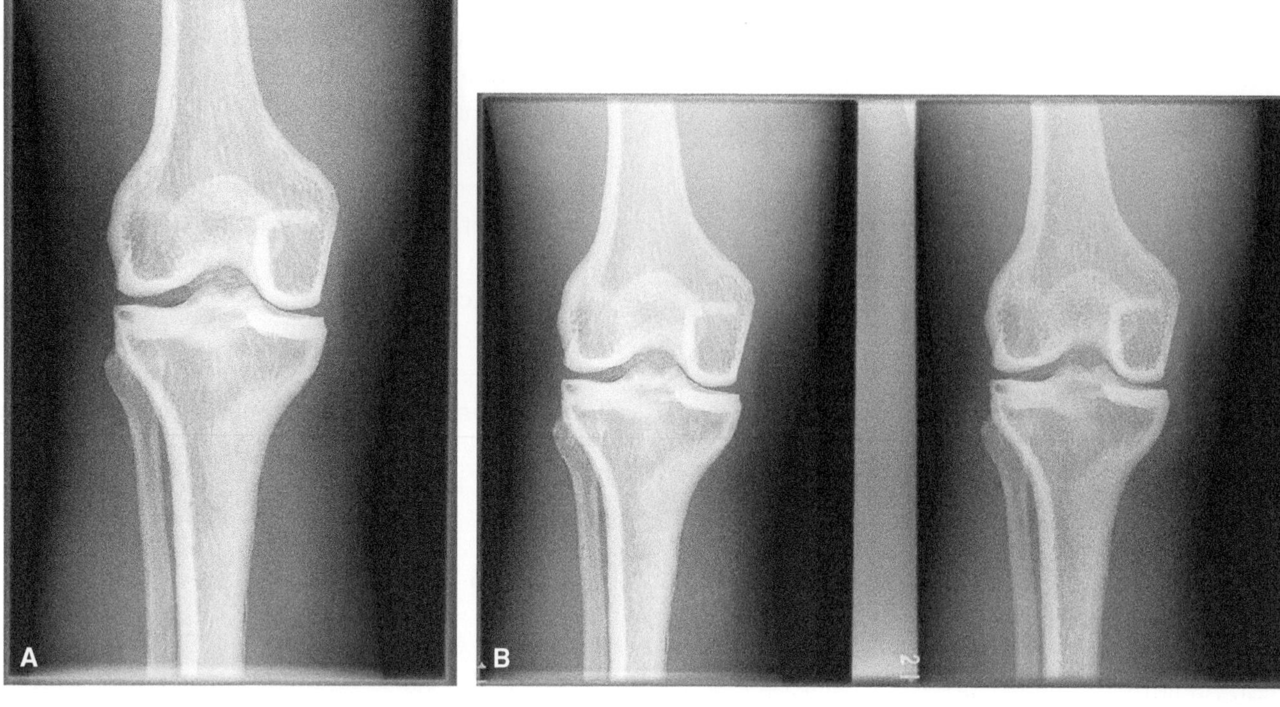

Figure 21.1. **Multiple fields. (A) Knee phantom was taken on one IR. (B) The same technique was used as A, but with two fields positioned 1 inch apart. The fog between the two fields resulted in a histogram error, which caused a lengthened gray scale.**

must be parallel and equidistant from the edges of the plate. This helps the computer distinguish between bone and blank areas between the fields.

Asymmetric Fields

Asymmetric distribution of multiple fields will contribute to field recognition errors. This is especially true when the field has no margins at the edge of the plate. Figure 21.2 illustrates collimated fields on a CR plate. Note how **A** has two fields that are correctly aligned and are equidistant from each other and the edges of the plate. **B** and C each have a single edge, which extends beyond the edge of the CR cassette. **D** has only one field on the CR plate; however, it is not centered in the middle. E has a field that has been angled and is not parallel with the CR cassette edges. Each of these images has **off-centering** errors that can cause exposure field recognition errors to occur. The industry has seen a persistent level of processing errors because of these alignment errors, which has led technologists and departments to develop a "new" practice where only one image is exposed on an IR. Traditionally, technologists had various procedures where two fields were exposed on one IR but with the need for repeat exposures, because of field recognition errors, technologists have had to adapt how they image some anatomy.

With CR, there is no compelling reason to attempt multiple fields on one cassette. Film-screen radiography

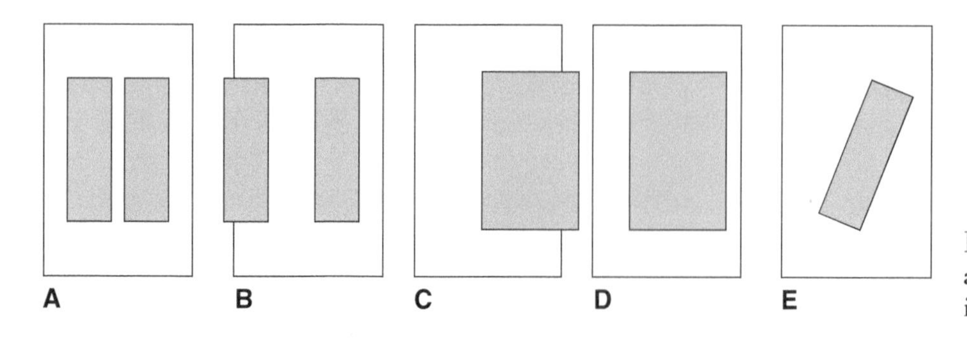

Figure 21.2. **Illustration of symmetric and asymmetric fields on one CR image receptor.**

used the multiple fields on one cassette as a cost-saving measure to reduce the amount of film and chemicals used. This is no longer the case with reusable CR plates. It has been found that by using one field on a CR plate, it produces more consistent image quality within the department.

Overcollimation

Collimation continues to be vital in improving the quality of an image. With digital imaging, exposure indicator errors are likely to occur, and at least 30% of the plate must be exposed to greatly decrease the possibility of exposure indicator errors. The 30% rule can be problematic when a collimated view of a finger or thumb is taken on a 10 × 12 plate. It is recommended that for these small digits, two or three views are placed on one plate to ensure the minimum 30% plate coverage. Each view must be evenly spaced and well centered on the plate. Large 14 × 17 plates should not be used for single extremity images such as AP ankle or AP foot.

Reducing Patient Exposure

One of the primary goals of producing an image is to keep the dose to the patient as low as reasonably achievable (ALARA). This was true in the film-screen era and is equally true today with digital imaging. Computerization of the industry has provided the opportunity to adjust our technical factors to further reduce patient dose by 20% to 50%. This may not be much of a consideration for a single image, but over the life of the patient, this amount of dose reduction is huge!

Sadly, the opposite has been seen in clinical practice. In film-screen imaging, an overexposed image has more radiographic density, and it is quite easy to see that an error has been made. Digital imaging almost always produces a good image even when the image is overexposed. In practice today, technologists have become complacent in changing factors between images. When imaging the lateral view first, the techniques are often left the same for the AP view when the images are taken back to back. The result should be obvious: the AP view is produced with more dose than is needed, and patient dose is increased. In digital imaging, this practice is called "**dose creep.**" In this section, students will learn about proper practice and how to avoid "dose creep."

Converting to Digital Imaging

Many CR systems operate at a 200-speed class, which is only one-half the speed of rare-earth 400-speed class for film screen. In making the conversion from rare-earth screen systems to CR, many radiology departments doubled mAs for Bucky exams, while more was often used. The result was a doubling of exposure to the patient having pelvis, abdomen, and head procedures where sensitive organs and tissues are located.

Digital imaging systems measure exposure to the IR, the 200-speed class effectively reduces the exposure to the IR by one-half. When using the established film screen, kVp levels found on technique charts will lead to insufficient exposure to the IR. The remedy is to increase kVp for more penetration of the x-ray beam through the anatomy and to the imaging plate. This does result in sufficient exposure to the detectors and allows the unit to operate at the 400-speed class.

The question becomes how much should kVp be increased? Because units measure exposure to the plate, the best practice is to use the **15% rule** across the board for all exposures. Remember that when kVp is increased 15%, the mAs can be decrease by one-half. This combination of factors keeps patient exposure consistent with rare-earth screen systems.

Some technologists argue that digital detectors are highly sensitive to scatter radiation and increasing the kVp will only produce more scatter and degrade the image. This is true when discussing the physics of the detector, but it doesn't consider the outcome of the final image. Manufacturers recommend higher kVp settings for CR and DR and discourage using <60 kVp for extremity images.

The primary cause of scatter radiation is patient size coupled with lack of appropriate collimation. Decreasing the field size to the area of interest reduces the amount of scatter radiation reaching the IR. As seen in Figure 21.3, two images of an ankle look remarkably similar. In film A, the AP ankle was produced with 65 kVp and 6 mAs, LGM 1.91. For film B, the kVp was increased 15% to 75% and mAs was lowered to 3, LGM 2.02. Both images are diagnostic images with the correct scale of

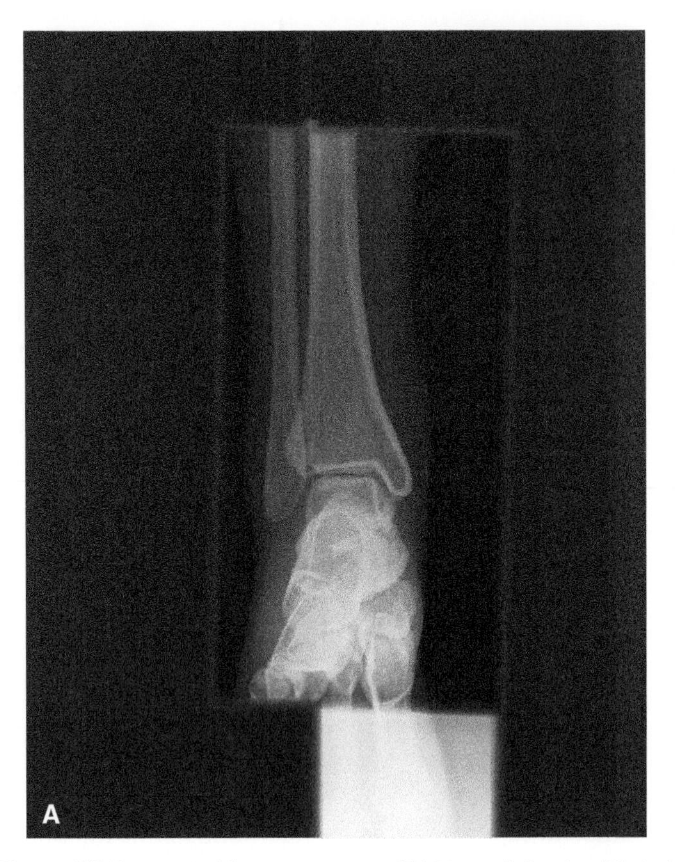

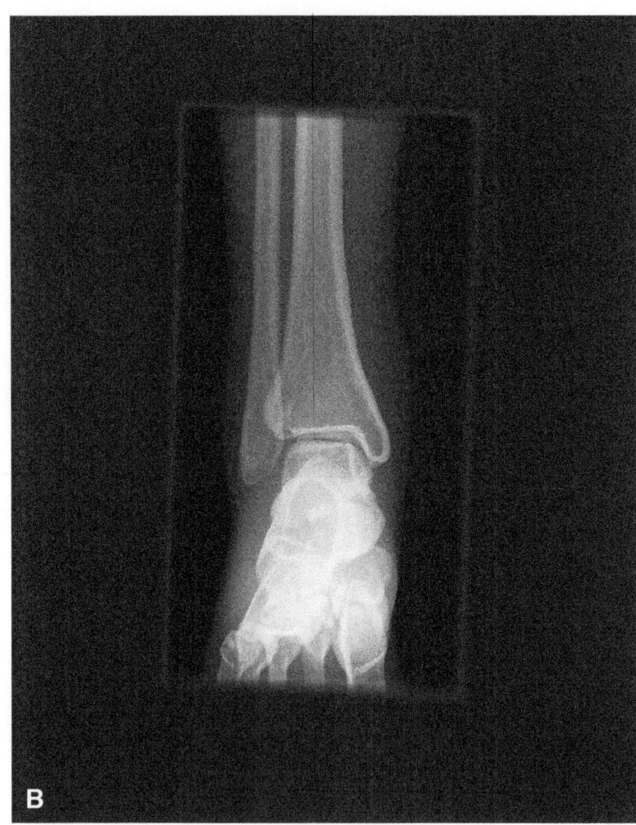

Figure 21.3. **(A) Ankle image using 65 kVp and 6 mAs. (B) Ankle image using 75 kVp and 3 mAs. Both images appear to have the same gray scale with appropriate visualization of anatomy. Image A is also demonstrating a segment recognition failure.**

contrast. This is proof that sufficient penetration of the x-ray beam reached the IR to produce an acceptable image.

As a profession, we must continually be aware of the radiation dose we are delivering to patients. We must strive to restore patient exposure to previous levels by establishing new "optimum kVp" settings. A department may not want to make a sweeping change to all procedures but should seriously consider changing the kVp levels for special circumstances like barium studies, morbidly obese patients, or pediatric imaging. For example, a scoliosis procedure is primarily performed on adolescents whose bodies and tissues are undergoing rapid change. In adolescents who have frequent, whole-spine exposures, there is an increased risk of breast and bone cancer from the multiple exposures. In an effort to decrease the radiation dose to adolescent patients, the 15% rule should be used because it will allow the mAs to be cut in half while increasing kVp. This change will result in the overall image quality and will be maintained.

Comparative Anatomy and Manual Technique Rules

Chapter 17 presented comparative anatomy process for deriving techniques from one body part to another. The development of CR and DR introduces fascinating possibilities for this approach. Gone are the days of having multiple speeds of cassettes and film that need to be matched, all procedures use the same speed because CR and DR systems only have one speed. Using the proportional anatomy approach and determining technical factor, combinations should be much easier. The rules discussed in Chapter 17 still apply; however, minor adjustments may need to be made, but generally, the rules are still accurate.

For example, a lateral skull, AP cervical spine, and AP shoulder can be imaged with 80 kVp and 6 mAs; the key is to use the minimum kVp needed for each image. An AP abdomen, AP lumbar spine, and AP pelvis all use the same technical factors of 80 kVp and 24 mAs. This method works very well for thicker body parts. Most discrepancies are in technical factors for extremities and need to be refined. Comparative anatomy is still a valid starting point to derive technical factors and to build new technique charts for CR and DR equipment.

Developing and using manual technique skills is essential! The foundational skills of measuring the part and changing factors when there is a 4- to 5-cm change in thickness still works very well. We have discussed the importance of using the 15% kVp rule, but it cannot be stressed too much. When SID is changed, there must be a corresponding change in technical factors to accommodate the increase or decrease in distance in order to have adequate penetration of the x-ray beam through to the IR. Though these rules are not as popular as they once were, the rules have potential to save the technologist a lot of grief when selecting new techniques.

Overexposure

CR and DR have greater exposure latitude than film-screen imaging. Film screen has a latitude of −30% to +50%. In comparison, CR/DR has latitude of −50% to +400%; the linear response provides a wider range for error especially in the direction of overexposure. In Chapter 13, the shape for the characteristic curve for film-screen imaging was described. Figure 21.4 demonstrates

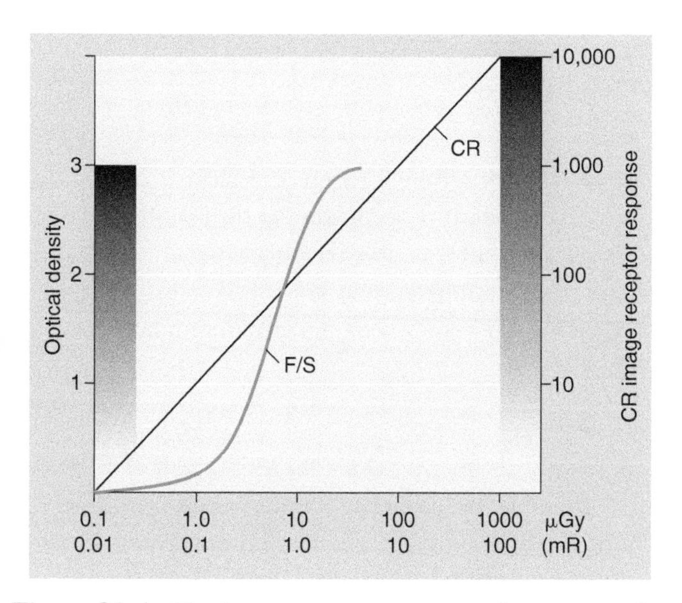

Figure 21.4. The image receptor response for computed radiography is compared to the characteristic curve of a film-screen image receptor.

the "characteristic curve" for a CR image receptor. In CR and DR imaging, it is not a curve but an image receptor response function. As seen in the illustration, there are several differences between CR and film-screen image receptors. The response of film screen ranges in OD from 0 to 3 because OD is a logarithmic function. Recall that film-screen images can only display ~30 shades of gray when viewed on a view box.

CR imaging is characterized by an extremely wide latitude. The CR image receptor response ranges from 0 to 10,000 levels of gray; each can be evaluated visually by postprocessing. Selecting the proper radiographic technique and exposure are critical for producing a diagnostic quality image in film-screen imaging. As evidenced by the following discussion, this is not the case with CR imaging.

A digital image, which is produced with greater amounts of exposure, can reach a point of saturation where the image is very dark (Fig. 21.5). Saturation requires 8 to 10 times the normal exposure that corresponds to an exposure index number higher than 3,000 on Kodak and an "S" number <25 on Fuji. Fortunately, saturation is rare and often happens when the technologist forgets to change technical factors from a previous patient.

In Figure 21.6, three knee phantom images were taken; the kVp remained the same and the mAs was changed incrementally. Image A used 80 kVp and 8 mAs, image B was 80 kVp and 6 mAs, and image C used 80 kVp with 24 mAs. The Agfa LGM was 2.5, 2.4, and 2.8, respectively. These images demonstrate how the CR system will compensate for the change in technical factors, and the final processed image is nearly unchanged. In film screen, image B would have been considered underexposed and would have appeared light, while image C used four times the mAs and would have been very dark or overexposed. This again demonstrates the dangers of using very high mAs settings, which result in unacceptable radiation dose to the patient.

Adjusting kVp while maintaining mAs is a useful method for producing images. In Figure 21.7, image A was taken using 70 kVp and 6 mAs. This is a common set of exposure factors for the knee images and is considered the starting point when making adjustments to kVp or mAs. In an effort to demonstrate the effect kVp changes will have on a digital image, three additional

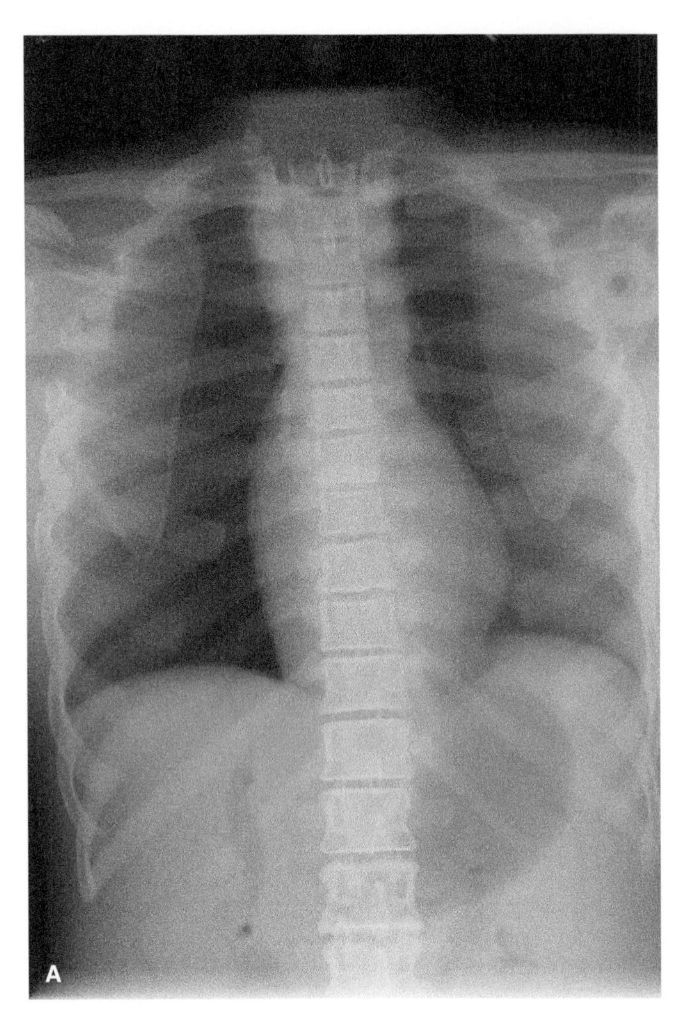

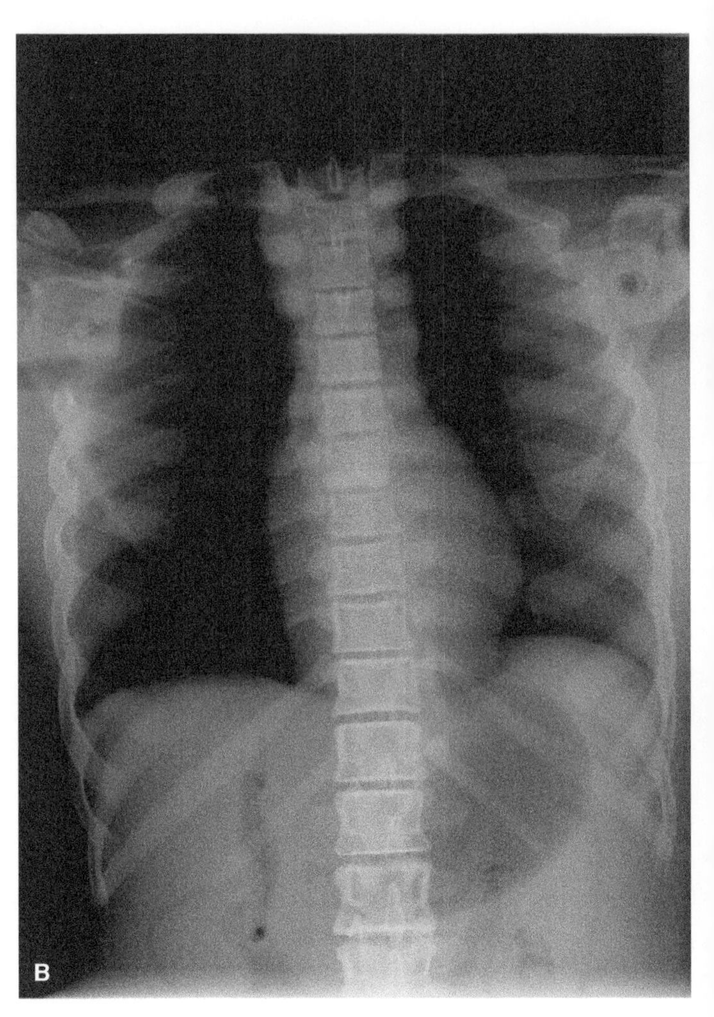

Figure 21.5. **Saturation. (A) This AP chest x-ray was taken using 120 kVp and 6 mAs, which is 200% more mAs than is typically used. (B) This image was taken with 24 mAs, which is 400% higher than normal. Notice the dark lungs fields that do not demonstrate any anatomy; this is called saturation.**

exposures were taken. For each exposure, 6 mAs was used.

- Image B kVp was increased 30% to 91 kVp.
- Image C used 59 kVp, which is 15% lower than the original kVp.
- Image D was produced with 49 kVp, which was a 30% reduction.

Images C and D note a progressive decline in density with image D demonstrating quantum mottle, which is most apparent on the magnified images. The very low 49 kVp was not able to effectively penetrate through the tissue and reach the image receptor, resulting in a lack of exposure to the image receptor. Lower exposure limits are easy to discern because quantum mottle or noise becomes apparent very quickly as techniques are reduced (Fig. 21.7). Quantum mottle or noise is a concern in digital imaging and is seen as density fluctuations on the image.

Underexposure

Underexposure occurs when there is insufficient exposure to the IP or IR. Even slight underexposure causes visible mottle in the image. The fear of repeating an image for underexposure has resulted in many technologists developing a habit of using more mAs than needed, which leads to overexposure. Unfortunately, there has

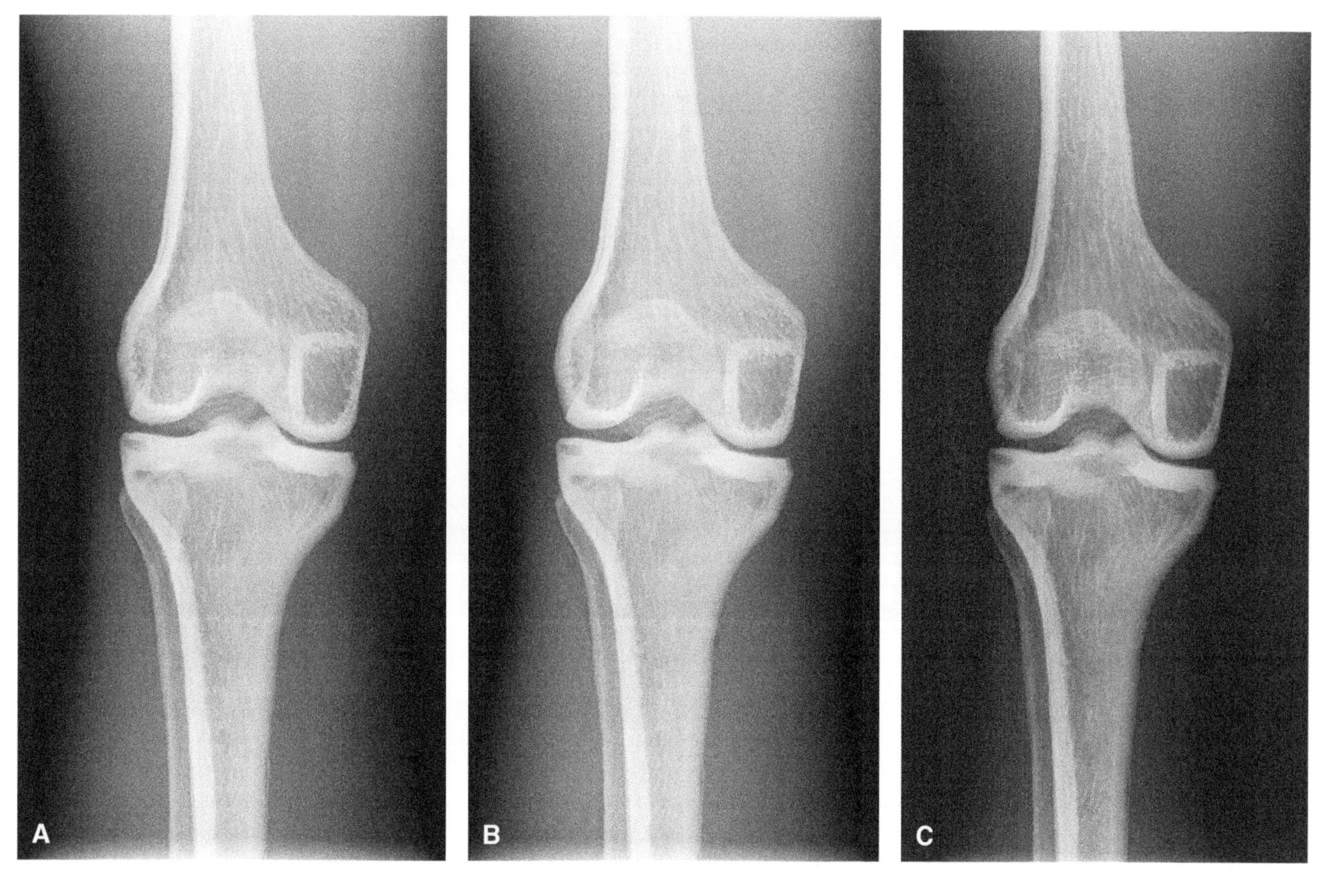

Figure 21.6. **Three knee phantoms were taken with normal technique A (80 kvp @ 8 mAs), B was taken using one-fourth the mAs, while C was taken using four times the mAs. The CR system compensated for the overexposure and produced a diagnostic image.**

been a lack of consequences for chronic overexposure patterns.

Remember that there is already a doubling of typical exposures while using the 200-speed class digital systems. When traditional kVp settings are used for a given anatomical area, the mAs is automatically doubled. This practice has steadily increased the radiation exposure to patients, which is a serious issue in diagnostic imaging. In other words, "dose creep" has become a common issue.

Dose Creep

As we have discussed, dose creep has become a problem, and it is necessary to understand the factors that are causing it to happen. There are at least four combined factors that are pushing technologists toward unacceptable levels of patient exposure. These factors include:

1. 200-speed class for CR/DR instead of 400-speed class.
2. Resistance to using increased kVp across the board. This is due to the long held view that increased kVp produces unwanted scatter, which degrades the image quality.
3. Legitimate fear of mottle from underexposure.
4. Inherent ability of CR/DR to correct for overexposure.

Students and technologists must use critical thinking to determine dose reduction strategies. One such strategy is that a repeat exposure should not be performed because of brightness or contrast of an image. These are easily manipulated with postprocessing. Another strategy is to always use the optimal kVp to provide sufficient exposure to the IP or IR. This results in decreased or eliminated quantum mottle in the image, and therefore, no repeat images will be needed. It cannot be stressed enough that digital systems are sensitive to exposure, which can be in the form of kVp instead of higher mAs settings.

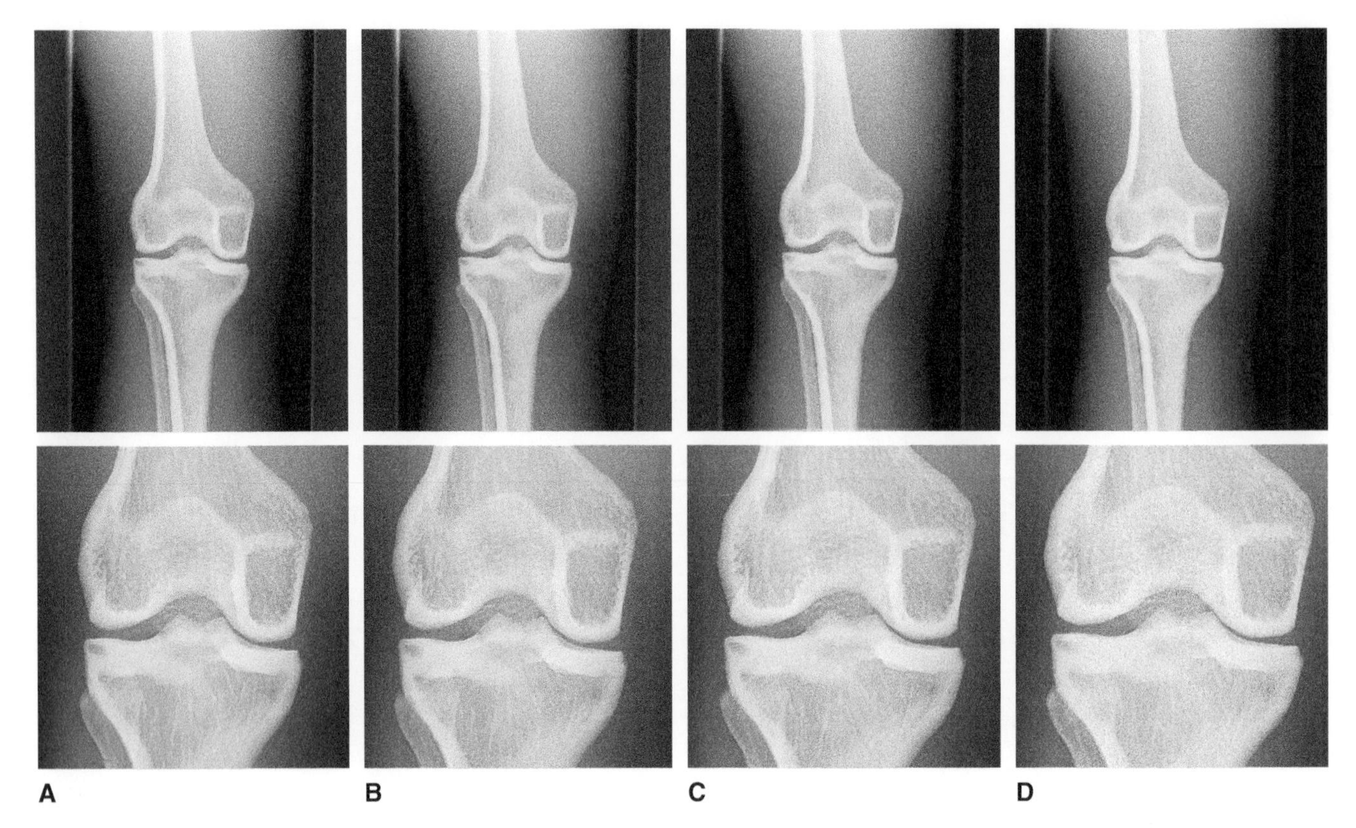

Figure 21.7. **Effects of extreme changes in kVp on CR images. Image A was taken using 70 kVp @ 6 mAs; image B was taken with 30% higher kVp; image C was taken with 15% lower kVp than image A; with this small change, quantum mottle is starting to be seen. Image D was taken with a 30% reduction in kVp and demonstrates severe quantum mottle. These effects are clearly seen on the magnified images.**

A third strategy is that overexposed images should never be repeated. Of course, it goes without saying that all anatomical information is on the image and the only reason for the repeat would be to change the technical factors. The habit of consistently using more mAs than needed should be stopped! It does not improve the image but only increases dose to the patient. Remember that with overexposure, the information is in the image, and the computer algorithms will automatically adjust the image to the appropriate visual levels. Table 21.1 summarizes dose reduction techniques.

TABLE 21.1. **HOW TO AVOID "DOSE CREEP"**

- Start by using the 15% rule. Increase kVp and decrease mAs.
- Computer algorithms measure exposure and process data to provide adequate image. Remember that kVp is seen as exposure and provides adequate data to the computer.
- Increasing kVp will maintain contrast resolution while decreasing patient dose.
- Very low kVp results in quantum mottle, which compromises bone and soft tissue resulting in a repeat image. Always use optimal kVp for all anatomical areas.

Automatic Exposure Control

AEC units, which are used for film-screen radiography, will have to be recalibrated for all new installed CR or DR units. Using optimal kVp, the AEC will receive the exposure to the detectors and will stop the exposure when the correct amount of exposure is read.

Some technologists have reported a mottled appearance when using the AEC; the correction is to use manual techniques. The likely cause of the mottled appearance is the obstinate use of low kVp levels because many technologists are afraid the higher kVp levels will result in a longer scale of gray than is needed.

With digital systems, technologists must get rid of obsolete thinking and must embrace the new way of thinking about kVp; higher kVp levels must be used to assure adequate penetration of the beam all the way through to the AEC detectors as well as adequate signal for the system to process. Many technologists and radiologists prefer a high-contrast appearance; often, this leads to images that lack detail and information. Using a long scale of contrast will improve visualization of detail and information in the image.

The correct detector cells will still be selected for the anatomy; this practice will not change. Density settings are not needed because their use unnecessarily increases mAs and patient exposure. If mottle is a problem, adjust kVp higher until sufficient signal reaches the detector cells. Positioning the anatomy properly over the detector cells is important; the anatomy must completely cover the selected detector cells. AECs traditionally have three detectors cells, while some newer DR systems have five detector cells, which provide more flexibility in positioning the patient. As with film-screen imaging, any time the AEC is used for CR or DR off-centering of the anatomy can cause premature termination of the exposure. For digital imaging, this will likely cause mottle to appear.

Exposure to IR/IP

For each imaging exam, it is of paramount importance that sufficient penetration occurs. No amount of mAs will compensate for inadequate kVp or penetration. This is true for any imaging method that is used: CR, DR, or film screen. The signal must reach the receptor by penetrating through the anatomy. Using the optimal kVp for the anatomical part still applies. It cannot be overstressed that although computer systems are able to compensate and adjust the brightness of the image for reduced kVp, the use of kVp that is too low is not an ethical practice. This results in increased patient exposure as mAs values are increased in an attempt to bring the exposure index numbers into range.

A better practice is to slightly overpenetrate the part than to underpenetrate. It is better to use higher kVp to ensure that the part is properly penetrated, the higher kVp will increase the exposure to the IR. Computer algorithms can adjust the image for slight overexposure, adequate signal is present, and the anatomical information is in the image to adjust. An image that is underpenetrated has a loss of information; no CR or DR system can replace or adjust information that is simply not there.

Effects of kVp Changes on the Image

Figure 21.7 demonstrates the effects of moderate and extreme changes in kVp on the CR image. Extreme underpenetrated images demonstrate obvious quantum mottle. Slight underexposure results in exposure index numbers in the low end of the acceptable range with some mottle present in the image.

Overpenetration does not result in obvious fog or degradation of image quality. In film screen, when the kVp was too high, the image was overpenetrated, and the radiographic density was increased because of the additional scatter radiation that "fogged" the image. This is not the case with digital imaging, and the technologist must adjust their thinking regarding the use of higher kVp levels and overpenetration. Anytime there is an acceptable increase in kVp, the computer algorithms produce a diagnostic image with no fog present. This means that applying the 15% rule with higher kVp will decrease patient dose for CR and DR imaging without reduction in image quality.

The imaging plate and computer system recognize exposure to the plate and use this to formulate the image. The exposure is a combination of kVp and mAs; the algorithms will process the data and display an acceptable image. Because CR systems recognize exposure to the IR, the technologist can use the higher kVp and lower mAs to produce a diagnostic image. The key is to always use established guidelines for making the changes, hence the 15% rule.

Technique Myths

As with any new technology, there are myths that take on a life all their own, and many believe the myth to be true. Some common myths are:

"Never use <70 kVp," "Never use more than 80 kVp," "System is mAs driven, only adjust mAs," "System is kVp driven, only adjust kVp," "Can't collimate with CR," and "Can't use grids with CR or DR." All of these statements are not accurate. The selection of the appropriate kVp and mAs are based on the same principles as conventional radiography; all the rules still apply. It is recommended for the kVp range for adults to be from 60 to 120, and for pediatric patients weighing <100 pounds, the kVp range is 50 to 90. Higher kVp displays more anatomical data with decreased patient dose. Radiologists can use window functions to increase image contrast when necessary. It is still highly recommended to develop technique charts for each radiographic unit as no two pieces of equipment are identical.

Effects of Scatter on Digital Images

As previously stated, film-screen radiography made it very easy to distinguish a diagnostic image from a nondiagnostic image. If the technical factors were not correct, the image quality suffered. As a result, the technologists had to be very careful when selecting kVp and mAs for the patient body habitus and part being image. No one wanted to produce an underexposed or overexposed image!

Digital equipment is resilient to the effects of scatter radiation caused during exposure. The systems have considerable latitude in selecting exposures including nongrid imaging. Only extreme deviations in exposure will result in computer errors. This only occurs when incredibly high exposure settings are used, which of course would be unethical. The extremely high exposure settings can cause saturation of the image to occur. Saturation of the detectors requires 8 to 10 times the normal exposure! The computer system can compensate when 30 kVp more than normal is used; this equates to four times mAs.

When the computer reads the data from the IR or IP, it will compensate for any scatter by using processing algorithms. As seen in Figure 21.8, a series of KUB images

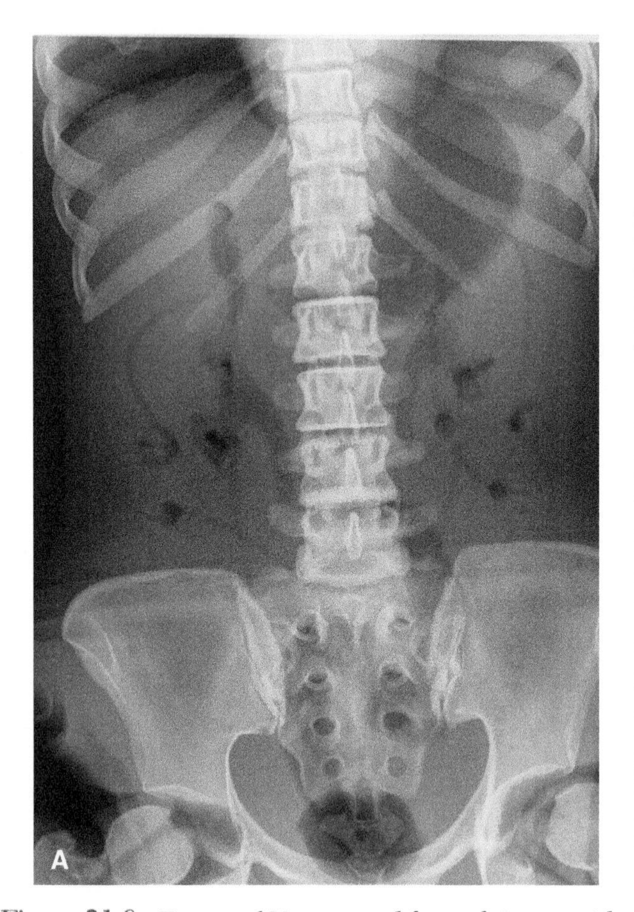

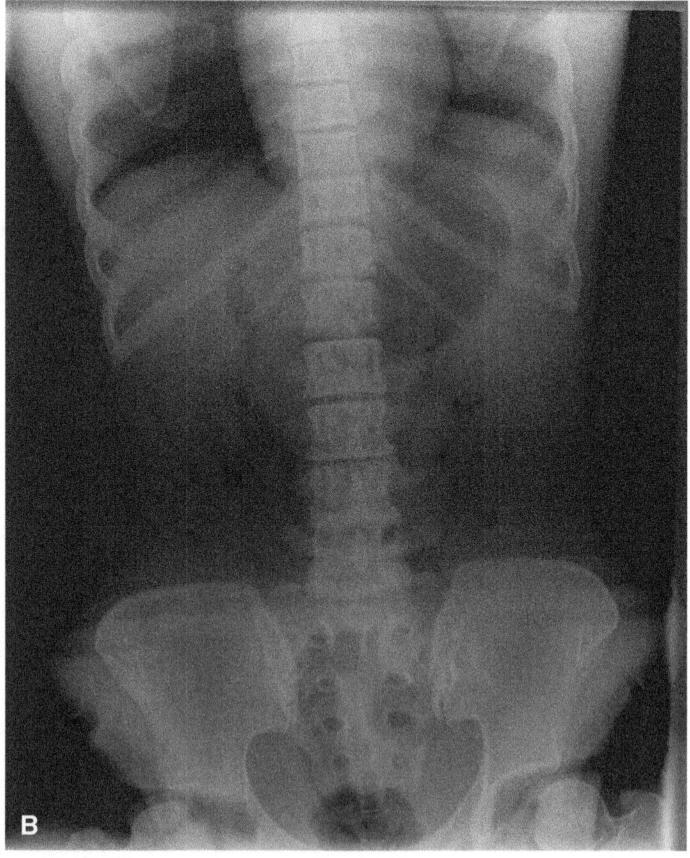

Figure 21.8. Extreme kVp was used for each image with nongrid technique. 105 kVp was used for each image, while 1 mAs was used for image A and 5 mAs for image B. The extremely high kVp results in large scatter production, and the computer processing cannot completely compensate for the effects of scatter radiation especially in image B.

were taken using a nongrid plate to maximize the effects of scatter on the image. It is easy to distinguish the progressive darkening from the additional scatter radiation density on the plate.

CR plates, which have been in storage or left in the imaging room during an exposure, are very sensitive to background and scatter radiation. CR plates can become "fogged" prior to the exposure resulting in a fogged image. Figure 21.9 demonstrates an abdomen image that has a very long scale of contrast because of fog in the image. This underscores the importance of erasing CR plates prior to use if there is any question of their condition. DR image receptors are not vulnerable to prefogging so a fogged image is rare.

Grids are still a viable piece of equipment with digital imaging. Grids are recommended for CR imaging for chest larger than 26 cm or any anatomical part larger than 10 cm. The purpose of the grid is to improve the data of the input signal. DR systems have a grid in place, which is used for all procedures including small extremities.

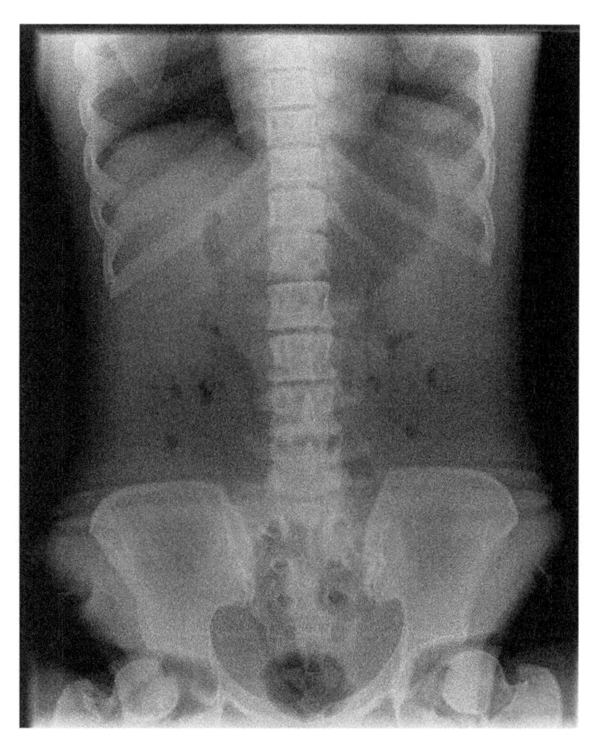

Figure 21.9. **Fogged IR. IR left in room while exposures were taken. The KUB was imaged with 70 kVp @ 20 mAs in the Bucky. The fog on the IR is seen as densities on the image.**

Chapter Summary

1. Optimum kVp and adequate penetration of the x-ray beam through to the imaging plate or imaging receptor are critical in producing a diagnostic image. Underpenetrated images simply do not have the anatomical data for CR and DR systems to create an acceptable image.
2. Increasing kVp 15% for all procedures can be done with CR and DR without substantial scatter radiation. The benefit in using the 15% rule is a reduction in mAs by one-half thereby greatly decreasing patient dose.
3. Radiographic rules still apply to digital radiography. A skilled technologists will continue to use manual technique especially when using the comparative anatomy method in addition to distance rules, 4 to 5 cm rule and the 15% rule.
4. The practice of increasing mAs to avoid potentially underexposed images has become common in digital radiography. Dose creep has become an issue based on the fear of image mottle and the ability of CR and DR systems to adjust the image for overexposure.
5. When using the AEC, correct centering of the anatomy is even more critical because off-centering quickly results in premature termination of the exposure, which leads to an image with mottle.
6. Multiple views can be performed in a CR plate; however, the anatomy must be centered in the middle of the area to be exposed, and there must be symmetrical distribution of the exposed fields on the plate. There must be sufficient separation between the fields to avoid exposure field recognition errors.
7. It is still recommended to use grids when the part is over 10 cm thick, which improves the input data to the computer system.

Case Study

Justine was called to the emergency department to perform mobile extremity images on a trauma patient who was secured on a spine board and was not able to move. The imaging department uses computed radiography and only has 14 × 17 image receptors. All the images were of diagnostic quality except for a PA wrist image. The image receptor was placed next to the patient and the wrist was positioned along one side; Justine collimated the field size to the wrist. Upon review of the final image, there were exposure indicator errors.

Critical Thinking Questions

1. Did aligning the wrist on one edge of the image receptor contribute to the errors?
2. Although Justine collimated properly to the part, was this a factor in the errors?
3. How much of the plate needs to receive an exposure to decrease the chance of an exposure error occurring?
4. Which steps can be taken to assure that exposure indicator errors are minimized?

Review Questions

Multiple Choice

1. **When considering field centering and collimation variables, which was most likely to result in analysis error?**
   a. Attempting bilateral projections of the lower extremity
   b. Using a diagonal field centered in the plate
   c. Collimating the field smaller than the imaging plate
   d. Having one side of the collimated field off the edge of the plate

2. **When should grids be used with CR?**
   a. Grids are never used with CR.
   b. Grids are used for the same procedures as film-screen imaging.
   c. They are used for all procedures.
   d. Grids are only used when the anatomical part measures 20 cm or larger.

3. **__________ is displayed in the image when there has not been sufficient exposure to the CR plate.**
   a. Quantum mottle
   b. Loss of density
   c. Loss of brightness
   d. Enhanced radiographic contrast

4. **Which of the following assists the computer in avoiding field recognition errors when multiple fields are exposed on a CR plate?**
   a. Center the anatomy within each field.
   b. Have the fields parallel to each other.
   c. The fields must be equidistant from each other.
   d. Equalization.
   e. a, b, and c only.

5. **What adjustment is recommended for all procedures to allow for the CR system to operate at a 400-speed class with reduction in patient dose?**
   a. Reduce all kVp levels by 15%.
   b. Double all mAs values.
   c. Increase all kVp levels by 15%.
   d. Cut all mAs values in half.

6. **Which statement is true in regard to CR systems?**
   a. Only mAs is adjusted because they are "mAs-driven" units.
   b. Never use <70 kVp.
   c. Process can typically compensate for scatter caused during the exposure.
   d. Grids are not used with CR systems.
   e. Collimating the field size smaller than the plate size is not possible.

7. **How much overexposure is required before a digital system becomes overwhelmed with data and reaches saturation levels?**
   a. 2 to 3 times
   b. 8 to 10 times
   c. 6 to 8 times
   d. 15 to 20 times

8. **The dawn of digital image has made the use of:**
   a. manual techniques outdated
   b. comparative anatomy methods for technique obsolete
   c. 4 to 5 cm rule as outdated
   d. all of the above
   e. none of the above

9. **For CR and DR systems, a strict lower limit for exposure to the receptor is demonstrated by:**
   a. the appearance of quantum mottle
   b. images with excessive contrast
   c. the appearance of fog in the image
   d. images turning out too light

10. **Scatter radiation resulting from the exit x-ray beam always results in a dark image on CR or DR systems?**
    a. True
    b. False

Short Answer

1. **Why is it important to have adequate separation between multiple fields on a CR plate?**

2. **What is the minimum amount of the CR plate, which should be exposed to avoid exposure indicator errors?**

3. **List the four factors, which contribute to "dose creep."**

4. **Can the CR or DR system correct the image for a long gray scale from overpenetration of the beam?**

5. **List the foundational rules, which still apply to digital radiography.**

6. **Will a CR or DR system correct the image for underpenetration?**

7. **What image characteristic are radiographers trying to avoid when a higher dose than needed for an image?**

8. **What "across-the-board" adjustment in techniques is recommended to reduce patient exposure and avoid image mottle?**

22

Digital Image Processing Operations

Objectives

Upon completion of this chapter, the student will be able to:

1. Describe the formation of an image histogram.
2. Analyze the use of an image histogram in digital imaging.
3. Discuss rescaling the image for improved brightness and contrast.
4. Explain how preprocessing is used to improve an image.
5. Identify the three types of look-up tables.
6. Describe postprocessing parameters that are used to improve an image.

Key Terms

- annotation
- gradient processing
- histogram
- histogram analysis
- look-up table
- low-pass filtering
- normalization
- postprocessing
- preprocessing
- region of interest (ROI)
- segmentation
- spatial frequency
- spatial location
- volume of interest (VOI)

Introduction

Once x-ray photons have been converted into electrical signals, the signals are available for processing and manipulation. Both photostimulable phosphor systems and direct capture systems have the capabilities for preprocessing and postprocessing. The processing parameters and image manipulation controls are similar for CR and DR systems. The technologist is able to select the parameter, which will be manipulated to improve the digital image. Although the algorithms are vendor specific, the basic principles of processing and manipulation are consistent. The primary advantage of digital imaging over film screen imaging is the ability to manipulate the image before display (preprocessing) and after display (postprocessing). The purpose of using preprocessing and postprocessing is to alter the image appearance, typically for the purpose of improving image contrast. Each type of processing will be discussed for a more in-depth knowledge.

Preprocessing

Preprocessing takes place in the computer where the raw digital image data are corrected for flaws that are inherent in the x-ray beam, the elements and electrical circuitry of the particular imaging system, or the physical elements and electrical circuitry of the processor. Preprocessing may also be called image acquisition processing. During the preprocessing stage, the components and characteristics of the image must be identified and analyzed. The processes for accomplishing this include segmentation, exposure field recognition, histogram construction and analysis, and normalization.

Segmentation

Segmentation is also called partitioned pattern recognition; this software will cause the system to scan across the plate and determine the number and orientation of views on one image receptor. Multiple views can be obtained on a single image receptor; however, the views must be arranged in a symmetrical manner with careful centering and collimation. The imaging system can recognize even numbered (2, 4) exposure fields that are centered and properly collimated. Demonstrating four-sided collimation is best with margins between each field. This method of partitioning or segmenting allows two or more images to be projected on a single IR. Restrictions for the use of multiple views on one IR are discussed in Chapter 19.

If the views are in a nonsymmetrical pattern, the system will be prone to segmentation failure, which typically results in a repeat exposure to accurately image the part of interest. Because of segmentation failures, many technologists prefer to place one image centered in the IR for each view. In this way, they do not need to be concerned for segmentation failures.

Even with one exposure field centered for direct capture digital radiography (DR), the computer must recognize the collimated borders of fields smaller than the image plate. Computer software must be capable of recognizing borders of the x-ray field so that data outside the field can be disallowed in constructing the image histogram. To obtain the most accurate information, the densities outside the field must not be included in the data for histogram rescaling.

Exposure Field Recognition

Exposure field recognition errors are caused by a field that is not properly collimated, sized, or positioned. The computer must distinguish between relatively "pitch" black areas of background density and very dark areas within anatomy such as the lung fields. Exposure field recognition software searches for anatomy recorded on the IR by finding the collimated edges and then makes the distinction between usable densities in the area of interest and scatter densities out of the field. The background densities (scatter) are then eliminated from the histogram. Failure of the system to find the edges of the image can result in incorrect data collection resulting in images that are too bright or too dark. Before we can fully discuss how the histogram for an image is analyzed, we must first discuss how the histogram is constructed.

Histogram Construction

A **histogram** is a graphic representation of optimal densities within a collimated area. The histogram is constructed by counting the number of pixels within the image at each density or brightness level as the computer scans across the image. The horizontal axis represents the value of each gray level, while the vertical axis is the number of pixels in each level. The values to the left represent white areas in the image. As the values vary toward the right, they get darker with the middle area representing the medium values. To the extreme right are the black values. Within the graph are many peaks and valleys, which are the variations in anatomical structures in the image. The scale of brightness or density is from white to black and read from left to right. An image that contains bone with a prosthesis and soft tissue will be represented on the histogram with some areas to the far left representing the white appearance of the metal prosthesis and bone. In the center, the medium values will represent the soft tissue, and if there are any areas with fat and gas or air, these dark densities will be to the far right. When an image has an overall darker appearance, the majority of values will be toward the right side of the graph. Conversely, light images will have the majority of values toward the left.

A typical histogram of a pediatric chest or extremity will have a bell-shaped curve followed by a spike toward the right side. The bell-shaped curve contains the variations in anatomy with a few very light densities to the left

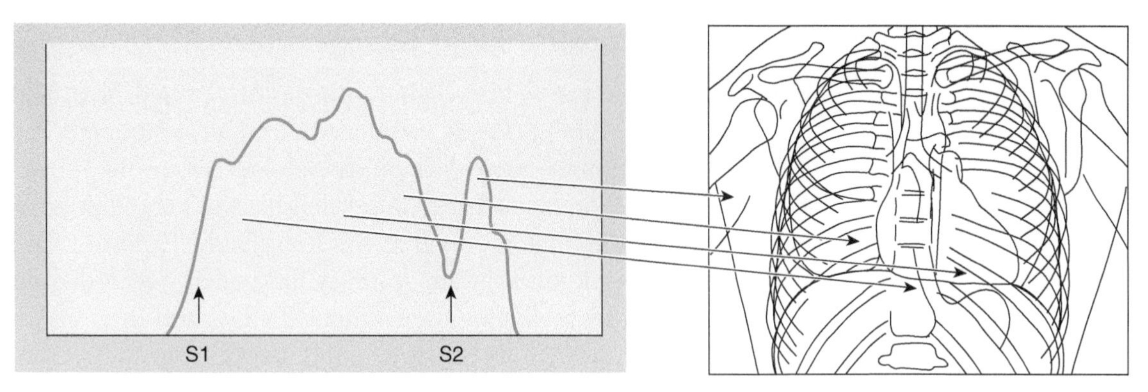

Figure 22.1. **Histogram of a chest x-ray. The left portion of the curve represents bone densities, the midportion represents soft tissues, the right portion is the aerated lung, and the "tail" is the background densities. The computer must recognize the area from S1 to S2 and analyze the information when processing the image.**

of the curve and a few very dark densities to the right of the curve, while most tissues are displayed as intermediate shades of gray or midpeak. The spike portion represents background density on the image and is outside of the anatomy, usually appears as pitch black. The spike is referred to as the "tail" of the graph (Fig. 22.1). When the anatomy such as the abdomen covers the entire IR, there is no "tail" because there are no background densities on the image. The computer must identify the "tail" portion and eliminate it from the **histogram analysis**. If the "tail" is included in the analysis, the image will be skewed away from the desired brightness and contrast levels. Only data from the anatomy must be used.

There are variables that can skew the histogram analysis, which includes positioning and collimation errors, unusual pathologies, and removed or added anatomy and prosthesis. Images that contain a lead shield, large bolus of barium, or a large prosthesis within the field of view can cause a histogram analysis error to occur. The computer tries to identify normal anatomical densities within the bell curve, extending from S1 to S2 (Fig. 22.2). If the area under the lead strip, prosthesis, or barium bolus receives enough scatter radiation to produce a signal, it can be included in the bell portion of the histogram. The result would be that S1 would move to the left, which would widen the analyzed area.

Figure 22.3 shows the appearance of scatter fog along the collimated field and how it can be included in the analysis, again widening the curve and throwing off calculations for the final image. The same effect can be seen in a chest image when a significant portion of the abdomen is included in the field. Because the abdomen has a different composition of tissues, it will show up much

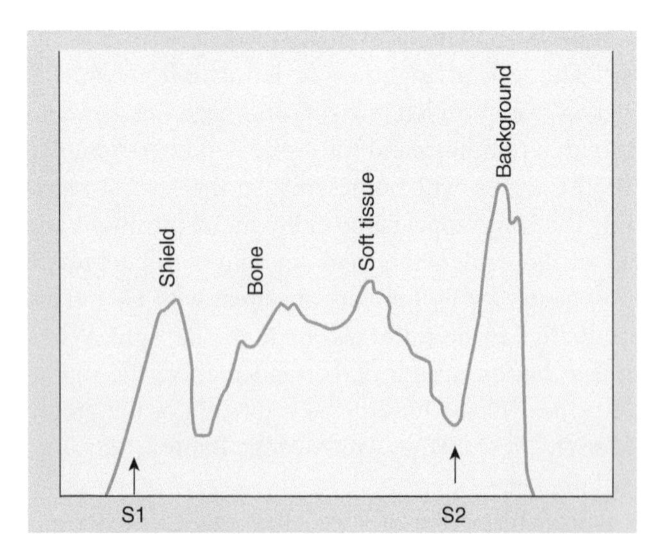

Figure 22.2. **Lead apron. When the scatter radiation goes under the lead strip, it can result in an incorrect placement of S1, widening the analyzed area and leading to histogram errors.**

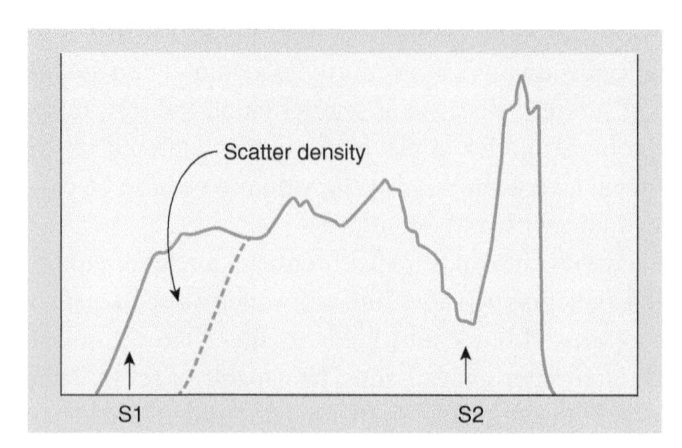

Figure 22.3. **Collimated borders. Excessive scatter radiation between or around collimated fields can result in S1 being located too far to the left. This widens the analyzed area and leads to histogram errors.**

lighter on the image. For each of these circumstances, the inclusion of lighter densities causes the computer to rescale the displayed image too dark.

There are dozens of causes for rescaling errors, which will result in a displayed image that has excessive gray scale or excessive contrast, an image that is too dark or too bright. These types of rescaling errors are less common with DR systems because only exposed pixels are included in the image database. CR systems scan the entire plate and then try to sort out exposed fields from unexposed portions of the plate.

Look-Up Tables and Types of Histogram Analysis

The computer stores the shape of the preset or reference histogram characteristics of each anatomical projection: chest, abdomen, extremity, etc. Each image that is produced is measured against the "ideal image" of the particular anatomy. Systems can store and analyze histograms for each projection. Depending upon the manufacturer, data are accumulated from 50 histograms, and the computer averages the value of each frequency interval, a representative histogram can be produced for each image receptor. The representative histogram can be updated regularly from new images.

A **look-up table (LUT)** lists the parameters that are used to produce the particular shape of an ideal histogram for the anatomy imaged. In order to rescale an image, different types of LUTs will treat the data differently in order to get the very best results in image quality for a particular body part being imaged. The goal is to accentuate the tissues for a sharp, crisp image. As seen in Figure 22.4A, the LUT is accentuating the bony anatomy; the computer focuses on closely aligning the left portion of the actual histogram and referenced histogram (LUT) curves. The bone densities are defined as **volume of interest (VOI)** or the **region of interest (ROI)**. Because the image is processed to accentuate the bone, the soft tissue densities are somewhat compromised. If the same image is processed with a soft tissue algorithm, the ROI will be the right portion of the bell curve representing tissues from dense organs to skin (Fig. 22.4B). The soft tissue algorithms align the bell curve at the expense of bone densities.

Types of LUTs

There are three types of LUTs that are based upon specific assumptions about the histogram that is used for image input. Each type of LUT expects to have a particular bell curve–shaped histogram for the anatomical area, and the LUT performs its calculations based on this assumption. It is important that each of the three types of histograms be properly aligned with the actual histograms acquired to avoid processing errors.

Type 1 histogram analysis is created to expect a direct exposure area on the image, meaning a "tail" or spike will be seen to the right of the graph as seen in Figure 22.4. Data from the spike must not be fed into the LUT; it is important that the computer identify the location of S2. Excessive background radiation and scatter can cause histogram analysis to include the "tail" within the main lobe and S2 will not be in the correct location.

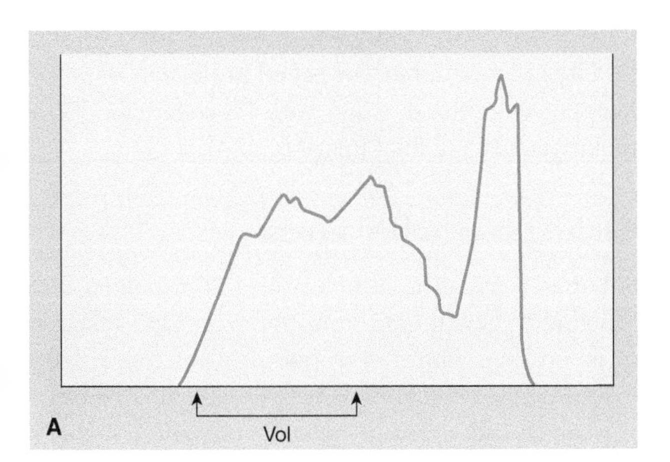

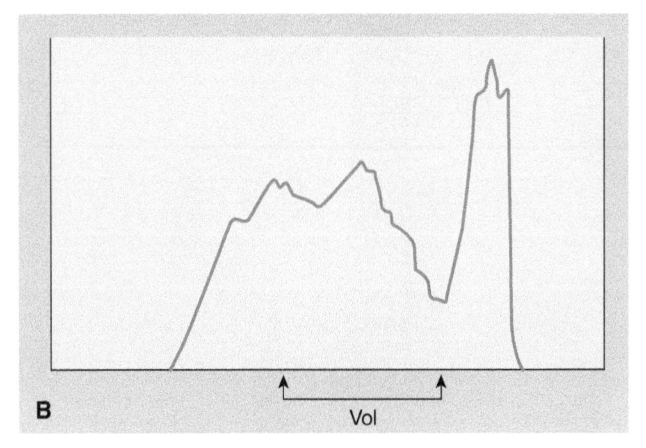

Figure 22.4. Histogram A illustrates the application of an LUT designed to emphasize bony anatomy by repositioning S1 and S2 farther to the left. Histogram B illustrates the repositioning of S1 and S2 to emphasize soft tissue anatomy. The area between S1 and S2 is called the volume of interest (VOI).

Type 2 histogram analysis assumes there is no "tail" or background radiation present. Prior to applying an LUT, histogram analysis must attempt to localize S2 without expecting any direct exposure area to be included in the bell curve. The Type 2 analysis tends to result in over-saturation in the least dense soft tissue areas, such as the skin. It is essential for projections of large body parts like the abdomen or pelvis to cover the entire IR and leave no background density to work with.

Type 3 histogram analysis allows for large prosthesis or bolus of barium to be included in the image. It also allows for lead shielding to be used and identified as part of the image. S1 must be identified as the point between the metal or barium densities and the normal tissue curve. The point just before the spike (S2) must also be identified during the histogram analysis. All data outside S1 and S2 must be eliminated from calculations used to produce the final image.

An average gray scale is typically included with the histogram. The gray scale is seen as an "S"-shaped curve overlaying the actual histogram. This "S"-shaped curve is similar to the H&D curves used to analyze response of film screen to x-rays. The gray scale curve is built by plotting output "densities" in the final processed image as illustrated in Figure 22.5. Similar to film screen, a digital image with a steep gray scale represents a high contrast or a short gray scale image. As exposure increases, the darkness of the pixel rapidly goes up. Long gray scale or low-contrast images are indicated by a curve with a shallower slope that gradually rises. It is best to achieve a balanced gray scale by applying the proper LUT for the image.

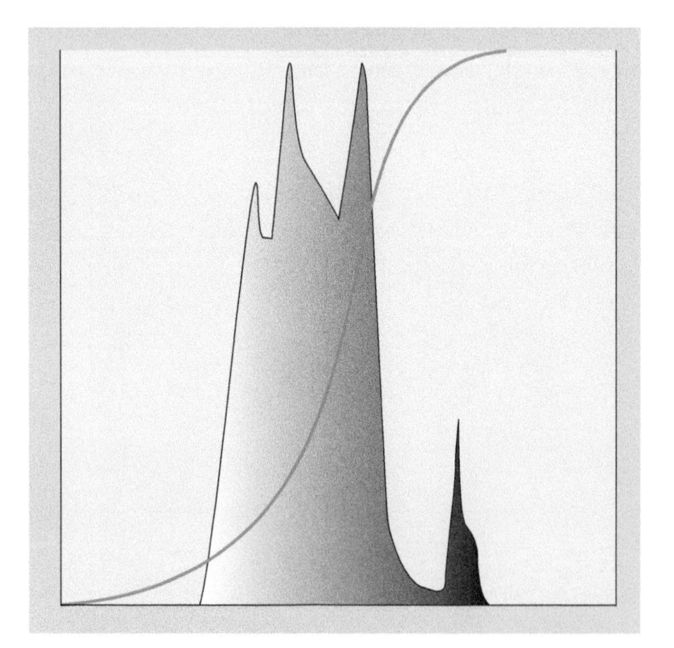

Figure 22.5. **Typical histogram with a superimposed gray scale curve.**

Normalization

The initial image captured by the detector system consists of gray levels, which would appear as washed out on the display monitor. The "raw" data must go through an initial round of default processes called **normalization**. The processes are designed to make the "raw" image appear like a conventional radiograph. Simple alignments of brightness and gray scale of the image are involved to produce the necessary contrast to visualize the anatomy. These processes are referred to as gradation or gradient processing.

Gradient Processing

Gradient processing refers to making simple adjustments in the brightness and contrast of the image. A gradient curve is plotted on a graph showing the various densities in the image; the average brightness of the image is where the curve is centered left to right. The contrast is how steep the slope (or gradient) of the curve is. The densities and contrast are also in film screen on the H&D curve, although the image capture method is different for digital versus film screen, the concept is the same. For digital imaging, the correct term of gradient processing describes the manipulation of both the centering and the steepness of the curve.

We can also consider gradient processing as an effort to conform the position and shape of the acquired images histogram to the ideal reference histogram for the specific anatomy. The position of the histogram, left to right, corresponds to the overall average brightness or density, while the shape corresponds to image contrast or gray scale. The histogram from the actual projection is moved and reshaped to closely align with the reference histogram and results in a final image to display.

Rescaling Image Brightness

In automated rescaling of image brightness, algorithms are applied to actual data from the projection taken to align its position with that of the ideal reference histogram. Automated rescaling can fail when the exposure field edges are not correctly detected by pattern recognition software, called Stage 1. Stage 2 failure occurs when unexpected material, like a metal prosthesis, is within the exposure field and distorts the data from exposure field recognition. Rescaling adjustments are algorithms that are very complex and carried out by the computer. These adjustments may be expressed as graphical changes, making it easier to visualize and understand. The goal of the adjustments is to make the curve of actual exposure identical to the curve of the reference histogram.

As illustrated in Figure 22.6, curve A is the ideal histogram resulting from the LUT for a specific radiographic image, and curve B represents an overexposed image. We know that curve B is an overexposed image because the curve is farther right, which indicates higher values. The first and easiest step would be to align the center points of the two curves by moving curve B right to left on the graph. Curve B can be moved to the left by simply subtracting a fixed amount.

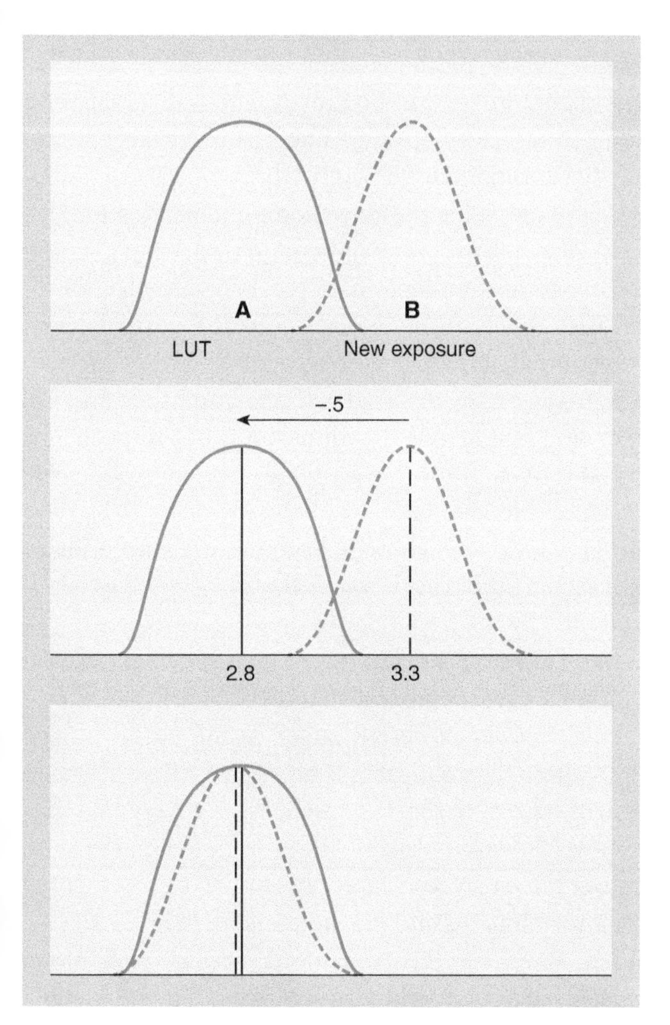

Figure 22.6. **Rescaling of brightness. (A) The dashed line represents the histogram for an overexposure compared to the ideal LUT in the system. (B) An algorithm measures the average pixel values for both curves then subtracts the difference from curve B. This aligns the brightness of the overexposure with the LUT. The aligned curves have a different shape indicating a difference in gray scale. Further postprocessing operations will be used to correct the gray scale.**

To determine the fixed amount, we must first locate the midpoint of each curve, which represents the average pixel value; this is also used as the exposure indicator number. A technologist can have the computer find the difference between these two average pixel values by subtraction. Then the computer subtracts that amount from all the pixels in the overexposed image. The formula to represent this is:

$$B-(B-A)=Bn$$

where Bn is the new position for curve B. The result of subtracting the fixed amount from each pixel in the original image is to achieve an identical overall brightness or average density in both curves. The rescaling of brightness effectively produces an image that appears to have been produced with the appropriate technical factors when in actuality more radiation was used than was necessary. In film screen, the image would appear too dark, while in digital imaging, the image would have the appropriate amount of density.

Rescaling Image Contrast

The dynamic range is the number of gray levels or brightness levels in the displayed image. It is synonymous with the gray scale seen in the image. In an image that has not undergone postprocessing manipulation, the standard radiographic techniques will demonstrate bony anatomy, while the soft tissue will appear too dark and will not be of diagnostic value. In conventional radiography, the technical factors would be adjusted to soft tissue techniques to improve visualization of the soft tissue; however, the bony anatomy would appear too light.

In digital imaging, the computer can use dynamic range compression (DRC) or tissue or contrast equalization to improve the contrast in the digital image. In Figure 22.7, the graph represents the concept of DRC, which will result in a shorter gray scale vertically. The computer defines the midpoint average brightness or density level. With mathematic manipulation, the computer progressively reduces pixel values above this point while progressively increasing values below it. Consider the original curve in Figure 22.7, the curve has the toe portion, which represents the extreme light densities and the shoulder or extremely dark areas. The toe portion is progressively compressed upward toward the average pixel

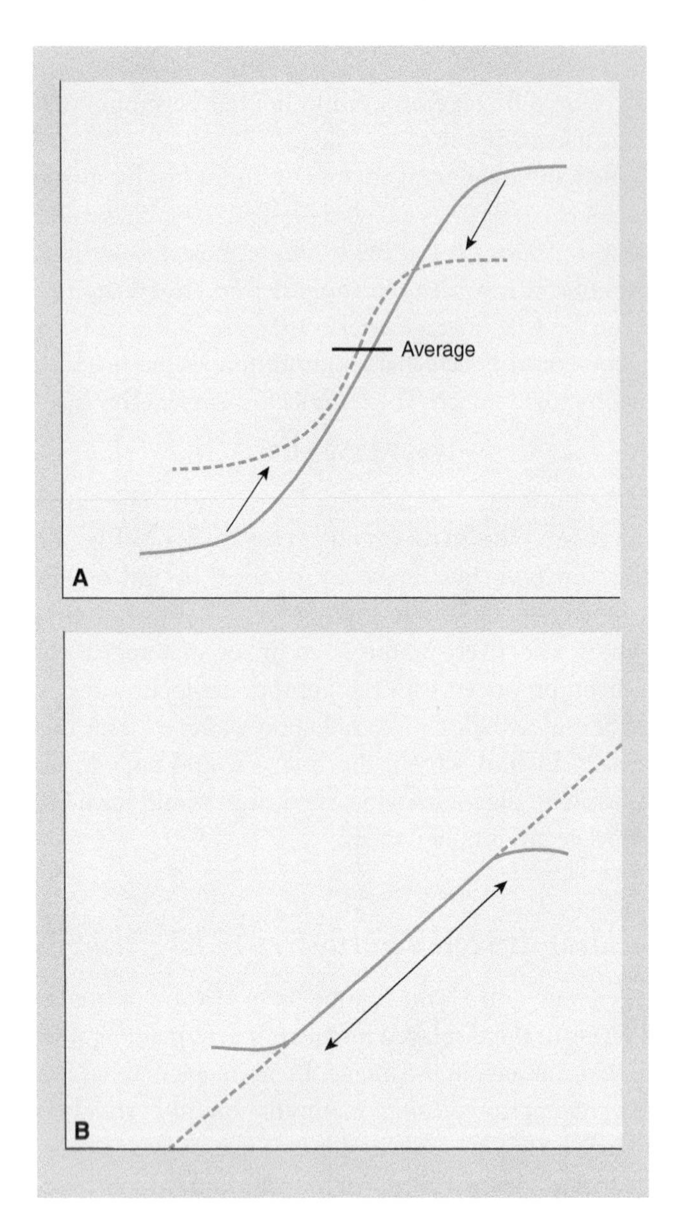

Figure 22.7. **Dynamic range compression. (A) The toe is demonstrated at the bottom of the range while the shoulder is at the top of the range. (B) Pixel values above the average pixel value are progressively compressed downward, while pixel values below are progressively compressed upward. The result is an equalization of tissue where the whole image can be lightened or darkened.**

value, effectively bringing the densities up to a darker level. The shoulder portion is progressively compressed downward toward the average pixel value, making the extremely dark areas lighter so that details can be seen.

The areas in the image that are white or pitch black do not add any diagnostic information to the image and are useless. Making the darker areas lighter can make those details visible. Recall that anatomical details that are absent from the image because of underpenetration of the x-ray beam can never be restored; the details are simply not there. On the opposite end, DRC is useful in bringing out anatomical details, which are hidden by excess density.

Postprocessing

Postprocessing includes all manipulation and adjustments of the digital image after corrections have been made in the preprocessing stage. These adjustments are aimed at refining and improving the appearance of the image. Although they may occur as part of the default processing of the image, they are subject to the personal preference of the person viewing the image.

Any digital image can be broken into individual components in two distinct ways. The first is breaking it into the spatial components or pixels, which are easy to understand. The second is the wave components or sine-wave functions, which are more difficult to understand. Think of an image as a collection of pixels or a collection of waves with different frequencies. Recall that particles in the electromagnetic spectrum also have a wave function. Waves are basically broken down into amplitude and frequency, the height and length of the wave, respectively. The pixels in each row have variable amounts of density based upon the attenuation of the x-ray beam. The density or gray level of each pixel becomes the amplitude or height of the sine waves, while the number of pixels is represented by the frequency of the sine wave.

When viewing a single row of pixels, one can assume that shorter waves represent smaller details in the image and longer waves represent larger details. In an image where extremely small details are represented, the sine wave will have very short wavelengths and very high frequencies. Mid-sized objects will have frequencies in the middle of the range. Very large objects will be represented by long wavelengths and low frequencies (Fig. 22.8).

What does all this mean? It means two broad approaches can be used for processing a digital image—the spatial domain and frequency domain. Processing operations can be performed with either spatial domain or frequency domain to achieve similar effects in the image. The choice is based upon comparing the efficiency of the two approaches in achieving the desired result. Let us consider the noise, which can degrade an image. The periodic noise caused by electronic malfunctions and occurs at regular intervals within the image is

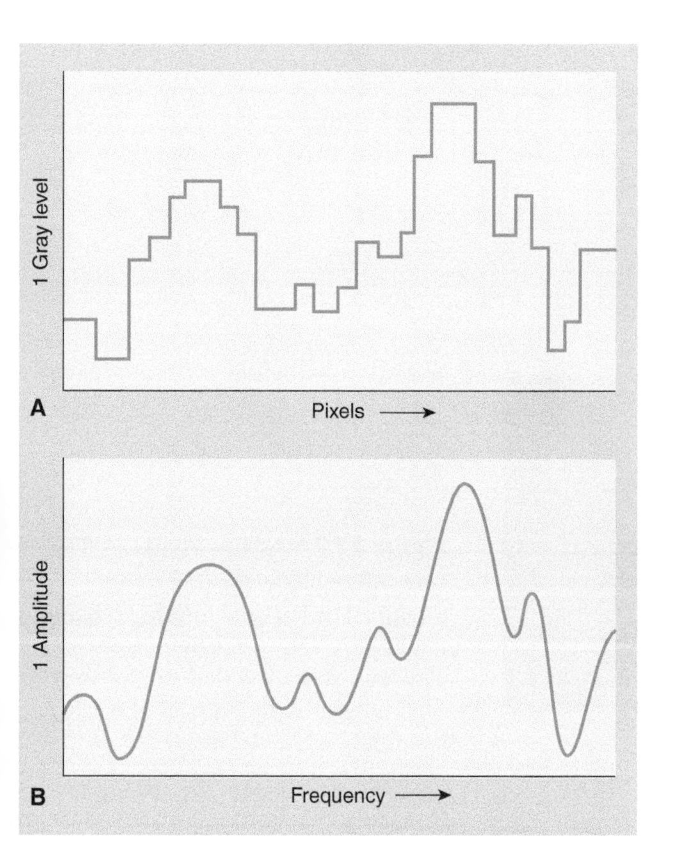

Figure 22.8. **Spatial and frequency components. (A) Graph representing the discrete density or gray level of each pixel in one row. (B) Using algorithms to average pixel density, a sine wave is formed to represent frequency.**

best reduced by using the frequency domain. The other type of noise, quantum mottle, occurs randomly and is best reduced by using the spatial domain.

Image Enhancement

Image enhancement is used to generate an image that is more pleasing to the observer. Image characteristics like contours and shapes can be enhanced to improve the overall quality of the image. Image enhancement includes the following: contrast, edge, spatial and frequency filtering, image combining, and noise reduction. Contrast enhancement (gradation processing) is used to optimize image contrast and density to enhance diagnostic interpretation. The pixels are normalized and rescaled using an LUT.

Windowing

The purpose of windowing is to make changes in the contrast and brightness of an image. A digital image is made up of numbers: window width is the range of numbers and window level is the center of the range. Window width controls contrast and window level controls brightness. A narrow window width provides an image with higher contrast or short scale. Conversely, a wide window width produces a lower contrast or long scale. When the window level is increased, the image will appear darker or less bright.

Edge Enhancement (High-Pass Filtering)

High-pass filtering is also known as edge enhancement; its purpose is to sharpen a blurred input image in the spatial domain. With this type of processing, algorithms adjust and control the sharpness or detail of an image by adjusting the frequency components of the image. This includes both high spatial frequency (detail information) and low spatial frequency (contrast information). **Spatial frequency** is a type of filtering that will affect the appearance of the edges of an image.

The Fourier Transform (FT) is a rigorous mathematical computation, which will not be covered in this text. The FT converts a function in the time domain to a function in frequency domain. The algorithm first identifies the **spatial location** of the image and converts it into spatial frequencies followed by a high-pass filter that suppresses the low spatial frequencies to produce a sharper output image.

Smoothing (Low-Pass Filtering)

Low-pass filtering is also called smoothing. The low-pass filter operates on the input image with a goal of smoothing. The output image will appear blurred. Smoothing is intended to decrease noise in the image as well as the displayed brightness levels of the pixels. An unfortunate consequence is that image detail is compromised.

Unsharp Masking

This type of spatial frequency processing uses the blurred image produced from low-pass filtering process. The computer system takes the blurred image and subtracts it from the original image to produce a sharp image. In this way, the original image that had the decreased noise levels can be sharpened. The result is an output image that is much improved compared to the original image (Fig. 22.9).

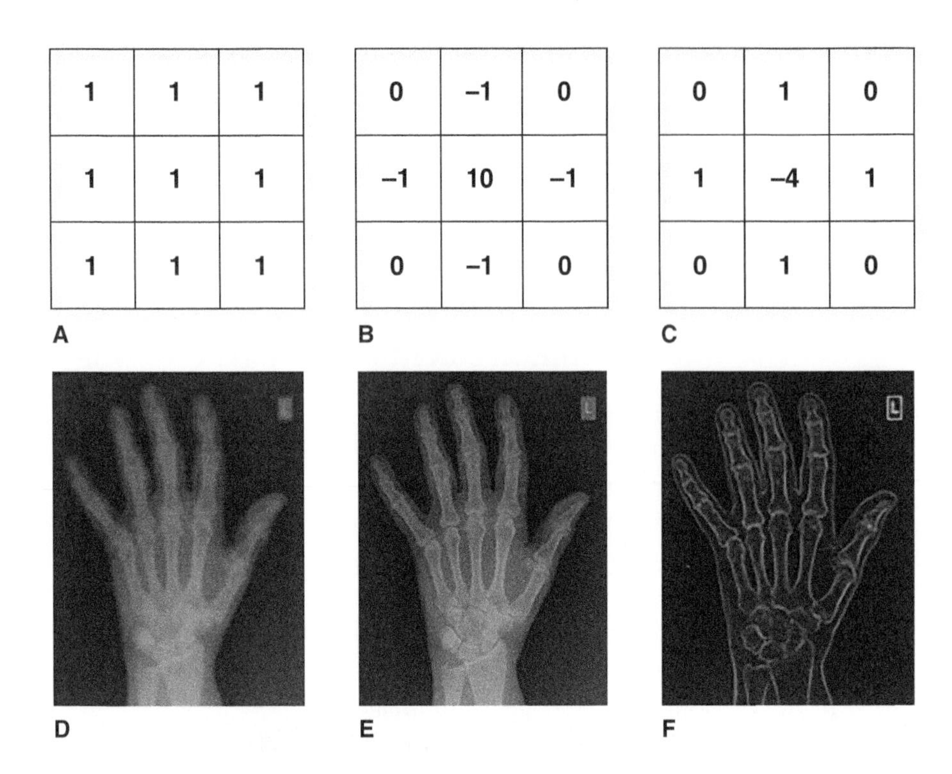

Figure 22.9. Unsharp masking. The computer system takes the image produced by low-pass filtering (D) and masks it over the original image (E). The large structures that are the same in each image will be subtracted resulting in a final high-detail image (F).

Operator Adjustments

One major disadvantage with film screen images is the lack of postprocessing capabilities; the final image could not be changed. Digital imaging has provided many opportunities for technologists to make operator adjustments to the image. The computer system has various icons on the display where the technologist can selectively choose the type of postprocessing adjustments, which is needed to improve the image. These adjustments include windowing for brightness and contrast, applying edge enhancement and other features to the image, adding annotations, magnifying areas of the image, and making global geometric changes such as translating the image right-to-left, rotating, or resizing the image.

Annotation is a very useful tool for adding text to an image. Depending upon the manufacturer, the image can be marked with a right or left along with the technologist's initials or number if the lead marker was not present in the image (Fig. 22.10). This capability has led to a common practice where technologists no longer use markers on an image. There is an ongoing debate of the legality of an image where the marker is not embedded in the image at the time of exposure. The best practice

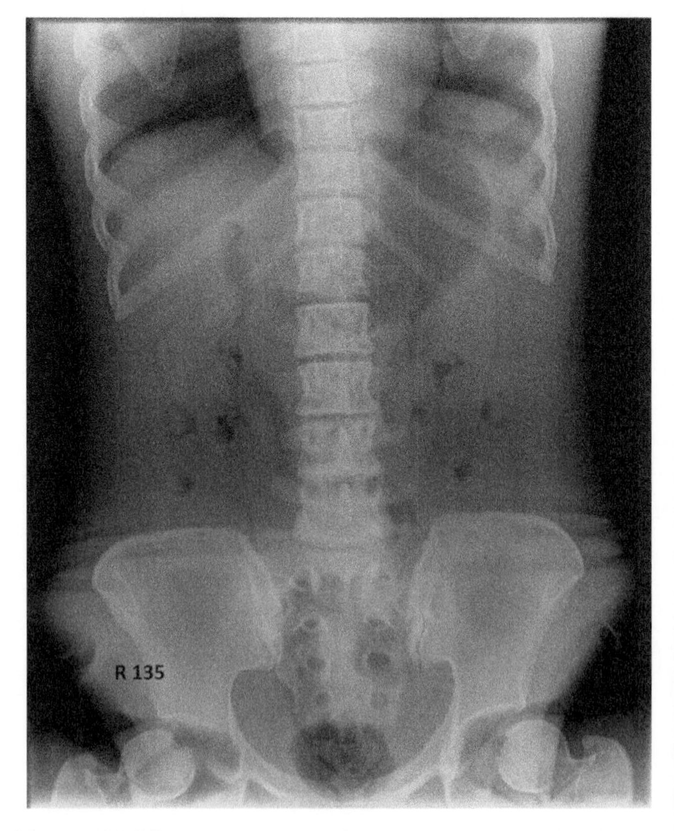

Figure 22.10. Annotation. The right marker (R) and technologist number (135) have been added to the image.

is to always use lead markers within the collimated light field. Adding text to an image, such as anatomy labels, is preferred by some physicians and can assist in their interpretation of the image.

Magnification is another useful tool of the digital system. When the radiologist or another physician sees an area of concern, the magnification tool can be used to magnify that ROI to make small details visible.

There are occasions where the image is not displayed in the correct orientation. Global changes can be made to flip the image right-to-left (horizontally) or top-to-bottom (vertically). These changes do not alter the appearance of the image aside from placing them in the standard viewing order.

Another global change is image inversion. This change is used to reverse black and white in the image; bone will be black and soft tissue white. Inversion is made possible by reversing the gradation curve where all the brightness values in the image are reversed. This inversion makes pathology more visible. Some physicians also prefer this type of orientation to assist in diagnosing areas of interest.

Digital image postprocessing involves a range of techniques that allow the user to change the appearance of the image displayed on the monitor. These techniques allow for enhanced images for improved viewing and interpretation. Image postprocessing is a common practice in the realm of digital imaging; technologists and radiologists are actively involved in using the various tools of image processing.

Chapter Summary

1. Preprocessing consists of corrections for errors in the acquisition of the input image, image analysis, and normalization.
2. Image analysis includes segmentation, exposure field recognition, histogram construction, and analysis.
3. When the correct exposure field is recognized, the proper type of LUT can be matched with the histogram for images that contain background densities, or a prosthesis or large bolus of barium, which might be confused with collimated borders.
4. Normalization is the initial gradient processing, which is designed to give the "raw" image brightness and contrast consistent with a conventional radiographic image.
5. Look-up tables are part of the computer memory and are specific for each type of anatomy. When these tables are applied to the original digital image, the position and shape of the acquired image histogram are aligned with those of the reference histogram (LUT) to produce an "ideal" output image.
6. Tissue equalization or dynamic range compression is used to adjust the brightness in an image. Darker areas can be lightened, while light areas can be darkened. An advantage of DRC is that it allows soft tissues to be better demonstrated while maintaining proper density for bone detail.
7. Operator-applied postprocessing includes detail processing, noise reduction, gradation process of the final display, adjustments in image appearance, and operator adjustments of annotation, etc.
8. The spatial domain operations are performed on pixels, while frequency operations are performed on particular structure sizes in the image.
9. High-pass filtering only leaves high frequency or small details in the image. Low-pass filtering leaves low frequency or large details in the image.
10. Unsharp masking is a process, which subtracts the low-pass–filtered image from the original input image to enhance the image details when performed in the spatial domain.

Case Study

A "raw" image of the pelvis demonstrated a long scale of contrast, which made it difficult to visualize the bony anatomy. Using the concept of rescaling the image contrast, answer the following questions.

Critical Thinking Questions

1. Which processing method will improve the contrast in the image?
2. How will DRC create a shorter gray scale?
3. What happens to the toe and shoulder portions of the gray scale curve?

Review Questions

Multiple Choice

1. **The term preprocessing best describes all the computer algorithms, which are designed to:**
   a. prepare the acquired data for entry into the computer system
   b. refine the characteristics of the image
   c. correct for errors and limitations in the image acquisition system
   d. prepare the image for display according to the parameters of the person viewing the image

2. **The expectation of segmentation software in all digital imaging systems is to recognize the:**
   a. difference between soft tissues and bone
   b. main lobe of the image histogram
   c. differences between bones and background densities within the field
   d. collimated borders on the x-ray field

3. **In a histogram graph of a digital image, the vertical height of a data point along the plotted curve indicates the:**
   a. number of pixels possessing the value
   b. S2
   c. image contrast
   d. S1
   e. pixel brightness

4. **__________ requires the greatest amount of preprocessing functions.**
   a. Conventional film screen radiography
   b. Direct digital radiography (DR)
   c. Computed radiography (CR)
   d. Digital fluoroscopy

5. **On an image histogram, an unusual spike to the right of the main bell-shaped lobe of the curve most likely represents:**
   a. bone pathology
   b. a large metallic object
   c. fog density
   d. air in the lungs
   e. background density

6. **When a large abdomen completely covers the image receptor plate, the expected shape of the original histogram will be:**
   a. a single spike to the right of the main lobe
   b. with a spike on either side of the main lobe
   c. no spikes will appear, only the main lobe
   d. a single spike to the left of the main lobe

7. **A main reason for the dynamic range to be much greater than the actual gray scale used in the image is to prevent data clipping when the:**

   a. image is compressed
   b. image is rescaled for brightness or contrast
   c. image is acquired
   d. histogram is constructed

8. **Periodic noise in an image that is caused by electronic malfunctions and occurs at regular intervals is best eliminated from the digital image by using:**

   a. processing in the frequency domain
   b. histogram analysis
   c. processing in the spatial domain
   d. gradation processing

9. **To display bone as black, which inverts all brightness values within the image, the gradation curve must be:**

   a. shifted to the right
   b. shifted under the *x* axis of the graph
   c. reversed
   d. shifted to the left of the *y* axis of the graph

10. **High-pass filtering only allows __________ to pass through processing to the output displayed image.**

   a. high frequencies
   b. low pixel values
   c. low frequencies
   d. high pixel values

Short Answer

1. **List the four general processes of preprocessing.**

2. **In unsharp masking, the creation of the "blurred" mask is a form of __________-pass filtering.**

3. **For histogram analysis, the desired lobe of the histogram is between S1 and S2. It is referred to as:**

4. **On a histogram, as we read from the left to right, the __________ of the pixels is changing from __________ to __________.**

5. **Describe the type of histogram analysis that is applied when a large area of lead shielding is expected within the field of view.**

6. **__________ results in conforming the shape of the acquired image histogram to the reference histogram.**

7. **Which is best suited for suppressing random noise like quantum mottle, spatial filtering, or frequency filtering?**

8. **A steeper gray scale curve on a displayed histogram indicates higher __________ in the image.**

9. **What is the visual effect of unsharp masking on a digital image?**

23

Digital Exposure Indicators

Objectives

Upon completion of this chapter, the student will be able to:

1. Explain the use of exposure indicators for digital imaging.
2. Differentiate between dose-area product and detective quantum efficiency.
3. Identify the role of kVp, mAs, and geometric factors for digital imaging.
4. Describe the various exposure indices based on manufacturer design.
5. List the myths and facts of digital exposure indicators.

Key Terms

- brightness
- detective quantum efficiency (DQE)
- dose-area product (DAP)
- exposure index
- inversely proportional scales
- logarithmic scales
- look-up table (LUT)
- proportional scales
- target (EI_T)

Introduction

In digital imaging, there are several concepts that must be understood for the radiographer to effectively and safely expose patients to radiation. Digital imaging has new terminology to explain the exposure to the image plate or image receptor as well as explain how efficiently the plate produces an image. The cassette-based digital systems use an exposure indicator value, which represents the exposure level to the photostimulable phosphor plate (PSP). The exposure indicator value can be confusing with the various types of exposure index numbers, which are specific to manufacturers. Fuji and Konica use sensitivity (S) numbers, and the value is inversely related to the exposure to the plate. CareStream uses exposure index (EI) numbers, and the value is directly related to the exposure to the plate. Philips has equipment, which uses either the S numbers or EI numbers. The concepts related to both types of exposure indicators will be presented. In this chapter, we discuss these concepts and dispel the myths that the foundational knowledge of film screen does not apply to the digital world.

Dose-Area Product (DAP)

Cassetteless systems use **dose-area product (DAP)** as the indicator for exposure. DAP is an actual measurement of patient dose that reflects the volume of tissue irradiated. It is an indication of total effect on or harm to a patient. Anytime an exposure is made, the radiographer must be aware of the potential harm to a patient's tissues. We know that an abdomen image delivers more dose to the patient than a hand image. The concept of DAP takes this into account and is determined by multiplying the dose by the field size.

$$\text{Patient A receives } 5\text{ mrad} \times 8'' \times 10'' = 5 \times 80\text{ inch}^2 = 450\text{ mrad} - \text{inch}^2$$

$$\text{Patient B receives } 5\text{ mrad} \times 10'' \times 12'' = 5 \times 120\text{ inch}^2 = 600\text{ mrad} - \text{inch}^2$$

Therefore, the DAP increases with increasing field size even if dose remains unchanged. It is easy to see that the total effect on or harm to the patient increases when a larger field size is used (Fig. 23.1). Using a smaller field size by collimating to include only the target anatomy will lower the DAP and therefore reduce the risk because a smaller amount of tissue is exposed.

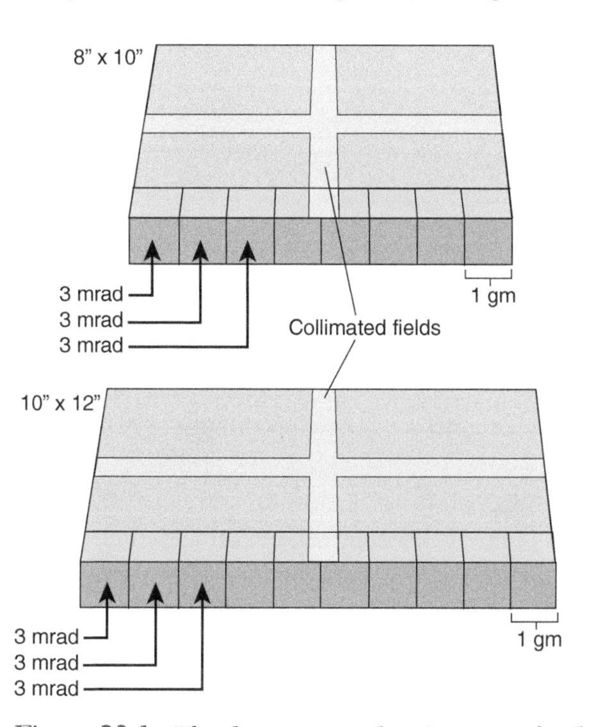

Figure 23.1. The dose-area product is greater for the larger IR even though the measured dose per gram of tissue is the same. DAP is a better indicator of biologic effect to irradiated tissues.

DAP may be used to monitor radiation output from radiographic and fluoroscopic units. A DAP meter is a radiolucent device that is placed near the x-ray source and embedded in the collimator before the beam enters the patient. The DAP meter is an excellent device to measure skin dose. The data collected from the DAP monitor help to implement radiation management procedures to keep patient exposures low.

Detective Quantum Efficiency (DQE)

Detective quantum efficiency (DQE) of the digital detector is a measurement of the overall efficiency with which the detector can convert the x-ray input signal into a useful output image. It is the expression of the exposure level that is required to produce an optimal image. Basically, it *predicts* patient dose. At the time an exposure is made, the x-ray beam must have sufficient energy to reach the image receptor. The probability the x-ray photons will interact with the IR is determined by the thickness and atomic composition of the capture layer. DQE is related to the absorption ability of the capture layer and the spatial frequency of the x-ray beam as it exits the patient.

Digital imaging uses barium fluorobromide (BaFBr), cesium iodide (CsI), and amorphous selenium (a-Se) in the detectors. Each has a high atomic number, which makes the detector more efficient at absorbing x-ray photons. It is also important to consider the K-shell binding energy; recall that most x-ray photons have energy that matches the K-shell binding energy. This directly relates to greater x-ray photon absorption at that specific energy. Table 23.1 presents the atomic number and K-shell binding energies for Barium fluorobromide, Cesium Iodide, and amorphous Selenium. The value of DQE for various systems is strongly dependent on x-ray energy, which means that fewer x-ray photons are required for higher DQE receptors to produce an image. Ultimately, this reduces the dose delivered to the patient.

TABLE 23.1 ATOMIC NUMBER AND K-SHELL BINDING ENERGY

Image Receptor	Capture Element	Atomic Number	K-Shell Binding Energy
Barium fluorobromide (BaFBr)	Barium (Ba)	56	37
Cesium iodide (CsI)	Cesium (Cs)	55	35
	Iodide (I)	53	33
Amorphous selenium (a-Se)	Selenium (Se)	34	12

As seen with digital receptors, higher DQE values result in higher-quality images and decreased patient dose. Amorphous selenium (a-Se) has high DQE because there is no light conversion step and consequently no light spread during the formation of the image. The importance of no light spread is that there is no light to blur the recorded signal output and a higher-quality image is produced. Consequently, a-Se delivers a lower dose compared to the other types of detectors.

When comparing computed radiography (CR), digital radiography (CR), and film screen, it is important to distinguish which method of capturing the image produces the higher DQE. DR has been shown to have the highest DQE and requires the fewest number of x-rays to produce an image. CR has the second highest DQE and is slightly higher than film screen. Film screen has the lowest DQE, which means it is the least efficient in creating an image. There is a point where the DQE is too high and very low dose is used; the result is an image with lots of mottle because of insufficient quantity of radiation reaching the image plate or image receptor. It is admirable to always be mindful of using the least amount of mAs for an exposure, but the tradeoff is the risk of repeating the image because of quantum mottle.

DQE Latitude

The linear and wide latitude of the input and output signal of digital systems lead to wider DQE latitude, which implies that a photostimulable phosphor has the ability to convert incoming x-rays into useful output signal over a much wider range of exposures. Although the DQE is higher in digital systems compared to film screen, no system can ever achieve a perfect DQE of 100%. As the DQE percentage increases, it indicates an increase in absorption efficiency with an optimal output signal. The DQE percentage depends on the x-ray beam uniformity, x-ray beam energy, latitude response of the system, sampling methods specific to the unit, quality of image display, and viewing conditions.

To determine the percentage of DQE, one must take the ratio of the SNR^2 output from the system to the SNR^2 input signal into the system. The formula for DQE percentage is:

$$DQE = \frac{SNR^2 \text{ out}}{SNR^2 \text{ in}}$$

where SNR^2 is the photons incident upon the system. The formula provides an excellent description of the dose efficiency of an x-ray detector system or how well the system converts SNR^2 incident on the detector into the SNR^2 in the image. The DQE compares the image noise of a detector to a "perfect" detector with the same signal response characteristics. This is a measure of how well the signal-to-noise ratio is preserved in the image. Remember that signal-to-noise ratio is used to describe how clearly a faint object appears in an image.

Exposure Index

All CR and DR images have been manipulated by the computer before a final image is displayed. Image-processing algorithms are used to compare measured histogram values (after exposure) with a predetermined value for the anatomy imaged. The measured histogram distribution on the image is used to determine the incident radiation exposure to the detector and to provide an **exposure index** value. Anatomically relevant areas in the image are segmented meaning areas where no patient attenuation is seen (high values) and collimated regions (low values) are excluded from the measurement. A histogram is generated from the relevant image area and is compared to an exam-specific (e.g., chest, abdomen, skull, etc.) histogram shape. Gray areas in the raw image are then digitally transformed using a **look-up table (LUT)** to provide desirable image contrast in the displayed image.

A median value is used to determine a proprietary exposure index (EI), which is dependent upon each manufacturer's algorithms and detector calibration method. EI indicates the amount of radiation reaching the detector and is not an indicator of dose to the patient, only an indication of exposure to the detector. There is a wide range of methods to calculate the EI of an image.

Because the final image is the result of computer algorithms upon the acquired raw data, neither the brightness nor contrast of the image can be entirely credited to the exposure factors used to produce the image. When a radiographer selects radiographic technique that is within the normal ranges, the only digital image quality that is directly affected by the set techniques is noise in the form of quantum mottle. The mottled appearance indicates the image was underexposed. With digital systems, nearly each image visually "turns out right," which makes it very difficult to tell if the correct techniques were set.

In order to prevent "dose creep," the radiographers must be motivated to carefully consider using techniques to reduce cumulative radiation exposure to the public. While patient exposure is generally considered an important issue in practice, the attitude of "out of sight, out of mind" is prevalent in the imaging field. The original goal for every image is to produce diagnostic high-quality images while keeping patient exposure to a minimum. This is such an important issue that various campaigns have been implemented to remind radiographers and students of the importance of reducing dose for all patients whether adult or pediatric.

Guidelines for CR and DR Technique

A set of guidelines for producing diagnostic images using either a CR or DR system include:

1. Insufficient techniques resulting in low EI numbers can cause unacceptable levels of mottle.
2. A high EI reflects unacceptable level of exposure to the IR/IP.
3. Achieving EI's in range; it is essential that high kVp and low mAs technique combinations be used. High kVp ensures adequate penetration of the anatomy and minimizes patient dose.

Each manufacturer uses a target median pixel value, which represents the "perfect" amount of x-ray exposure to the detectors. The target median pixel is located at the center point of the EI scale. After the exposure, the radiographer must review the EI number to determine whether the technique fell within acceptable range of exposure. **target (EI_T)** and range of acceptable EI's are all generally based upon the median pixel value in the image, determined by each manufacturer's particular method. There has been no standardization in how EI's are presented to radiographers, but committees are working on a solution to this important issue. For now, the radiographer must learn how to interpret the format for EI's for each piece of radiographic equipment in the facility.

Exposure Indicator Scales

Three broad approaches for exposure indicator scales are currently in use:

- Logarithmic scales
- Proportional scales
- Inversely proportional scales

One consistent factor for any logarithmic scale is that a 0.3 change or some multiple thereof represents a change in exposure by a factor of two. If EI goes up 0.3, it equates to a doubling in exposure, while an EI that goes down 0.3 means the exposure is halved. Table 23.2 provides a quick

TABLE 23.2 SUMMARY OF MANUFACTURERS AND EXPOSURE INDICATORS

Manufacturer	Exposure Indicator	Symbol
Agfa	Log of median	LgM
Alara CR	Exposure indicator value	EIV
Fuji	S value	S
General Electric	Detector exposure index	DEI
CareStream	Exposure index	EI
Konica	Sensitivity number	S
Philips	Exposure index	EI
Siemens	Exposure index	EXI

reference to the types of manufacturers and exposure indicators each uses.

Logarithmic Scales

CareStream use an exposure index that is abbreviated as EI. This EI is derived from an *average* pixel value in the area of interest. The formula is:

$$1{,}000 \times \log(\text{exposure in mR}) + 2{,}000$$

2,000 is the center of the scale that indicates 1 mR of exposure was received at the imaging plate using 80 kVp with 1.5 mm aluminum filtration and 0.5 mm copper of added filtration. Because it is a **logarithmic scale**, every change of 300 EI represents a change in actual exposure by a factor of 2, whether positive or negative. For example, an EI of 2,300 indicates twice the ideal exposure level and EI of 1,700 indicates one-half the ideal level.

Alara CR uses an EIV or exposure indicator value, which is nearly identical to CareStream. Alara CR uses a slightly different formula to determine the EIV:

$$\frac{1{,}000 \times \log(\text{SC} \times \text{mR})}{2}$$

where SC is the speed class the processor is operating at. After the anatomical region of interest on the image has been identified, the *mean* pixel value is calculated and converted to mR. Measurements are calibrated at 70 kVp with 21 mm aluminum filtration. As with the CareStream system, every change of 300 EIV correlates to a change by a factor of 2 in the actual exposure. The EIV target is 2,000 and a change in 300 either doubles of cuts exposure in half.

Agfa also uses an EI that is obtained from the central portion of the histogram. This is identified as the region of anatomical interest after eliminating the high and low spikes from background radiation and the collimated areas. The values from most pixels in the entire central portion are used to find the *median* value. Agfa uses the abbreviation LgM, which stands for log of median. The LgM is calibrated on exposure of 20 micro-Grays being received at the imaging plate using 75 kVp and 1.5 mm copper of added filtration. The range for LgM is 1.9 to 2.5 with 1.9 at the low end of the range for an acceptable image. The center of the scale is set at 2.2 LgM. Below 1.9, the image is considered to be underexposed while above 2.5 is overexposed. Because this is a logarithmic scale, a change of 0.3 will either increase or decrease exposure by a factor of 2. If an image is exposed and results in a 2.5 LgM, this indicates twice the ideal exposure was received. An LgM of 1.9 would then indicated one-half the exposure was received.

Proportional Scales

Siemens uses the exposure index abbreviated as EXI, which is independent of the anatomical menu selection made by the radiographer for processing and other processing parameters. The exposure field is divided into a 3 × 3 matrix, and the EXI is derived as an *average* pixel value in the center segment. The average pixel value is multiplied by a calibration factor while adjusting for 70 kV and 0.6 mm copper filtration to obtain an estimated exposure in micro-Gray units. One advantage of the **proportional scale** system is the read out is directly proportional to actual exposure to the patient. The micro-Gray is a standard unit of measurement for radiation dose.

General Electric new units use a detector exposure index or DEI, which has upper and lower limits that are determined by the user. The AEC is used to make exposures of acrylic phantoms to define the target pixel value range. After the anatomical area on the image is defined, the DEI is derived from the *median* anatomy value. The median of the pixel values in the raw image after preprocessing functions has been applied.

Inversely Proportional Scales

Fuji and Konica units use a scale called the sensitivity number (S number). Fuji was the first to use the S number to indicate exposure. The S number is taken from the image histogram after it has been normalized electronically. The center of the scale actually indicates the speed class at which the system is being operated to achieve an exposure of 1mR to the image plate using 80 kVp. CR and DR units using a 200 speed class have an S number of 200 that indicates proper exposure. **Inversely proportional scales** use a linear scale that is *inverted* relative to the actual exposure received by the image plate. For instance, when operating at 200 speed, an S number of 100 indicates that twice the amount of exposure was received. An S number of 400 indicates the exposure was one-half of the perfect exposure. High S numbers indicate the exposure factors were not sufficient enough to create the image, and there is a risk of image quantum mottle. The opposite is true for very low S numbers; these indicate an excessive patient exposure was received. The grossly overexposed image (S number 75) will still appear normal on the display monitor with the appropriate shades of gray.

Philips has designed newer units that derive an estimated x-ray exposure by averaging the original pixel values in one of two ways. First, using the areas of the activated detector cells of the AEC when it is activated and second from the central 25% area of the image called the "quarter field" when manual technique is used. The average is then adjusted according to the kVp used because this affects the sensitivity of the DR detectors. Using this method ensures the validity and accuracy of the EI are more reliable and consistent. The Philips EI readout uses rounded values (100, 125, 160, 200, and so on) in steps of ~25%. The 25% increment corresponds to scales conventionally used for film screen speeds and "exposure point" systems known to many radiographers. This scale is *inverted* to represent a relative speed class that would accommodate that exposure level in producing a medium optical density using conventional film screen. When compared to an EI 100, an exposure resulting in an EI 50 indicates two times the exposure was received by the patient.

Recommendations

It is easy to see why it can be very confusing to determine if an image was under- or overexposed with digital radiography. With film screen, one only had to hang the film on the view box to immediately determine if the film was under- or overexposed. Now with computer algorithms correcting for poor exposure, it can be very difficult to distinguish diagnostic from nondiagnostic images. In an effort to standardize exposure index numbers across manufacturers, the American Association of Physicists in Medicine task force #116 recommends a standardized EI be adopted by all manufactures. The task force stated "Different DR detectors require different technique factors due to differences in energy dependence of the detector materials in use. This inconsistency among DR systems may cause confusion and suboptimal image quality at sites where more than one type of system is in use. Operators need a clear set of rules based on the image receptor exposure provided and actively monitored by the system." The task force further recommended the exposure indicator be called the *Indicated Equivalent Air Kerma* (K_{IND}) to be expressed in units of micro-Gray. Requiring all manufacturers to use the same exposure indicator would provide a clear, straightforward indication of actual exposure. This practice would remove any arbitrary system that is difficult to remember.

The International Electrotechnical Commission (IEC) recommends an international standard for an exposure index for digital radiographic systems be developed. IEC 62494-1 describes "Exposure Indices" and "Deviation Indices" along with a method to place these values in the DICOM header of each radiographic image. Manufacturers would have the following responsibilities:

1. Calibrate detectors according to a detector-specific procedure.
2. Provide methods to segment pertinent anatomical information in relevant image region.
3. Generate an EI from the histogram data that is proportional to detector exposure.

The dose index standard would require target EI values for each digital radiographic system and for each procedure. A deviation index (DI) value of 0 (zero) would indicate correct exposure; a positive number would indicate overexposure, while a negative number would represent an underexposure. The DI range would then be −1 to +1 for all procedures. It is important to track values with respect to equipment, and the radiographer can be useful in maintaining high image quality for radiography at the facility.

Myths and Facts

Digital radiography has become common in radiography departments, and on the job training on the new equipment has occurred in a limited capacity when a new unit is installed. The limited information radiographers have received has created many myths regarding the differences between film screen and digital imaging. In this section, the myths and facts will be presented.

Myth #1

- mAs no longer controls density in the image.
- ***Fact***: mAs does not affect density but will affect IR exposure because mAs still represents the quantity of radiation in the beam.

In film screen, the film both captures the remnant radiation and after processing displays the image. With digital imaging, the capture and display are separate. Whether cassette-based or cassetteless, the detector captures the remnant beam and the computer monitor displays the image. The computer that displays the image adjusts density, which is now called **brightness**.

Myth #2

- mAs plays a prominent role in creating a digital image.
- *Fact*: Digital systems measure the exposure to the imaging plate or detector. The exposure is a combination of mAs and kVp; both are equally important to producing a diagnostic image.

Quantity of radiation represents patient dose and the amount of radiation available to form the image. Too little radiation results in excess noise or quantum mottle. Film screen images are also susceptible to quantum mottle when the optimum mAs has not been used. Sadly, a common practice has developed where excessive mAs is used to avoid repeat images. This practice has occurred because of the limited training and lack of understanding of the digital detectors. It is never acceptable to use excessive mAs for any reason because the practice is not based on sound logic. Furthermore, it is a violation of the ARRT and ASRT Code of Ethics and the ALARA principle.

Myth #3

- Digital systems must only have mAs adjusted to increase the amount of exposure to the image plate.
- *Fact*: Kilovoltage peak (kVp) can be used to adjust exposure to imaging plates or detectors.

Digital image receptors or image plates are sensitive to the overall amount of exposure that is received. IRs and IPs have a wider dynamic range and a linear response to exposure, meaning more shades of gray are displayed. The primary factor influencing contrast is the LUT; these are histograms of luminance values used as a reference to evaluate input intensities and assign predetermined grayscale values for the anatomical region selected.

Myth #4

- If the image has the correct appearance on the display monitor, then the exposure index doesn't need to be reviewed.
- *Fact*: A radiographer must always review the exposure index to determine if the exposure was correct.

A digital image should be viewed using two different perspectives: Review the image to determine if it has the proper appearance for the anatomy of interest. Review the exposure index to determine if the proper exposure was made.

The computer program rescales the image by adjusting the image to a predetermined image brightness. The image that is overexposed is rescaled lighter, and the underexposed image is rescaled to appear darker. The display computer presents a consistent and uniform image over a wide range of exposures.

Digital receptors can dramatically improve image quality and provide additional tools to make adjustments to the image, but sound physics and ethics still apply. While producing images, the radiographer must pay close attention to the EI values as indicators of patient exposure. It is not acceptable practice to send an underexposed image for interpretation; although the image appears normal on the display monitor, it may have signs of mottle or noise on the high-definition monitors the radiologists use to interpret the images. When the EI falls significantly under the range, the image must be repeated.

Myth #5

- Using high kVp must be avoided because there will be a longer scale of gray that may produce a less than diagnostic image.
- *Fact*: kVp can be increased one or two steps with a corresponding decrease in mAs; the image will not be degraded by this change.

A foundational principle has always been that kVp can be increased, within certain parameters, in an effort to reduce patient dose. By using the 15% rule, kVp can be increased and mAs lowered by one-half while still maintaining proper exposure to the image receptor. When kVp is changed by three steps or more with a further lowering of mAs, there will be a resultant lack of photons in the beam.

The importance of using optimum kVp is crucial with digital imaging. Optimum kVp must be used for adequate penetration of the anatomical part with sufficient mAs to create the image. Excessive kVp (more than two steps) will result in excessive scatter and loss of contrast, while insufficient mAs will increase noise in the image, which is seen as quantum mottle. Scatter control is more important in digital imaging because the receptors capture and record low-energy scattered photons and the image quality suffers.

The two primary ways to control scatter are the same for film screen and digital imaging: collimation and grid use. Precise collimation limits the area of exposed tissues, which reduces effective dose and the amount of scatter produced. Grids absorb scatter while allowing useful photons to pass through to the image receptor. In digital imaging, a fairly high-frequency grid is recommended.

Myth #6

- Radiographers should not to be concerned with geometric factors such as focal spot size, SID, and OID.
- ***Fact***: Geometric factors continue to be relevant in digital imaging as each is a cornerstone in producing a diagnostic image.

Geometric factors include small focal spot size results in a sharper image, OID must be minimized, and maximum SID must be used within reason. The importance of accurate positioning and proper part alignment with the AEC is critical whether using film screen or digital imaging. The computer algorithms cannot correct for poor positioning of the anatomical part.

Myth #7

- mAs must be increased to prevent repeating exposures because of quantum mottle.
- ***Fact***: The flawed logic of increasing mAs to prevent a repeat exposure because of quantum mottle has no basis. Because the digital receptors are sensitive to exposure, the radiographer can adjust kVp and lower mAs accordingly to prevent exposing the patient to unnecessary radiation.

Radiographers must review possible factors, which may cause histogram errors: exposure field recognition errors, collimation, excessive scatter, processing under the correct menu, and proper technical factor selection.

Finally, the radiographer must evaluate the image for proper positioning and tube-anatomic part-image receptor alignment. Many of these are foundational principles that are valid for film screen and digital imaging. The importance of all these factors does not change with the advent of new digital equipment.

Chapter Summary

1. In cassette-based systems, the exposure indicators must be monitored as a guide for optimal technical factor selection. Cassetteless systems use the DAP for the same purpose.
2. DQE is a measure of the overall efficiency with which the detector can convert the x-ray input signal into a useful output image. It is the expression of the exposure level that is required to produce an optimal image.
3. In digital systems, mAs no longer controls density. The display computer fulfills this role, and density is now called brightness. mAs is still important because it still determines the quantity of radiation exposure to the patient and the amount of radiation available to produce the image.
4. Optimum mAs should be selected to provide a sufficient number of photons in the x-ray beam and to avoid quantum mottle.

5. Contrast is still influenced by kVp, but digital systems have a much wider dynamic range, which means they can display a much wider range of gray scale. kVp can be increased by 15% and mAs decreased by one-half to maintain contrast in the image while minimizing patient radiation dose. Optimum kVp must still be selected for the anatomical part to be imaged to ensure adequate penetration of the part.
6. Excessive kVp results in the production of excess scatter radiation, which will result in a loss of contrast and degradation of the image.
7. Geometric factors of OID, SID, and focal spot size along with proper alignment of the tube-part-image receptor affect digital imaging in the same manner as for film screen imaging.
8. There is no standardized method in digital imaging for exposure indices. Each manufacturer has their proprietary method for determining the exposure index for their equipment.

Case Study

Tomi's department is wanting to buy a new x-ray unit for the department. She has been tasked with researching the unit made by Philips. Tomi is to locate specific information about this digital system and share it with her supervisor.

Critical Thinking Questions

1. Does the system use an inverted or logarithmic scale?
2. What type of exposure indicator is used?
3. How does the system determine the EI value?

Review Questions

Multiple Choice

1. **In digital imaging, a strict lower limit for exposure to the image receptor is imposed by:**
   a. the appearance of quantum mottle
   b. images appearing too light
   c. the appearance of additional fog density
   d. image with excessive contrast

2. **Quantum mottle is more likely to appear in the digital image when the:**
   a. density is low
   b. brightness is low
   c. contrast is low
   d. exposure indicator is low

3. **The acceptable range of exposures for the Agfa system is:**
   a. 100 to 400
   b. 50 to 230
   c. 1.9 to 2.5
   d. 1,700 to 2,300

4. **The manufacturer that uses the S number to adjust brightness in the image is:**
   a. Fuji
   b. Kodak
   c. General Electric
   d. Agfa

5. A high original S number indicates __________ for systems that use an inverted scale for the exposure index.

   a. too high displayed brightness
   b. too low original exposure
   c. too high original exposure
   d. too low displayed brightness

6. Quantum mottle in a CR or DR image can result from:

   a. improperly calibrated AEC
   b. insufficient kVp
   c. insufficient mAs
   d. none of the above
   e. all of the above

7. __________ is the manufacturer that uses *exposure index* to refer to its exposure indicator.

   a. Fuji
   b. Agfa
   c. Kodak
   d. Philips

8. Which of the following measures the efficiency of a system to convert the x-ray input signal into a useful output signal?

   a. MTF
   b. DQE
   c. Exposure latitude
   d. Spatial resolution

9. __________ is the actual measurement of patient dose that reflects the volume of tissue irradiated.

   a. DAP
   b. DQE latitude
   c. EI
   d. EIV

10. The CareStream system uses 2,000 EI as the ideal exposure. What does it mean when an image has a 2,300 EI?

   a. One-half exposure was used
   b. Triple amount of exposure was used
   c. One-fourth the exposure was used
   d. Two times the exposure was used

Short Answer

1. The measure of an imaging detector's overall efficiency, expressed as a ratio for the SNR output over the SNR input, is called its:

2. For digital images, the only indication the radiographer has that the technical factors used to produce an image have resulted in an overexposure is the __________.

3. For a logarithmic scaled exposure indicator, if the EI reads 0.3 or a multiple thereof below the target value, the actual exposure to the detectors was what ratio of the target exposure level?

4. The AAMP task force #116 recommends what general unit be used as a standardized unit for all exposure indicators?

5. Which manufacturer refers to its exposure indicator as the *log median value*?

6. What is the formula for determining DQE percentage?

7. Explain how the 15% rule can be used for digital imaging.

8. Which manufacturer uses rounded numbers for their exposure indicators?

24

Digital Image Evaluation

Objectives

Upon completion of this chapter, the student will be able to:

1. List the seven criteria for producing quality images.
2. Discuss noise in an image and how it is created.
3. Identify methods for improving the signal-to-noise ratio in an image.
4. Evaluate an image for noise.
5. Discuss the Moire artifact and aliasing.
6. Discuss the importance of using grids to improve signal-to-noise ratio.
7. Identify common errors in positioning and tube/Bucky alignment.

Key Terms

- aliasing
- Moire artifact
- signal-to-noise ratio

Introduction

The advancements in digital technology have brought the medical imaging field a long way away from the traditional film screen imaging. The many concepts of film screen imaging are just as relevant today as they have been over the past few decades. In this chapter, we will discuss the importance of critically evaluating the digital image.

Digital Image Qualities

The qualities we seek in a digital image should be consistent with producing a diagnostic quality image. As students have already learned, there are many facets to consider from pixel/matrix size, the brightness and contrast in an image to selecting the appropriate kVp and mAs for the anatomical area to be imaged.

Seven Criteria

There are seven criteria, which are essential in the production of a quality image.

1. Pixel brightness: All pixel brightness levels should have an intermediate level of gray ranging from very light gray to very dark gray. The brightness levels may need to be adjusted to achieve the best level of brightness.
2. Image contrast: Image contrast should be balanced with the gray scale to improve visualization of all anatomical tissues in the image. This will result in maximum visualization of detail within the image. Contrast or gray scale may be adjusted to strike the correct balance.
3. kVp: Sufficient kVp must be used to ensure proper penetration of the signal through the patient to the detector. High kVp techniques ensure proper penetration while allowing a lower mAs technique; this saves radiation dose to the patient. High kVp techniques also ensure sufficient signal-to-noise ratio (SNR) resulting in a displayed image with no evidence of mottle or electronic noise.
4. Spatial resolution: Maximum spatial resolution or sharpness must be apparent in the digital image. To maximize sharpness, the resolution should be 8 lp/mm. The geometric factors utilized in film screen radiography are just as relevant for digital imaging. The horizontal and vertical resolution capabilities of the display monitor will also affect the spatial resolution when the image is viewed.
5. Artifacts: To the extent possible, all artifacts must be absent from an image. This includes all removable objects such as jewelry, IV lines, oxygen tubes, etc. (Fig. 24.1). Other items that can be considered artifacts include anatomical structures that are superimposed over the area of interest or electronic noise.

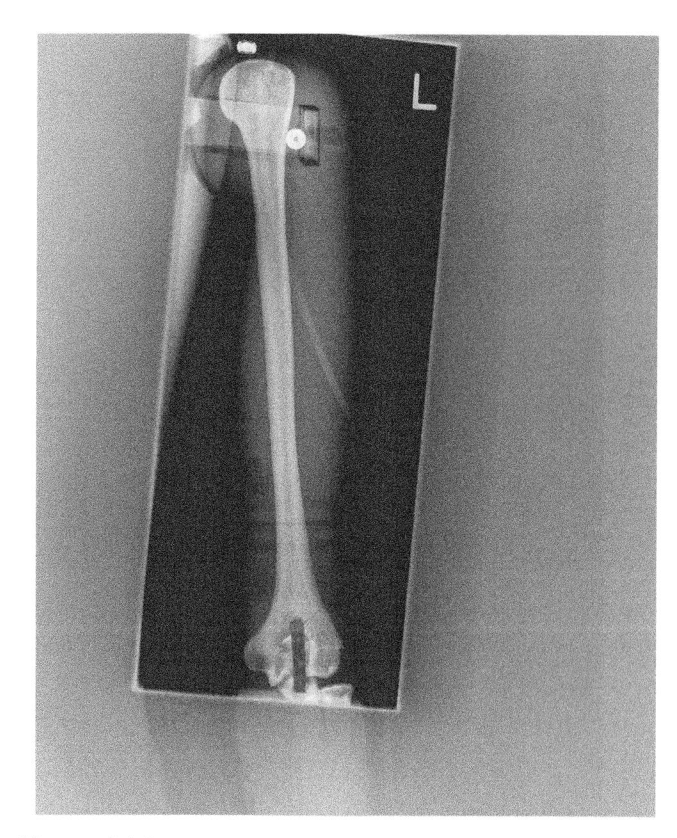

Figure 24.1. **IV line and snap artifacts in humerus image. Collimated field is not properly centered in the IR.**

6. Shape distortion: The accurate representation of the anatomical region must be free of shape distortion. If this is not possible, then shape distortion should be minimized when possible.
7. Size distortion: Size distortion or magnification of the digital image is affected by the display screen size. Magnification has its benefits, but when the image becomes very pixelated, where individual pixels can be seen, the sharpness of the edges in the image is lost.

Demonstrating Anatomical Structures

By now, we all know the primary goal of producing an image is to accurately demonstrate the anatomical region of interest. There are many imaging criteria to follow based on the projection and position of the body part. We will not have an exhaustive discussion of positioning as that is outside the realm of this text; however, it is relevant to at least briefly discuss it in relation to digital imaging.

Proper Positioning

Proper positioning begins with following protocols for projections necessary to adequately image the part of interest. The central ray location is incredibly important for any type of imaging. When the central ray is off centered in either direction, the anatomy is not in the middle of the image. Figure 24.2 demonstrates excessive density where the beam was not attenuated by the tissue. The computer algorithms will include the density in determining the exposure indicator. Additionally, there is a lack of collimation to the part because of the off-centering.

Tube and Bucky Alignment

A common error occurs when the overhead tube is not in detent position. As seen in Figure 24.3, there is a dark strip where the x-ray beam stopped. Also seen is the humeral head, which is only partially seen, had the tube been aligned in detent position, the entire humeral head would have been demonstrated. When the tube is positioned closer to the technologist, the dark strip will be on the patient's left side as seen in Figure 24.3.

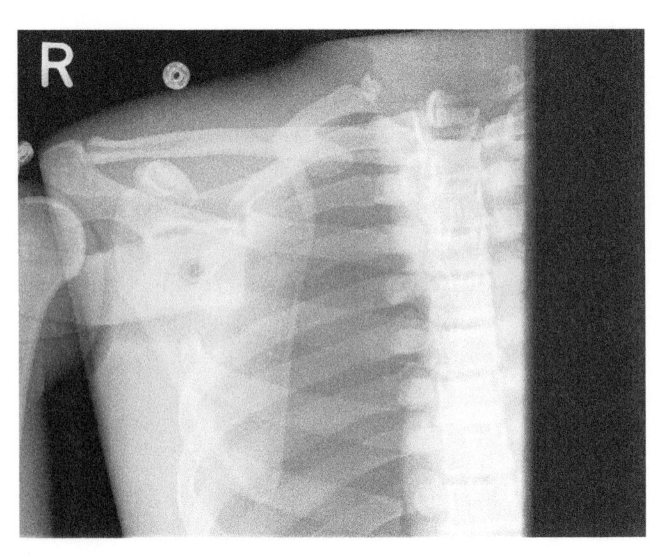

Figure 24.3. Common error where the overhead x-ray tube is not locked in detent to the table.

Figure 24.4 illustrates the importance of pushing the table Bucky completely into position. The x-ray tube was

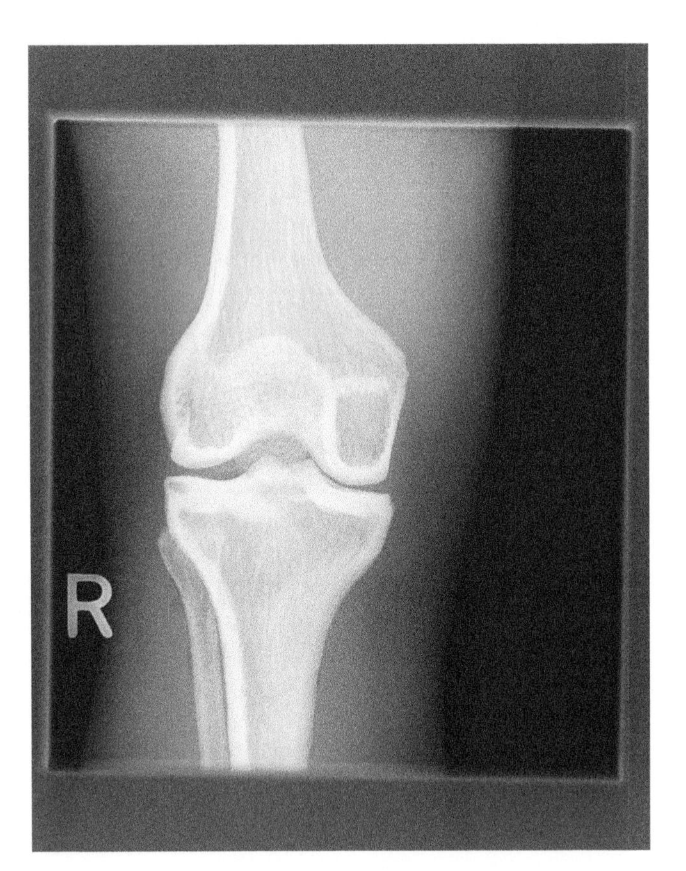

Figure 24.2. The central ray location is not centered on the bone. Computer algorithms will identify the excess density and use it to determine the exposure index.

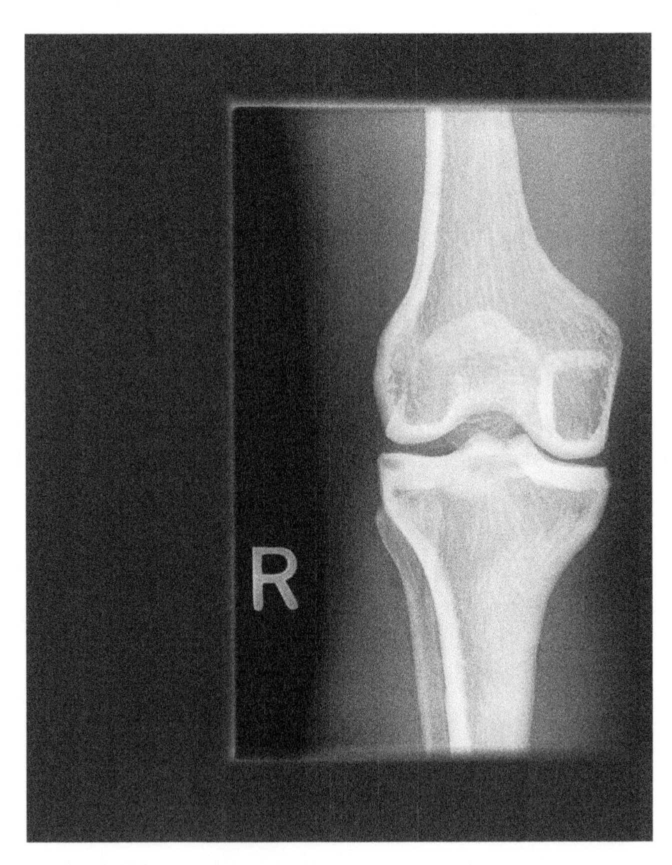

Figure 24.4. Table Bucky was not pushed in all the way. Resulted in the collimated field being projected to one side of the IR with a large area of density on the opposite side.

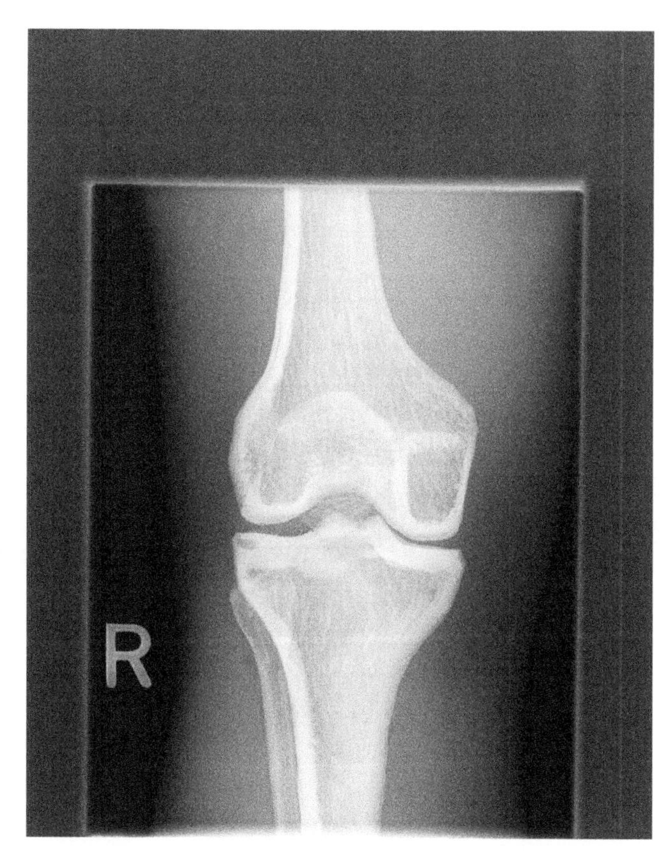

Figure 24.5. **The center of the x-ray beam was not correctly aligned with the IR. Resulted in an area of density with the collimated field toward the opposite end of the IR.**

locked in detent and the anatomy properly centered. The dark strip on the image detracts visually from the overall appearance of the image. More importantly, the additional density was used in determining the exposure index.

A final error with tube and Bucky alignment is seen when the Bucky center is not aligned with the center of the x-ray tube. The Bucky can be either toward the patient's head or feet. As seen in Figure 24.5, the wide strip of density is seen at the top of the image, which is seen when the Bucky is aligned toward the patient's feet. The anatomy is properly centered left to right with appropriate amount of collimation.

Each of these examples included an image that would be considered diagnostic with the exception of the shoulder image. The LgM for each image was within the range of 1.9 to 2.5. Although each image was diagnostic, there is something to be said for taking a bit of time to make sure all the components of the equipment is properly aligned so that the areas of density around the image are equal.

Mobile x-ray images are particularly challenging as it can be difficult to align the x-ray beam perpendicular to

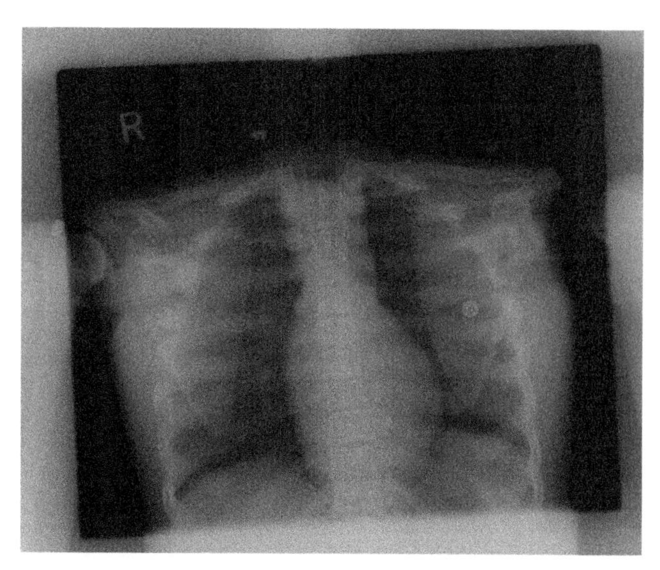

Figure 24.6. **Mobile x-ray image demonstrating common positioning errors. The collimated field is not perfectly parallel with the IR, and an artifact is seen in the lung field.**

the grid as seen in Figure 24.6. The light field was aligned with the chest anatomy; however, the grid was not placed in the same orientation. This image is also too dark for the lung field, and the clavicles are projected too far cephalic. A repeat image is in order to correct the errors in the image; this results in additional exposure to the patient.

Digital Image Noise

All electronic components in a digital imaging system are associated with the movement of electrons through the system; this results in electronic noise. This type of artifact is a random disturbance that obscures or reduces clarity in the image. The image will have a grainy or mottled appearance. Electronic noise produces regions of brightness that appear as "snow" on the displayed image. The snow-like appearance is seen on a TV monitor when there is a lack of signal strength. Another example is the static heard in a sound system when a radio station is not properly tuned in.

Electronic noise doesn't contribute to the image but only manages to degrade the image. If high noise levels are present in the system, they can significantly compromise the image details. Digital systems are very sensitive, which makes them extremely susceptible to all types of image noise.

Signal-to-Noise Ratio

Signal-to-noise ratio or SNR is a standard method used to express noise in comparison to signal strength. In electronic imaging systems, the signal strength is directly related to a given signal strength. The number of photons that strike the image receptor is considered the "signal" (mAs). High SNR is desirable in imaging because the signal is greater than the noise, which improves visualization of the low-contrast soft tissue structures. Low SNR is not desirable because a low signal accompanied by high noise obscures soft tissue detail and creates the mottled appearance.

Although high SNR is favorable, technologists must ensure the proper technical factors are used for the projection and must avoid exceeding recommended mAs so as not to overexpose the patient. As previously discussed in this text, overexposed images are not readily evident with digital processing and display. It is important to check the exposure index for each exposure to determine if the correct exposure index was reached.

When insufficient mAs (signal) is used for a projection, the image receptor will not receive the appropriate number of photons, which results in low SNR or a noisy image. The mottle may not be visible on the low-resolution monitors in the work station, but the exposure index should indicate if the exposure was in range or below the range. When noise is clearly visible on the image, the technologist should have it reviewed by a radiologist to determine if the image needs to be repeated. An SNR of 500:1 is considered acceptable for digital fluoroscopy, but CRT monitors used with digital systems require an SNR of 1,000:1.

Aliasing or Moire Artifact

Aliasing or the **Moire artifact** is seen in images when the sampling rate in line pairs per millimeter is the same as the line resolution of the image plate (lp/mm). Essentially, the two frequencies overlap. Another problem occurs when the line resolution is a multiple of the sampling frequency. When the plate resolution is 8 lp/mm and the sampling frequency is 4 lp/mm, pixel sampling will not be adequate and will result in every other line being missed.

The Moire artifacts are also caused by grids. The importance of using grids for body parts measuring 10 cm or more was discussed in Chapter 15. As a reminder, the purpose of a grid in digital imaging is to improve the SNR for the image data fed into the computer. When higher-quality data are available from the start, the chances of processing errors are reduced.

In CR imaging, the Moire or aliasing artifact is due to the Nyquist frequency, the sampling frequency at which the CR plate is scanned line by line with the laser beam. Short dimension or SD grids have grid lines running crosswise to allow for vertical off-centering when a horizontal beam is used for cross-table projections. When a short dimension grid is used with the grid lines running parallel to the scan direction of the reader and when the grid frequency closely matches the Nyquist frequency, the artifact will be created. This type of artifact is more common with stationary grids, the type of grid used for mobile x-ray imaging (Fig. 24.7).

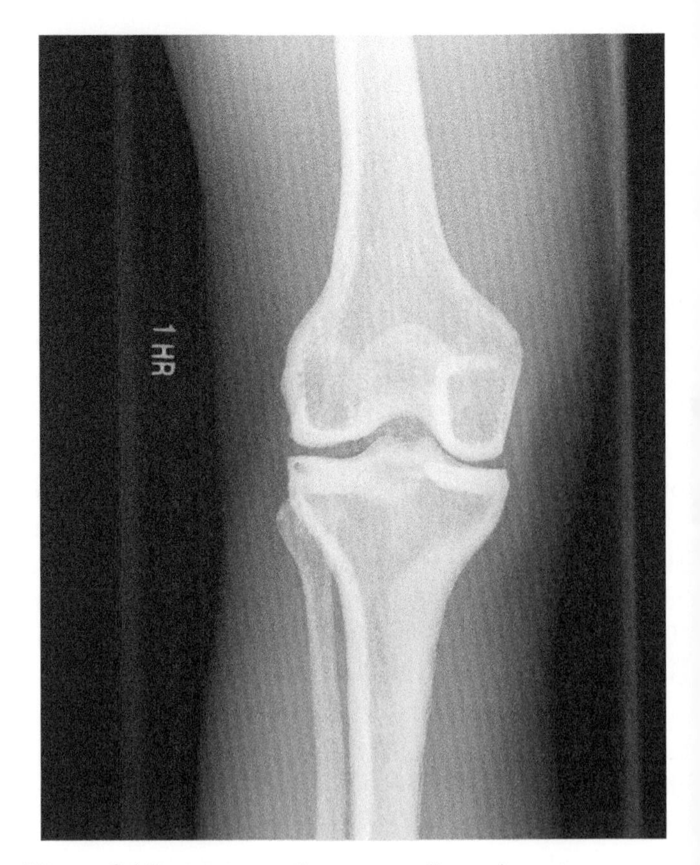

Figure 24.7. Moire artifact seen as lines obscuring anatomy.

Chapter Summary

1. Diagnostic images comprise an intermediate level of gray, ranging from very light gray to very dark gray.
2. Visualization is improved when the gray scale in the image is properly balanced.
3. Sufficient kVp must be used to ensure adequate penetration of the anatomical part.
4. Spatial resolution or sharpness must be maximized in all digital images. Geometric factors utilized in film screen are still relevant in digital imaging.
5. All removable artifacts must be identified and removed from the light field area so they do not obscure any anatomy.
6. Shape distortion should be kept to a minimum to most accurately represent the part of interest.
7. The display screen can affect the size distortion and magnification of an image.
8. When the sampling rate in lp/mm is the same as the line resolution in the image plate in lp/mm, the Moire artifact or effect is seen. The Moire artifact or aliasing also occurs when the line resolution is a multiple of the sampling frequency.
9. In CR imaging, the Moire artifact is caused by the Nyquist frequency.
10. Short dimension grids have grid lines, which run crosswise to allow for vertical off-centering. When a short dimension grid is used with horizontal beam imaging, the grid lines run parallel to the scan direction of the reader. If the Nyquist frequency matches the parallel grid lines, the Moire artifact will occur.
11. Centering the x-ray tube to the anatomy of interest produces an equal distribution of anatomy on the image plate.
12. Off-centering, poor tube and Bucky alignment, and a tube not locked in detent will create an area of excessive density on the image. The excess density is processed as part of the exposure indicator and has the possibility of creating an image with a long gray scale.

Case Study

Using Figure 24.1, critically evaluate the image for proper positioning and tube/Bucky alignment. Answer the following questions based on your critique.

Critical Thinking Questions

1. Is the humerus centered in the imaging plate?
2. Are there identifiable artifacts, which could be removed?
3. What changes would be made for the repeat image?

Review Questions

Multiple Choice

1. **To obtain maximum visualization of detail, it is necessary to have a balanced gray scale within the image.**

   a. True
   b. False

2. **Where would the x-ray field be located if the x-ray tube is not locked in the detent position over the table with the tube closest to the technologist?**

   a. At the top of the image
   b. On the right side of the image
   c. Toward the bottom of the image
   d. On the left side of the image

3. **Which technical factor setting ensures proper penetration of the anatomical part?**

   a. High mAs
   b. Low kVp
   c. High kVp
   d. Low mAs

4. **A "snow"-like appearance on the digital image means that:**

   a. a sufficient amount of kVp was used.
   b. electronic noise is evident in the image.
   c. the image has high signal-to-noise ratio.
   d. an aliasing artifact is present.

5. **Why is a low signal-to-noise ratio not preferred?**

   a. Because it is accompanied by high noise levels, which obscure soft tissue detail
   b. The low SNR demonstrates a balanced level of gray scale in the image.
   c. It will result in a Moire artifact.

6. **The SNR for a digital fluoroscopy display screen is:**

   a. 300:1
   b. 500:1
   c. 1,000:1
   d. 250:1

7. **The Moire artifact is caused when the ______ rate in lp/mm is the same as the line resolution of the image plate.**

   a. reading
   b. sampling
   c. scanning

Short Answer

1. **Explain the importance of size distortion in a digital image.**

2. **Why is it important to remove any nonpermanent artifacts from the anatomical area prior to imaging?**

3. **Where does electronic noise come from?**

4. **Describe what high SNR is and why it is desirable.**

5. **What is the Nyquist frequency?**

25

Digital Image Display

Objectives

Upon completion of this chapter, the student will be able to:

1. Distinguish differences between the CRT and AMLCD.
2. Identify the components of the cathode ray tube.
3. Explain how the raster pattern functions to produce an image.
4. Describe how the electron stream is shaped.
5. Differentiate between reflective and veiling glare.
6. Explain the construction of the liquid crystal diodes.
7. Discuss the features of an active matrix liquid crystal display.

Key Terms

- active matrix liquid crystal display
- cathode ray tube
- liquid crystal diode
- raster pattern
- refresh time
- response time

Introduction

Nearly all radiographic images are displayed electronically. Image display systems are used for viewing the images at control consoles of most x-ray units and also at all computer terminals. It is necessary for radiographers to have a base familiarity with electronic display systems and how each works. Types of display monitors include the cathode ray tube (CRT) and liquid crystal display.

Cathode Ray Tube

A conventional TV screen or monitor is easily recognized because of its front to back depth. The depth is needed because the monitor has an electron gun, which projects a thin stream of electrons onto the back of the fluorescent screen. Roentgen was experimenting with a CRT, which directed a stream of electrons across a vacuum tube toward a positively charged anode. The rays that were emitted from the cathode to the anode were called cathode rays. The name caught on and even today the TV tube is referred to as a **cathode ray tube** or CRT.

The CRT is one type of monitor used to display the digital image. It consists of a vacuum tube, an electron gun (cathode) with focusing and accelerating grids, and a deflecting coil for steering the electron beam (Fig. 25.1). It has an anode assembly with a coating of fluorescent phosphor crystals on the inside of the front screen. When the phosphor crystals are struck by the electron stream, they will glow. The crystals have a linear shape and are aligned perpendicular to the glass support; this configuration minimizes lateral light dispersion. On the back of the phosphor layer is a very thin layer of aluminum, which the electrons can penetrate; the aluminum also forms a reflective backing for the light from the phosphor layer.

The electron gun emits a stream of electrons, which must go through three modifications to control the shape, direction, and quality of the electron stream.

- Modification #1: The control grid attached to the electron gun modulates the intensity up and down over 1 million times per second. This modulation of intensity will ultimately determine the brightness with which the phosphors will glow when struck by the electron stream.
- Modification #2: The focusing and accelerating grids use negative repulsion to keep the electrons in a very tight, narrow beam.
- Modification #3: The electron stream passes through a deflection coil, which uses alternating degrees of charge to steer the stream in a pattern of lines indexing across the phosphor surface.

The electron gun, control grid, and focusing and accelerating grids are located inside the neck of the glass envelope while the deflecting coils are outside the CRT, surrounding the neck of the glass envelope. The electron beam scans across the phosphor screen in a left to right manner with a slight diagonal angle called a **raster pattern** (Fig. 25.2). The scan begins in the upper left corner and moves to the upper right corner. This single line is called an active trace meaning the phosphor crystals are activated to varying degrees of brightness. The beam turns off as it indexes or returns to the start of the third line, this is called the horizontal retrace. The beam makes an active trace on the third line and continues in a series to scan all the odd lines until it reaches the bottom of the screen. The beam then retraces vertically to the top of the screen and begins at line number two and all the even lines are scanned in the raster pattern. Each scan from the top to bottom of the screen is called a television field and each pair of interlaced fields produces one frame image.

Units using 60 Hz electrical current will have 60 fields scanned per second, which translates to 30 frames per second. The human eye requires a frame rate of at least

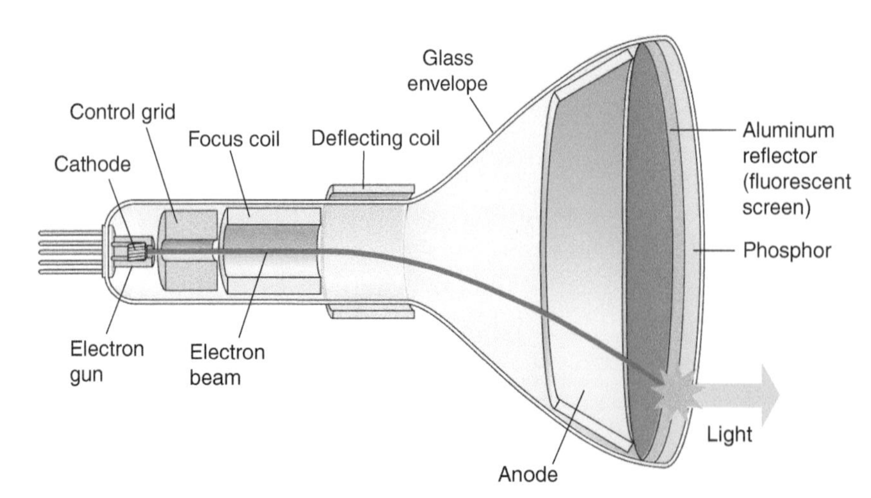

Figure 25.1. **CRT and its components.**

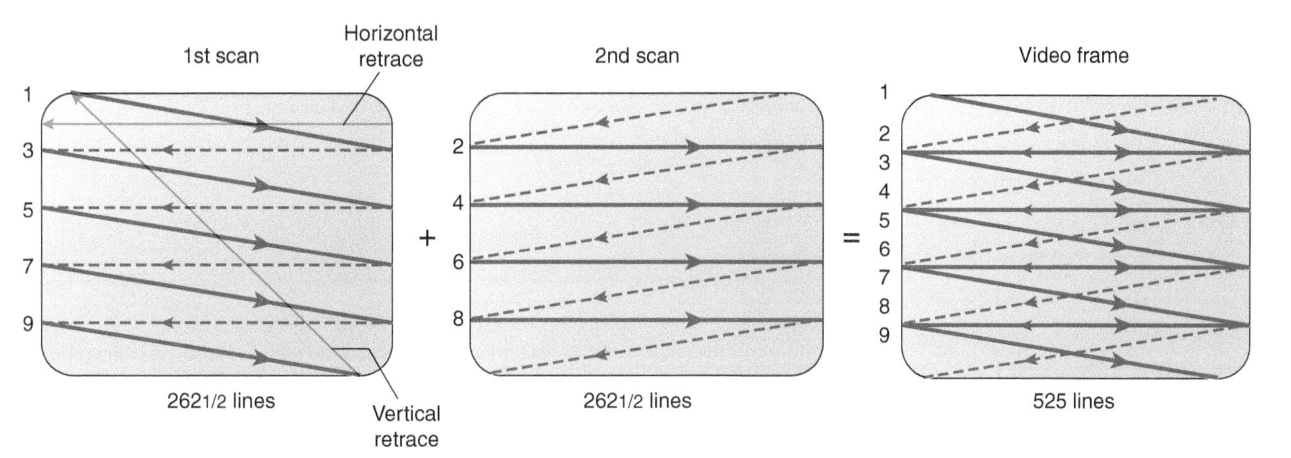

Figure 25.2. **A video frame raster scan pattern. The electron beam scans the diagonal lines as active traces and the horizontal lines as inactive traces. The horizontal lines set up the position of the electron beam for the next scan. The electron beam scans 262½ odd number lines until it reaches the bottom of the screen where one complete television field is seen. To prepare for the next television field, the screen is vertically retraced from bottom right to top left at which point the raster pattern scan takes place again. The set of 262½ even number lines are scanned. The two scans are interlaced together to provide the 525 active trace line or raster pattern.**

20 frames per second to avoid the appearance of flicker. Although old movies may be fun to watch, the image flashes rapidly because the frame rate was lower than 20 frames per second. In modern TV monitors, the light from the activated phosphor crystals in the screen quickly fades, but it is refreshed every 33 ms, which appears as a seamless image to the human eye.

Vertical Resolution

The number of lines in the raster pattern controls the vertical resolution of the CRT. Standard TV screens have a raster pattern that consists of 525 active trace lines, which produces a spatial resolution of <2 LP/mm. Newer CRTs are available with up to 2,000 active lines resulting in a resolution of up to ~8 LP/mm.

Horizontal Resolution

The horizontal resolution is determined by the number of times the electron stream can be modulated, which is changing the magnitude of a video signal. Recall the electron stream is refreshed every 33 ms. This is stated as a frequency, modulations per second, and is expressed in units of Megahertz (MHz). The frequency modulations, called bandpass, directly determine the number of bits of information, which can be stored on each line in the raster pattern. Therefore, the bandpass determines the number of bits in the frame, which is a measurement of image resolution, similar to the number of pixels in each line in an image matrix.

The majority of standard broadcast TVs operate at a bandpass of 4.5 MHz, which is far below the requirement for digital imaging applications. Fluoroscopy requires a bandpass of 20 to 40 MHz to match the vertical resolution with the horizontal resolution in a 1,000 or 2,000 scan line system. Fluoroscopy will be discussed in greater depth in Chapter 27.

Signal-to-Noise Ratio

In Chapter 24, signal-to-noise ratio (SNR) was discussed in relation to electronic imaging system components, which includes CRT monitors. When high noise levels are present, they can significantly degrade image details. To offset the high noise levels, the CRT monitor must have a high SNR. Standard broadcast TV sets have an SNR lower than 200:1, which produces a poor-quality image. A modern fluoroscopic system uses an SNR of 500:1. The CRT monitors used with digital imaging systems require an SNR of 1,000:1; this will provide a sharp, crisp image where tiny details will be easily detected.

Reflective and Veiling Glare

There are two types of glare, which affect the ability of technologists and radiologists to view the digital image. Reflective glare occurs when ambient or room lighting reflects off of the surface of the monitor or display screen. The room lights need to be turned down to minimize reflection of the ambient light off of the monitor. Reflective glare is a problem when viewing an image on any monitor screen, especially on a CRT screen.

CRT monitor screens have an internal glare called veiling glare. Internal processes within the monitor cause veiling glare: electron backscatter, lateral leakage of light from the phosphor crystals, as well as other scattering light within the phosphor layer. Each of these can cause veiling glare, which degrades the contrast of the image.

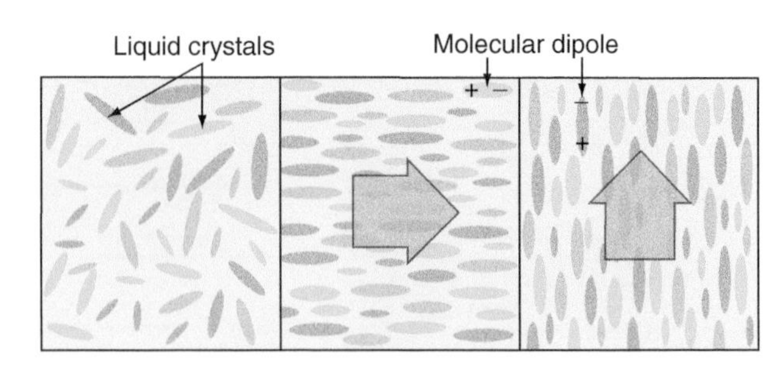

Figure 25.3. Liquid crystals are oriented in a random manner in their natural state and are aligned in the same direction when under the influence of an external electric field.

Liquid Crystal Diode

Liquid crystal diode (LCD) displays have many design characteristics, which makes them preferred over CRT monitors. LCD displays are lightweight, portable, less expensive, and available in many sizes. They have a flat shape and take up much less space than a CRT and they generate less heat and have a longer life. LCD monitors do not produce veiling glare and have much lower reflection of room lighting. Because of their small size and superior image display, LCD monitors have replaced the CRT monitor in medical imaging departments.

One disadvantage of the LCD monitor is the screen cannot be viewed from multiple angles. In order to get the best view possible, a person must stand directly in front of the screen to see the full detail in the image. This can be a problem when two or more individuals are looking at and discussing the image.

Display Characteristics

Liquid crystal compounds are materials that have the properties of both a liquid and a solid. The liquid crystal compounds are in a crystalline configuration of molecules and have the property of viscosity, which allows the crystals to flow like a liquid. The liquid crystal material is considered a nematic liquid crystal material, such as hydrogenated amorphous silicon. Nematic means the crystal molecules are linearly shaped and are electrically charged. The electrical charge makes the crystals a natural molecular dipole. Subsequently, the long axes of the liquid crystals can be aligned through the action of an external electric field. As seen in Figure 25.3, the liquid crystals are randomly aligned in their natural state and become aligned when under the influence of an external electric field.

LCD displays are constructed of two thin flexible glass plates with the liquid crystal material sandwiched between the glass plates. Each glass plate has transparent conductors (electrodes), which act like flat-shaped wires that transmit the electricity through the system. One glass plate consists of rows of these transparent conductors, while the other glass plate has columns of vertical conductors. The individual locations where these rows and columns intersect make up a pixel.

Active Matrix Liquid Crystal Display

Medical imaging display monitors must be much brighter and have sharper resolution and high-speed response times. To accomplish this, the **active matrix liquid crystal display** (AMLCD) was developed. The term *active* refers to the ability to individually control each pixel of the digital display. The AMLCD is created pixel by pixel. In the AMLCD system, each pixel consists of two glass plate substrates that are separated by spherical glass beads, which are embedded in the glass plates and act as spacers. Conductors called bus lines control each pixel with a thin-film transistor (TFT).

The TFT allows each column to access a pixel simultaneously to form a row; this speeds up response and refresh times. The **response time** is the amount of time the pixel requires to change its brightness and the **refresh time** is the amount of time it takes to reconstruct the next frame. Even if the refresh rate is low, the LCD monitors do not have any flicker because the pixels remain turned on between frames. The capacitor in each TFT prevents any charge from leaking out of the liquid crystal cells, which maintains the brightness and continuity of each pixel. The display has a very intense white backlight that illuminates each pixel. Individual pixels contain light-polarizing filters and films to control the intensity and color of the light transmitted through the pixel.

AMLCDs can be either in color or monochromatic. The difference is in the design of the filters and films. Color AMLCDs have red-green-blue filters inside each pixel, which are formed into subpixels, and each subpixel has three filters. Medical flat panel digital image displays are monochromatic, and images are displayed in shades from white to black. Figure 25.4 illustrates the design and operation of a single pixel. An intense light is emitted by the backlight illuminating the pixel and the light is either blocked or transmitted based on the orientation of the liquid crystals.

The resolution in the AMLCD is commonly expressed by the total number of pixels on the entire screen in width and length, for example, 480 × 640. LCD monitors may have resolution of up to 3 to 5 megapixels. Recall that pixel pitch is the distance from the middle of one pixel to the middle of an adjacent pixel. Smaller pixel pitch results in less graininess in the image and sharper image resolution.

AMLCDs have many positive characteristics including better grayscale definition; they are not limited by veiling glare or reflections in the glass plate, which results in better contrast resolution. The internal noise of an AMLCD is less than that of the CRT, which also results in better contrast resolution.

Great care must be taken when using the LCD monitor because the electrodes making up the pixels are embedded in the screen and the flexible glass is extremely thin. This design is very easily damaged with improper daily use. It is very easy to apply pressure to the screen when pointing to anatomy, but this can damage the LCD screen and will eventually destroy the pixels; this is called "dead" pixels and cannot be repaired.

Viewing Conditions

Throughout the medical imaging department, there are various workstations for technologists and radiologists to view a digital image. Display workstations are considered either primary or secondary. Primary workstations are used for official interpretation of medical images and must follow established guidelines to include maximum luminance levels of at least 171 candelas per meter squared, contrast response that meets AAPM Task Group 18 requirements, 8 bit or greater luminance resolution, minimal veiling glare, and minimal levels of room light.

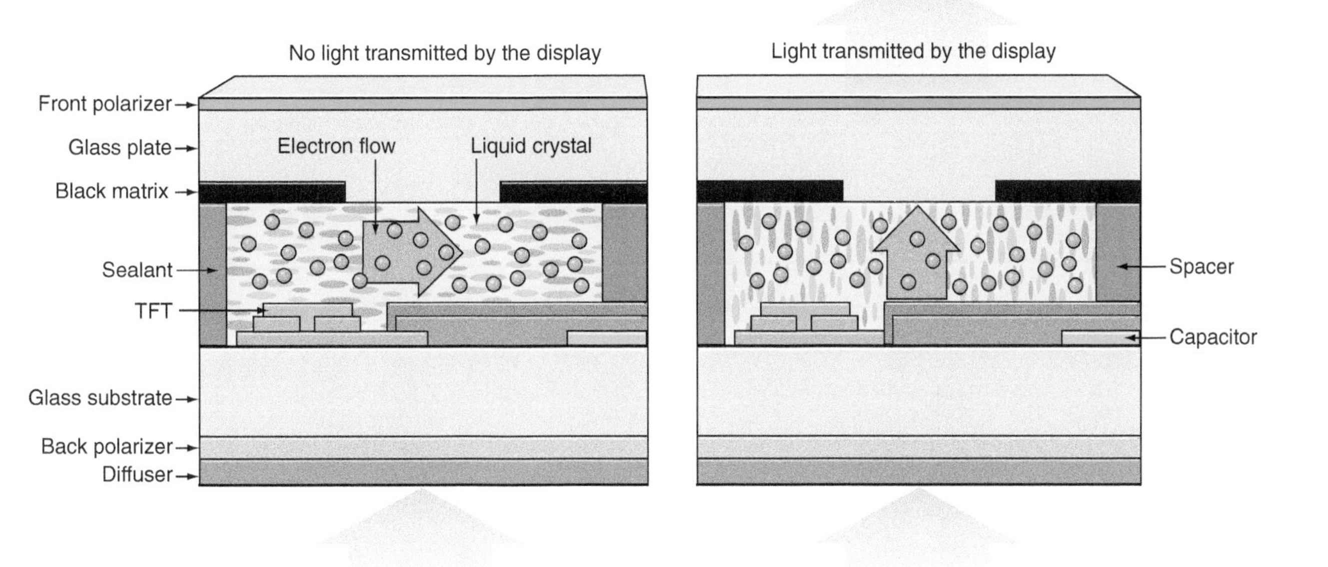

Figure 25.4. Cross-sectional illustration of one pixel in an active matrix liquid crystal display.

Secondary workstations are used by technologists to view a digital image. The monitors have a significantly lower quality compared to monitors used by the radiologists. The viewing conditions are very different because the workstation is often in a brightly lit work area while the radiologist's high-resolution monitors are in a dimly lit reading room. The secondary workstations do not have to adhere to the established guidelines as they are not used for interpretation. A word of caution is warranted when postprocessing an image prior to sending it to the PACS system for the radiologist to interpret. The postprocessing changes should be carefully considered by the technologists before sending the images for interpretation as these changes may limit the radiologist's abilities to manipulate the images in the manner necessary for the official interpretation.

Chapter Summary

1. The CRT uses an electron gun, focusing and accelerating grids, and deflection coils to shape the electron stream.
2. Medical viewing systems, CRTs have a higher vertical resolution, bandpass, and signal-to-noise ratio than consumer televisions.
3. The electron stream strikes the fluorescent phosphor crystals in a raster pattern starting with the odd number lines and then the even number lines. Each line is called an active trace because the phosphor crystals are activated to varying degrees of brightness.
4. Frequency modulations directly determine the number of bits of information, which can be stored on each line in the raster pattern. This is called bandpass.
5. CRT monitors are subject to high noise levels both internal and external. To offset the noise levels, the CRT monitor must have a high signal-to-noise ratio.
6. Veiling glare is caused by internal processes within the monitor.
7. Liquid crystal diode displays are quickly replacing CRTs because of their efficiency and compact size.
8. AMLCDs have a high response and refresh times, which provide constant brightness and improved continuity of the image.
9. Advantages of the LCDs include uniform brightness, contrast and sharpness, minimal reflectance of ambient light, and no glare. Disadvantage is limited off-angle viewing.

Case Study

Donovan is a first year student in a radiologic technology program. He was given an assignment to explain the CRT and the process it uses to form an image.

Critical Thinking Questions

1. What are the internal components which make up the CRT?
2. How is the electron stream controlled for shape, direction, and quality?
3. What is a raster pattern and how does it affect the image on the CRT monitor?

Review Questions

Multiple Choice

1. In a cathode ray tube, which device is responsible for the proper location of the electron stream as it strikes the back of the fluorescent screen?
   a. Signal plate
   b. Control grid
   c. Accelerating grid
   d. Deflection coils

2. The pattern of lines formed on the CRT is called a(n):
   a. signal
   b. interlacing scan
   c. raster
   d. active matrix array

3. The standard frame rate for television images is __________ frames per second.
   a. 30
   b. 60
   c. 120
   d. 15

4. For the CRT monitor, which of the following consists of 262.5 lines?
   a. A field
   b. A frame
   c. A scan
   d. A latent image

5. The CRT monitors used for a digital radiographic unit will require a minimum signal-to-noise ratio of:
   a. 50:1
   b. 100:1
   c. 200:1
   d. 1,000:1

6. The molecules of a nematic liquid crystal material:
   a. have a linear, threadlike shape
   b. tend to keep their axes aligned
   c. flow like a liquid
   d. b and c only
   e. all of the above

7. For an active matrix liquid crystal display, each pixel has its own __________ to provide much higher brightness and continuity along with faster response and refresh times.
   a. LED
   b. TFT
   c. CRT
   d. signal plate

Short Answer

1. What range of bandpass is required in CRT monitors to match a 1,000 to 2,000 scan line system?

2. How many raster lines make up one field as the electron gun scans the raster pattern?

3. In consideration of viewing quality, what is the greatest disadvantage of an LCD monitor when compared to the CRT monitor?

4. **State the purpose of the deflecting coils which surround the neck of a CRT.**

5. **What is the frame rate for a typical CRT and why does it have to be this high?**

6. **__________ is the distance between the center point of two adjacent pixels.**

26

Digital Image Management

Objectives

Upon completion of this chapter, the student will be able to:

1. Describe the use of image storage in relation to short- and long-term storage.
2. Explain the function of the image manager.
3. Define Digital Imaging and Communications in Medicine (DICOM).
4. Describe what a picture archiving and communication system (PACS) is and how it is used.
5. Compare a radiology information system to a hospital information system.
6. Explain the purpose of the Health Level 7 communication system.

Key Terms

- archives
- archive server
- compression ratio
- Digital Imaging and Communications in Medicine (DICOM)
- digital versatile disk (DVD)
- display workstation
- electronic medical record (EMR)
- health level 7
- hospital information system (HIS)
- image manager
- image storage
- magnetic disk storage
- magneto-optical disk (MOD)
- picture archiving and communication system (PACS)
- radiology information system (RIS)
- redundant array of independent disks (RAID)
- ultra density optical (UDO) disk

Introduction

The **picture archiving and communication system (PACS)** has become an integral component in hospitals and imaging clinics because administrators understand the importance of serving patients and physicians. Initially, a PACS is very costly to implement but the benefits far outweigh the costs. In this chapter, the student will learn about the basic concepts of a PACS and its components, DICOM and electronic archives, radiology and hospital information systems, and the need for integrating all facets of the digital exam. The purpose of this chapter is to present a broad overview of the components and technologies involved in PACS; however, to obtain a deep knowledge of PACS, students must immerse themselves in a dedicated PACS course.

Picture Archiving and Communication System

A PACS is a networked group of computers, servers, and **archives** that are used to manage digital images (Fig. 26.1). The archives store images from multiple modalities, which can be accessed from various locations within the hospital. A PACS also integrates images with patient demographic information, facilitates hard copy management of images, and displays both images and patient information at workstations throughout the network.

The first PACSs were used in the early 1980s and generally served a single modality. Research institutions developed and housed early systems. As medical imaging vendors became more involved, each developed their own unique proprietary systems that were specific to their modalities. As physicians and facilities became interested in utilizing the PACS, it became clear that a standardized method must be developed. Early PACSs lacked the ability to interface with information systems such as radiology information systems (RIS) and hospital information systems (HIS), this created workflow problems with delivering data to locations at a specific time. In modern day, the problems have been solved; however, PACS are always evolving and improving efficiency for all users.

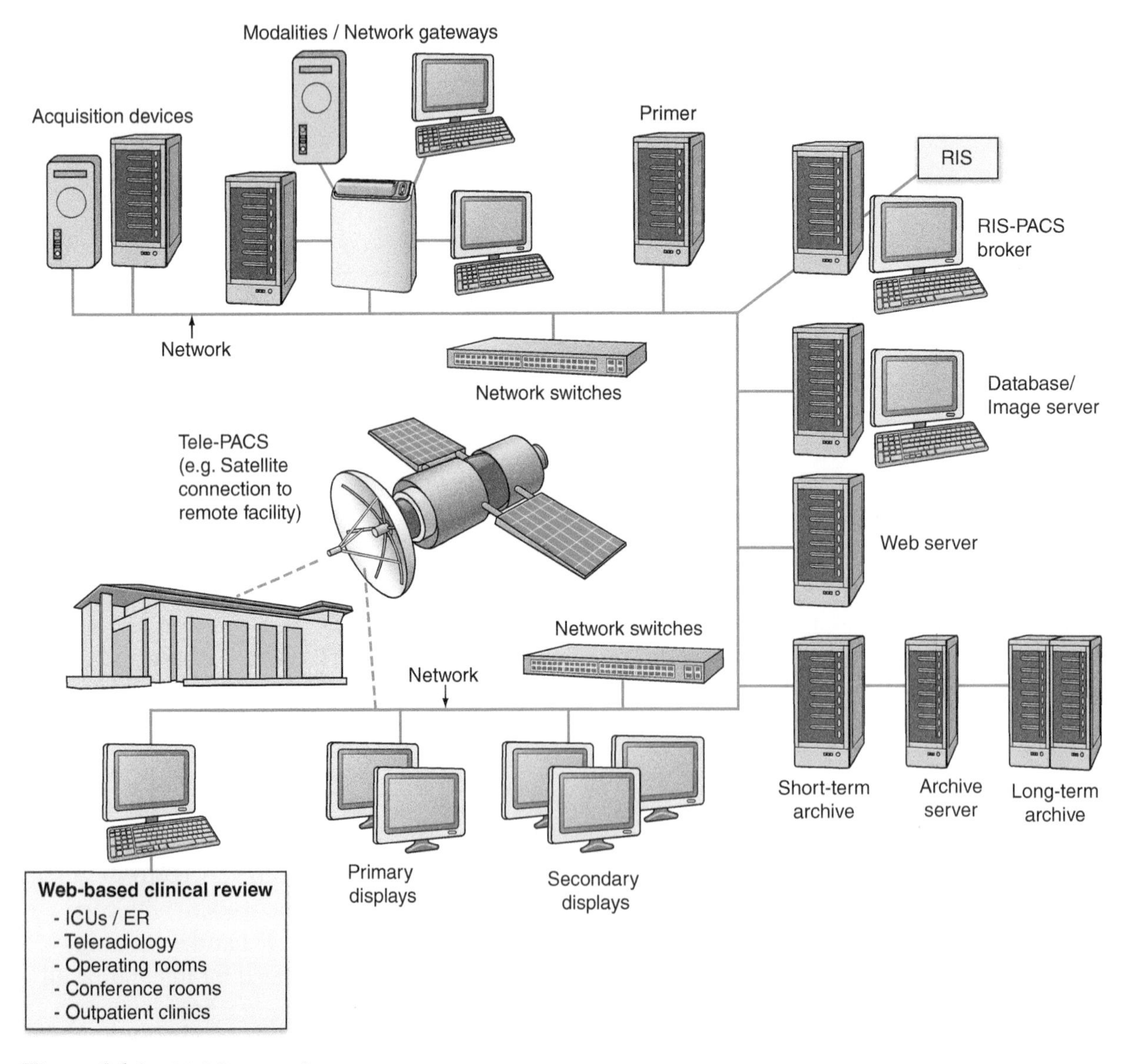

Figure 26.1. **PACS network.**

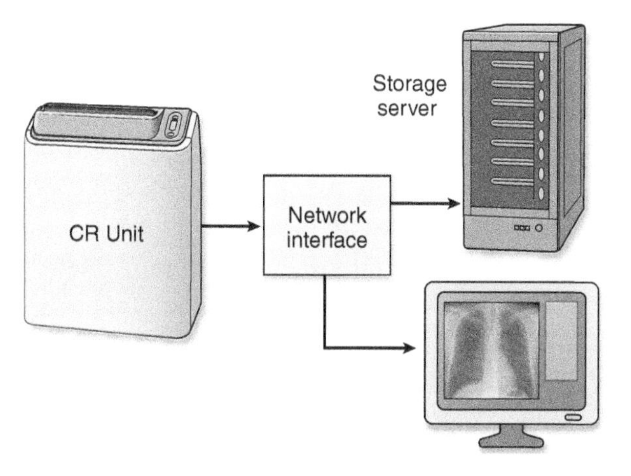

Figure 26.2. **Mini-PACS, a single imaging modality (CR) is connected to the storage server and viewing workstation by a local area network.**

PACSs vary widely in size and in scope. A PACS may be designed for a single modality such as nuclear medicine, ultrasound, mammography, or computed tomography. A small single PACS is often called a mini-PACS (Fig. 26.2). CT and MRI exams have become larger because of the increased number of cross-sectional images per patient exam. A large medical facility may have several mini-PACS along with an enterprise-wide PACS. Radiologists routinely viewed the images in the modality, but this became a hindrance to the technologists as well as the radiologists. To address this issue, vendors designed workstations that were connected to the modalities and served as a console where the radiologist could view the images and perform simple image manipulation.

Foundational Concepts

Before we delve further into a PACS, we must revisit the importance of radiographic foundational concepts of patient demographics, technologist markers, and preparing the image for interpretation by the radiologist.

Patient Demographics

When a patient's demographics is entered into a computer system, great care must be taken to properly and accurately input all the information. Patient demographics include such items as the patient's name, date of birth, hospital identification number, date of exam, facility where exam is performed, and ordering physician. The information is manually input into the system and verified each time the patient has an exam. Problems arise when the patient name is entered differently from visit to visit. For example, if the patient's name is Jon P. Doe and is entered that way, that name must be entered exactly the same for each subsequent exam. If the name is entered as Jon Doe, the system will save it as a different patient. The patient's demographic information must be included on each image. In digital imaging the information can be placed on the image by using a barcode scanner which acts as a mechanism to initialize the patient demographic information on each image. Merging the files can be very difficult or impossible especially if several versions of the name are used. The correct exams must be placed in the correct data files for each patient so that no valuable information is lost.

Technologist Markers

Digital imaging systems provide a method to add anatomic side identification markers along with other demographic information after the exposure. Because of the construction of digital image receptors and processing software, it is very easy for the image to be upside down, backward, or both. This makes it incredibly difficult if not impossible to distinguish the left side from the right side. Errors in using digital markers can occur and the result can be disastrous for the patient. Every effort must be made to place the anatomic side markers within the light field area or on the image receptor before the exposure.

Preparing the Image for Interpretation

With film screen systems, the processed image was reviewed for errors and if deemed diagnostic additional labeling can be placed on the film. Technologist notes indicating special circumstances during the exam or relevant patient history were added to the file, transported to the radiologist for interpretation, and finally stored in a film library. In digital imaging, all the relevant information is attached to the digital file. This includes position indicators (upright, supine, AP, etc.), acquisition markers (cross-table, portable, etc.), or other symbols like arrows. Many systems also have an option to make notes or annotate the image with text.

PACS Components

To understand what a PACS is and how it is used, it is helpful to look at the systems individual components. A PACS has three fundamental components: image acquisition, display workstations, and archive servers. Each will be covered in this section.

Image Acquisition

In modern medical imaging departments, the majority of images are acquired in a digital format meaning the images can be transferred by a computer network. Computed tomography (CT), ultrasound (US), magnetic resonance imaging (MRI), and nuclear medicine (NM) have been digital for many years and have been using a PACS. General radiography has finally joined the digital realm and has been enjoying the advantages of using PACS! Now, the conversion to a completely digital medical imaging department is a reality.

Digital modalities include CT, MRI, US, NM, computed radiography (CR), digital radiography (DR), digital fluoroscopy (DF), digital mammography (DM), and film digitizers. Digital image acquisition is the first step where data and images are entered into a PACS. It is crucially important that all entries must be error-free because any error will spread throughout the system adversely affecting all clinical aspects.

There are two types of digital image acquisition modalities: those modalities that are fundamentally digital such as CT and US where the raw image data is obtained from the equipment with full spatial resolution and bit depth (grayscale). The second type are modalities that use frame grabbers. A frame grabber digitizes the analog signals received from the image receptors; the images are then sent to the display device such as an liquid crystal display (LCD) for viewing. An example is digital fluoroscopy where the CCD output signal is digitized, processed, and sent to the display monitor. The frame grabber will "grab" the output signal and convert it into a digital signal, which is then sent to the display monitor.

Digital Imaging and Communications in Medicine

Digital Imaging and Communications in Medicine (DICOM) is the universally accepted standard for exchanging medical images among the modality, workstations, and the archive. Early in digital imaging, there were many problems when connecting imaging devices to a PACS, and the images were not transferred along with related information. The files could be transferred, but the manufacturers of imaging equipment and the PACS vendors often used proprietary formats, which did not "communicate" with each other. Some facilities solved this problem by purchasing all their equipment from one vendor; other facilities had specialized software written, which would translate one vendor's format into another vendor format. To overcome these problems, the American College of Radiology and the National Electrical Manufacturers' Association worked together to set standards known as DICOM to facilitate the transfer of images and related information between various vendors. DICOM has become the recognized standard for all countries worldwide.

DICOM has specified standard formats for information objects, such as "patients," "images," and "examinations." This information is compiled into composite information objects such as DICOM computed radiography (CR) image object; this is accomplished for each medical imaging modality. DICOM specifies standards for how these information objects are searched, stored, retrieved, print management, and media storage.

DICOM provides standards for workflow management. Modality worklist is a listing of patients and which modality will be used for imaging, Performed Procedure Step to communicate the status of a procedure and Presentation State. DICOM Presentation State is a standard for capturing and storing adjustments of the image and annotations on the image, whether made by the technologist or radiologist. These adjustments include cropping, flipping, windowing, leveling, zooming, and annotations of clinical notes or symbols like arrows. Each of these is stored with the image set in PACS, and when the images are viewed, the adjustments and annotations will be on the image.

DICOM is compatible with common computer network protocols. It adopts the Internet protocol suite (TCP/IP) and will function on any local area network (LAN) or wide area network (WAN) as long as the intermediate network layer protocol is TCP/IP. Currently, the products of most vendors of medical imaging and PACS equipment allow exchange of information that conforms to the DICOM standard. Every vendor and modality boasts DICOM compatibility but each DICOM *conformance statement* must be read carefully to fully understand the specific implementation of the DICOM standard. There are 20 different parts ranging from image display to media storage. Every device does not conform to every part of the DICOM standard, but rather a device will conform to the parts, which are necessary to perform tasks it is assigned based on what the user wants the system to do.

Image Compression

Digital imaging modalities are responsible for creating large files of information for nearly each exam, which is performed. This large amount of data causes delays in transmission and challenges in storage of all the images. An effective way to manage the size of image files for transmission and storage is to compress the image data. DICOM provides an outline for the use of compression on digital images. The purpose is to speed up the transmission of text and images while reducing the amount of storage that is needed for the exam. Compression can either be:

- Lossless compression: This is called reversible compression because no information is lost in the compression process. This is the most commonly used in hospitals because there is no image degradation when viewing the image after compression.
- Lossy compression: This is called irreversible compression because there is some loss of information. This type of compression is used when images are to be sent to an outside hospital; it is often necessary to shrink the file size to work with outside networks.

DICOM accommodates the Joint Photographic Experts Group (JPEG) lossless compression of 2:1. The **compression ratio** is the part that reduces the size of the image file and affects image quality. The compression ratio is the ratio between the computer storage required to save an original image and the storage required for the compressed data. Lossless compression results in a 2:1 to 3:1 compression ratio, and lossy compression ratios range from 10:1 to 50:1. As the compression ratio increases, the image requires less amounts of storage, and the image can be transmitted much faster; however, this is done at the expense of image quality. High-quality digital images are critical for a radiologist to make an accurate diagnosis. At low compression ratios, the overall loss of image quality is within an acceptable range, which means the image is still visually acceptable to the radiologist (Fig. 26.3).

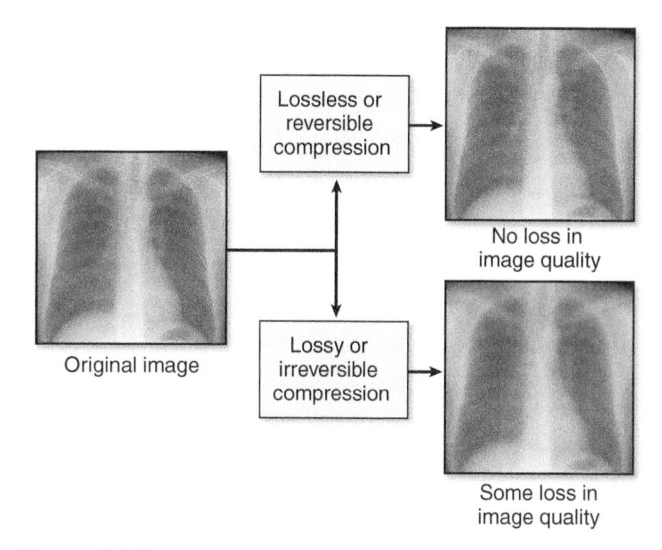

Figure 26.3. **Image compression. Lossless or reversible image compression where there is no loss of image quality. Lossy or irreversible image compression where there is some loss of image quality.**

Display Workstations

A **display workstation** is any computer that health care personnel can use to view the digital image. This is a highly interactive part of a PACS, and the workstations are located in the medical imaging department and throughout the facility. The workstations consist of a monitor, computer, keyboard, and mouse. The display workstation allows a user to search for and receive images from the archive or to display images from any of the modalities (Fig. 26.4).

The display workstations are designed to accommodate the needs of the person viewing the image. Technologists must be able to review the image prior to sending it to the PACS, the computer the technologist uses allows for minor image manipulation. A 1 megapixel (Mp) monitor is sufficient for general viewing by physicians and health care personnel. Radiologists

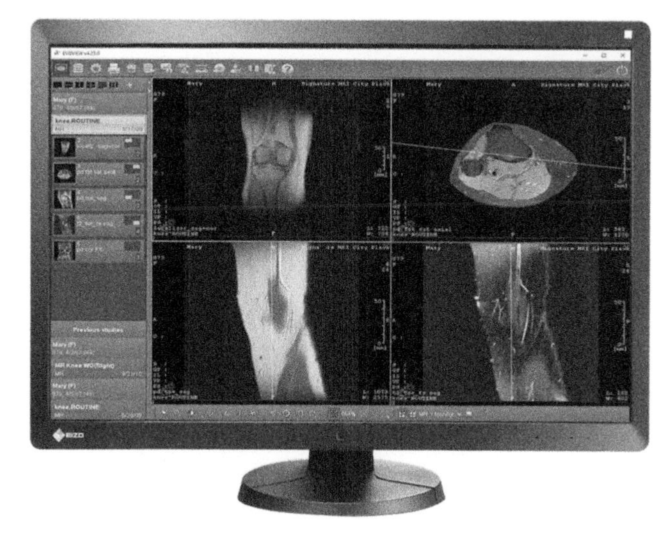

Figure 26.4. **Workstation with the capability of multiple screenshots. (Reprinted from UMG/Del Medical, Bloomingdale, IL, with permission.)**

require a 2 Mp monitor to better visualize the detail in an image, which is necessary for interpretation or for quality control by the technologist. The display workstations have a PACS application software that provides versatility in performing image manipulation techniques to enhance the image. For general viewing by noninterpreting physicians and technologists, a very basic software package allows minor adjustment. Select workstations used for quality control and interpretation have software permitting more advanced manipulation of the image such as windowing and leveling, annotation, cropping, magnification, edge enhancement, and patient demographic information. Depending on the duties of the technologists, each may have access to different functions, which are protected by a login and password; these functions are limited in the effort to prevent accidentally damaging or negatively altering the image or patient record.

At one point, the CRT was the monitor used in medical imaging departments, but it has been replaced with the LCD monitor. The LCD is superior in quality and has become popular because the monitor has a more ergonomic size, has better resolution, and does not produce heat compared to a CRT display. Another advantage of the LCD is that it gives out more light and can be viewed in areas with a high amount of ambient light.

Archive Components

One of the biggest challenges of a PACS is storage. Modalities have the capability of producing complex sets of image data, which requires a large amount of storage and the need to more storage in consistently increasing. The archive component in a PACS has an **image manager** that contains a database that handles the workflow of the system by moving images from storage to viewing or work stations and then back to the archive. It also controls the DICOM processes running within the archive. The image manager also interfaces with the RIS and HIS, which allows the PACS to collect additional patient information for effective operation in routing the images to various locations throughout the PACS. The image manager also assists in populating image information into the patient's electronic medical record (EMR).

The image manager database contains the DICOM header information: patient name, identification information, date of the procedure, ordering physician, and location. The fields are organized in the database and a person can use a workstation to run a query for an examination. The image manager will locate the searched data fields and locate the images that are being searched. The database has indicators associated with each image on the **archive server** that points back to the data fields in the database. The process is summarized as:

- Order is placed in the RIS for a medical imaging examination.
- The images are obtained and sent to the archive.
- The image manager removes the image header from each image and assigns a pointer to each image. It can also assign a pointer to a series of images.
- The database files the image and textual information in a variety of fields and communications back to the RIS to verify information.
- The examination is queried and the indicators locate the image on the archive server, the images are sent to the workstation.

Image Storage

The **image storage** component is part of the system that stores or archives the data on a physical storage device such as magnetic tape, optical disk, or server. Types of storage include short and long term. Short term means the data is online and available very quickly, usually a few seconds. Long-term means near line or images that must be retrieved from a tape or jukebox (**magnetic disk storage** device) and brought to a **redundant array of independent disks (RAID)**, which can take several minutes. A RAID is several magnetic disks or hard drives that are linked together in an array. The size can range from several hundred gigabytes to several terabytes.

Short-term storage commonly uses a RAID to store data across the array. The array is set up to have several disks where the information is stored; if one disk fails, the data from that disk can be regenerated using the redundancy of data from the remaining disks. When the information is transmitted, errors can occur, which means data will be lost, the RAID is able to detect these errors and make a correction, and the data will be regenerated based on the information from the remaining disks.

Long-term storage also uses a RAID, as technology has advanced the cost of the arrays has decreased making it possible for hospitals to use a RAID for both short- and long-term storage. There are other forms of long-term storage that are still in use today. Magnetic tape is the oldest storage technology; these tapes are kept in a tape library, which can hold hundreds of terabytes of data. Tape technology has continually improved to expand its storage limits. Magnetic tape is a low-cost archive medium and comes in a variety of sizes. The tapes are contained in a jukebox or library that has multiple drives and a robotic arm that moves the tapes in and out of the drives. A tape library can hold over 1,400 tapes with the capability of adding on other libraries to the original library. The tapes can be used multiple times, but with increased use, the tapes can get damaged and become unreliable.

Optical disks are another common storage technology. There are several types of optical disk: **magneto-optical disk** (MOD), **digital versatile disks** (DVDs), and **ultra density optical** (UDO) disks. The MOD is similar to a compact disk (CD) or DVD because it is read with an optical laser and the disk is contained in a plastic cartridge. CDs were used in the early years of PACSs, but the CDs were not able to hold enough data to make a CD archive cost effective. DVDs were initially used for videos, but their storage capabilities were an advantage over CDs. DVDs have a much higher capacity up to 17 GB and are very economical in price. The UDO disk is the newest generation of the MOD. The UDO disk uses blue laser technology to both write and read the data. The cost of the UDO is less than the MODs and is competitively priced with DVDs.

Application Interfacing

Radiology Information Systems and Hospital Information Systems

In a medical facility, it is beneficial to have communication between the PACS, **radiology information system (RIS)**, **hospital information system (HIS)**, and the **electronic medical record** (EMR). The RIS is an information system that supports functions within a medical imaging department such as ordering and scheduling examinations, maintaining a patient database, transcription, reporting, and bill preparation. The RIS can provide worklists of scheduled examinations to the consoles of various imaging equipment so that the information does not have to be manually entered into the system; this decreases the opportunity for improperly identified examinations. The RIS can be a separate system or it can be part of the PACS or HIS.

The HIS contains the patient's full medical information from hospital billing to inpatient ordering systems, basically any service that has been provided to the patient. The EMR houses the patient's private health records including prior imaging or medical procedures, laboratory results, pathology reports, and notes from physicians and nurses just to name a few. The EMR interfaces with most ancillary services systems to pull reports so they can be viewed in a common format. The EMR also interfaces with PACS, RIS, and HIS systems to manage all subsequent procedures and services the patient will have at that facility.

Modality worklists permit prior imaging exams, which are relevant to the current exam to be used for comparison by the interpreting physician. The network interfaces to the RIS, and HIS also provides the interpretations of those prior exams and the EMR to a PACS workstation; this saves valuable time for the physician. The interface of all the systems allows the referring physician to view medical images and reports along with other patient-specific information; ultimately, this enables all medical professionals who interact with the patient to have valuable information easily accessible when making decisions regarding the patient's health.

Health Level 7

Health Level 7 (HL7) is a communication standard configured for information systems where the PACS, RIS, HIS, and EMR can exchange alphanumeric data. It addresses the communication of textual data like patient demographics, admission and discharge orders, and types of medical imaging procedures and radiology reports, administrative information, and clinical data. HL7 has multiple parts and is used at many levels in the hospital. HL7 to DICOM is a step where the RIS and HIS can provide worklists to imaging devices.

Chapter Summary

1. The PACS is an integral part of the digital medical imaging department and is divided into acquisition, display, and storage systems.
2. PACS is an electronic network for communication between the modalities, which acquire the images, the display stations, and the archival systems. Each component uses a common language called DICOM.
3. The role of DICOM is to allow for the display and storage of medical images and all information related to the images.
4. Workstations are computers that allow for the retrieval and viewing of medical images from one of the modalities or from the archive. The quality and available functions are determined by the end user.
5. PACS storage is classified as online or near line.
6. DICOM standards make PACS and RIS system widely compatible.
7. RAID systems protect archives of medical images from accidental loss.
8. The HL7 is a communication standard configured for information systems where the PACS, RIS, HIS, and EMR can exchange alphanumeric data.

Case Study

Kaitlyn has been learning about performing radiographic exams and submitting the images to the PACS. She is unsure about the role of the image manager and how it is used to archive and search for images. Answer the questions to assist Kaitlyn in gaining knowledge about the image manager.

Critical Thinking Questions

1. What is an image manager?
2. Which patient information does the image manager contain?
3. How does the image manager search the archive server for images?

Review Questions

Multiple Choice

1. **What does the acronym PACS stand for?**
   a. Picture access computer system
   b. Permanent access communication system
   c. Permanent archival computer system
   d. Picture archiving and communication system

2. **The type of monitor and how it is configured is of no concern when implementing a PACS in a medical imaging department.**
   a. True
   b. False

3. **Of the following, which cannot be transmitted through a PACS?**
   a. Digital projection images
   b. Analog fluoroscopy images
   c. Digitally reconstructed CR images
   d. Photostimulable storage phosphor images

4. **The DICOM standard was developed for which purpose?**
   a. Consistency in the computerized diagnostic process for mammography
   b. Radiographic image quality and consistency
   c. Compatibility between medical systems that store information
   d. Compatibility between analog systems and computerized imaging systems

5. **When patient demographics are entered into the computer system, it is crucial that the patient's name is spelled exactly the same for each instance.**
   a. True
   b. False

6. **The display workstation technologists' use has which components?**
   a. 1 Mp monitor
   b. Keyboard for text
   c. Mouse
   d. a and b
   e. a, b, and c

7. **Once the medical images are acquired, they are sent to the:**
   a. archive server
   b. local hard disk on the workstation computer
   c. radiologists workstation computer for storage

8. **Long-term storage of images is accomplished by which methods?**
   a. Optical disk.
   b. Magnetic disk.
   c. Ultra density optical disks.
   d. Each can be used based on the needs of the facility.

Short Answer

1. **Define the term "compression ratio."**

2. **What is image compression and what is its purpose?**

3. **Explain the differences between lossless and lossy image compression.**

4. **What is DICOM and what is its purpose in medical imaging?**

5. **List the types of storage devices.**

6. **How is an RIS different from a HIS?**

PART V

Specialized Imaging Techniques

27

Fluoroscopy

Objectives

Upon completion of this chapter, the student will be able to:

1. Identify the components of a fluoroscopic system.
2. Identify the components of an image intensifier.
3. Describe the purpose of an automatic brightness control circuit.
4. Identify the factors that influence patient dose during fluoroscopy.
5. Explain the effects of flux and minification gain on total brightness gain.
6. Discuss the factors that affect fluoroscopic image contrast, resolution, distortion, and quantum mottle.

Key Terms

- automatic brightness control (ABC)
- brightness gain
- camera tube
- carriage
- charge-coupled device
- cine
- conversion factor
- electrostatic focusing lenses
- entrance skin exposure
- fluoroscopy
- flux gain
- image intensifier
- input phosphor
- magnification
- minification gain
- output phosphor
- photocathode
- photoemission
- photospot camera
- source-to-skin distance
- vignetting

Introduction

Fluoroscopy is a live, moving x-ray technique that is used to localize potential abnormalities without recording the images on film. It gives a real-time or dynamic image as the x-rays pass through the patient. An **image intensifier** converts x-ray energy into visible light energy. The image intensifier is used during fluoroscopy for increasing sensitivity and brightness, thus reducing the patient radiation dose. Inside the image intensifier, the pattern of x-rays is converted into an electron pattern, and the electrons are accelerated onto an **output phosphor** and converted into a brighter visible light image. In this chapter, we cover the construction and application of an image intensifier and the automatic brightness circuit of a fluoroscopic system.

Historical Perspective

Thomas A. Edison invented the fluoroscope in 1896, the year after Roentgen's discovery of x-rays. The original fluoroscope was held by hand above the patient's body in the path of the x-ray beam. The radiologist had to stand directly in front of the fluoroscope to view the patient's anatomy, which meant the radiologist's head and eyes were in the direct path of the primary beam. The fluoroscope emitted a very faint fluorescent image, which required the radiologist to "dark adapt" his or her eyes. This meant the radiologist had to wear red goggles for up to 30 minutes prior to the examination to adjust his or her eyes to viewing the faint image and the examination had to be performed in a completely dark room. These conditions permitted the radiologist to see the faint fluoroscopic image. Obviously, there were many hazards to the radiologist when viewing the fluoroscopic image. Eventually, the fluoroscopic screen was replaced with an image intensification tube, video cameras, and monitors for viewing the image.

Eye Physiology

Early fluoroscopic systems employed a phosphor coating on a lead glass plate. The image brightness of these systems was so low that they could be viewed only with a dark-adapted eye. The retina of the human eye has two types of light receptors, rods, and cones. Cone vision requires bright light or daylight, which is called photopic vision. Rod vision is used in dim light or complete darkness, which is called scotopic vision. Cone vision has excellent spatial resolution with high visual acuity because the cones are concentrated near the center of the retina. Cones are also better able to distinguish the difference in brightness levels, are sensitive to a wide range of wavelengths of light, and can perceive color. Rod vision has poor spatial resolution and is color blind.

During a fluoroscopic examination, maximum image detail is necessary and image brightness must be high. The image intensifier was developed by Bell Laboratories during the 1950s to increase the brightness of the image so that the image could be viewed with cone vision.

Fluoroscopy

Fluoroscopy is a dynamic imaging modality designed to observe moving structures in the body, in contrast to conventional radiography that produces static images of body structures. During fluoroscopy, a radiologist views the fluoroscopic image to obtain a diagnosis. Static digital images of the fluoroscopic image can be obtained whenever a permanent record is needed. Fluoroscopy is currently used for examinations that require observation of physiologic functions such as the movement of barium through the gastrointestinal tract, injection of contrast medium into a joint or blood vessels.

Most fixed fluoroscopic rooms also have an overhead tube for conventional radiography and are called radiographic and fluoroscopic rooms or "R and F" rooms. The fluoroscopic x-ray tube and image intensifier are connected in a C-arm configuration that allows synchronous movement (Fig. 27.1).

X-ray Tube

Fluoroscopic x-ray tubes have the same design and construction as conventional x-ray tubes, but they are operated for several minutes at a much lower milliampere (mA) value. An x-ray room that can only perform conventional or static imaging is called a radiographic room, while a unit that has live x-rays is called a fluoroscopic room. A room, which is capable of both static and live imaging, is called an R and F room. Figure 27.2 shows a modern "R and F" room. Most of these rooms have digital capabilities; therefore, spot film devices are not necessary. Typical fluoroscopic tube currents are 0.5 to 5 mA, whereas radiographic tube currents are 50 to 500 mA. Fluoroscopic kilovoltage peak or kVp is adjusted on the control panel. High kVp is usually selected with low fluoroscopic mA. This kVp selector is separate from kVp used for conventional x-ray imaging. All fluoroscopic and radiographic rooms have separate mA and kVp controls, depending upon the selection of fluoroscopy or conventional x-ray imaging. The fluoroscopic tube can be operated by a foot switch that allows the radiologist to use both hands to move the fluoroscopic tower and to position the patient. There are fluoroscopic units with the operator switch on the fluoroscopic tower; this configuration allows the radiologist to collimate, to select the mode of operation, and to turn on the fluoroscopy beam.

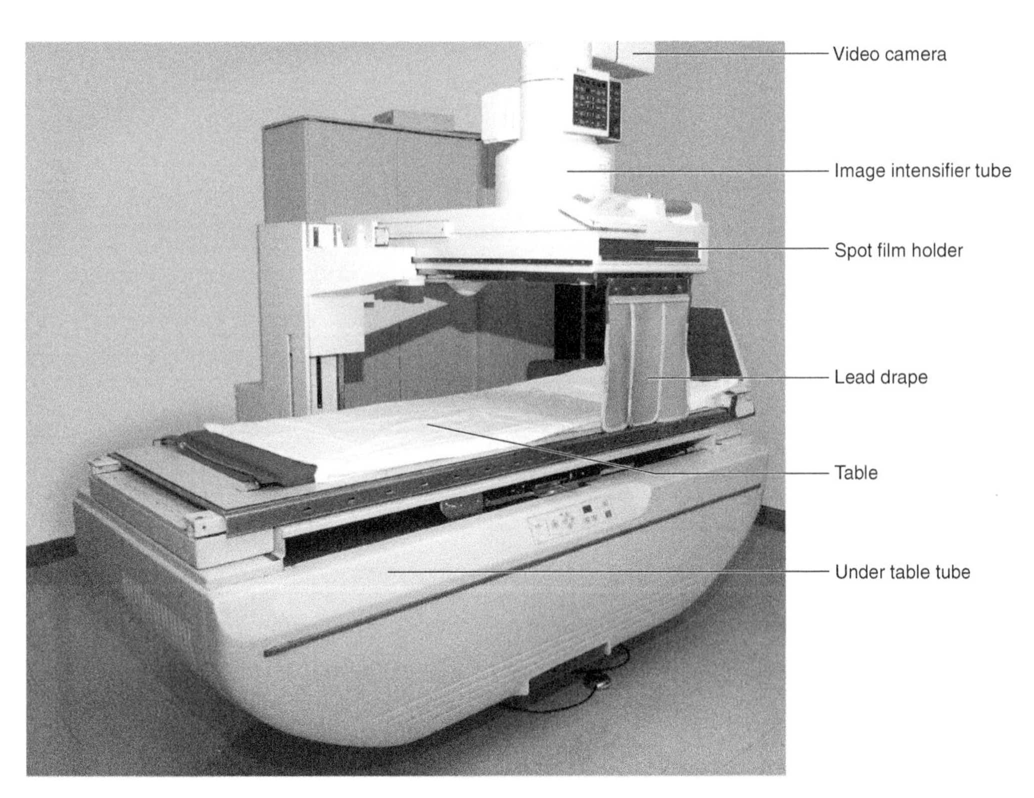

Figure 27.1. Shows a typical older model fluoroscopic room.

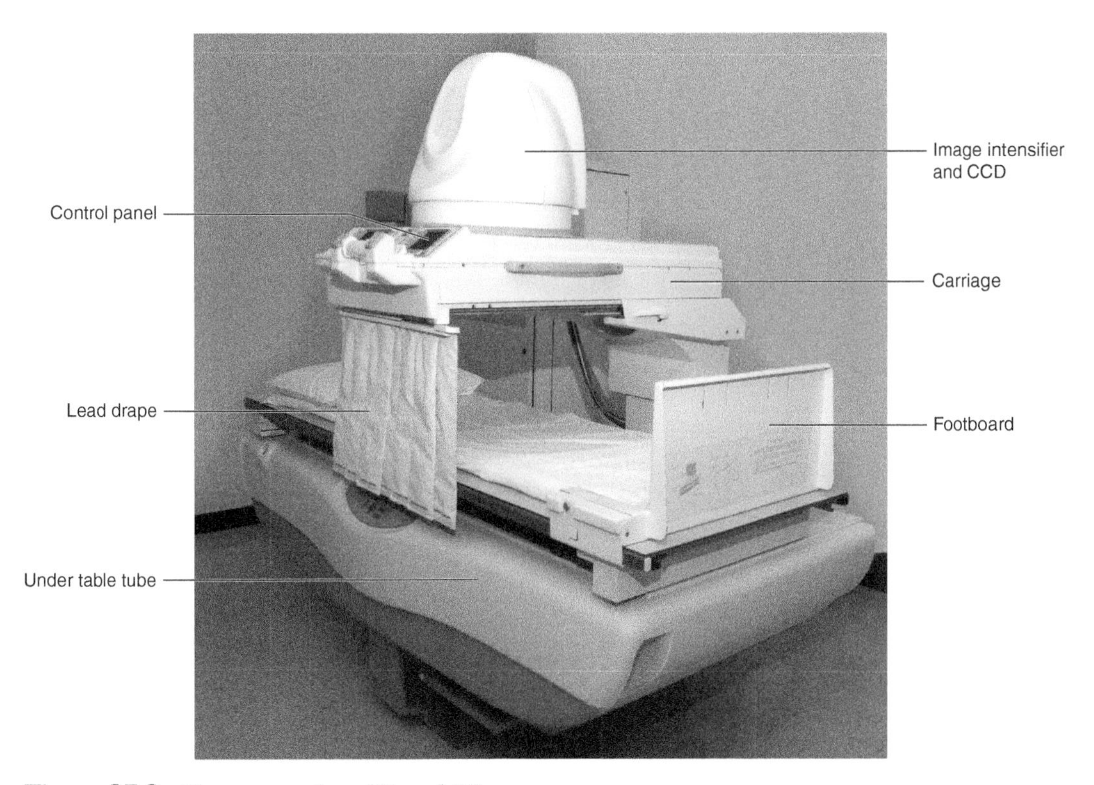

Figure 27.2. Shows a modern "R and F" room.

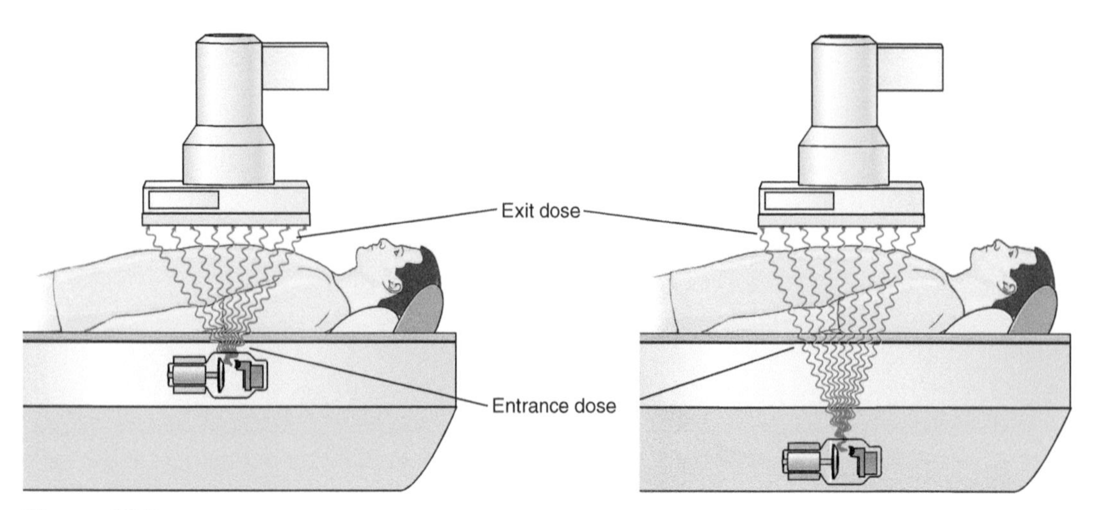

Figure 27.3. **When the x-ray tube is placed close to the tabletop, the patient will have a higher skin entrance dose.**

When the equipment is set up for fluoroscopy, care must be taken to avoid stepping on the foot switch or pressing the operator switch and inadvertently exposing the patient and personnel to unnecessary radiation.

The fluoroscopic tube is usually located beneath the patient support table. Tube shielding and beam-limiting collimators are also located in the tube housing beneath the table. The collimators adjust the size of the x-ray beam and restrict x-rays to the image receptor, which is the image intensifier. The **source-to-skin distance** (SSD) of a fixed fluoroscopic tube must be at least 38 centimeters (cm) or 15 inches. If the fluoroscopic tube is <38 cm below the table, the patient could experience a higher skin entrance dose. Increasing the distance between the fluoroscopic tube and the patient will ultimately result in a lower patient dose.

C-arm and portable fluoroscopic units must have an SSD of at least 30 cm or 12 inches between the focal spot and the patient skin entrance. This is to limit the radiation dose to the skin during fluoroscopic procedures (Fig. 27.3).

X-ray Beam Intensity

Fixed fluoroscopy units must have dose rates of <100 mSv/min (10 R/min) at the tabletop, unless there is an audible alarm that sounds during the high dose rate mode. The high dose rate fluoroscopy unit has a maximum tabletop intensity of 20 R/min.

Table

The table that supports the patient can be changed from a horizontal position into a vertical position for upright examinations. Some tables are constructed of carbon fiber materials, which have great strength and reduce attenuation of the x-ray beam by the tabletop, thus reducing patient exposure. The table is equipped with a removable footboard for routine radiographic procedures. Care must be taken to properly secure the footboard on the table for fluoroscopic examinations.

Total Filtration

The total filtration of the fluoroscope must be at least 2.5 mm aluminum equivalent. The total filtration includes the tabletop and any material located between the x-ray tube and tabletop.

Bucky Slot Cover

The table Bucky must be moved to the foot of the table for the fluoroscopic exam. A Bucky slot shielding device of at least 0.25 mm lead equivalent should automatically cover the Bucky slot. This shielding provides the radiologist and radiographer with protection at the gonadal level.

Protective Curtain

The image intensifier carriage has a protective curtain or panel of at least 0.25 mm lead equivalent that is positioned between the fluoroscopist and the patient. Without the use of the protective curtain and the Bucky slot cover, the exposure of radiology personnel exceeds 100 mR/h at 2 ft from the beam (Fig. 27.4). Using these devices decreases the exposure to 5 mR/h.

Image Intensifier Tower

The image intensifier carriage acts as a primary protective barrier and must have a 2-mm lead equivalent. The

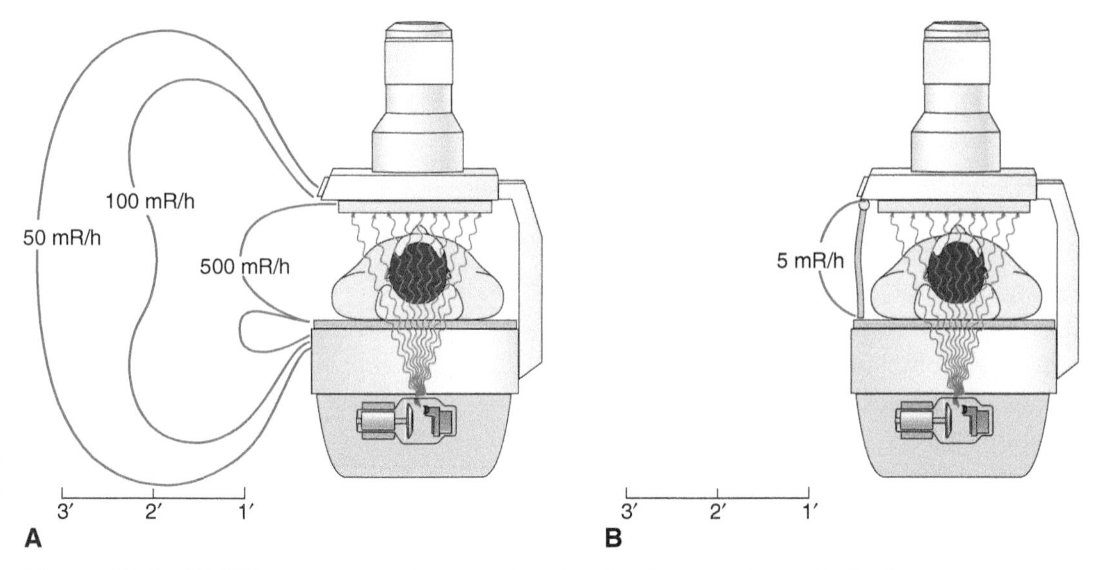

Figure 27.4. **(A) When no protective curtain or Bucky slot cover is used, the fluoroscopist will receive a significant dose of radiation. (B) With the protective curtain and Bucky slot cover properly used, the radiation dose is significantly decreased.**

carriage must be attached to the x-ray tube and include a safety design that prevents the x-ray tube from operating when the carriage is in the parked position.

The image intensifier tower contains the image intensifier and a group of controls that allow the operator to adjust the field size, move the x-ray tube and table, and make spot film exposures. A lead drape hangs from the image intensifier tower to attenuate radiation scattered from the patient. This lead drape has 0.25 mm Pb (lead) equivalent. The video camera is mounted at the top of the image intensifier tower. The tower is connected to the x-ray tube mount, so that both move together as a unit. The x-ray tube can be pushed away from the table to allow access to the patient; however, it must be locked in place for the beam to be energized and directed toward the image intensifier.

Image Intensifier Components

The image intensifier is a sophisticated piece of electronic equipment, which greatly increases the brightness of the image. Modern image intensifiers can increase image brightness up to 8,000 times. Figure 27.5 demonstrates the components of a typical image intensification tube, which are input phosphor, photocathode, electrostatic focusing lenses, accelerating anode, and output phosphor.

Input Phosphor

The **input phosphor** of the image intensifier tube is made of glass, titanium, steel, or aluminum and coated with

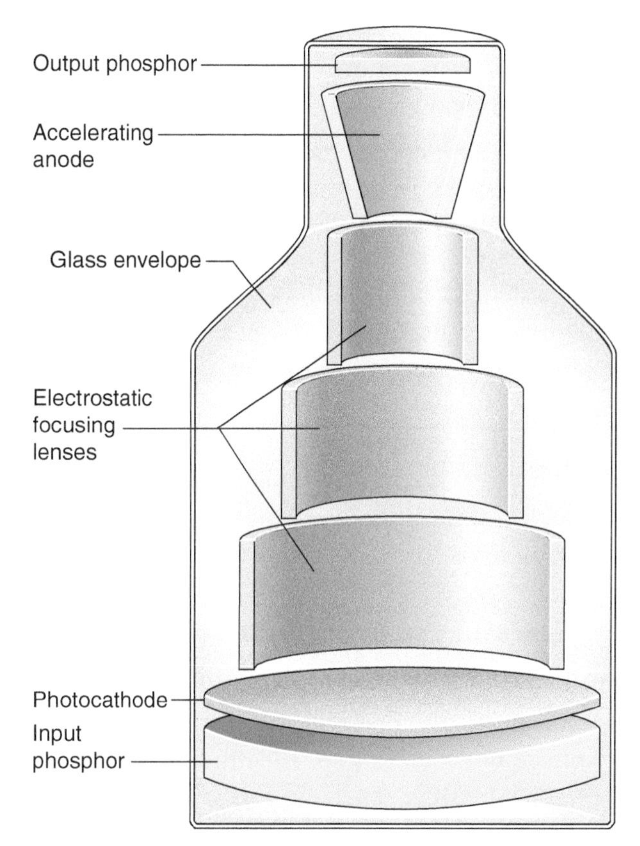

Figure 27.5. **Illustrates a cross-sectional view of a typical image intensifier tube.**

cesium iodide (CsI) crystals because CsI has high x-ray photon absorption and light emission characteristics. The interactions in the input phosphor are similar to the interactions in an intensifying screen. The input phosphor is ~10 to 35 cm in diameter and absorbs about 60% of the exit radiation leaving the patient.

The input phosphor is concave to maintain the same distance between each point on the input phosphor and its matching location on the output phosphor. The concave surface enhances the sharpness of the image. The phosphor emits light in a vertical line, which improves image detail and spatial resolution. The light emitted is proportional to the absorption of the photons. Each x-ray photon produces between 1,000 and 5,000 light photons.

The input phosphor and photocathode are bonded together. The input phosphor is coated with a protective coating to prevent a chemical interaction with the photocathode materials. The photocathode is made of cesium and antimony, which emit electrons when stimulated by light.

Photocathode

The **photocathode** is located on top of the input phosphor and also has a concave surface. The photocathode is made of compounds of cesium and antimony that emit photoelectrons when struck by light. This phenomenon is known as **photoemission**. Light from the input phosphor ejects photoelectrons from the photocathode. The number of photoelectrons is proportional to the amount of light striking the photocathode. Bright regions of the phosphor cause the photocathode to emit many photoelectrons. Dark regions of the phosphor result in the emission of few photoelectrons. The pattern of x-ray photons at the input phosphor is converted into a similar pattern of electrons leaving the photocathode. The pattern of photoelectrons carries the latent image of the patient's anatomy.

Electrostatic Focusing Lenses

The **electrostatic focusing lenses** are located along the inside of the image intensifier and are charged with a low voltage of 25 to 35 kVp. Electrostatic lenses inside the image intensifier repel and focus the negative photoelectrons from the photocathode toward the output phosphor. The concave surface of the photocathode reduces distortion by maintaining the distance between all points on the input screen and the output phosphor. As the photoelectrons travel to the output phosphor, they will cross at the focal point where the image is reversed, so the output phosphor image is reversed from the input phosphor. The focal point is the precise location where the photoelectrons cross; this location is changed when the image intensifier is used in normal or magnification mode (Fig. 27.6).

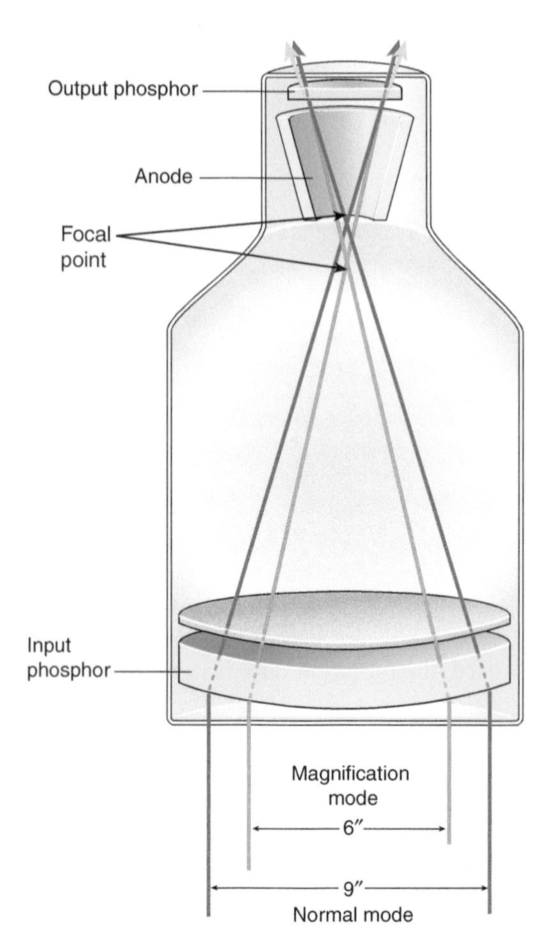

Figure 27.6. **Illustrates the image intensifier focusing for a normal and a magnified image.**

Accelerating Anode and Output Phosphor

Photoelectrons from the photocathode are accelerated toward the positively charged anode by low voltage ranging from 25 to 35 kVp; this kVp accelerates the photoelectrons even more. This allows the photoelectrons to have high kinetic energy. The photoelectrons pass through the anode and strike the output phosphor. The output phosphor is ~2.5 to 5 cm in diameter. The output phosphor is made of silver-activated zinc cadmium sulfide (ZnCdS), which efficiently converts photoelectron energy into visible light. Each photoelectron that reaches the output

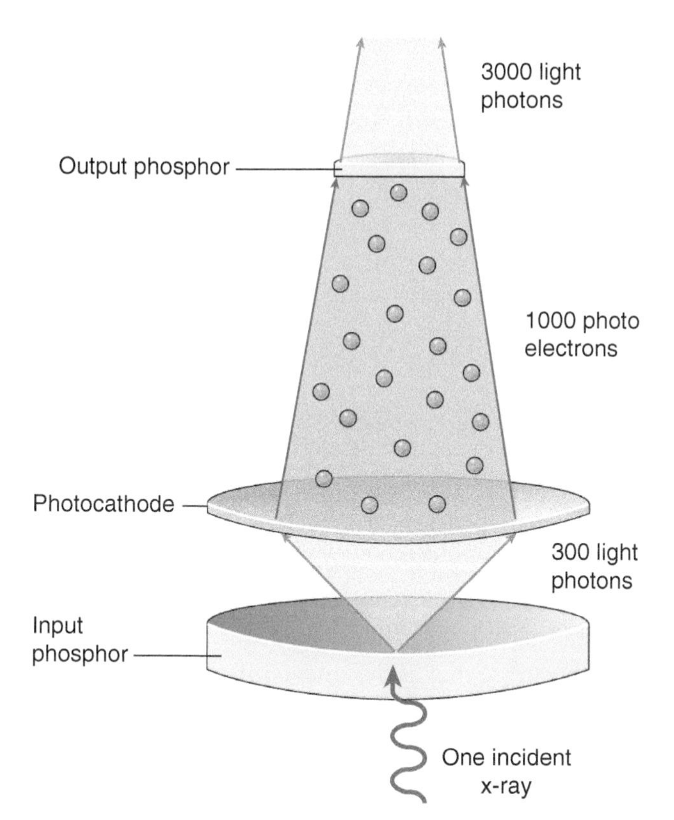

Figure 27.7. **In the image intensifier tube, one incident x-ray photon that interacts with the input phosphor results in a large number of light photons at the output phosphor. This figure demonstrates the flux gain of 3,000 light photons.**

phosphor converts into 50 to 75 times more light photons (Fig. 27.7). The end result is an increase in image intensity and brightness. The light photons are emitted in all directions, which risks some light photons being emitted toward the input phosphor, which would degrade the image. The output phosphor has a thin aluminum coating that prevents the light photons from leaking back across the image intensifier, thereby decreasing the image noise and improving the resolution of the image (Fig. 27.8).

Intensification Principles

Brightness gain is a measurement of the increase in image brightness or intensification achieved by the conversions in the image intensification tube. The increased illumination of the image is due to the multiplication of the light photons at the output phosphor compared to the incident x-ray photons, which interact with the input phosphor. Traditionally, brightness gain was determined by multiplying **flux gain** by minification gain.

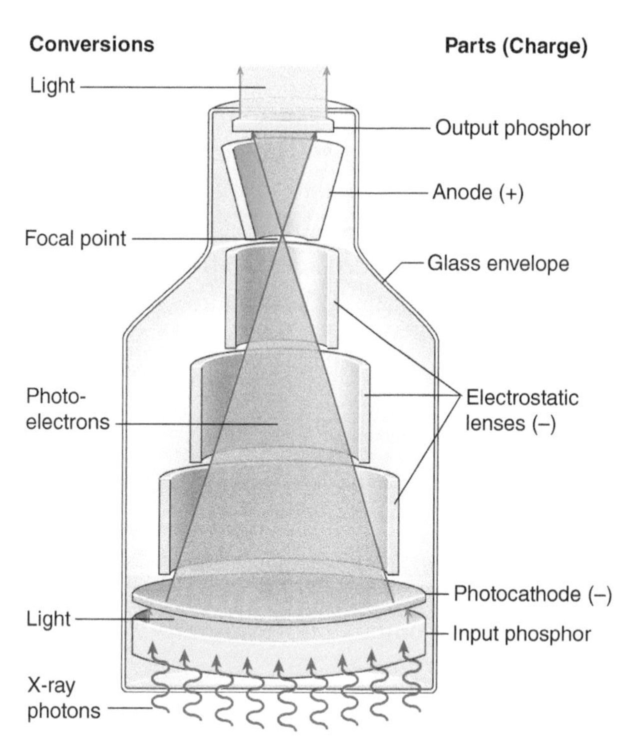

Figure 27.8. **Summarizes the components of the image intensifier and the process of converting remnant radiation with the latent image into light photons at the output phosphor. A thorough knowledge of these concepts is critical in understanding how an image intensifier works.**

Flux Gain

Flux gain is the ratio of the number of light photons at the output phosphor to the number of x-ray photons at the input phosphor, thus producing the conversion of the electron energy into light energy. If the output phosphor produces 100 light photons for each photoelectron that strikes it, the flux gain would be 100.

$$\text{Flux gain} = \frac{\text{Number of output light photons}}{\text{Number of input x-ray photons}}$$

CRITICAL THINKING BOX 27.1

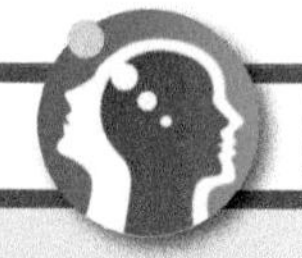

What is the flux gain if there are 50 x-ray photons at the input screen and 4,500 light photons at the output phosphor?

Minification Gain

Minification gain is the ratio of light from input phosphor to light at the output phosphor, thus producing concentrated light from the larger input phosphor onto the smaller output phosphor. The result is an image that has been *minified* or made smaller. Minification gain is an increase in brightness or intensity of the image because the same number of electrons is being concentrated onto a smaller surface area; it is not an improvement in the quality or number of photons making up the image, as this information is contained in the latent image as the x-ray photons exit the patient. Minification gain is determined by dividing the square of the diameter of the input phosphor by the square of the diameter of the output phosphor:

$$\text{Minification gain} = \frac{\text{Input phosphor diameter}^2}{\text{Output phosphor diameter}^2}$$

In general, the input phosphors are 15 to 30 cm in diameter, and the output phosphors are 2.5 cm in diameter.

CRITICAL THINKING BOX 27.2

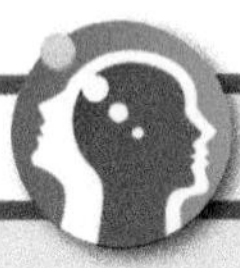

What is the minification gain when the input phosphor diameter is 30 cm and the output phosphor diameter is 2.5 cm?

Total Brightness Gain

Total brightness gain is obtained by multiplying flux gain by minification gain. Typical image intensifiers have brightness gains of 5,000 to 30,000. The output image at the output phosphor is over 5,000 times brighter than the image at the input phosphor. The image intensifier will have decreased brightness as it ages, resulting in increased patient dose to maintain brightness. The formula to determine the total brightness gain is:

$$\text{Brightness gain} = \text{flux gain} \times \text{minification gain}$$

CRITICAL THINKING BOX 27.3

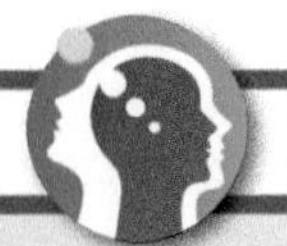

What is the total brightness gain when the flux gain is 70 and the minification gain is 100?

The International Commission on Radiation Units and Measurements recommends the evaluation of the brightness gain of the image intensifier based on the **conversion factor**. The conversion factor is defined as the ratio of the luminance of the output phosphor to the input x-ray exposure rate:

$$\text{CF} = \frac{\text{Candela/meter}^2}{\text{mR/s}}$$

The candela is the unit for the direct light measurement of light intensity or luminance. The conversion factor is ~0.1 times the brightness gain. Image intensifiers have conversion factors that range from 50 to 300, which correspond to brightness gains of 5,000 to 30,000. The ability of the image intensifier to increase brightness will deteriorate as the image intensifier ages. The radiographer should be aware that as the image intensifier ages, higher doses of radiation will be necessary to maintain the level of output brightness, resulting in increased patient dose.

Automatic Brightness Control

The automatic brightness gain or the **automatic brightness control** (ABC) maintains the fluoroscopic image density and contrast at a constant brightness by regulating the radiation output of the x-ray tube. A detector monitors the brightness level of the image intensifier output phosphor. The ABC allows the radiologist to select an image brightness level that is subsequently maintained by varying the kVp, mA, or both to maintain a constant output brightness regardless of the thickness or density of the body part being examined. Fluoroscopic mA is increased or decreased to compensate for various body thicknesses.

The ABC has a relatively slow response time, which temporarily affects the image on the monitor. During a fluoroscopic examination, rapid changes in body thickness can cause the ABC to lag behind for a moment or two before the kVp, and mA is adjusted to provide the appropriate amount of brightness for the tissue thickness. ABC is also called automatic brightness stabilization (ABS) and automatic gain control (AGC).

Magnification Mode

Electrostatic lenses can change the **magnification** of the image by changing the focal point of the photoelectrons. Dual- or multifield mode image intensifiers provide different magnification modes for different applications. Magnification is an increase in the image size of an object, which allows for better visualization of small structures. The operator can change the magnification mode through the controls on the image intensifier tower. Selection of a smaller portion of the input phosphor produces a magnified image but results in a higher patient dose because there is less minification gain in the magnification mode.

When the magnification mode is selected either on a dual-focused or trifocused image intensifier, the voltage supplied to the electrostatic focusing lenses inside the image intensifier is increased, which causes the focal point to move closer to the input screen and the image to be magnified. Figure 27.9 illustrates the area on the input phosphor that is used in the magnification mode. Notice how the focal point has moved closer to the input phosphor; this movement causes the magnification of the image.

Only the electrons from the center area of the input phosphor and photocathode are accelerated to the output phosphor. In the magnification mode, the minification gain is reduced because there are fewer photoelectrons reaching the output phosphor, resulting in the appearance of magnification. For example, a 30/23/15 cm trifocus image intensifier can be operated in any of the three modes. When the 15-cm mode is used, only the electrons from the center 15 cm of the input phosphor will interact with the output phosphor. The remaining electrons will not contribute to the image. The same process is true for the 23-cm mode. When selecting a magnification mode, the x-ray beam is automatically collimated to include only the displayed tissue image. Tissue that does not appear in the image is not irradiated.

Magnification image intensifiers are capable of 1.5 to 4 times magnification. The spatial resolution of the image refers to the ability to see the smallest structure detected in the image. Spatial resolution is measured in line pairs per millimeter (Lp/mm) with typical systems having 4 to 6 Lp/mm when the magnification mode is selected. To calculate the magnification factor, the following formula is used:

$$\text{Magnification factor} = \frac{\text{Input screen diameter}}{\text{Input screen diameter during magnification}}$$

This will cause the fluoroscopic mA to be automatically increased to maintain the same brightness level, but it will also cause an increase in patient dose. In a dual-focused mode, selection of the magnification can increase patient dose by two times. The increased patient dose will result in

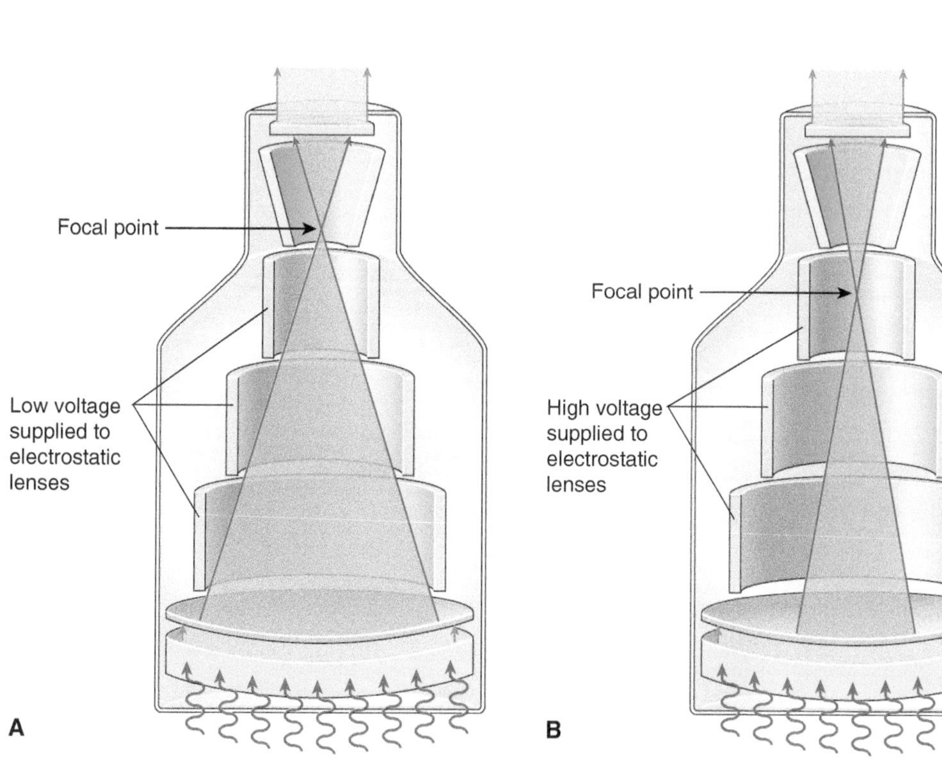

Figure 27.9. Voltage supplied to the electrostatic lenses controls the location of the focal point. (A) Low voltage supplied to lenses. (B) High voltage supplied to lenses. As the focal point gets closer to the input phosphor, the size of the area of the input phosphor decreases.

better image quality because more x-ray photons make up the latent image, which lowers image noise and increases contrast resolution. The ABC increases the fluoroscopic mA to compensate for the reduced minification gain.

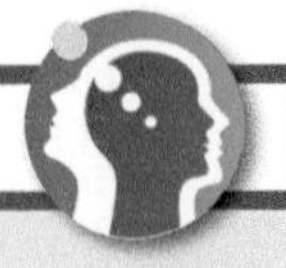

CRITICAL THINKING BOX 27.4

What is the magnification for an image view with an image intensification tube where the input screen diameter is 9 inches and a 6-inch diameter is used in magnification mode?

Image Quality

Creating a fluoroscopic image is a complex procedure with many factors. Fluoroscopic images must also be evaluated for contrast, resolution, distortion, and quantum mottle.

Contrast

Contrast in fluoroscopy is affected by the same factors as in static radiography. The contrast is affected by the scattered radiation coming from the patient, light scatter at the input and output phosphors, and light scatter within the image intensifier itself. Scattered radiation produces scatter photons at the input phosphor and also produces limited background fog from incident x-ray photons, which are transmitted through the image intensifier tube to the output screen. The output phosphor has an aluminum filter that is designed to prevent backscatter from the output phosphor to the input phosphor, but in reality, it does not block 100% of light photons from leaking back toward the input phosphor. Each of these combine to create background fog that increases the base density of the image. These principles are the same as discussed in film screen processing where the base plus fog affects image contrast. In a fluoroscopic image, the visible contrast is decreased.

Resolution

The resolution of the fluoroscopic image is directly affected by the video monitoring system. Many video monitoring systems are limited to a 525-line raster pattern where fluoroscopic geometric factors affect the overall resolution of the image. The fluoroscopic geometric factors include minification gain, flux gain, focal point, input and output phosphor diameter, size and thickness of the anatomy being imaged, viewing system resolution, and object-to image receptor distance (OID).

Distortion

Distortion in fluoroscopy has the same considerations as distortion in routine radiography. Size distortion, caused by OID, makes the image appear to be more magnified under fluoroscopy especially when the image intensifier is in magnification mode. The size distortion is the same whether the image has been magnified or not, there just appears to be more distortion because the image is larger and the distortion is easier to see.

Shape distortion is caused by the design of the image intensifier tube. The concave curve of the input phosphor was designed to provide each electron with the same distance of travel to the output phosphor. In fluoroscopy, distortion is a result of inaccurate focusing of the electrons released at the periphery of the photocathode and the concave shape of the photocathode. The combined result is unequal magnification (distortion) of the image, creating a "pincushion appearance" (Fig. 27.10).

The "pincushion appearance" also causes reduced brightness at the edges of the image; this effect is called **vignetting**. Vignetting also causes greater image intensity at the center of the image, which minimizes distortion and improves contrast. Vignetting can be used to our advantage when using the magnification mode of

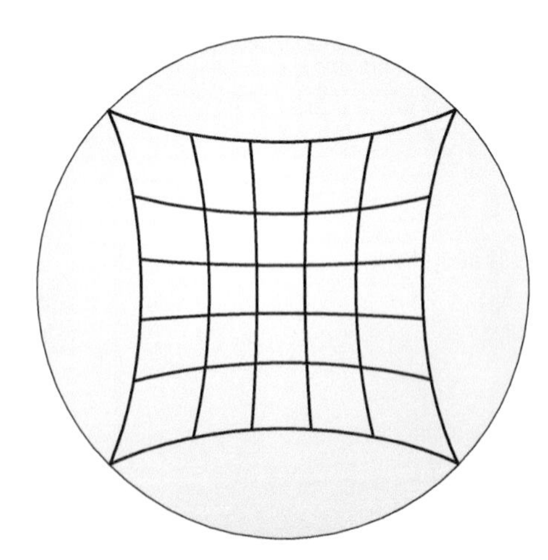

Figure 27.10. Example of pincushion distortion.

the image intensifier. Remember that when using the magnification mode, the center of the input phosphor is used. The resulting image has less shape distortion and improved spatial resolution.

Quantum Mottle

Quantum mottle is the grainy appearance, which is caused by insufficient radiation to produce a uniform image. Quantum mottle is controlled by mA and time. In fluoroscopy, a minimum number of photons are used to activate the fluoroscopy screen; this can create noise on the video image and the grainy appearance. Various factors influence quantum mottle, and increasing the efficiency of any of the factors will assist in reducing quantum mottle. The factors are radiation output, beam attenuation by the patient, the conversion efficiency of the input phosphor, minification gain, flux gain, total brightness gain, and the viewing system. Although several of these factors are out of the control of the radiographer, the most useful solution is to increase the mA setting to the fluoroscopy tube.

Fluoroscopic Displays

The most commonly used method of viewing the fluoroscopic image is the television monitor. Before the image can be viewed, it must go through various types of equipment to make the electrical signal visible to the human eye. The output phosphor of the image intensifier can be coupled to a camera tube for TV monitor viewing or to a spot film camera or **cine** camera. A closed-circuit video signal is sent to a TV monitor for visualization of the dynamic imaging; cine and spot film images provide permanent records of the examination. Figure 27.11 illustrates how the image from the output phosphor of the image intensifier can be viewed or recorded in different ways. A beam-splitting mirror sends the output phosphor image to both the spot film camera and the camera tube for viewing on the TV monitor system.

Figure 27.12A and B shows an illustration of the target assembly. The target assembly of a typical **camera tube** shows a large video signal produced by a large amount

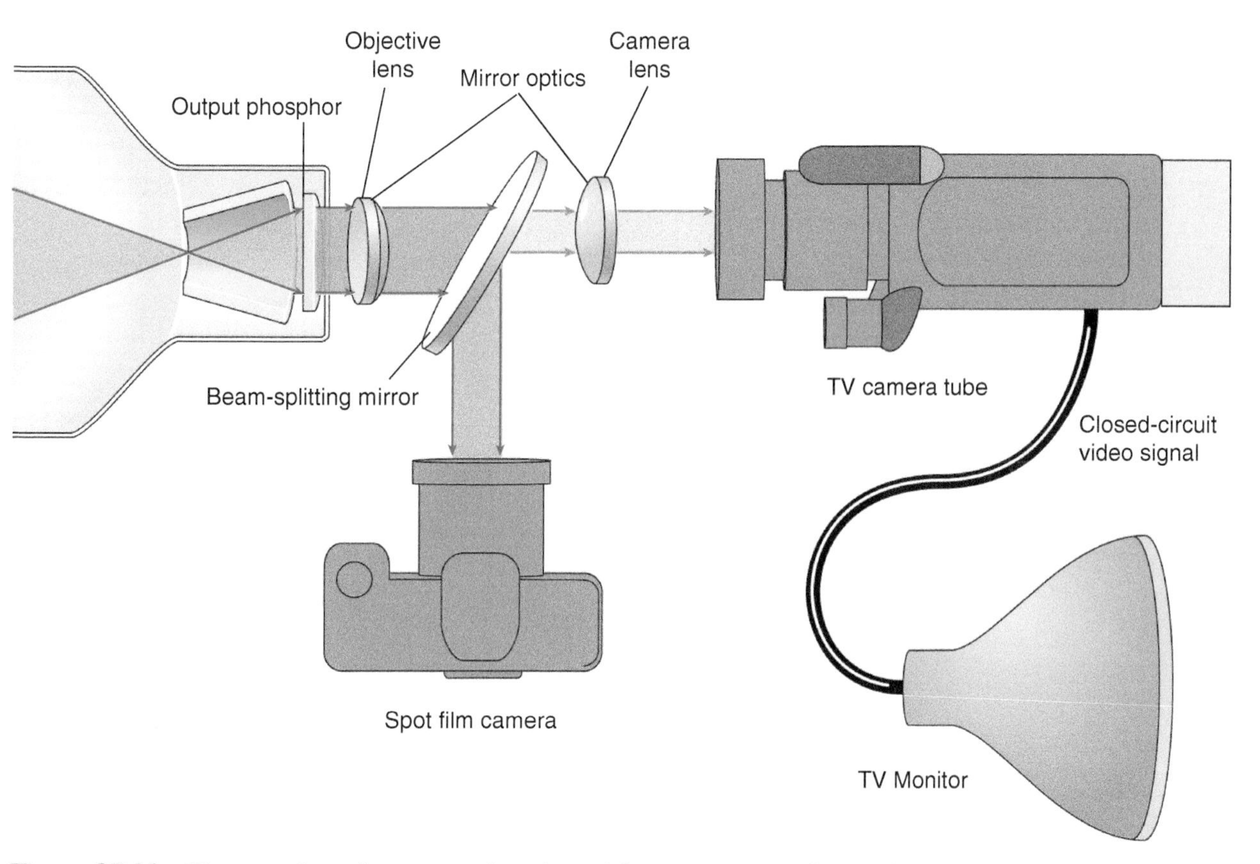

Figure 27.11. Illustrates how the output phosphor of the image intensifier can be viewed or recorded in different ways.

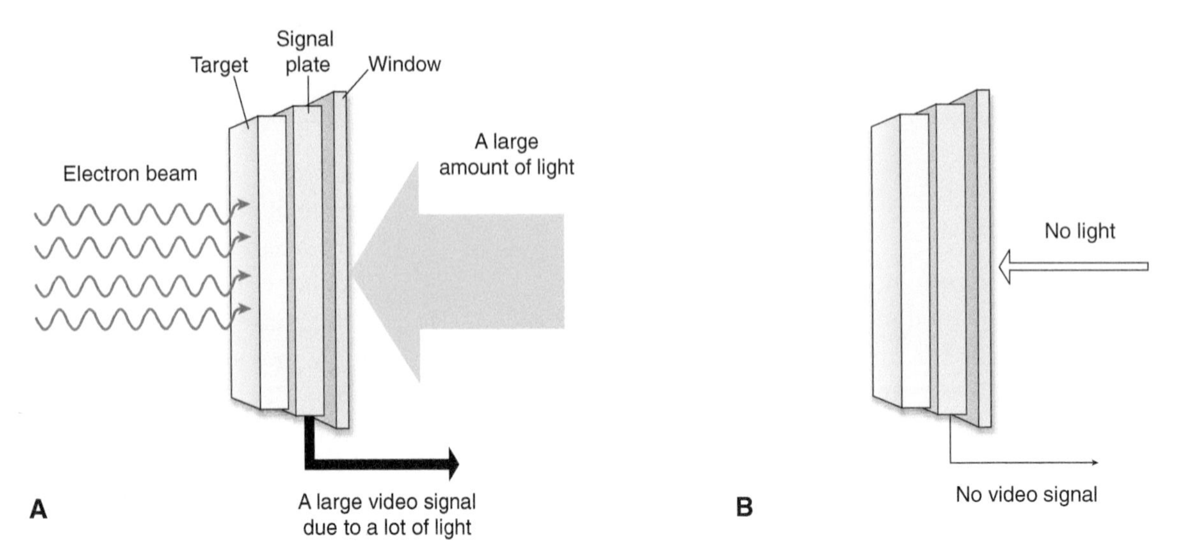

Figure 27.12. **(A) and (B) demonstrate an illustration of the target assembly when illuminated and the resulting video signal.**

of light striking the window compared to no video signal generated from no visible light striking the window of the target assembly.

The synchronized image intensifier is viewed with a camera tube and displayed on a TV monitor. The camera tube is similar to a home video camera. The camera tube converts the light image from the output phosphor into electrical signals that are displayed on a standard TV monitor. There are two devices used today to accomplish the viewing of the fluoroscopic image: the camera tube and the charge-coupled device.

Camera Tube

The camera tube most commonly used is the vidicon. Occasionally the plumbicon camera tube is used. The vidicon and plumbicon tubes are similar in operation; however, the plumbicon tube has a faster response time. The tubes have a glass envelope, which maintains a vacuum and provides support for the internal components (Fig. 27.13). Inside the camera tubes are a cathode and an electron gun, electrostatic grids, and the target assembly that is also the anode.

Cathode

The cathode has a heating assembly, which forms an electron gun through the process of thermionic emission. The cathode consists of an electron gun that provides a continuous stream of electrons and a control grid that forms the electron stream into an electron beam. The tube is surrounded by focusing and accelerating grids

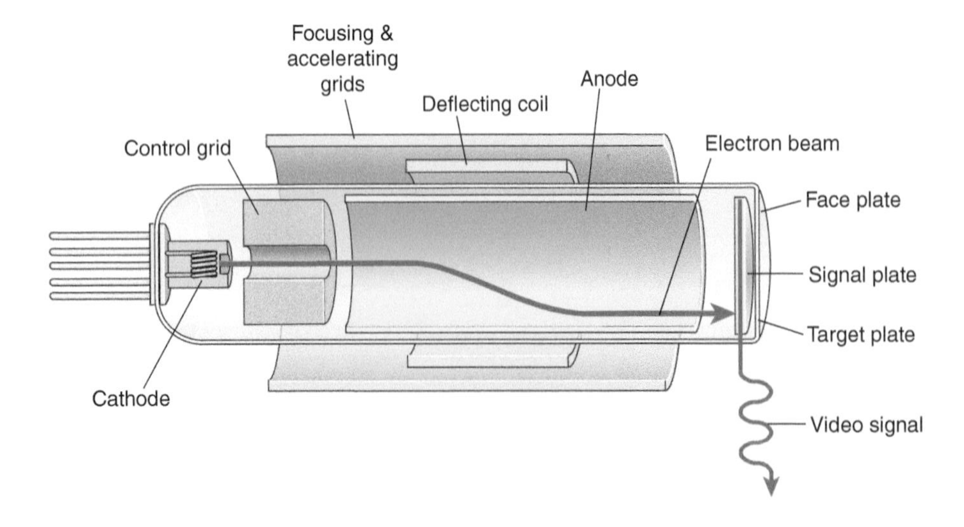

Figure 27.13. **A camera tube and the internal components.**

and deflection coils. These coils accelerate and control the electron beam toward the anode. The coils make the beam sweep across the anode from top to bottom in a pattern known as a raster pattern.

Anode

The anode in the vidicon or plumbicon tubes has a target assembly comprised of three layers: the faceplate, signal plate, and target plate. The faceplate acts as the window and is the thinnest part of the glass envelope, which is closest to the output phosphor on the image intensifier; this allows the transition of light from the output phosphor to the camera tube. The signal plate has a thin coating of graphite material on the inside of the glass window that conducts electricity; the signal plate is bonded to the faceplate. The graphite layer is thin enough to transmit light, which is traveling through the faceplate but thick enough to be an efficient electrical conductor to conduct the electronic signal that is generated in the camera tube out of the tube and into the external video circuit.

The target plate is coated with a photoconductive layer, vidicon tubes use antimony trisulfide, and plumbicon tubes use lead oxide. The photoconductive layer is capable of absorbing light photons and releasing the amount of electrons, which are equivalent to the intensity of the absorbed light, thereby making up the video signal. At the target, the electron beam passes through a wire mesh control grid and interacts with the target assembly where the beam is slowed down. The control grid also aligns the electron beam so that it is oriented properly when it interacts with the anode.

Now that you know the various parts of the camera tube, let us discuss the whole process of making the image visible on the monitor. The electron beam is activated and starts sweeping the anode target plate. Light from the output phosphor of the image intensifier travels through the faceplate and signal plate to the opposite side of the target layer. When the electron beam and light from the output phosphor strike the same place at precisely the same time, the electrons will be transmitted (conducted) through the target plate to the signal plate. The signal plate then carries the electron beam as an electric signal via cables to the television monitor where it is reconstructed to form a visible image. When the electron beam is in a different location in its sweep than a particular photon of light from the output phosphor, the target plate will act as an insulator. This action of the target plate, conducting or insulating, modulates the electronic signal. This means that the greater the light intensity, the greater the number of electrons being transmitted and the greater the magnitude of the electronic signal. This all provides variations in brightness to different parts of the television image in order for the various shades of gray to be visualized.

Coupling Devices to the Image Intensifier

The vidicon tube is connected to the output phosphor of the image intensification tube by either fiber optics or an optical lens system. Of these methods, the fiber optics is only a few millimeters thick and contains thousands of glass fibers. The small size of the fiber optics is an advantage when manipulating the image intensification tower. The fiber optics coupling allows the use of cassettes to record spot films, but it doesn't allow the use of cine or spot film cameras. Cine and spot filming requires the optical lens system. Spot filming requires the use of beam-splitting mirrors, which permit the image to be recorded while being viewed. As seen in Figure 27.14, optical lens systems are much larger than the fiber optics coupling and are easily identified by the large size of the housing on top of the image intensification tube. Careful handling to avoid trauma is essential to keep the mirror and lens system precisely balanced.

Charge-Coupled Device

Some fluoroscopy systems use a **charge-coupled device (CCD)** instead of a camera tube. The CCD is a light-sensitive semiconducting device that generates an electrical charge when stimulated by light and is capable of storing a charge in a capacitor. When light strikes the photoelectric cathode, electrons are released in response to the intensity of the incident light. The CCD has a series of metal oxide semiconducting capacitors; each capacitor represents a pixel. The electric charge is stored in rows of pixels, and each pixel is comprised of three polysilicon gates. To digitize the charge, the gates of each pixel are charged in sequence thereby moving the signal down the row where it is transferred into a capacitor. The charge then leaves the capacitor and is sent as an

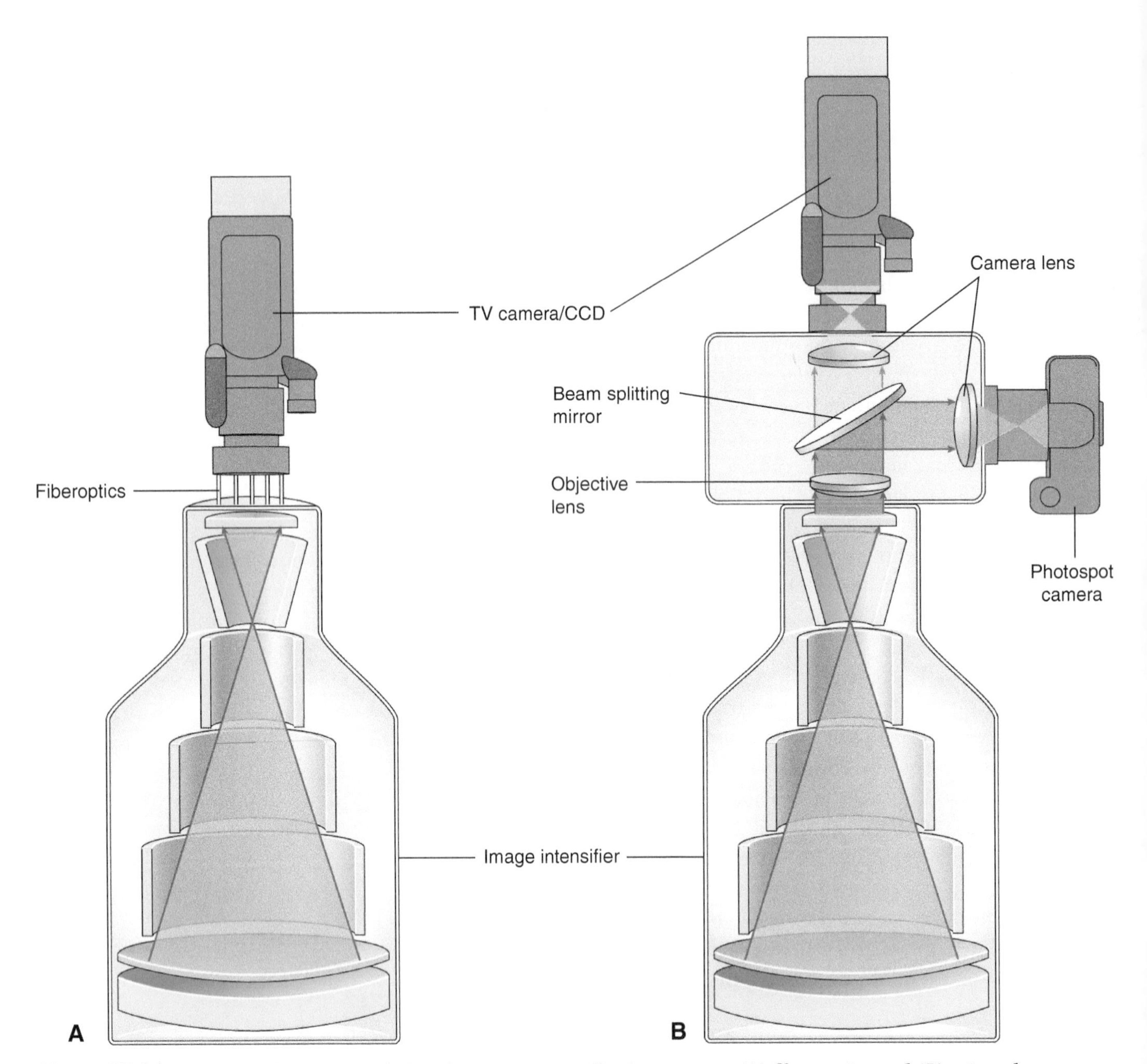

Figure 27.14. **Camera tubes are coupled to the image intensifier in two ways, (A) fiber optics and (B) mirror lens system.**

electronic signal to the television monitor. A video signal is then emitted in a raster pattern by discharging the stored electrons as pulses.

The video signal is amplified and transmitted by cable to the television monitor where it is transformed back into a visible image. The process of constructing the image on a television monitor is explained in Chapter 25. The main advantage of the CCD is the extremely fast discharge time, which is useful in cardiac catheterization where high-speed imaging is critical to visualizing blood flow. The CCD operates at a lower voltage, which prolongs its life, it is more sensitive than camera tubes, and its resolution is adequate for imaging structures in the body.

Digital Fluoroscopy

As with other advancements in digital imaging, digital fluoroscopy has evolved over time. Early versions added an analog-to-digital converter to the conventional fluoroscopy unit and placed a computer between the

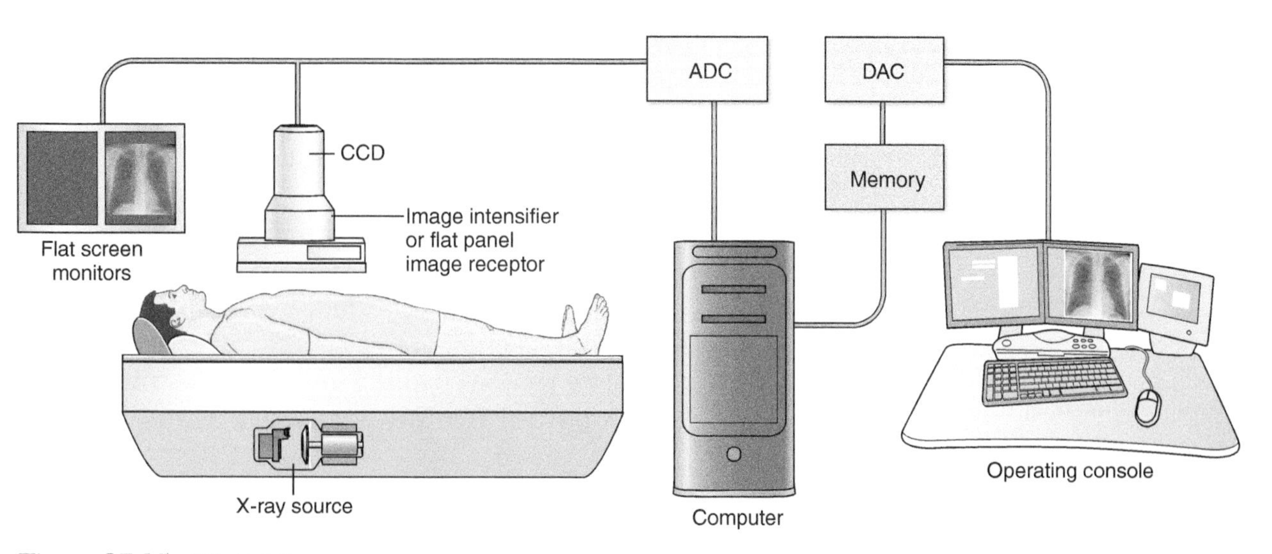

Figure 27.15. **Digital fluoroscopy system components.**

camera tube and monitor. Recall that the ADC takes the video signal and converts it to binary code the computer can understand. The computer can then process and display the digital image (Fig. 27.15). The digital image can then be postprocessed and stored in the archives.

Incorporation of the CCD further improved fluoroscopy and helped to bring it into the digital era. Compared to the camera tube, the CCD is more light sensitive (higher detective quantum efficiency [DQE]), has a low level of electronic noise, has no spatial distortion, has higher signal-to-noise resolution, has better contrast resolution, and requires less radiation. All of these provide the patient with a higher-quality examination and lower radiation dose.

The CCD is mounted to the output phosphor of the image intensifier tube and is coupled through either fiber optics or a lens system (Fig. 27.16). Notice the device labeled "ABS sensor." With this system, a sample of light from the image intensifier is measured and is used to determine if the ABS system needs to make any adjustments in kVp, mA, or both to compensate for fluctuations in the signal.

CCD's main advantage is their compact size and durability. The size of the CCD and the number of pixels determine the spatial resolution of the system. Systems with a 1,024 matrix produce images with 10 Lp/mm spatial resolution. Unlike camera tubes, which can have spatial distortion that is described as a "pincushion appearance," the CCD has no such distortion. The advantages of a CCD for use in medical imaging are located in Table 27.1.

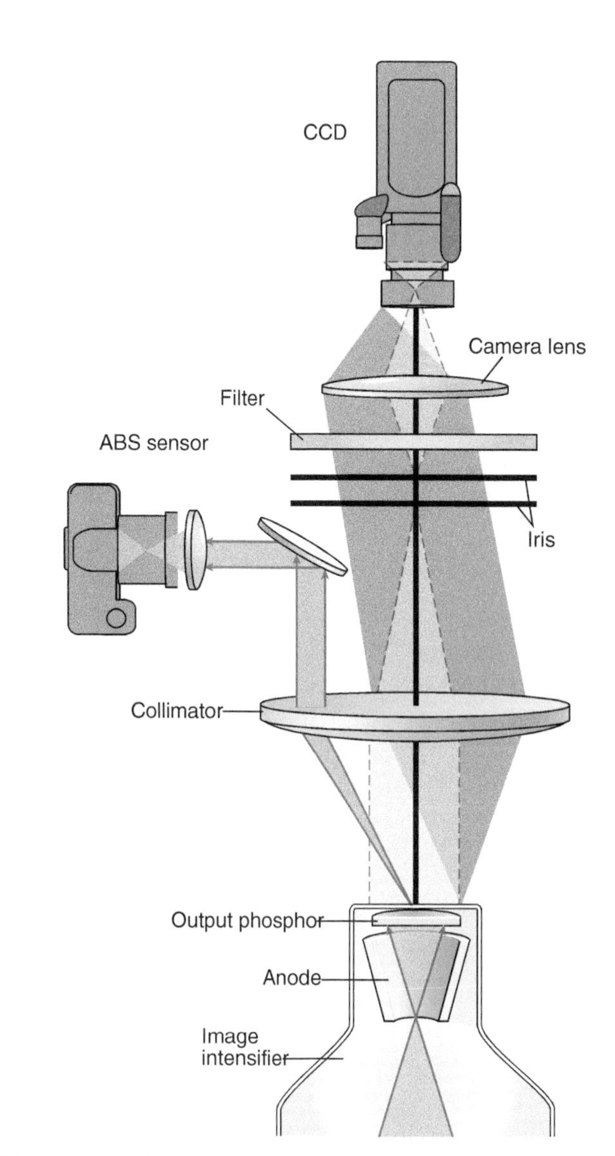

Figure 27.16. **Illustration of a lens-coupling system for a charge-coupled device to an image intensifier.**

TABLE 27.1 **ADVANTAGES OF CCDs FOR MEDICAL IMAGING**

- High spatial resolution
- High signal-to-noise resolution
- High DQE
- No warm-up required
- No screen lag
- No spatial distortion
- No maintenance
- Unlimited life span
- Lower patient radiation dose

Dynamic Flat Panel Detectors

A recent advancement in digital fluoroscopy is the replacement of the image intensifier with dynamic flat panel detectors (DFPD). There are two types of dynamic FPDs: an indirect-capture detector using a cesium iodide phosphor coupled to an active matrix array (AMA) of amorphous silicon TFTs and a direct-capture detector using an AMA of amorphous selenium TFTs. Each of these are described in Chapter 20, refer back for a refresher of the mechanics of each detector. The DFPDs have several differences compared to those used for routine radiography.

The DFPDs have larger physical dimensions and larger matrix sizes up to 2,048 × 2,048 pixels. Pixel sizes of 200 to 300 μm are used in digital fluoroscopy detectors, twice as large as those used for digital radiography detectors (100 to 150 μm). The DFPDs must respond in rapid sequences to create a dynamic image. The dynamic FPDs can operate in either continuous or pulsed x-ray modes. The readout electronics must be able to handle high frame rates up to 60 frames per second. This is accomplished by the active matrix processes, which rapidly process the image data; the flat panel is a two-dimensional rectilinear array of pixels that is processed line by line in a fraction of a second.

For digital fluoroscopy applications, a very low noise dynamic FPD system is needed. Fluoroscopy typically operates with a low-dose output, which means that any operational noise will degrade the fluoroscopic image. Unfortunately, this makes noise a greater factor in digital detectors. The active matrix uses application-specific integrated circuits (ASIC) to minimize noise and amplify the signal. These circuits are especially critical in fluoroscopy because they minimize noise, maximize readout speed, and allow for switching between low-dose and high-dose inputs for spot imaging.

Most dynamic FPDs are also capable of a zoom feature, equivalent to the magnification mode for the image intensifier.

In dynamic FPDs, a light-emitting diode array is located below the detector, which produces a bright microsecond flash of light to erase images between frames to prevent "ghosting" caused by residual exposure charge from the previous frame. The LED erases the detector panel between each frame to prevent this phenomenon from occurring.

Dynamic FPDs have other advantages over conventional fluoroscopy including their contrast enhancement of low subject contrast anatomical structures, high DQE and dynamic range across all levels of exposure, and no appearance of distortion. DFPDs are also smaller in size and bulk, which make it easier to manipulate the unit; it has greater flexibility of movement and allows easier access to the patient throughout the procedure.

Archiving the Fluoroscopic Image

Fluoroscopic images can be recorded using cassette spot filming, photospot camera, digital display, a standard videocassette recorder (VCR), or a digital image recorder. VCRs and cine cameras record dynamic images. VCR images are analog images recorded on magnetic tape. Cine cameras record the images on a 35-mm movie film. Digital images provide a permanent static image of the anatomy viewed during fluoroscopy. Fluoroscopic images can also be digitized and stored as digital data.

Cassette Spot Film

Cassette spot filming is necessary when a permanent image of the fluoroscopic examination is needed to document the anatomy. Cassette spot filming is used with almost every fluoroscopic examination when the information is necessary to diagnose and has been the standard for many years. During the fluoroscopic examination, it is possible to use cassette spot filming to rapidly record a series of static images so that when viewed, they

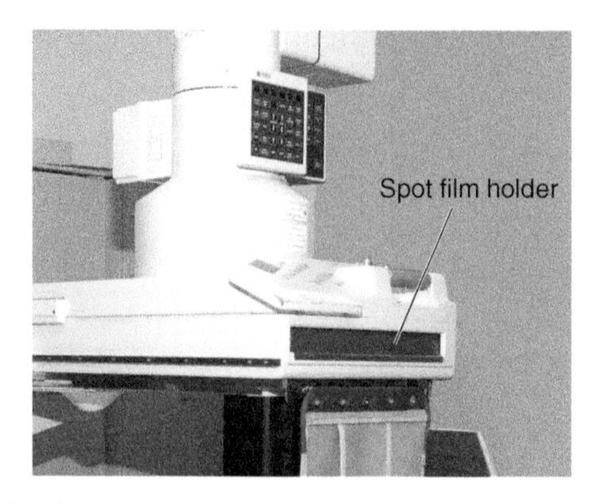

Figure 27.17. **Demonstrates the image intensifier with a slot film device for a standard radiographic cassette.**

provide a comprehensive record of the patient's anatomy and potential pathology. There are several methods for recording a spot film, including standard cassettes.

Standard radiographic cassettes allow the radiologist to record one image or multiple images on a film. Selections include 1-on-1, 2-on-1 vertical, 2-on-1 horizontal, or 4-on-1. Standard cassette sizes include 8 × 10 inch, 9 × 9 inch, or 10 × 12 inch. The image intensifier has a lead-lined compartment where the cassette is stored (Fig. 27.17). At the time of a spot film exposure, the radiologist must activate the control located on the fluoroscopic **carriage**, which moves the cassette into the primary beam between the patient and the image intensifier. The carriage controls allow selection of the area of the cassette to be exposed and automatically collimates the spot image mask shutters to the correct size. The radiologist must also change the operation of the tube from low fluoroscopic mA to high radiographic mA.

After an exposure or set of exposures is made, the radiographer is responsible for replacing the cassettes that have been exposed with new cassettes for further imaging. Cassette spot filming is a slow process due to the time required to place the cassette for the exposure. This type of imaging causes the highest dose to the patient due to the increased mA necessary to produce a diagnostic image.

Photospot Camera

Photospot cameras or film cameras have also been commonly used with conventional fluoroscopy. The photospot camera is similar to a movie camera except it exposes one frame at a time; it uses a 70-mm roll film or 105-mm "chip" film. The photospot camera can also be used to obtain static images where an optical lens system with a beam-splitting mirror is used. When the spot film exposure switch is activated or pressed, the beam-splitting mirror is moved into place. The fluoroscopic beam will strike the mirror diverting some of the beam toward the photospot camera and exposing the film, while the remainder of the beam produces an image on the television monitor. This allows the fluoroscopist to view the image while it is being recorded. This device receives the visible light from the output phosphor and is exposing the film photographically. This system allows for very rapid imaging of up to 12 frames per second. Because it is using the image directly off the output phosphor, it requires approximately half the radiation dose of the cassette spot-filming system.

Video Recording

Video recording makes a permanent record of the dynamic fluoroscopic images on magnetic tape. VHS and high-resolution VHS-S videotape recorders are used to create the dynamic images. The VHS-S system requires high-resolution cameras, recorders, tape, and monitors, which offer a significant increase in resolution that is desirable for viewing fluoroscopic examinations. During the fluoroscopic examination, the record button is pressed on the system, and it records the "moving" images from the monitor. It is very useful for physicians to be able to view functional examinations of the esophagus or placement of central lines or medical devices.

Cine Recording

Fluoroscopic images can also be recorded on a 16- and 35-mm movie film. Such recording is referred to as cinefluoroscopy, or simply cine. The output phosphor image is directed to the cine camera by a beam-splitting mirror. Cine image recording uses a 16- or 35-mm film to record static images at a high speed typically at 30 or 60 frames per second. Special x-ray tubes and generators that pulse the x-rays so that the x-ray beam is on only when the cine film is in position and the camera shutter is open are required. Cine imaging is common in angiography and cardiac catheterization. The cine film can be viewed as both a movie and stop-action film. It must be shown at 16 frames per second for smooth motion to occur. The principal advantage of cine recording is the improved spatial resolution; however, radiation exposure rates are about ten times greater than in conventional fluoroscopy.

Although it is necessary to understand different methods of capturing a fluoroscopic image, the use of cine, VHS, and VHS-S is rapidly becoming obsolete with the advancement of digital fluoroscopic technology.

Mobile C-arm Fluoroscopy

Mobile C-arm units are portable fluoroscopy systems that are used in the operating room, the emergency room, and many other areas when it is not possible to bring the patient to the radiology department. Figure 27.18 shows a typical C-arm unit. The name comes from the physical connection between the x-ray tube and the image intensifier, which looks like a "C." The tube and image intensifier can be moved to provide anteroposterior, posteroanterior, oblique, or lateral fluoroscopic examinations as needed. C-arm fluoroscopes are equipped with last image hold and digital recording capabilities.

Last Image Hold

Some fluoroscopic units can display the last image when x-ray production is stopped. This is also known as "freeze frame" capability. The output image is digitized and continuously displayed on the output monitor. Most portable C-arm fluoroscopic units have this capability. It allows the operator to study the image without continuously exposing the patient and staff to additional radiation.

Patient Dose

The patient dose during fluoroscopy depends on the patient thickness, the exposure rate, and the duration of exposure. Higher exposure rates, thicker patients, and longer fluoroscopic examinations produce higher patient doses.

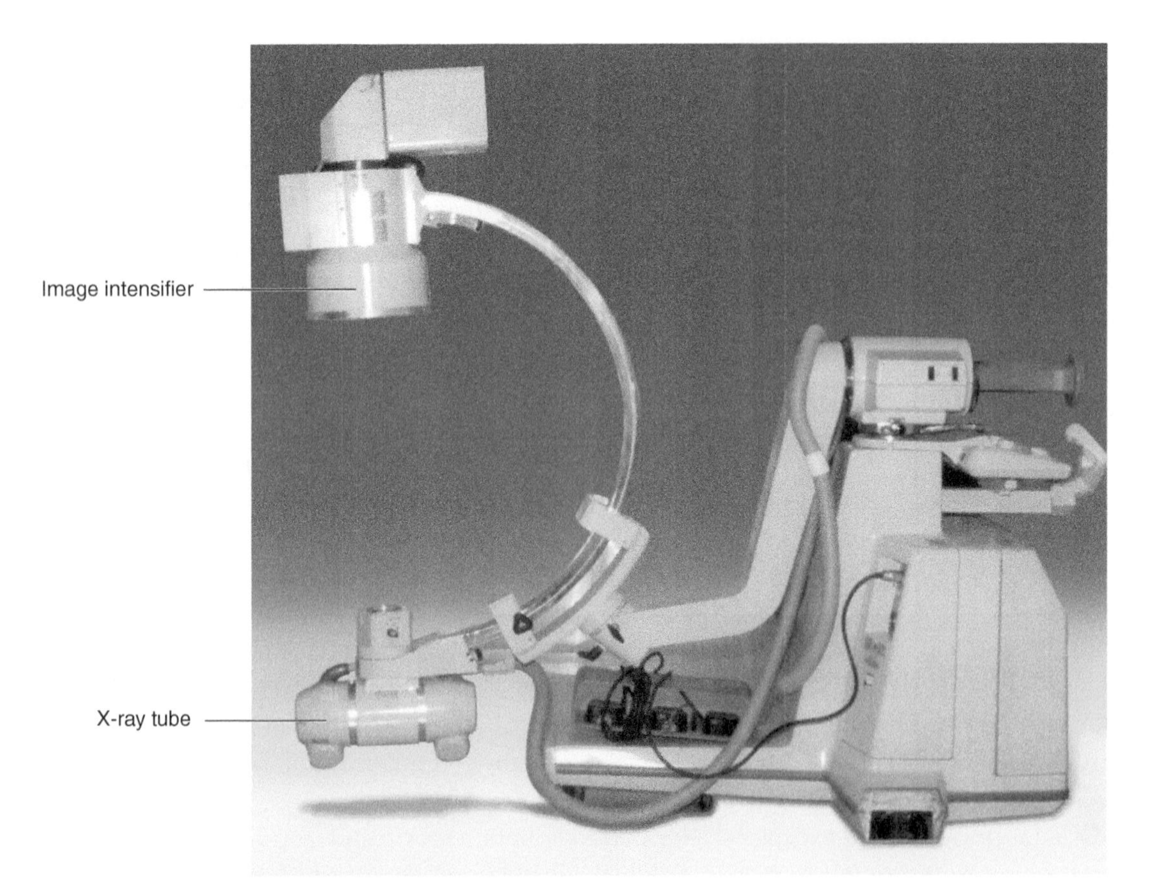

Figure 27.18. **Shows a typical C-arm unit.**

The exposure of the patient depends on the thickness and density of the body part being examined, the distance from the image intensifier to the patient, and the image intensifier magnification. A change in any of these factors changes the exposure rate because the ABC circuit adjusts the mA to maintain constant output brightness. This mA adjustment changes the patient dose. Thicker, dense body parts are more difficult to penetrate and require higher exposure rates, resulting in higher patient doses.

The x-ray intensity at the image intensifier depends on the source to image receptor distance (SID). Moving the image intensifier closer to the patient decreases the SID and increases the beam intensity at the surface of the input phosphor. This results in the ABC decreasing the mA and producing a lower patient dose.

In addition to patient dose, other factors must be considered when using a fluoroscopic system. The **entrance skin exposure** (ESE) for the patient is that part of the patient that is closest to the x-ray source. For units with the x-ray tube under the table, the ESE is measured from the patient surface next to the tabletop. With the x-ray tube over the table, the ESE is measured from the patient surface closest to the fluoroscopy carriage. The tabletop exposure rate should not exceed 10 R/min, with most units averaging from 1 to 3 R/min. The minimum source to skin distance for mobile fluoroscopic equipment (C-arms) is 12 inches, while 15 inches is standard for stationary fluoroscopic equipment.

Fluoroscopic Timer

All fluoroscopic systems are equipped with a timer as required by law. The timer must indicate the amount of time that has elapsed while the fluoroscopic beam is on. The timer can either use an audible signal or temporary or permanent interruption of the live beam when 5 minutes of fluoroscopy has elapsed; this serves as a reminder to the fluoroscopist of how much exposure time has been used. There is no limit to the number of times the signal may be reset; however, this does not reset the timer. At the end of the procedure, the total amount of time will be displayed on the control console. Some departments record the fluoroscopy time in the patient's record so that the total fluoroscopic dose can be calculated as necessary.

Chapter Summary

1. Fluoroscopy is a method of viewing dynamic moving structures. A fluoroscopic system contains an x-ray tube, a patient support table, and an image intensifier.
2. The image intensifier produces a brighter image by converting x-ray photons into visible light at the input phosphor, converting visible light into electrons at the photocathode, accelerating and focusing the electrons onto the output phosphor, and finally converting the electrons into visible light at the output phosphor.
3. An ABC circuit maintains the brightness of the output phosphor at a constant level by adjusting the fluoroscopic mA.
4. Brightness gain is a combination of flux gain and minification gain. The output phosphor is brighter than the input phosphor because of brightness gain.
5. Flux gain is produced by the acceleration of electrons in the image intensifier tube.
6. Minification gain is produced because the output phosphor is smaller than the input phosphor.
7. A camera tube views the output phosphor image and displays the image on a standard TV monitor.
8. Distortion, pincushion appearance, vignetting, and image noise are common problems with image intensifiers.

9. The CCD is another method of coupling the image intensifier to the TV monitor. It is a light-sensitive semiconducting device that generates an electrical signal when stimulated by light and stores the charge in a capacitor.
10. Digital fluoroscopy systems use flat panel detectors to capture the dynamic image. The detectors are either indirect capture or direct capture.
11. Compared to conventional fluoroscopy, flat panel detectors have many advantages including reduction in size and bulk, easier manipulation, ability to capture more frames per second, etc.
12. Digital fluoroscopy uses LEDs to "erase" residual exposure on the frames to prevent "ghosting" from being seen on subsequent images.
13. Fluoroscopic images can be recorded on spot films, videotape, or cine film.
14. Patient dose is affected by patient size, the amount of magnification, and the distance between the patient and the image intensifier input surface.
15. All fluoroscopic systems must have a timer to audibly indicate when 5 minutes of fluoroscopic beam on time has elapsed.

Case Study

Tami is the lead radiographer in her radiology department. She is researching fluoroscopy equipment so she can advise administration on an upcoming purchase. She discovered that there are many different types of machines, but they were all very similar. The information Tami discovered included image intensifiers with variable magnification modes, different video camera tubes and CCDs, types of image display, and how to archive the image. In her report, Tami will answer the following questions.

Critical Thinking Questions

1. How does image intensifier compare in size?
2. How is magnification achieved? Which video camera tube or CCD will meet the department's work flow?
3. What types of archiving are available?

Review Questions

Multiple Choice

1. Changing from standard to magnification mode on an image intensifier:

1. increases the patient dose
2. decreases the patient dose
3. produces a magnified image
4. decreases the minification gain

a. 2, 3, and 4
b. 1 and 3
c. 1, 3, and 4
d. 2 and 4

2. Brightness gain is the product of the ________ gains.

a. magnification and minification
b. minification and flux
c. flux and magnification
d. confiscation and flux

3. The ________ have good spatial resolution and are used for viewing in bright light.

a. rods
b. cones
c. optic discs
d. olfactory bulbs

4. Multiplying the flux gain by the minification gain in the image intensifier will equal the total:

a. input phosphor size
b. image size
c. output phosphor size
d. brightness gain

5. The TV camera converts the light image from the output phosphor into a(an):

a. brighter image
b. high-resolution image
c. magnified light image
d. electrical signal

6. The input phosphor of an image intensifier is coated with which material?

a. Zinc cadmium sulfide
b. Calcium tungstate
c. Cesium iodide
d. Iron oxide

7. Light photons are converted into electrons by which part of the image intensifier?

a. Input phosphor
b. Anode
c. Output phosphor
d. Photocathode

8. The focusing electrostatic lenses in the image intensifier:

a. force photoelectrons to converge on the output phosphor
b. convert photoelectrons into light photons
c. convert light photons into photoelectrons
d. force photoelectrons to converge on the input phosphor

9. The lead drape on the image intensifier tower must have a minimum of:

a. 50 mm Pb equivalent
b. 10 mm Pb equivalent
c. 25 mm Al equivalent
d. 25 mm Pb equivalent

10. What is the flux gain if the input phosphor has 100 x-ray photons and the output phosphor has 6,000 light photons?

a. 6
b. 60
c. 0.16
d. 16

11. What is the total brightness gain if the flux gain is 47 and the minification gain is 80?

a. 2,500
b. 1.7
c. 3,760
d. 1,880

12. The minimum distance between the source and the patient skin surface for a mobile fluoroscopic unit is __________ inches.

a. 15
b. 10
c. 25
d. 12

13. Which flat panel detector uses cesium iodide amorphous silicon?

a. Direct capture
b. Indirect capture

14. A fluoroscopy system using a CCD and a 1,024 pixel matrix will produce images with __________ of spatial resolution.

a. 5 Lp/mm
b. 15 Lp/mm
c. 10 Lp/mm
d. 20 Lp/mm

15. Which of these is not considered an advantage of using a CCD in a fluoroscopy system?

a. There is no screen lag while moving the tower.
b. No warm-up is required.
c. Unlimited life expectancy.
d. Increased patient dose.

Short Answer

1. Draw a diagram of an image intensifier tube and discuss the function of each part.

2. What is vignetting?

3. The electron gun in a vidicon is a heated filament that supplies a constant electron current by:

4. During a fluoroscopic examination, the radiologist sees something and would like to preserve that image on a 2-on-1 __________.

5. What is the formula to determine brightness gain?

6. What are the basic components of the tube used in a video camera?

7. What is the difference between rod and cone vision? When is visual acuity greater? Define photopic and scotopic vision.

8. The cassette spot film is placed between the __________ and the __________.

9. What is the purpose of the ABC?

10. What are the types of dynamic and static filming systems used to record the fluoroscopic image?

11. What are the advantages of digital fluoroscopy over conventional fluoroscopy?

28

Imaging Equipment

Objectives

Upon completion of this chapter, the student will be able to:

1. Describe the principles of linear tomography.
2. Recognize the variations between mobile and dedicated units and linear tomography.
3. State the purpose of dedicated units and identify their unique features.

Key Terms

- exposure angle
- focal plane
- fulcrum
- linear tomography
- mobile
- object plane
- panoramic tomography (panorex)
- pivot point
- section interval
- section thickness
- tomographic angle

Introduction

Medical imaging has a variety of specialized equipment that is used to improve visualization of anatomic tissue. The improved visualization makes it easier to identify pathologic processes. Radiographers need to be familiar with the unique features of the specialized equipment used in the radiography department. Additional education and applications training may be required to operate this equipment in a safe and competent manner.

Linear Tomography

thePoint® *An animation for this topic can be viewed at http://thepoint.lww.com/Orth2e.*

In a conventional radiographic image, all the structures are seen with equal clarity even though the structures are superimposing each other. The three-dimensional objects are imaged in only two dimensions, making it very difficult to locate pathologies or small anatomic structures. **Linear tomography** is a special technique used to improve the visualization of selected objects by blurring structures located above and below the objects of interest. Tomography overcomes superimposition by utilizing principles based on the synchronous movement of two elements: the x-ray tube and the image receptor.

With linear tomography, the x-ray tube and Bucky are connected either by a vertical rod or electronically. The x-ray tube and Bucky are moved in synchronous but opposite directions. The movement of the Bucky and tube creates motion on the image that blurs structures above and below the focal plane, an area of relatively clear anatomical structures that lie in the plane of interest. In this specialized imaging technique, motion makes it easier to visualize structures. Tomographic exposures employ longer exposure times with lower mA values. In addition to selecting the appropriate technical factors, the radiographer must select each of the following to produce a tomographic image:

- Fulcrum: pivot point of the tomographic image
- Object plane or focal plane: area of tissue that appears in focus
- Tomographic angle: total distance the tube travels
- Exposure angle: distance the tube travels during the exposure
- Section thickness: width of the focal plane, controlled by tomographic angle
- Sectional interval: distance between fulcrum levels

Fulcrum

During movement of the x-ray tube and image receptor, there is a fixed point called the **pivot point** or **fulcrum**. The location of the fulcrum lies within the object plane or focal plane and corresponds to the center of the anatomic area to be imaged. Tomographic equipment has an adjustable fulcrum that moves up and down while the patient remains stationary.

Object Plane or Focal Plane

Structures that lie above and below the **object plane** appear blurred, while objects in the object or **focal plane** are relatively sharp and in focus in the tomographic images. The position of the object plane is defined by the level of the fulcrum. Changing the level of the fulcrum can be done by raising or lowering the table or the fulcrum. The level is measured in increments of millimeters or centimeters and is changed by the radiographer to set the body part being examined within the object plane (Fig. 28.1).

Tomographic Angle

The **tomographic angle** or arc is the total distance the tube travels. The tomographic angle determines the amount of tube and image receptor motion and is measured in

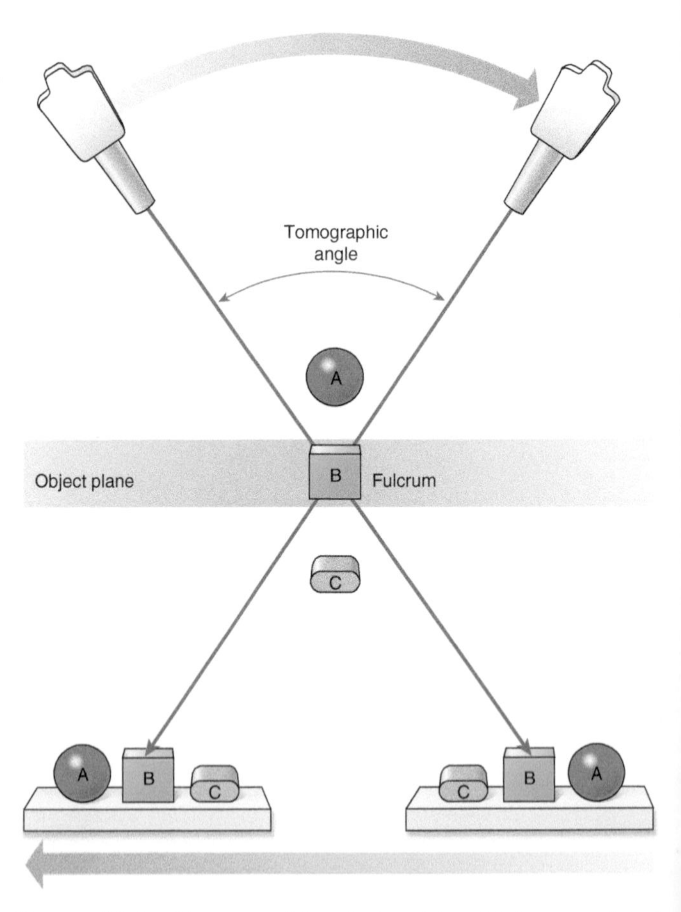

Figure 28.1. **Tomographic relationship of fulcrum, object plane, and tomographic angle.**

TABLE 28.1 TOMOGRAPHIC ANGLE AND RELATED SECTION THICKNESS

Tomographic Angle (Degrees)	Section Thickness (mm)
2	31
4	16
6	11
10	6
20	3
35	2
50	1

degrees. Larger tomographic angles produce thinner tomographic cuts. Smaller tomographic angles produce thicker tomographic cuts. A tomographic angle of 50 degrees produces a 1-mm-thick object plane, while a tomographic angle of 10 degrees produces a 6-mm thick object plane. Table 28.1 shows the approximate relationship between tomographic angle and section thickness.

The tomographic angle or arc also determines the amount of blur seen in an image. Increasing the tomographic angle increases the amount of blur, while decreasing the angle decreases the amount of blur. The location of structures in relation to the x-ray tube affects the amount of blur as well. To achieve maximum blurring, the area of interest should be perpendicular to the direction of x-ray tube movement. For example, when imaging the kidneys, the spine is a large structure that lies perpendicular to the x-ray tube. As the tube and image receptor move, the spine will be easily blurred. The kidneys lie parallel to the x-ray tube motion and will be demonstrated with less blur, which is needed to create a diagnostic image of the kidney structures.

Exposure Angle

The **exposure angle** is the distance the tube travels *during* the exposure. When the exposure switch is engaged, the x-ray tube will turn on the beam and will remain on during the entire exposure angle. The correct amount of time must be set to ensure the required amount of blurring will occur; typically, the exposure time must be increased. When the exposure time is too short, it doesn't allow for complete blurring and an exposure time that is too long will cause unnecessary exposure to the patient. As seen in Figure 28.2, the tomographic angle is longer than the exposure angle.

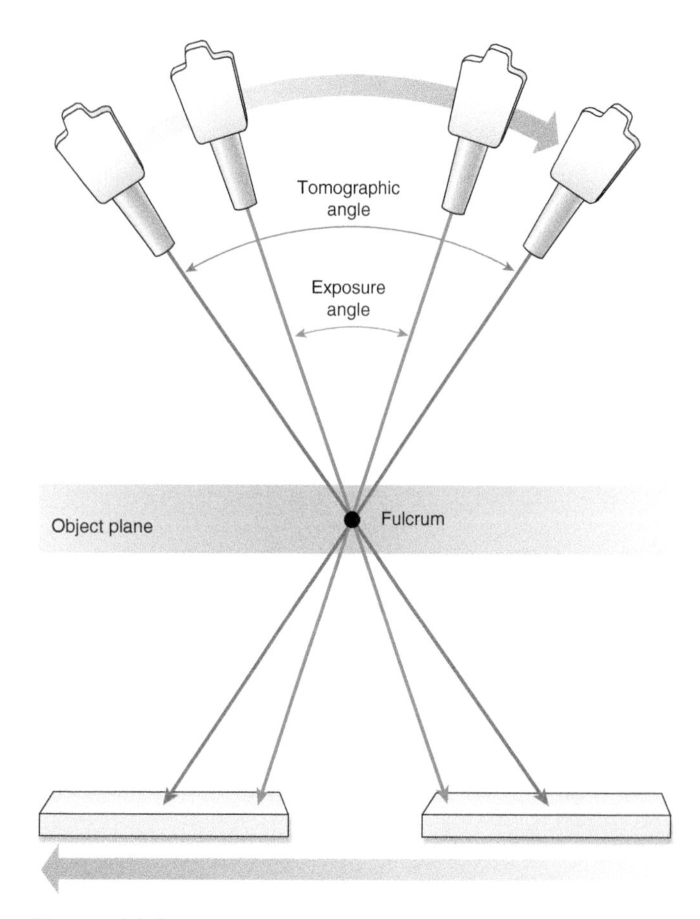

Figure 28.2. **Tomographic angle or amplitude in relation to exposure angle or amplitude.**

Section Thickness

Section thickness defines the width of the focal plane or the plane of tissue that will not be blurred. The section thickness is controlled by the tomographic angle. As stated under tomographic angle, long tomographic angles result in thinner cuts, which is preferred for small objects like renal calculi. Small tomographic angles result in thicker cuts, which demonstrates larger objects like vertebral bodies or the lungs (Fig. 28.3). Table 28.2 lists common tomographic examination and representative section thicknesses.

Section Interval

The **section interval** is the distance between fulcrum levels. The section interval should never exceed the section thickness. For example, when using a section thickness of 0.8 mm, the section interval should be 0.7 mm; as the fulcrum level is changed for subsequent tomographic slices, the tissue will overlap by 0.1 mm. This will provide a complete imaging sequence of the affected area without missing any tissue.

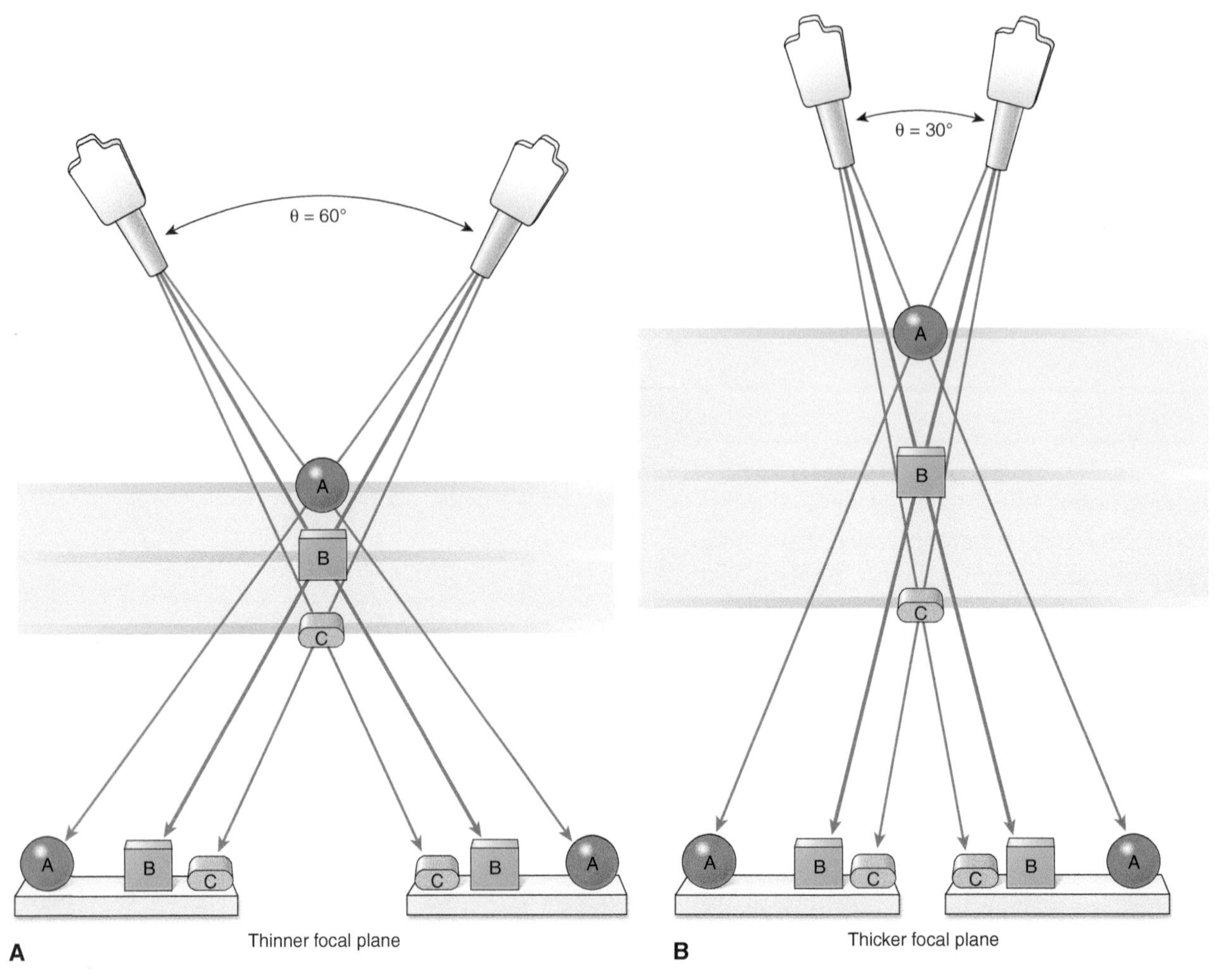

Figure 28.3. **Tomographic angle determines section thickness. (A) The large angle results in a thin slice of tissue. (B) The small angle results in a thick slice of tissue.**

Producing a Tomographic Image

Now that the fulcrum, tomographic angle, exposure angle, section thickness, and interval have been set, the radiographer is ready to produce an image. The tomographic examination begins with the x-ray tube and image receptor in a vertical orientation, positioned on opposite sides of the fulcrum. When the prep button is depressed each moves in a linear motion toward opposite ends of the table. Once the tube and Bucky are in position, the exposure switch is fully depressed and the exposure occurs at the same time the tube and Bucky move simultaneously over the patient. At the end of the exposure, the x-ray tube and Bucky return to the vertical position. The image of the anatomic object lying in the object plane will have a fixed position at the center of the image receptor throughout the tube movement. The images of structures, which lie above and below the object plane, will have varying positions on the image.

As seen in Figure 28.3, the images of points A and C are spread over the entire image receptor, while the position of B remains fixed on the image receptor throughout the

TABLE 28.2 **COMMON TOMOGRAPHIC EXAMINATIONS AND REPRESENTATIVE SECTION THICKNESSES**

Examination	Projection	Section Thickness
IV urogram	AP	1 cm
Wrist	AP	2 mm
Thorax	AP	2–5 cm
Cervical spine	AP	3–5 mm
Thoracic spine	AP	5 mm
Lumbar spine	AP	5 mm

tomographic motion. Consequently, the margins of A and C will be overlapped and will appear blurred. The blurring of objects lying outside the object plane is an example of motion blur caused by the motion of the x-ray tube. Of all the objects, object A has the greatest OID and will experience increasing motion blur with increasing distance from the object plane. Object C will experience less motion blur than object A and object B should have no motion blur.

Types of Tomography

The tomographic motion where the x-ray tube and image receptor move in a straight line is known as linear tomography. There are also more complicated motions such as circular, elliptical, hypocycloidal, and trispiral. These more complicated motions are used to image smaller structures and eliminate artifacts. The principal advantage of tomography is improved radiographic contrast due to the blurring motion of tissues outside of the object plane.

Dedicated Units

Dedicated units are radiographic units, which are designed for a specific imaging procedure. The use of these units may have limited applicability; however, radiographers must be familiar with each of these specialized systems.

Panoramic Tomography

Panoramic tomography (panorex) was first developed for use in dental practice. It has been increasingly used in diagnostic radiography to image curved structures such as the mandible. During the procedure, the x-ray tube and image receptor move around the patient's head (Fig. 28.4). The x-ray beam is tightly collimated to the center most portion of the beam. During the procedure, long exposure times are required to achieve the correct image. The tube and image receptor movement causes blurring of overlying and underlying tissues. The panorex is generally used for imaging the mandible because it provides a high-quality image with improved radiographic contrast.

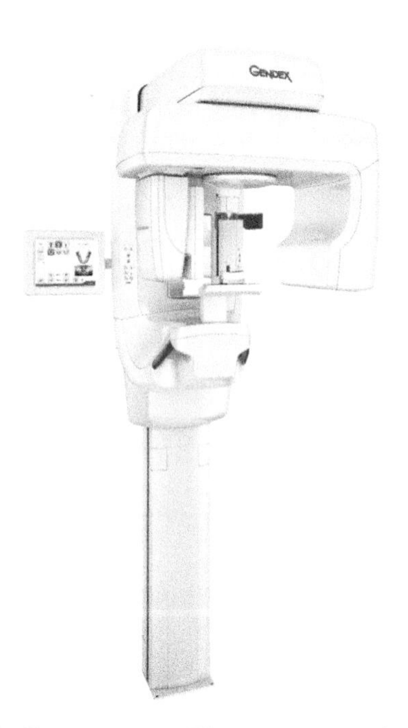

Figure 28.4. **Panorex unit. The unit moves the x-ray tube and image receptor around the patient. GXDP-700 Series Digital Panoramic Unit. (Image courtesy of KaVo Kerr Group.)**

Imaging the mandible can be challenging because of the curved nature of the bone. The panorex "straightens" the mandible and makes it appear flat on the image as seen in Figure 28.5. The advantage of the panorex image compared to a routine series of mandible images is that with one image, the entire mandible is seen with clarity.

Chest

Dedicated chest units are designed to image the thorax in the erect position. The Bucky mechanism is electronically connected to the x-ray tube; when the x-ray tube moves vertically, the Bucky automatically changes position to remain in alignment with the x-ray tube (Fig. 28.6). The image receptor can be a conventional film screen cassette, CR cassette, or DR plate. The conventional cassette uses radiographic film, which must be placed in an automatic processor. As discussed previously in this text, the image displayed on the radiographic film cannot be manipulated to improve the image; what you see is what you get. Digital imaging overcomes this problem, whether CR or DR was used, the images displayed on the monitor can be postprocessed to improve the image.

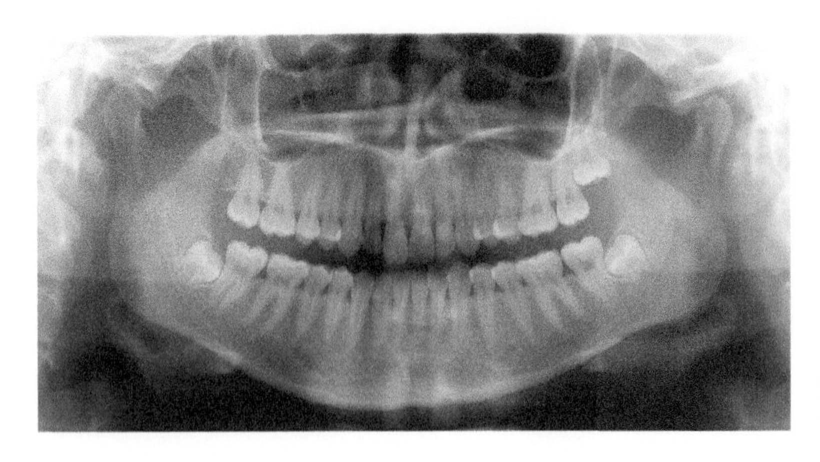

Figure 28.5. **Pan mandible image. (Image courtesy of KaVo Kerr Group.)**

The control panel is more compact with fewer preprogrammed exposure factor selections. Radiographers have the ability to use the AEC or manually set technical factors. Dedicated chest units improve efficiency and patients can be image more quickly. The use of such units improves workflow and patient care by standardizing a routine exam, that is, two-view chest x-rays.

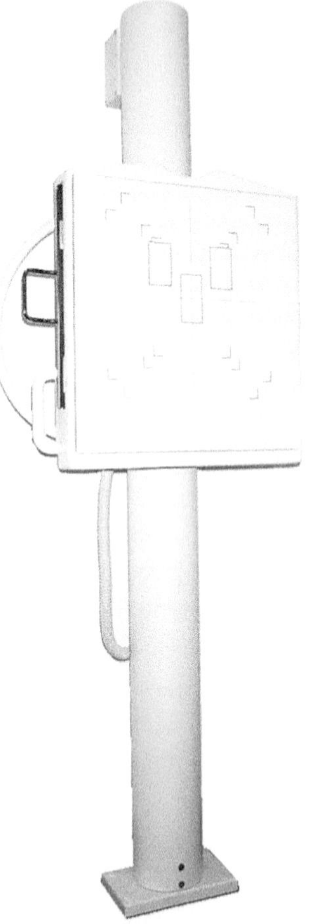

Figure 28.6. **Dedicated chest unit. (Reprinted from Virtual Imaging, Inc., a Canon company, with permission.)**

Mobile Radiographic Units

Mobile radiographic units are designed to be taken to a patient's room or surgery when a standard x-ray image is needed. Many patients are too ill or in critical condition, which makes it impossible to bring them to the radiology department for an exam. Mobile units are designed to provide the flexibility needed for imaging patients in unique settings (Fig. 28.7).

Mobile units are categorized in several ways: direct power, battery power, capacitor discharge, and high frequency. The direct power unit must be plugged into a wall outlet to make an exposure; this method is prone to power fluctuations, which affects the amount of radiation used. Battery units provide a more consistent exposure but have to be recharged. Capacitor discharge units must be plugged into a wall outlet during an exposure but provide a more consistent x-ray beam compared to direct power units. High-frequency units are lightweight and provide a consistent x-ray beam but must be plugged into a wall outlet during use. Exposure techniques can vary greatly depending on the type of mobile unit. Modern DR mobile units often use much less radiation compared to other mobile units.

Geometric Factors

The benefit of using mobile imaging is the flexibility to perform procedures in many locations. Imaging patients with a mobile unit presents many challenges.

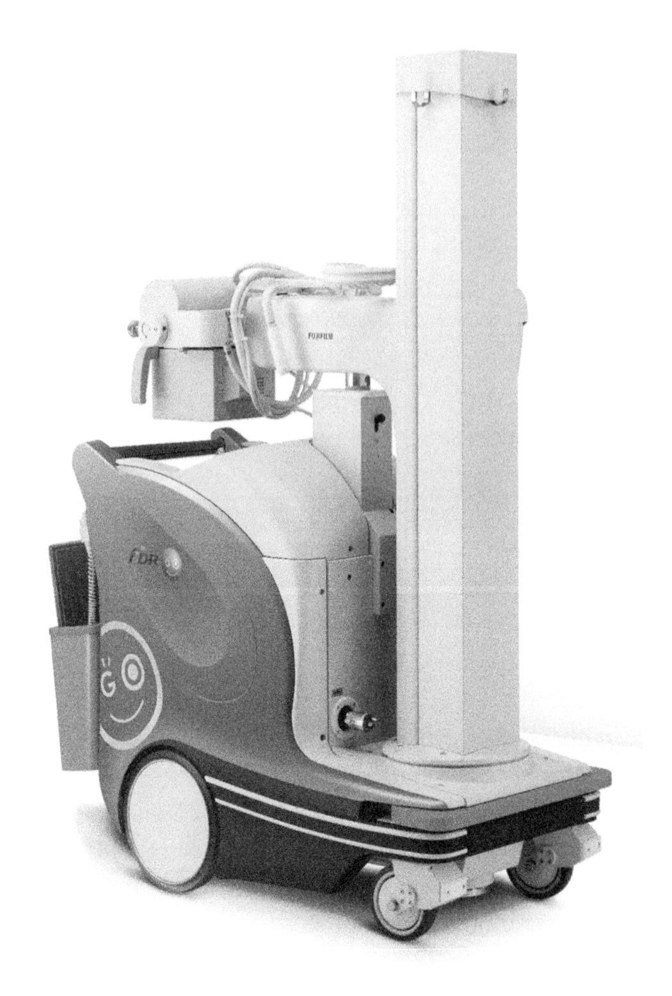

Figure 28.7. **Mobile radiographic unit. (Reprinted from FujiFilm Medical Systems USA, with permission.)**

Radiographers must assess the patient's condition to determine the correct alignment of the image receptor, x-ray tube, and patient. Radiographers often perform cross-table projections during mobile procedures, which can be challenging because of all the other equipment in the patient's room. The patient's room may have furniture, IV poles, and electrical cords, which may limit the use of the mobile unit.

The radiographer must be able to angle the tube in any conceivable direction while properly centering to the image receptor. It is crucial that the radiographer be able to manipulate the equipment to maintain proper image receptor and x-ray tube alignment. In the process, all distances and alignment must be preserved to maximize image sharpness while minimizing magnification and distortion.

SID Considerations

During a mobile procedure, the SID must often be estimated. If the unit has a tape measure that is attached to the tube or collimator, it should be used to assure the correct 40- or 72-inch SID is achieved. When a tape measure is not available, a 72-inch SID can be estimated as the distance from fingertip to fingertip of a 6-foot tall person. For a person of this height, both arms may be extended from the image receptor to the x-ray tube housing. For radiographers who have a shorter stature, they can extend both arms from the image receptor to the collimator. A 40-inch SID can be estimated by extending one arm and measuring to the opposite axilla.

The radiographer must make every effort to minimize the amount of OID between the image receptor and part being imaged. This can be accomplished by keeping the part in contact with the image receptor. If this is not possible, minimize the OID as much as possible and increase the SID that should be contemplated to compensate.

Any change in SID >10% requires compensation in the set technical factors. Another consideration is that any angle >15 degrees requires a compensation in SID, which will affect the set technical factors. Most mobile radiography units have preset steps in the mAs settings. The radiographer should use a rule of thumb that allows them to work around emergency room and intensive care equipment and to be able to compensate technique for various distances. The rule is quite simple: change one step in mAs for every 10 inch change in SID.

When performing a cross-table lateral image of the cervical spine with a horizontal beam, it is always wise to maximize SID. The maximum SID will assist in minimizing the shoulders from obscuring the C7 to T1 region. If you have a technique for a 40-inch SID but have achieved a 50-inch SID, just increase the mAs to the next higher step. For a 60-inch SID, increase by another step. Consider that you have a good technique for a 72-inch SID for the lateral cervical spine but because of the constraints of the room you can only get a 60-inch SID; the mAs would be reduced by one step. This simple rule has proven to work very well in a variety of situations for mobile radiography and should be memorized by radiographers.

Equipment Alignment and Positioning Considerations

The radiographer must become an expert at visually estimating the alignment of the x-ray beam to the patient and image receptor. It takes much practice with various patients in a variety of situations to become proficient with the alignment. This skill is essential to minimize shape distortion and to avoid superimposition of unwanted anatomy over the area of interest. The radiographer must observe the angle of the x-ray tube in relation to the patient; there are two types of angles that must be addressed.

The first is to check the side-to-side angle as observed by standing at the x-ray tube and visually inspecting the collimator to make sure it is level. Mobile chest radiographs often appear as if the patient was slightly rotated with the sternoclavicular joints not being equidistant to the sternum. In effect, the tube was angled toward the patient's left or right side. To prevent this from occurring, the radiographer must stand directly behind the x-ray tube and make sure that the tube is centered not only to the image receptor and patient's chest but also to the patient's feet. This will result in the central ray being centered and perpendicular to the anatomy.

The second type of angle to check is the cephalic/caudal angulation as observed from the side of the patient and x-ray tube. In order to properly visualize this angle, it is very helpful to stand back as far as possible because this relationship is easier to see from a distance. Ideally, the patient will be sitting in a semierect position; despite all positioning efforts, the patient's lower back is frequently not in contact with the image receptor. This means that the long axis of the patient's body and the image receptor are at different angles. Typically, the central ray is angled to be perpendicular to the image receptor or even to the bed; this results in a lordotic appearance of the thorax. A better practice is to angle the central ray until it is perpendicular to the patient's actual coronal plane. The chest anatomy will then appear in the correct orientation.

Additional Considerations

Low-ratio grids of 5:1 or 6:1 are very helpful for mobile imaging of larger body parts. The low-ratio grids allow a much wider margin for error in angulation, centering, and distance variations. Care must be used to align the x-ray tube to a grid to ensure grid cutoff will not occur. For all mobile procedures, watch for off-centering or off angling of the beam and tilt of the grid in either plane and use the proper SID for the grid radius and for grids placed upside down under the patient. In the surgical environment, the grid is placed in a sterile cover held by a nurse; it is not uncommon for the nurse to then place the covered grid upside down under the patient.

When manipulating the mobile unit in a patient's room or in surgery, the radiographer must use caution and care to make sure the unit or patient equipment are not damaged. In the mobile environment, the radiographer is the radiation safety expert! They are responsible for making sure radiation protection is used for themselves, the patient, or any person within close proximity. The greatest source of radiation exposure is the scatter radiation created when the x-ray beam is incident upon the patient. To minimize radiation exposure, the radiographer should wear a lead apron and stand at least 6 feet away from the patient. It is preferable for the radiographer to stand at a 90-degree angle to the patient to further decrease exposure to radiation.

Technique charts should be developed and attached to every mobile x-ray unit. The technique charts from one of the radiography rooms is not a suitable chart for the mobile unit. Recall that all x-ray units are not exactly alike and each should have its own unique technique chart. The technique chart must include adult and pediatric techniques. The charts can be laminated and taped to the unit for easy use. Mobile imaging is a challenge because the skill and knowledge of the radiographer are continually tested. The same high-quality standards for imaging and minimizing patient exposure applied in the radiography department should be implemented for mobile imaging.

Chapter Summary

1. Linear tomography is an imaging technique, which uses motion to blur out overlying and underlying structures to improve the image contrast of structures of interest.
2. The tomographic fulcrum is the imaginary pivot point from which the x-ray tube and the image receptor move.
3. The tomographic angle is the angle of movement that determines section thickness.
4. The tomographic angle is directly related to the amount of blurring, long angles result in more blur, while short angles result in less blur.
5. The section thickness is the width of the focal plane and is controlled by the tomographic angle. A thin section thickness is produced by a long tomographic angle and a thick section thickness is produced by a short tomographic angle.
6. The panorex unit uses tomography to produce a single image of the mandible. The curve of the mandible is "straightened" so that the entire mandible is seen as a flat structure.
7. Dedicated chest units are designed to use on patients who require an erect examination of the thorax.
8. Dedicated chest units have the capability of using the AEC to determine the exposure factors or the radiographer can manually set the technical factors for each patient.
9. Mobile radiographic units are used when images are required in areas of the hospital outside of the imaging department.
10. There are several types of mobile units: direct power, battery power, capacitor discharge, and high frequency.
11. During mobile imaging, the SID used for the exam must be measured with a tape measure if available. Obtaining a 40- or 72-inch SID is necessary; however, a shorter SID may have to be used because of exam room size.
12. A 10% change in SID requires a change in the technical factors.
13. Every attempt must be made to place the image receptor flush with the patient's anatomy. This prevents shape distortion due to OID.
14. In imaging the chest with a mobile unit, the central ray should be perpendicular to the patient's coronal plane.

Case Study

An Intravenous Urogram (IVU) with tomographic images was ordered to assess a patient's kidneys. Amanda is setting up the equipment and must determine the following:

Critical Thinking Questions

1. What tomographic angle will be used to adequately image the kidney?
2. What is the common section thickness used for IVU tomography?

Review Questions

Multiple Choice

1. The __________ is the pivot point for the tube and image receptor during a tomographic exposure.
   a. tomographic angle
   b. exposure angle
   c. section thickness
   d. fulcrum

2. As the tomographic amplitude becomes __________, a __________ slice of tissue will be imaged.
   a. larger, thicker
   b. smaller, thinner
   c. larger, thinner
   d. amplitude has no relationship to slice thickness

3. Which tomographic angle produces a focal plane thickness of ~6 mm?
   a. 10 degrees
   b. 20 degrees
   c. 35 degrees
   d. 50 degrees

4. Which type of mobile unit is not plugged into a wall outlet at the time an exposure is made?
   a. Direct power
   b. Capacitor discharge
   c. Battery power
   d. High frequency

5. The objective plane is the area in focus in the image.
   a. True
   b. False

6. The __________ is the point where the x-ray tube and Bucky pivot.
   a. exposure angle
   b. fulcrum
   c. section interval
   d. objective plane

Short Answer

1. Why are tomographic images used as an alternative to conventional radiographic images?

2. Define fulcrum, focal plane, and tomographic amplitude.

3. How are tomographic angle and section thickness related?

4. What is defined as moving the patient's body part in order to blur out superimposing anatomy?

5. The longer the exposure arc, the __________ the focal plane that is produced.

6. What is the typical focal plane thickness obtained with a 35-degree linear tube movement?

7. Describe the purpose of panorex imaging of the mandible.

29

Quality Assurance and Control

Objectives

Upon completion of this chapter, the student will be able to:

1. Describe factors included in radiographic quality control (QC).
2. State the factors included in processor QC.
3. Explain the types and sources of film artifacts.
4. Explain the various test patterns suggested by the AAPM TG18 and SMPTE.
5. State the factors included in fluoroscopic QC.
6. Describe various factors associated with the performance of digital display systems.
7. Identify concepts that are tested for AEC quality control.
8. Describe tomographic QC tests for section depth indicators and section thickness.
9. Explain quality control measures for electronic display systems.

Key Terms

- dichroic stain
- diffuse reflectance
- entrance skin dose (ESD)
- exposure linearity
- exposure reproducibility
- focal spot blur
- guide-shoe mark
- luminance
- photometer
- pi mark
- positive beam limiting (PBL)
- quality assurance
- quality control
- specular reflectance

Introduction

In the health care industry, the terms **quality assurance** and **quality control** have different meanings. Quality assurance deals primarily with personnel and their interactions with the patient and other staff. It is the term used to describe the process or program used to maintain high-quality imaging. It is a many-step process that involves identifying goals, formulating plans to achieve these goals, implementing the plans, and evaluating the success of the program. Quality assurance also includes outcomes analysis, such as how often the radiologist's report agrees with the patient's condition.

Quality control (QC) refers to the measurement and evaluation of radiographic equipment, together with the identification and correction of problems associated with the equipment. It includes periodic checks and monitoring of the operation of all equipment, initial acceptance testing of equipment, periodic testing of equipment performance, and the steps taken to correct deviations from expected performance. QC measurements often require specialized equipment. Often, regularly scheduled maintenance can detect and correct potential problems before they affect image quality. Documentation of all QC monitoring should include the date, the type of test, the outcome, and identification of the individual performing the monitoring test. This chapter discusses the factors that should be monitored and the frequency of monitoring for film screen and digital radiographic quality control.

Radiographic Quality Control

Radiographic quality control (QC) consists of periodic monitoring of the x-ray tube, the associated electric circuits, the accuracy of the exposure factors, and the film processor (Table 29.1).

Focal Spot Size

As the tube ages, the anode surface may become rough, resulting in a larger effective focal spot, because the rough surface leads to an increase in off-focus radiation. Degradation of the focal spot can produce blurred structures on the radiograph. This is known as **focal spot blur**. The focal spot size or spatial resolution should be measured annually or when the x-ray tube is replaced. For focal spots, the size should be within ±50% of the nominal or stated focal spot size.

There are three tools used to measure focal spot size: the pinhole camera, star test pattern, and slit camera. The pinhole camera is extremely difficult to set up and use and requires excessive exposure time. This test has significant limitations for focal spot sizes <0.3 mm. The star pattern uses an image of a star to determine the focal spot size by using a formula to relate the diameter of the star image to the size of the focal spot (Fig. 29.1).

The line pair resolution tool, an alternating series of metal strips with different separations, gives the spatial resolution of the system directly. The advantage of the line pair resolution tool is that it can readily detect degradation of image quality. The resolution of a film/screen system should be >8 line pairs per millimeter (Lp/mm).

Collimation

It is important that the light field and the radiation field coincide so that the x-ray field placement is correct. This is called light-radiation field congruence. When the fields are misaligned, anatomy in the light field

TABLE 29.1 ESSENTIALS OF A QUALITY CONTROL PROGRAM FOR RADIOGRAPHIC SYSTEMS

Factor	Monitoring Frequency	Limits	Test Tool
1. Focal spot size spatial resolution	Annual	±50%	Slit or pinhole camera Star phantom
2. Collimation	Semiannual	±2% of SID	Film + metal markers
3. kVp	Annual	±5 kVp	Penetrometer or step wedge
4. Filtration/HVL	Annual	≥2.5 mm Al	Aluminum sheets
5. Exposure time	Annual	±5%	Exposure meter or spinning top
6. Exposure reproducibility	Annual	±5%	Dosimeter
7. Exposure linearity	Annual	±10%	Dosimeter
8. AEC	Annual	±10	Exposure meter

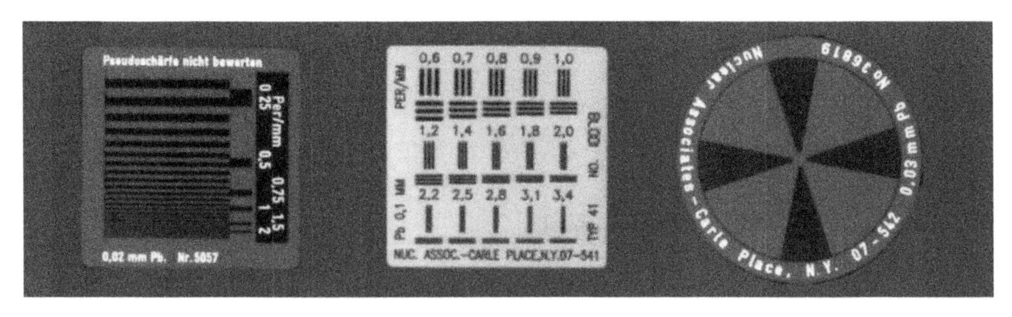

Figure 29.1. **Photographs of the star and line pair resolution tool together with the star and line pair resolution tool images used to measure the size of the focal spot or determine the resolution of the imaging system.**

will not be imaged, while anatomy outside the light field will be irradiated.

The alignment of the collimator that defines the x-ray beam and the light field must be checked annually and whenever the tube or field light is replaced. To measure the light-radiation field congruence, the image receptor is placed on the tabletop. The edges of the light field are marked on the cassette by placing metal markers such as coins or paper clips at the edge of the light field. An exposure is made, and the edges of the light and radiation fields are measured. The sum of the differences between the light and radiation field edges must be ±2% of the source to image receptor distance (SID).

As x-ray machines age, the SID and locking mechanisms tend to drift. These should be tested to determine if the distance, centering locks, stops, and detents are accurate. SID indicators can be checked with a tape measure, while centering indicators can be checked visually for the collimator light beam. SID indicators should be ±10% and centering indicators should be ±2%. If either of these indicators is not within limits, they will need to be adjusted.

Most systems are equipped with **positive beam-limiting (PBL)** collimators. These devices are automatic collimators that sense the size of the image receptor and adjust the collimating shutters to the exact size. These devices should never allow the light field size to be larger than the image receptor placed in the Bucky tray except when the override control is activated.

kVp Calibration

Technologists select the kVp for every procedure, which uses an image receptor. It is important to use the appropriate kVp for the anatomical part; therefore, the x-ray generator must be properly calibrated. If the kVp settings are incorrect, the patient dose may be increased and the image contrast compromised. When using film/screen, a measurement of the kVp can be made using a step wedge penetrometer. The optical density (OD) under the steps of the penetrometer is related to the penetrability of the beam because higher-kVp x-ray photons have greater penetration.

The same principle is used in modern electronic kVp meters (Fig. 29.2). Electronic detectors measure the penetration of the x-ray beam through two different attenuating filters. The ratio of the readings from the two detectors is used to calculate the kVp of the x-ray beam. Electronic kVp meters are more accurate than penetrometers and are the preferred method of measuring kVp for digital imaging systems. The kVp should be within ±10% and should be tested annually or when the high-voltage generator components have significantly changed. Electronic kVp meters are accurate to ±1 kVp and give the maximum, average, and effective kVp of the x-ray beam. kVp measurements are made by the service engineer or the medical physicist.

Filtration

Quite possibly the most important patient protection method of a radiographic system is the filtration of the x-ray beam. It is not possible to directly measure filtration so the filtration of an x-ray beam is reported in terms of its half-value layer (HVL), expressed in terms of aluminum

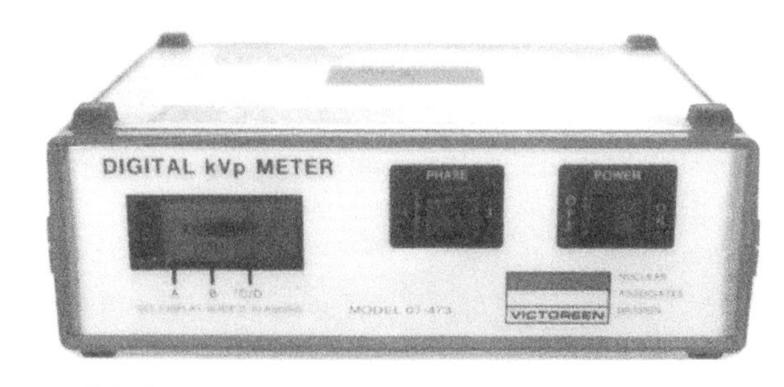

Figure 29.2. **Electronic kVp meter.**

thickness. The HVL is measured using thin sheets of aluminum (Al). A series of output measurements is made, first with no added aluminum in the beam and then with added thicknesses of Al. The HVL is calculated from the decrease in output as the Al thickness is increased. A minimum HVL of 2.5 millimeters (mm) Al equivalent is required. The HVL of the x-ray beam is measured annually or at any time after a change in the x-ray tube or tube housing. Testing is to ensure that the penetrability of the beam has not been degraded.

Exposure Time

The length of exposure time is selected on radiographic control consoles. Although the automatic exposure control (AEC) is used or milliampere stations (mA) are set, the exposure time is still the responsibility of the technologists. This setting is directly responsible for patient radiation dose and image optical density. There are several ways to assess the accuracy of the exposure timer. Most medical physicists use one of several commercially available devices that measure the duration of the exposure time of an ion chamber or photodiode assembly. If the timer settings are not accurate, the mAs values may be incorrect, resulting in poor quality images and potentially more patient radiation dose. Timer accuracy should be checked annually or when a component of the operating console or high-frequency generator has undergone major repairs. Timer accuracy must be within ±5% for exposure times >10 ms and within ±20% for exposure times <10 ms.

Exposure Linearity

Milliamperage settings tend to drift over time as a result of tube aging. The accuracy of the ma settings is essential to maintaining image quality because exposure cannot be predicted unless the mA station is accurate. Many combinations of mA and exposure time produce the same mAs output. The ability of the unit to produce a constant radiation output from various combinations is called **exposure linearity**. A radiation dosimeter is used to measure radiation intensity at various combinations of mA and exposure time.

Table 29.2 demonstrates various mA and exposure time settings, which will produce 10 mAs. Each combination would be set and the resultant radiation intensity would be measured. The radiation output per mAs (mR/mAs) should remain the same within ±10% as the mA stations are changed. Prior to testing for exposure linearity, it is necessary to test the exposure timer to be certain it is accurate; if it is not, it needs to be corrected before the linearity test can be performed.

TABLE 29.2 EXAMPLES OF EXPOSURE TIME AND mA COMBINATIONS EQUAL TO 10 mAs

Time Set	mA	mAs	Radiation Output (mR)
0.02	500	10	40
0.033	300	10	42
0.05	200	10	41
0.1	100	10	40
0.2	50	10	40
0.4	25	10	39

Exposure Reproducibility

When a technologist selects the correct kVp, mA, and exposure time for an exam, they expect the optical density and contrast in the image to be optimal. If any or all of these factors are changed and then returned to the previous setting, the radiation exposure should be exactly the same. **Exposure reproducibility** means that the radiation output (measured in milliroentgens [mR]) should be the same for a series of exposures in which all the technical factors are the same.

Exposure reproducibility should be measured annually using one of two methods that both rely on a precision radiation dosimeter. The first method is to make a series of at least three exposures with the same technical factors; these factors will be changed and reset between exposures. If the subsequent exposures do not produce the same radiation output, it is usually an error in the kVp control. The second method is to set a combination of factors and make ten exposures, the resultant radiation output should remain the same. If either test fails, the system lacks reproducibility and should be serviced by qualified personnel.

The differences in exposure as measured by the output in milliroentgens arise from slight differences in the calibration of the time and mA stations. The unit demonstrated in Table 29.2 meets the exposure reproducibility requirements because all mAs values are within ±5% of the average.

Intensifying Screens

Intensifying screens should be checked periodically for dust or other particles that enter cassettes when they are opened for loading and unloading radiographic film. These particles will cause an artifact to appear on the image. Periodic cleaning of the screens with a soft, lint-free cloth and cleaner from the manufacturer should be performed in accordance with the work load of the imaging department but should be performed at least every other month. When cleaning the cassette, it should be inspected for signs of wear at the corners and edges or for deformity of the screen. Film/screen contact should be evaluated once or twice a year. A wire mesh test pattern must be performed to evaluate any areas of damage or blurring. If there are areas of blurring or excessive damage seen on the wire mesh test image, the cassette should be taken out of service.

Cassette Cleaning

Radiographic cassettes and intensifying screens are exposed to dust and foreign objects during normal use. Periodic cleaning of the outside of the cassette will remove dirt and grime, which can lead to artifacts. The intensifying screens on the inside of the cassettes must also undergo periodic cleaning with a specially formulated antistatic solution to remove artifacts. In addition to the special solution, the cassettes should be cleaned with a lint-free cloth. At the time the cassettes are being cleaned, they should also be inspected for wear at corners, edges, and hinges. After the cassettes are cleaned, they must be placed vertically on a surface and allowed to air dry. Once the screens are dry, the cassette can be reloaded with radiographic film and placed in the film bin for use.

Each cassette must be labeled with a number on the outside and on the intensifying screen on the inside. This will allow technologists to identify the cassette that produced an artifact on an image. At this time, the cassette is cleaned to remove the artifact and inspected for any structural problems.

Viewbox

Viewbox illumination testing should be performed annually. The test is performed with a **photometer**, which measures the light intensity at several areas of the viewbox. The intensity should be at least 1,500 cd/m^2 and should not vary by more than ±10%. If it is determined that the bulb is defective and needs to be replaced, then all the bulbs should be replaced in the viewbox. All viewboxes in a department should be consistent and should use the same bulbs from the same manufacturer.

Automatic Exposure Control

The AEC is designed to compensate for differences in patient size by adjusting the time. The AEC measures the exit radiation and adjusts the exposure time to produce a proper density image. The AEC circuit is tested annually to verify that the mAs increases with increasing patient thickness.

Exposure Reproducibility

The reproducibility standards for the AEC are the same as diagnostic radiography. Radiographs must be produced using a phantom, and the densitometer readings of the images produced with the AEC should be within OD ±0.1%. If the readings are not within limits, the AEC generator must be tested and recalibrated.

Ion Chamber Sensitivity

AECs have three ion chambers and permit activation of many combinations of the chambers during an exposure. Each ion chamber must be tested for its sensitivity, and all three chambers must be equally sensitive. All three chambers are tested with a reproducibility test utilizing very low kVp. The next step is to block two chambers and produce an image with the unblocked chamber. This test must be done on each chamber. Each chamber must respond within ±10% from the other's chambers to be considered within range.

Density Variation Control

AEC units have density variation controls to increase and decrease the density of the image by changing the sensitivity of the ion chamber. A mR/mAs measurement is taken to verify the intensity differences for each control. Each unit is unique and the percentage of change is different in each unit. The equipment manuals must be referenced to know the exact range for the given unit.

Response Capability

Each AEC has a minimum response time, and if it cannot respond by the minimum time, the radiographer cannot be sure the image will be produced with diagnostic quality. The response capability is measured by using a Lucite phantom with multiple layers. Multiple exposures are made with the phantom thickness being reduced for each exposure. The AEC should produce images with intensity within ±10% of one another until a time below the minimum exposure is used. If the minimum response time is longer than specified, the AEC should not be used until the error has been corrected.

Backup Timer Verification

The AEC backup timer is used to terminate exposures when the x-ray beam has been activated for too long a time. To test the backup timer, a lead plate is placed over the AEC ion chamber and an exposure is made. The backup timer should terminate the exposure and a warning alarm should sound. If the timer or alarm fails, the AEC should not be used until the problem has been fixed.

Tomography Quality Control

In addition to standard radiography, QC testing units with tomographic capabilities are required to have additional tests.

Uniformity and Completeness of Tube Motion

Tomography relies on the motion of the tube to make a sectional image of the object during the exposure. QC tests must be completed to assure the smooth movement of the tube and to be sure the tube path is a complete path. To test tube movement, a lead mask with a pinhole is placed several centimeters above the fulcrum and centered to the image receptor. A tomographic exposure will take place, and the resultant image should have demonstrated a dot with a blurred line running through it. If the tube motion were not complete, there would not be a full length tracing. If the tube motion were erratic, there would be uneven densities along the pinhole exposure (Fig. 29.3).

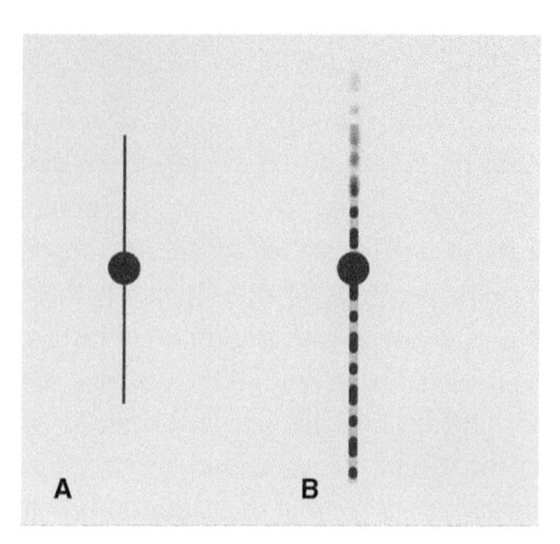

Figure 29.3. **Tomographic uniformity and completeness of tube motion tested with a pinhole tracing image. Notice how the line in A is smooth and has uniform density. Line B has uneven densities along the pinhole exposure representing a problem with the tube motion.**

Section Depth Indicator

The area of interest that is placed at the fulcrum level should appear sharp and in relative focus on the tomographic image. All other structures above and below the fulcrum level should appear blurred. The section depth indicator test is performed to assess the accuracy of the fulcrum level. Using a commercial test tool with numbered levels, the fulcrum level is set and a tomographic image is made. The number at the level of the fulcrum should appear sharp; if it does not appear sharp, the fulcrum level must be adjusted. This way the radiographer can be sure that the anatomy of interest at specific fulcrum levels will be imaged.

Section Thickness

The section thickness of a tomogram is determined by the arc of the tomographic motion. The equipment manual will indicate the section thickness for each type of arc available on the unit. The arc and resulting section thickness are measured by using an angled wire mesh. When the angled wire mesh is imaged, the section thickness is determined by measuring the region of sharpness on the image. If the section thickness is not accurate, a qualified service engineer must be notified.

Resolution

Tomographic resolution is tested by imaging a resolution test pattern. The test pattern is placed at the fulcrum level, this is crucial because this is the only part of the image that is not blurred by the motion of the tube. The image is then inspected to determine the resolving capability of the unit. If the resolution is not adequate, diagnostic QC tests should be performed to determine the nature of the problem.

Processor Quality Control

Processor QC is necessary to ensure that the processed films produce consistently high-quality images. Processor QC consists of daily monitoring and periodic cleaning and maintenance of the processor. All efforts expended in obtaining an excellent latent image are wasted if the latent image is not processed in a reproducible manner (Table 29.3).

Processor Cleaning and Maintenance

Current automatic processors are fast-action systems that can process a film in 90 seconds. These processors can handle up to 500 films per hour, but this requires a high concentration of chemistry, high development temperatures of 35°C (95°F), and developer immersion time of 22 seconds. The wash water temperature should be 31°C (87°F). Current processors include a thermostatically controlled heater to maintain the temperature of the wash water. This fast-action system coupled with automatic processors requires weekly cleaning procedures to maintain a properly operating processor.

High temperatures and concentrated chemistry cause wear and corrosion of the transport system and can contaminate the chemistry with processing sludge. When sludge and other debris build up on rollers, it comes into contact with film as it is moved through the rollers. This can be prevented by daily cleaning of the crossover racks. The crossover racks are very easy to remove and clean. Proper cleaning prevents the sludge from building up, and it also facilitates the movement of the films through the rollers.

The processor must also have a weekly cleaning to remove the transport rollers and crossover racks. The processing tanks are cleaned and rinsed as well. This is a fairly simple task to perform and should only take a few minutes. When the processor is reassembled, sensitometric levels must be reestablished. Records of all cleaning must be maintained. A clean processor will produce high-quality radiographs that are free from artifacts and will also increase productivity because there will be no processor downtime due to jammed films.

Processor maintenance should be scheduled at regular intervals in addition to daily and weekly cleaning. Scheduled maintenance is performed on a weekly or monthly basis where the mechanical parts are observed for wear and adjustment of belts, pulleys, and gears for proper operation. Automatic processors should have a planned maintenance program where parts are replaced at regular intervals before the processor experiences failure and downtime. Unexpected failure can lead to processor downtime, which severely affects productivity of the radiography department. A proper program of scheduled and preventative maintenance will ensure the proper operation of the processor and will keep unexpected failures to a minimum.

TABLE 29.3 ESSENTIAL PROCESSOR QUALITY ASSURANCE FACTORS MONITORING FREQUENCY

Factor	Monitoring Frequency
Sensitometry/densitometry	Daily
Temperature (chemicals/ water)	Daily
Crossover racks cleaning	Daily
Replenishment rates	Daily
Tanks and transport roller cleaning	Weekly

Processor Monitoring

The overall operation of the processor is most easily monitored by preparing a sensitometric strip and processing it in the processor. The most accurate results will be

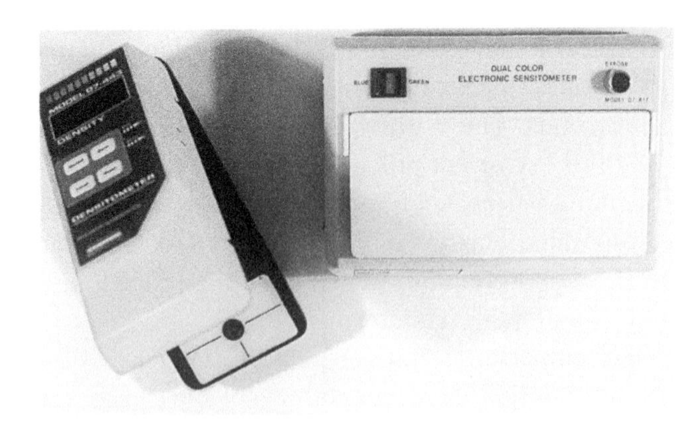

Figure 29.4. **Sensitometer and a densitometer.**

obtained when the monitoring is done at the same time each day.

The sensitometer is an instrument that exposes a test film to light through a series of filters (Fig. 29.4). Sensitometer eliminates any variations due to x-ray output variations. The output of the sensitometer is a film with a series of densities extending from base plus fog level to completely black in discrete steps (Fig. 29.5). For this reason, this process is also called a step wedge exposure.

A densitometer is used to measure the OD of each step. The background density (which is the base plus fog density), average speed, and contrast in the middensity range are calculated from the measured OD values. These values are then recorded and compared with previous measured values. The OD values from the daily sensitometric strip must be within acceptable limits, which are set by the department. The base plus fog value must be <0.05 OD. If the readings are outside the acceptable limits, the processor cannot be used clinically until the problem is corrected.

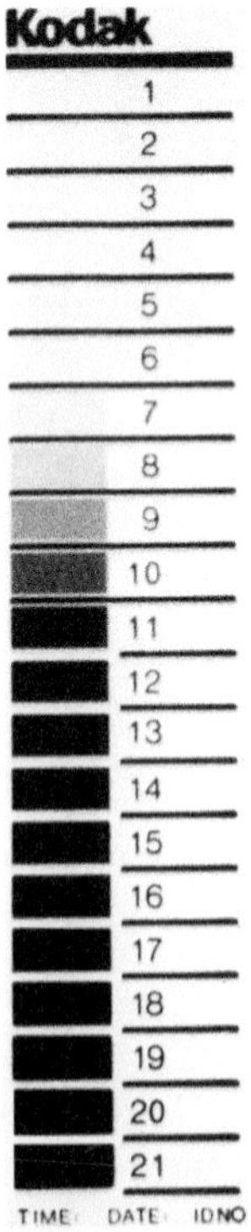

The temperatures of the processor solutions, developer, fixer, and wash water should be checked with a digital thermometer and recorded daily. Slight changes in the temperature of the developer solution will produce significant density changes in the final radiograph. The developer temperature should be maintained within ±2°F of the set value. The developer and fixer replenishment rates should be monitored and recorded.

Figure 29.5. **Sensitometer strip image.**

Film/Screen Artifacts

An artifact is an unwanted density or image on the radiograph. Film artifacts can be divided into three categories based on their source. The major sources of artifacts are exposure artifacts, handling artifacts, and processor artifacts.

Exposure Artifacts

An exposure artifact occurs during the exposure of the patient. The artifacts can be present with both film and digital image receptors. Exposure artifacts are caused by improper positioning, technical factors, or patient motion. Grid cutoff due to improper alignment of the grid to the x-ray tube can produce artifacts; these appear as lighter areas on one or both sides of the image. Exposure artifact can also be caused when the imaging receptor is not loaded with the correct film for the intensification screen, poor film/screen contract, double exposure, warped cassettes, and improper positioning of the grid.

Lack of patient preparation can also be a significant source of exposure artifacts. Failure to remove eyeglasses, jewelry, rings, watches, and hair clips will produce exposure artifacts. Hair, especially if braided or wet, can cause exposure artifacts. Exposure artifacts can be reduced or eliminated by careful attention to details before taking the exposure. Using excellent communication skills can prevent motion artifact caused by breathing or patient movement (Fig. 29.6).

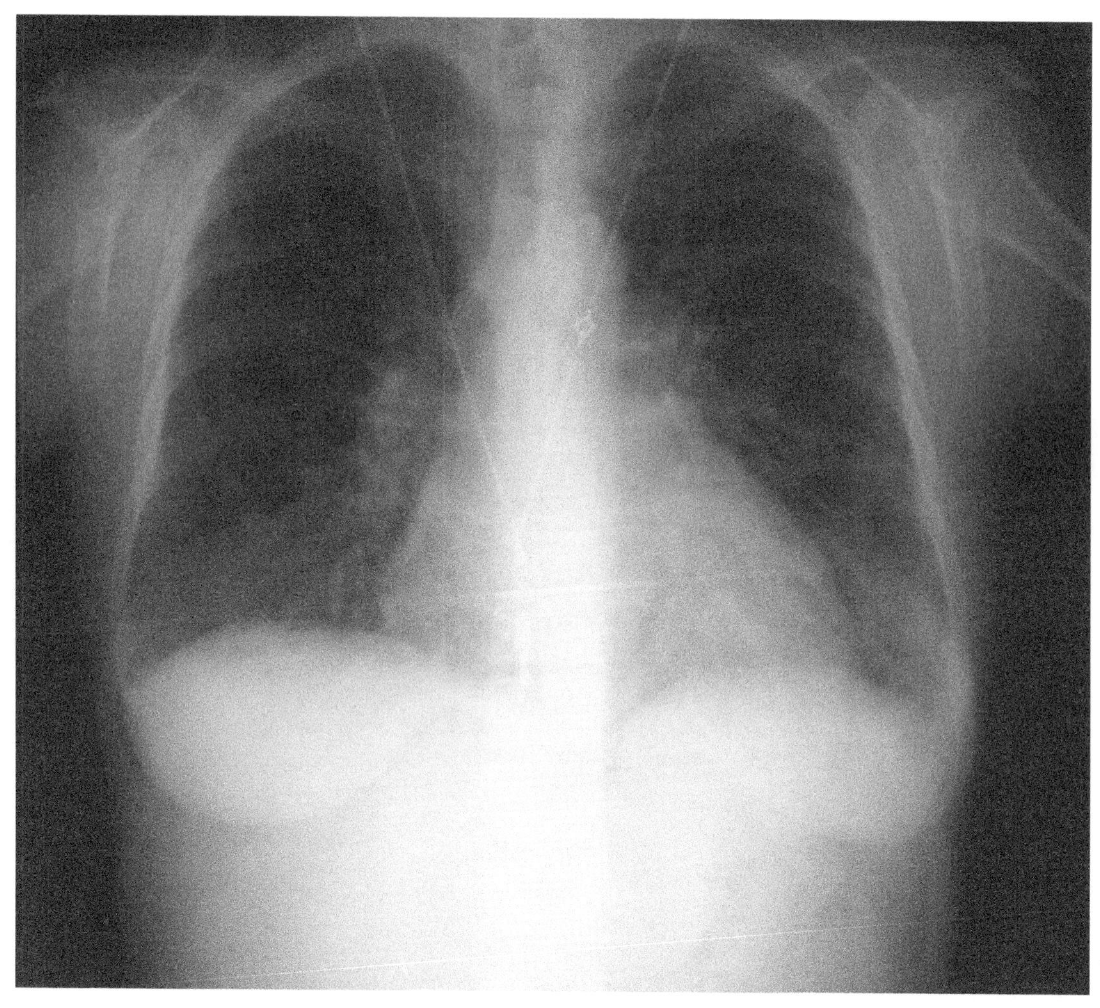

Figure 29.6. **Presents an example of an exposure artifact due to a necklace.**

Handling and Storage Artifacts

Handling artifacts occur because of improper handling and storage of the film. Handling artifacts include light leaks, static streaks, crease marks, and fingerprints. The source of handling artifacts is usually easy to identify because the cassettes must be light tight; any physical damage or rough handling may destroy the light-tight integrity. Light leaks appear as positive-density areas, darker areas on the image. Light leaks can also occur in the darkroom if the safelight has an improper filter, if the safelight is too bright, or if the safelight is too close to the processing tray of the automatic processor. White light leaks can occur if the darkroom door allows light to leak through the perimeter of the door or underneath the door. This white light will cause fog on the film as it is loaded into the cassette or as the film is placed on the processing tray. Safelight fog and radiation fog look alike on an image.

Screens should be cleaned monthly with a special cleaning fluid and lint-free wipes to remove any potential dust and to prevent static buildup. Static artifacts are caused by electrical discharges and appear as positive dark lines on the image. They are most common in winter, when the air is dry and relative humidity is low. The three types of static artifacts are tree, which appear with branches; crown, which have many lines radiating from a common area; and smudge, which appear as slightly positive areas on the image. Film should be stored under conditions where the relative humidity is between 40% and 60% and the temperature is below 72°F.

Rough handling of the exposed, undeveloped film can produce crease or kink marks, sometimes called fingernail marks because they resemble fingernail clippings. These positive-density marks result from bending or creasing of the film during loading, unloading, or processing. Handling the film with damp, greasy, or oily hands can result in negative-density areas, or lighter areas, in the form of fingerprint marks on the film (Fig. 29.7).

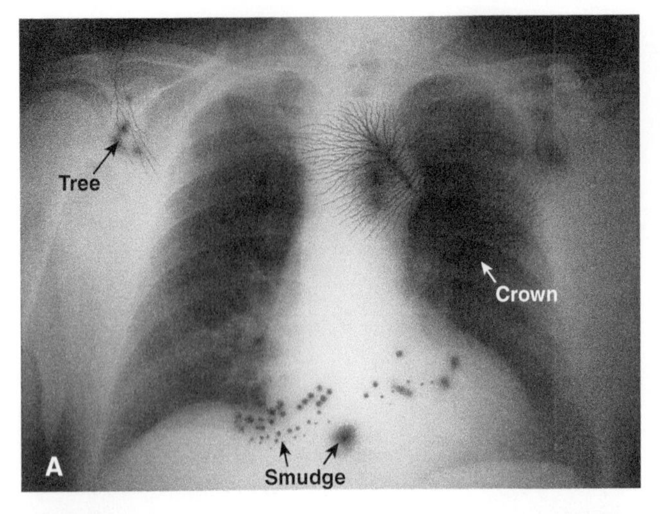

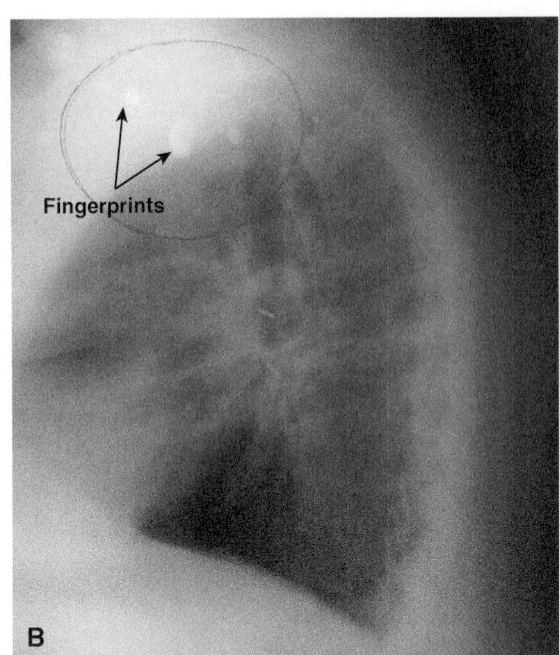

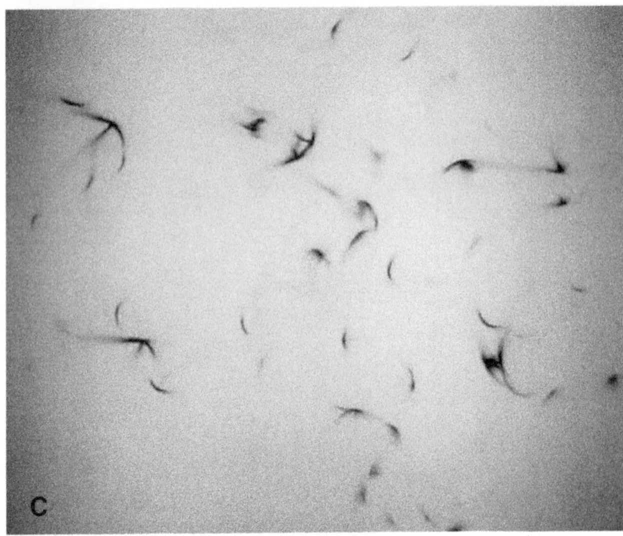

Figure 29.7. **(A–C) Presents examples of handling artifacts.**

Processor Artifacts

Processor artifacts occur as a result of improper processor QC of the transport system. Processor artifacts include pi marks, guide-shoe marks, chemical stains, emulsion pick-off, and gelatin buildup.

A deposit of dirt or chemicals on a portion of a roller will make a dark or positive mark on the film on each revolution. These **pi mark** artifacts are perpendicular to the direction of film travel through the processor and are spaced at pi, or 3.14-inch intervals. Typical transport rollers are 1 inch in diameter, so pi marks are 3.14 inches apart and represent one revolution of the roller. Regularly scheduled processor cleaning will eliminate pi marks and many other processor artifacts. It is essential to clean the crossover racks daily.

Guide-shoe marks are caused by the guide shoes, which are used to reverse the direction of the film at the crossover rack assembly. Guide-shoe marks indicate that the guide shoes are misaligned and are scratching the film emulsion. These marks appear as light lines or negative densities parallel to the film direction. Realignment of the guide shoes will eliminate guide-shoe marks (Fig. 29.8).

Chemical fog can occur when there is improper chemistry in the processor. The chemical fog appears similar to light or radiation fog and has a dull gray appearance. The chemical fog is called a **dichroic stain** and typically is comprised of two colors. The stains can appear as yellow, green, blue, or purple on the film. The chemical stains occur when a slow processor does not properly remove chemicals from the film and the excess chemicals run down the leading or trailing edges of the film.

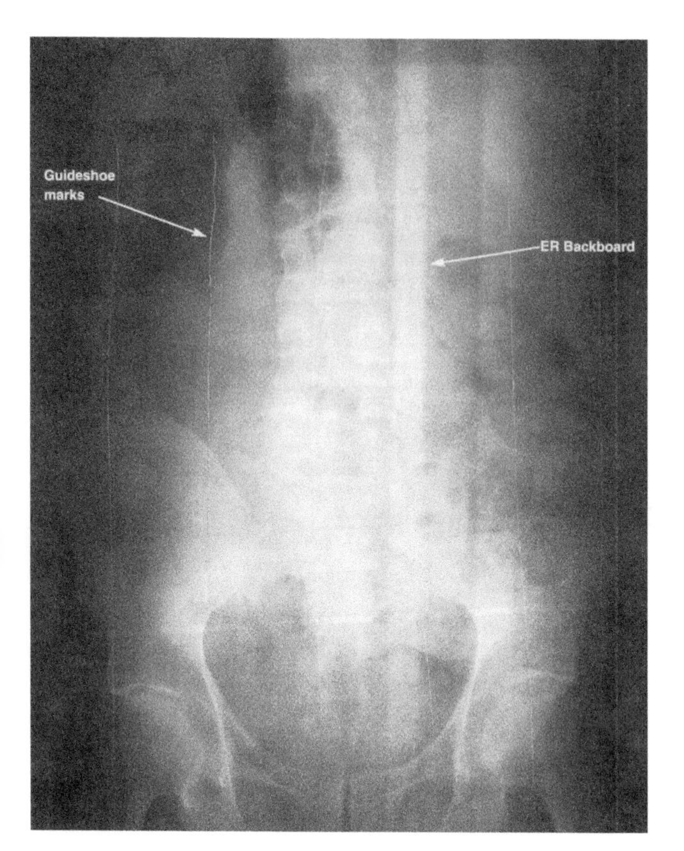

Figure 29.8. **Image demonstrates guide-shoe marks.**

Fluoroscopy Quality Control

Fluoroscopic procedures can result in high patient radiation dose. The **entrance skin dose (ESD)** or entrance skin exposure for an adult averages between 30 and 50 mGy/min (3 to 5 R/min) during fluoroscopy. The resultant skin dose can reach 100 mGy (10 rad) for many fluoroscopic procedures. Interventional radiology procedures commonly reach a skin dose of 1,000 mGy (100 rad), but these levels should be avoided. Stationary fluoroscopic units must be installed with a source to skin distance (SSD) of at least 38 cm (15 inches) at tabletop. Mobile C-arm fluoroscopy units must have an SSD of at least 30 cm (12 inches). QC of fluoroscopic systems consists of monitoring the radiation output exposure rate, the spatial and contrast resolution, the operation of the automatic brightness control (ABC) of the system, and other factors necessary to produce a quality fluoroscopic image.

Radiation Output or Exposure Rate

The radiation output or exposure rate must be checked with an attenuation phantom placed in the beam to ensure that the measurements are made under conditions similar to those in clinical practice. State statutes and federal laws require that ESD rates shall not exceed 100 mGy/min (10 R/min). In interventional radiography, the fluoroscope may have a high-level control, which allows up to 200 mGy/min. Because the ESD is higher with higher magnification modes, it must be measured at all magnification modes. The ESD of a fluoroscopic system must be measured annually.

Resolution

The spatial resolution of a fluoroscopic system is checked by placing a resolution phantom in the beam and observing the system resolution. The resolution phantom consists of a series of lead bars of differing separation labeled in line pairs per millimeter. The higher the number of line pairs per millimeter visible, the better the resolution of the system. The resolution must be checked annually at all magnification modes (Fig. 29.9).

Automatic Brightness Control

ABC circuits are designed to maintain constant image brightness regardless of the thickness of the patient. The operation of an ABC circuit is measured by placing attenuators of made of Lucite, aluminum, copper, or lead filters in the beam. The mAs should increase with increasing attenuator type and thickness. The operation of the backup timer in the radiographic mode can be verified by placing a lead sheet in the beam. The beam should be terminated at the backup timer setting, usually about 500 mAs or 5 seconds. ABC circuits should be tested annually (Table 29.4).

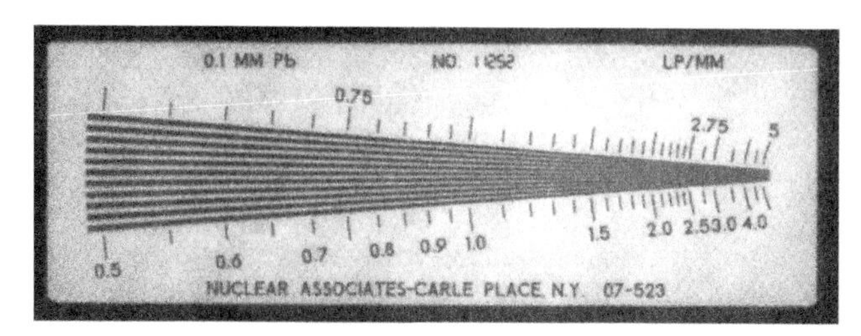

Figure 29.9. **Fluoroscopic resolution phantom.**

TABLE 29.4 FLUOROSCOPIC QC TESTS AND LIMITS

Factor	Frequency	Limits	Tools
Exposure rate	Annual	<10 rad/min	Exposure meter
Resolution	Annual	None	Resolution phantom
ABC	Annual	None	Exposure meter
Protective apparel	Annual	No cracks or gaps	Fluoroscope or film

Automatic Brightness Systems

All fluoroscopes are equipped with some type of ABC. The system operates as a phototimer to produce constant image brightness on the TV or flat panel monitor regardless of patient thickness.

Spot Film Exposures

Spot film images can be produced in two ways: cassette spot film and photofluorospot. Proper exposure of the cassette spot film depends on the kVp, mAs, and sensitivity of the film/screen systems being used. ESDs vary widely (Table 29.5). The exposures were performed with a 10:1 grid and a 400-speed image receptor. This is due to the placement of the cassette between the patient and image intensifier. The cassette is exposed with remnant radiation, which has only passed through the patient. Subsequently, greater exposure factors are necessary to create a diagnostic image.

The photofluorospot images use film but require lower patient dose to create diagnostic images. Photofluorospot images are affected not only by kVp, mAs, and the sensitivity of the film/screen system but also by the characteristics of the image intensifier. These images are recorded on the film after the image has passed through the output phosphor of the image intensifier tube. The ESD for photofluorospot images is greatly reduced when compared to cassette spot films. The properties of the image intensifier, which brightens the image thousands of times, mean that the kVp and mAs used to create the image can be much lower. This equates to reduced dose to the patient and personnel.

TABLE 29.5 ENTRANCE SKIN DOSE FOR SPOT FILM WITH CASSETTES

Kilovolt Peak	Entrance Skin Dose (mGy)
60	4.5
70	2.7
80	1.7
90	1.5
100	1.3

Field Size and Beam Alignment

Fluoroscopic units use field size to image the patient, field size is the equivalent to collimation in diagnostic radiography. Just as in diagnostic radiography, fluoroscopic tubes should not be capable of irradiating tissue outside the field size area. The accuracy of the field size in fluoroscopy should be within 1 cm of the edges of the image intensifier tube. The primary beam from the under-the-table fluoroscopy tube must be aligned to the center of the image intensifier.

Intensifier Viewing System Resolution

Resolution for proper visualization of anatomy and pathology is critical in fluoroscopic imaging just as in radiographic or digital imaging. Fluoroscopic resolution is much poorer than radiographic resolution and must be checked periodically to ensure adequate resolution and to check for deterioration. A resolution pattern test tool or fluoroscopic mesh test tool can be imaged to visualize the resolution of the system.

Monitors and Recorders

Modern fluoroscopic units use video systems to display the image. The monitors and recorders must be tested periodically to assess the resolution of the image on the monitors. The fluoroscopic mesh test tool or wire mesh tool can be used to test for resolution. The test tool is imaged on the fluoroscope to allow visual measurement of the system resolution on the monitor and to assess for distortion of the image such as pincushion distortion.

Protective Apparel Quality Control

Protective aprons, gloves, gonadal shields, and other radiation shields must be checked for tears, gaps, holes, and voids at least annually. All protective apparel should be visually inspected and also tested radiographically. This inspection may be performed fluoroscopically or by taking radiographs of the apparel. Any apparel, which demonstrates defects, must be replaced (Fig. 29.10).

Digital Radiography Quality Control

With the arrival of digital imaging, the scope of quality assurance procedures has grown to include digital radiographic imaging quality control. Quality control requirements for digital radiography involve the reading environment and digital display device. In radiology reading rooms, viewboxes are being replaced with digital monitors for image review and diagnosis. Any component that malfunctions can produce image degradation, which can simulate or obscure pathologic processes. To ensure proper functioning of display devices, it is crucial to have a comprehensive QC program.

Monitoring of Digital Acquisition Systems

The medical physicist will perform sophisticated tests of all digital imaging systems such as detective quantum efficiency (DQE). In addition to this testing, technologists or QC technologists can perform several equipment checks. A baseline image or other data is established when the system is installed after which the unit can be monitored for any sudden or extreme deviations by performing simple, regular visual checks.

Field Uniformity

Digital detectors are inherently nonuniform. Depending on the equipment, uniformity corrections must be performed on a regular basis ranging from daily to semiannually. If a radiopaque artifact is seen on multiple images, a nonuniform detector field may be the reason. The following test procedure is performed: thoroughly erase the plate, place the image receptor on the floor to achieve a 78-inch SID, which will minimize the anode heel effect,

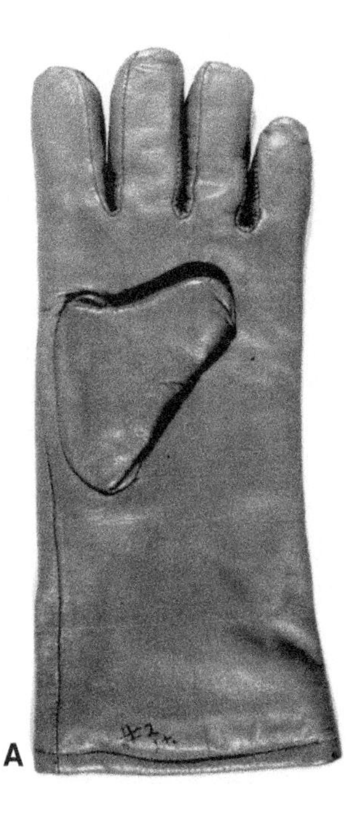

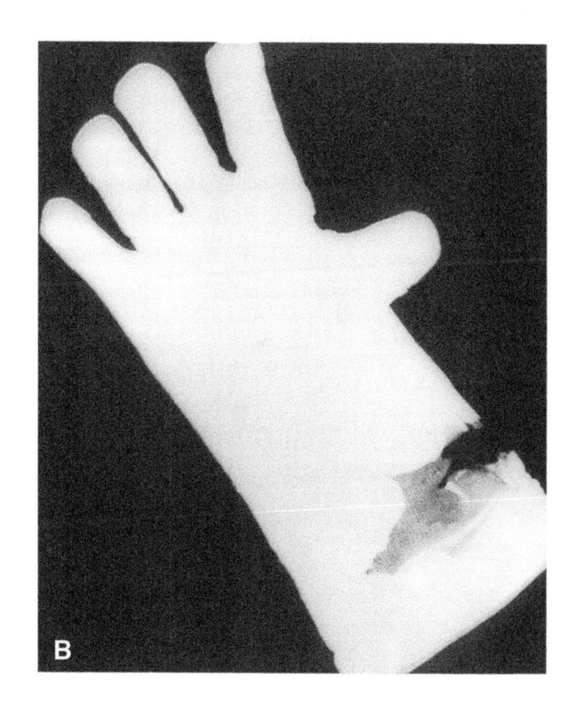

Figure 29.10. (A) Picture of a normal-appearing lead glove. (B) Radiograph of the same glove that shows a gap in the protection because the internal lead shielding is torn and shifted.

set moderate technique settings, and make the exposure. The resulting image may be visually scanned for any defects, which should be reported to the medical physicist.

Erasure Thoroughness

The erasure of the plate requires extremely bright light bulbs. When there is inadequate erasure on the CR system, it is likely from burned out bulbs in the erasing chamber of the processor, loss of bulb intensity, or the erasure time is too short. Even if there is proper erasure of the plate, extreme overexposure from a prior exam can leave residual signal on the plate. To test proper erasure, expose the imaging plate with an aluminum step wedge placed in the beam then process the plate. Immediately reexpose the same plate without the step wedge in the beam and with a 1-inch border of collimation on all sides of the cassette. Expose the plate again and process, and visually inspect the second image for any ghost image of the step wedge. This indicates inadequate erasure is occurring.

Ghosting or image lag in a DR system is visually checked in the same manner. On a DR plate, image lag is caused when electrical charge has been trapped in metastable states in the amorphous silicon or selenium during an exposure and is released only slowly over time. Indirect systems, which are silicon based, generally have a shorter image lag than direct systems.

Spatial Resolution

To test the sharpness of the image, a wire mesh is laid on the detector and an exposure is made. Visually review the image for any distortions or unsharp areas. Compare this image with a baseline image, which was obtained when the equipment was installed. To obtain the spatial resolution in line pairs per millimeter, a standard bar test pattern is used. A medical physicist may use a sharp-edged lead object or slit cut into a lead foil to test for edge-spread function or line-spread function, respectively.

Electronic Image Display System Monitoring

Nearly all radiographic images are viewed on an electronic image display. It is critical that a quality assurance program is established to monitor the quality of the digital image display. The display monitor is the weak link in the medical imaging chain and misdiagnosis can result from poor display quality. It is essential that display systems be regularly and carefully evaluated.

Diagnostic workstations often consist of two or more monitors; consistency between all the monitors on a workstation is critical; all monitors should have the same level of luminance and be set at the same contrast level. The workstation monitor must be cleaned at least monthly or when visibly soiled. The rate of testing will depend on whether the monitor is a CRT or an LCD, if the monitor is self-calibrating, and whether it is in a diagnostic workstation, technologist workstation, or display station.

Multiple scientific groups have published guidelines for monitoring the quality of electronic image display systems. Standards for medical images are found in DICOM Part 14. Guidelines and tests are available from the Society of Motion Picture and Television Engineers (SMPTE), American Association of Physicists in Medicine (AAPM), and the American College of Radiology (ACR) to name a few. The tests include maximum luminance, luminance response, luminance uniformity, contrast, resolution, noise, reflectance, etc. AAPM Task Group 18 and other scientific groups developed various test patterns that can be downloaded from their Web sites to check each type of monitor for specific quality. The SMPTE designed a generic test pattern, which includes elements for most of the image qualities in one comprehensive pattern (Fig. 29.11).

Recall there are two types of monitors at workstations: primary monitors, which are used for diagnosis and must follow more stringent guidelines for quality control, and secondary monitors, which are not used for diagnosis but for simple viewing of the images. Sophisticated quality control measurements are performed by a medical physicist; however, a QC technologist can determine if image deterioration is occurring over time. Anytime a new monitor is installed, baseline testing is performed using the SMPTE test pattern to establish the levels of brightness, contrast, and resolution. The testing results are logged and used for subsequent testing to compare new measurements against the original.

Luminance

Luminance is the rate of light emitted from a source such as a CRT monitor or LCD screen. The luminance

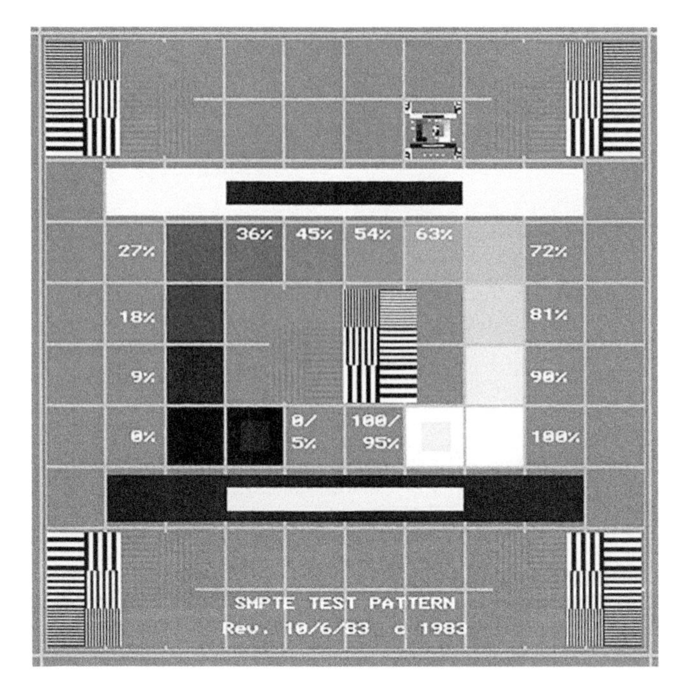

Figure 29.11. **The SMPTE pattern was adapted by adding an apparent smaller SMPTE pattern within the larger pattern. (CC BY-SA 2.5, Rich Franzen author.)**

response of monitors and luminance uniformity measurements require the use of a properly calibrated photometer. Most photometers are read out in units of lux, lumens, or candela/m^2 (cd/m^2). Many manufacturers of LCDs provide photometric instruments designed for their monitors, which the QC technologist or medical physicist may use in accordance with the manufacturer's instructions. Consistent methods for monitoring are to be followed each time the tests are performed so that the measurements can be validated.

The National Institute of Standards and Technology (NIST) established standards for the photometer, which states the luminance should measure in the range of 0.05 to 1,000 cd/m^2 with better than 5% accuracy and a precision of at least 0.01. The photometer should also comply with the Commission Internationale de l'Eclairage (CIE) standard photopic spectral response within a range of 3%.

An illuminance meter is used to measure monitor display reflection and to assess ambient light conditions. The illuminance meter is calibrated according to NIST standards and must have a response better than 5% at a 50-degree angulation. Over time, ambient light should be kept constant each time a test is performed; if it is not kept constant, the results will be skewed.

Luminance and Contrast Tests

The maximum luminance is checked at the same monitor setting over a period of time and a photometer is used to complete the test. New LCDs have self-correcting capabilities and are checked annually. CRTs are prone to rapid deterioration and must be checked monthly.

The luminance response refers to the monitor's ability to accurately display various shades of brightness from a test pattern. Because adjacent shades of brightness are compared, this is essentially identical to a contrast test, although different units of measurement are used. In order to test the sensitivity of the monitor, test patterns with adjacent dark gray squares at threshold contrasts are just visible. These squares will be resolved with a barely visible difference in density on a monitor with good contrast. On monitors with poor contrast, two adjacent squares will appear to form a rectangle of a single density.

The SMPTE test pattern seen in Figure 29.11 is an adaptation from the original test pattern. The adapted pattern has a ring of density squares in the middle of the test pattern. At the bottom are two sets of squares, one set marked 0/5% and the other set 100/95%. The 0/5% set consists of a black square with a 5% brightness square in the center. The 100/95% set consists of a 95% white square embedded within a 100% white square. The differences in each square should be distinguishable to the person performing the test.

DICOM standards include a grayscale standard display function (GSDF), which was developed to bring the digital values assigned to the dynamic range into alignment with human perception, in increments of JNDs for "just noticeable differences." The AAPM recommends the luminance response should be within 10% of the GSDF standard. To test the luminance response, the SMPTE pattern is again used. The SMPTE pattern has a ring of squares separated by 10% increments from white to black. Using a photometer, the measurements should all fall within 10% accuracy.

Luminance uniformity refers to the consistency of a single brightness level displayed across the screen. This test consists of measuring five areas of luminance: each of the four corners and the center of the screen. AAPM guidelines state that these measurements should not deviate more than 30% from their average.

Reflectance Tests and Ambient Lighting

In a reading room or in the control area of a radiography room the ambient light significantly contributes to the light reflected by the display monitor. There are two kinds of reflection or reflectance off the surface of any display monitor screen. Typically, the display reflection is characterized as diffuse or specular. **Diffuse reflectance** is light that is randomly scattered on the digital display device. **Specular reflectance** results in the mirror images of light sources surrounding the display monitor. To assess specular reflectance, turn off the monitor and look for sources of illumination within a 15-degree angle of viewing at an approximate distance of ~30 to 50 cm. Look for images of light sources such as lightbulbs or high-contrast patterns from the viewer's clothing or room furnishings.

The TG18-AD pattern consists of uniformly varying low-contrast patterns. To evaluate diffuse reflectance, the viewer must observe the threshold of visibility for low-contrast patterns with ambient lighting and total darkness. Both conditions should have the same visibility of the low-contrast patterns. If the ambient lighting changes the threshold, then the ambient lighting must be reduced. In other words, the ambient lighting within the room must be dimmed to the point where specular and diffuse reflectance is below any noticeable level that would interfere with full visibility of the image.

Display Resolution

The ACR and AAPM recommend a minimum resolution of electronically displayed images of 2.5 Lp/mm. As with film/screen, spatial resolution of the digital images is a measurement of the ability of the display system to produce differences between black and white bar patterns. The SMPTE test pattern has a series of high-contrast and low-contrast bars of decreasing widths to check for resolution; this is similar to the "slit camera" used to check focal spot. The bar patterns are inspected for any blurring of each white or black bar into adjacent bars. The TG18-CX pattern from the AAPM (Fig. 29.12) provides a check for resolution across the area of the digital display screen. The TG18-CX pattern is a very small pattern that consists of sets of squares with an x inside; this pattern is repeated across the entire screen. In the center of the test tool is a set of larger TG18-CX patterns that have been progressively blurred. The TG18-CX patterns in the middle and in the corners can be evaluated using a magnifying glass and compared to determine the resolution of the monitor.

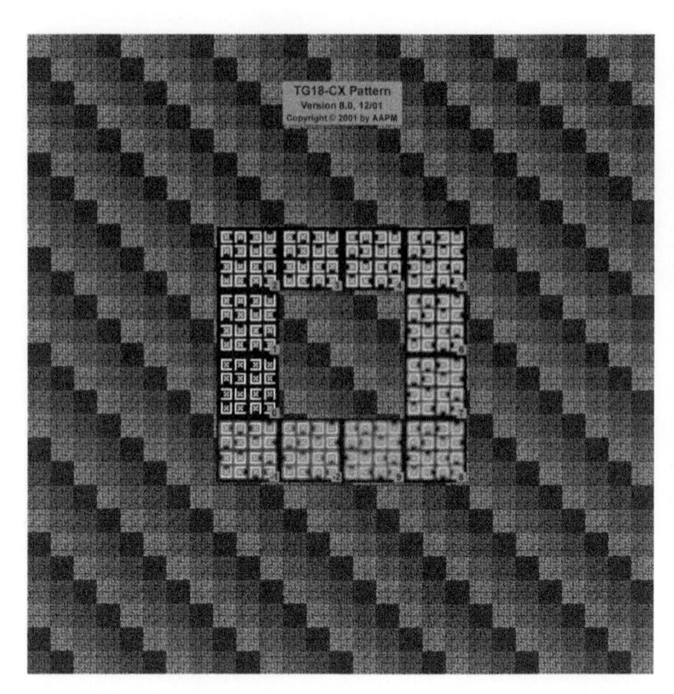

Figure 29.12. **TG18-CX pattern for display resolution evaluation. (Reprinted from Executive Summary of AAPM TG18 Report, Dr. Ehsan Samei, PhD, with permission.)**

Display Noise

Noise and image contrast are important factors in determining the visibility of objects in the image. Any patterns or electrical fluctuations that interfere with the detection of the true signal are called noise. The AAPM has made a test pattern (TG18-AFC) to measure noise levels in the electronic image. The TG18-AFC is based on the method used to determine just noticeable differences as a function of size.

As seen in Figure 29.13, the test pattern consists of a large number of regions with changing target positions. Size and contrast are held constant in the four quadrants to which the pattern is subdivided. Each quadrant contains a large number of regions with varying target positions. The observer should view the patterns from approximately a 30-cm viewing distance. The observer can subjectively evaluate the contrast size relationships for which they can confidently place the position of all targets within the test pattern. The target visibility in each of the regions may be quantified by counting the

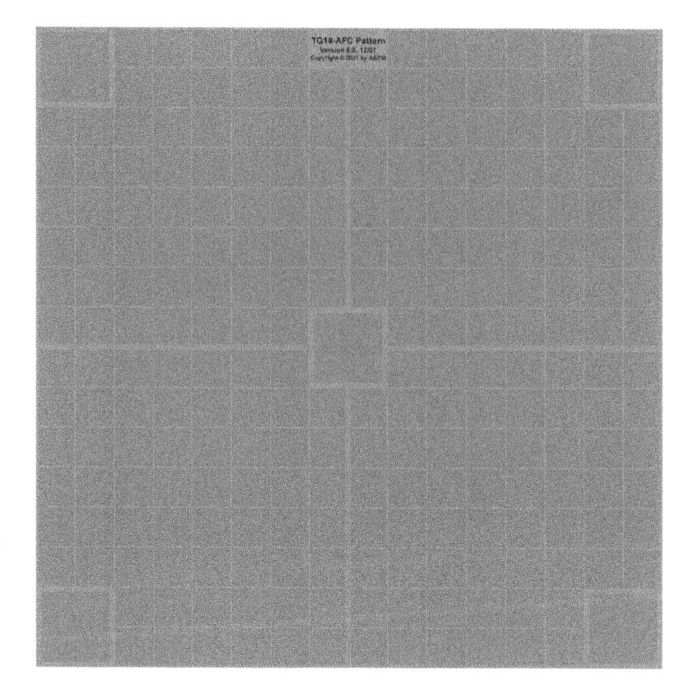

Figure 29.13. TG18-AFC pattern used to assess display noise. (Reprinted from Executive Summary of AAPM TG18 Report, Dr. Ehsan Samei, PhD, with permission.)

number of targets visible in each of the quadrants. The visual evaluation should render all the targets except the smallest one visible for primary display monitors and the two largest sizes visible for secondary display monitors.

Dead and Stuck Pixels

Dead and stuck pixels are seen on an LCD screen. The LCD screen can be examined visually to identify any bad pixels. Using a magnifying glass, the display is scanned for any areas where a pixel appears as a dot, similar to a period or the dot on an "i." Upon close inspection, failure of any segment of a pixel is apparent as a small defect in the image. Recall that in an LCD, the electric charge is applied to turn the pixel off so that it is dark against a light background. This means that a truly dead pixel is seen as a white spot on a solid black background. On the other hand, it is possible for a pixel to become "stuck" in the on state. These "stuck" pixels are seen as a black spot on a solid white field. Both tests should be performed for a complete check of the LCD monitor.

The AAPM guidelines for primary LCDs used for interpreting an image to determine a diagnosis include the following recommendations:

- Fifteen or fewer bad pixels across the entire screen
- Three or fewer bad pixels within any circle of 1 cm diameter
- Three or fewer bad adjacent pixels

Manufacturers recommend the primary LCD monitors must be "near perfect," and a secondary LCD monitor can be allowed two defective pixels per million.

Chapter Summary

1. Quality assurance deals with personnel and the performance of the team required to produce high-quality radiographs. Quality control deals with equipment performance.
2. Radiographic QC includes monitoring the components that affect radiologic image quality. These include focal spot size, kVp, the timer, exposure linearity, exposure reproducibility, and processor performance, including monitoring of processor temperature and replenishment rate.
3. The focal spot size or system resolution should be measured at least annually to detect gradual degradation of image resolution.
4. Regular processor QC tests are necessary to ensure that the processed films are of high quality.
5. An exposure made with a sensitometer and measured with a densitometer gives a good measure of processor operation.
6. Artifacts are unwanted densities or images on a radiograph. Pi marks are positive-density artifacts

perpendicular to the direction of film travel through the processor and separated by 3.14 inches. Guide-shoe marks are negative-density straight-line artifacts parallel to the direction of film travel through the processor.

7. Fluoroscopy QC involves monitoring the exposure rate and spatial resolution. The tabletop dose rate must be <0.01 Gy/min (10 rad/min).
8. The medical physicist will perform specific equipment checks, while technologists can perform several tests, including beam alignment and collimation, AEC density control linearity, focal spot, and many others.
9. The maximum luminance for CRTs used for diagnosis should be checked monthly; LCDs are checked annually.
10. Ambient lighting in a reading room must be low enough to deny specular and diffuse reflectance.
11. Pixels in an LCD can become either dead or stuck. The LCD will need repaired or replaced if there are more than 15 bad pixels present or more than three bad pixels within 1 cm.
12. Several visual quality checks for radiographic and digital imaging equipment can be performed by the technologist.
13. Several national scientific organizations have published protocols for assessing the quality of a digital display monitor. Assessment requires visual interpretation of a test pattern and photometric measurement of emitted light intensity.

Case Study

Recently, several radiographs have come out of the processor with static artifacts and guide-shoe marks. Tess is the QC technologist, and she is responsible for determining the causes of the artifacts and taking corrective action. After reviewing the various artifacts, Tess must answer the following questions.

Critical Thinking Questions

1. What QC tests should be performed?
2. What is the cause of static artifacts?
3. How can static artifacts be avoided?
4. What is the cause of the guide-shoe marks?
5. How frequently should the processor be cleaned?

Review Questions

Multiple Choice

1. **An x-ray rube operating above 70 kVp must have an HVL of at least __________ mm Al.**

   a. 1.5
   b. 2.5
   c. 3.5
   d. 5

2. **The developer temperature should be maintained within __________ °F of the set value.**

   a. ±2
   b. ±4
   c. ±5
   d. ±8

3. The __________ can be used to measure timer accuracy.

a. pinhole camera
b. optical densitometer
c. spinning top
d. line pair test pattern

4. A 4-min fluoroscopic examination with a 1.5-mA tube current results in a patient dose of __________ rad.

a. 4
b. 8
c. 12
d. 16

5. Which combination of temperature and humidity should be used for film storage?

a. 60% relative humidity, 10°F
b. 10% relative humidity, 10°F
c. 98% relative humidity, 68°F
d. 50% relative humidity, 68°F

6. Which QC test tool is used to determine blurring of an image?

a. Wire mesh test
b. Star test pattern
c. Pinhole camera
d. ERF

7. The light intensity of a viewbox should not vary by more than __________ when comparing several areas.

a. 1%
b. 20%
c. 10%
d. 15%

8. Exposure reproducibility for a radiographic unit should be within:

a. 8%
b. 25%
c. 5%
d. 1%

9. Pi mark artifacts run __________ to the direction of the film travel and at intervals of __________.

a. parallel, 3.14 inches
b. perpendicular, 3.14 inches
c. perpendicular, 2.58 cm
d. parallel, 2.58 cm

10. The ESD of a fluoroscopic system is typically __________.

a. 8 rad/min
b. 3 mrad/min
c. 3 mGy/min
d. 6 mGy/min

11. The actual kVp of any x-ray beam should not deviate by more than __________ of the readout from the kVp meter.

a. 8
b. 3
c. 1
d. 5

12. The size of the projected light field must be within ±__________ of the SID of the actual size of the x-ray beam.

a. 1%
b. 2%
c. 5%
d. 10%

13. Recommendations require that each mA station be linear to the two adjacent stations to within __________ accuracy.

a. 2%
b. 5%
c. 10%
d. 20%

14. Which of the following equipment calibration checks should fall with ±5%?

1. mAs reproducibility
2. X-ray beam alignment
3. Exposure timer
4. mA linearity
   a. 1 only
   b. 2 and 3 only
   c. 1 and 3 only
   d. 2, 3, and 4

15. Which QC tests for digital imaging can be reasonably performed visually by a technologist?

a. Field uniformity
b. Uneven spatial resolution
c. Erasure thoroughness
d. All of the above

16. A single CR plate is erased and then processed without exposing it to x-rays. This describes the test for:

a. lag or ghosting
b. erasure thoroughness
c. intrinsic noise
d. field uniformity

17. The device designed to directly measure luminance or the light intensity emitted from a display monitor is the:

a. densitometer
b. photometer
c. SMPTE test device
d. TG18-CX

Short Answer

1. Filtration is measured in radiography equipment using ___________.

2. The indicated kVp should fall within ___________ of the actual tested kVp.

3. The ___________ test is performed on intensifying screens and cassettes to check for proper screen/film contact.

4. The integrity of lead apparel should be checked how frequently?

5. The average skin dose during a fluoroscopic examination is ___________.

6. What is the importance of preventive maintenance for an automatic processor?

7. Name the three QC tools used to measure focal spot size.

8. Define linearity and provide the allowed variation.

9. Refer to Table 29.1, list the parts of the radiographic equipment that is tested regularly and give the tolerance specifications for each.

10. Quality control standards are more rigorous for primary monitors which are defined as those used for:

11. Luminance response for contrast for a display monitor should be such that the __________ percent and __________ percent areas on the SMPTE test pattern can be resolved.

12. The DICOM grayscale standard display function (GSDF) in incremented in steps called JNDs. This stands for:

13. On the SMPTE test pattern, resolution bars are provided in what five positions?

14. To check an LCD for an electronically dead pixel, what solid background color is used?

15. The American Association of Physicists in Medicine requires that not more than __________ defective pixels should be across a primary display monitor.

30

Computed Tomography

Objectives

Upon completion of this chapter, the student will be able to:

1. Compare the different generations of computed tomography (CT) scanners.
2. Describe the operation of a CT scanner.
3. Identify the components of a CT scanner.
4. Define CT numbers.
5. Identify the factors that influence spatial and contrast resolution.
6. Explain common CT artifacts.
7. Identify quality control tests performed on a CT unit.

Key Terms

- array processor
- computed tomography (CT)
- contrast resolution
- detector array
- edge response function (ERF)
- filtered back projection
- Hounsfield unit
- indexing
- interpolation algorithms
- maximum intensity projection (MIP)
- modulation transfer function (MTF)
- multiplanar reformation (MPR)
- multislice CT
- pitch
- predetector collimator
- prepatient collimator
- reconstruction time
- shaded surface display (SSD)
- shaded volume display (SVD)
- slip-ring technology
- solid-state detectors
- spatial frequency
- spatial uniformity
- translation
- voxel

Introduction

The invention of the computed tomography (CT) scanner revolutionized radiographic examinations because of the difference in appearance and sensitivity of CT scans. CT scanners produce cross-sectional images of the body with the tissues and organs displayed separately, instead of superimposed as in a conventional radiograph. CT scans are much more sensitive to small differences in tissue composition than are conventional radiographs.

Historical Perspective

The invention of the **computed tomography** (CT) scanner has revolutionized medical imaging. CT produces a dramatic increase in diagnostic information compared with conventional x-ray procedures. This extraordinary invention was made possible by Godfrey Hounsfield and Allan Cormack.

Godfrey Hounsfield was born in 1919 in Nottinghamshire, England. He studied electronics and electrical and mechanical engineering. In 1951, he joined the staff at Electric and Musical Industries (EMI) in Middlesex, England, where he worked on radar systems and computer technology.

In 1967, Hounsfield was researching pattern recognition and reconstruction techniques by using a computer. Through this work, he hypothesized that if an x-ray beam was passed through an object from all directions and measurements were made of the x-ray transmission data, that information about the internal structures could be obtained. His work used an apparatus with gamma radiation and a crystal detector. The apparatus required 9 days to scan an object and 2.5 hours to process the information to produce a single-section image.

In 1971, the first clinical CT brain scanner was installed at Atkinson-Morley's Hospital in England. Under the direction of Dr. James Ambrose, clinical studies were conducted resulting in modifications of the scanner to reduce processing time for the picture to 20 minutes. With the introduction of minicomputers, the processing time was further reduced to 4.5 minutes. During this time, Allan Cormack was developing solutions to the mathematical problems in CT. Cormack was a physics professor at Tufts University in Medford, Massachusetts, and he worked on solving the mathematic formulas used to reconstruct the CT image. He published articles in the *Journal of Applied Physics* in 1963 and 1964, respectively. Hounsfield and Allan Cormack were awarded the Nobel Prize in Medicine or Physiology in 1979 for their contributions to the development of computed tomography.

Principles of Operation

In CT, the scan produces a transverse or transaxial image. This image is perpendicular to the long axis of the body. Digital processing of the transverse data produces images in sagittal and coronal sections (Fig. 30.1). Using postacquisition reconstruction algorithms, various images can be produced without the need to rescan the patient and expose them to additional radiation.

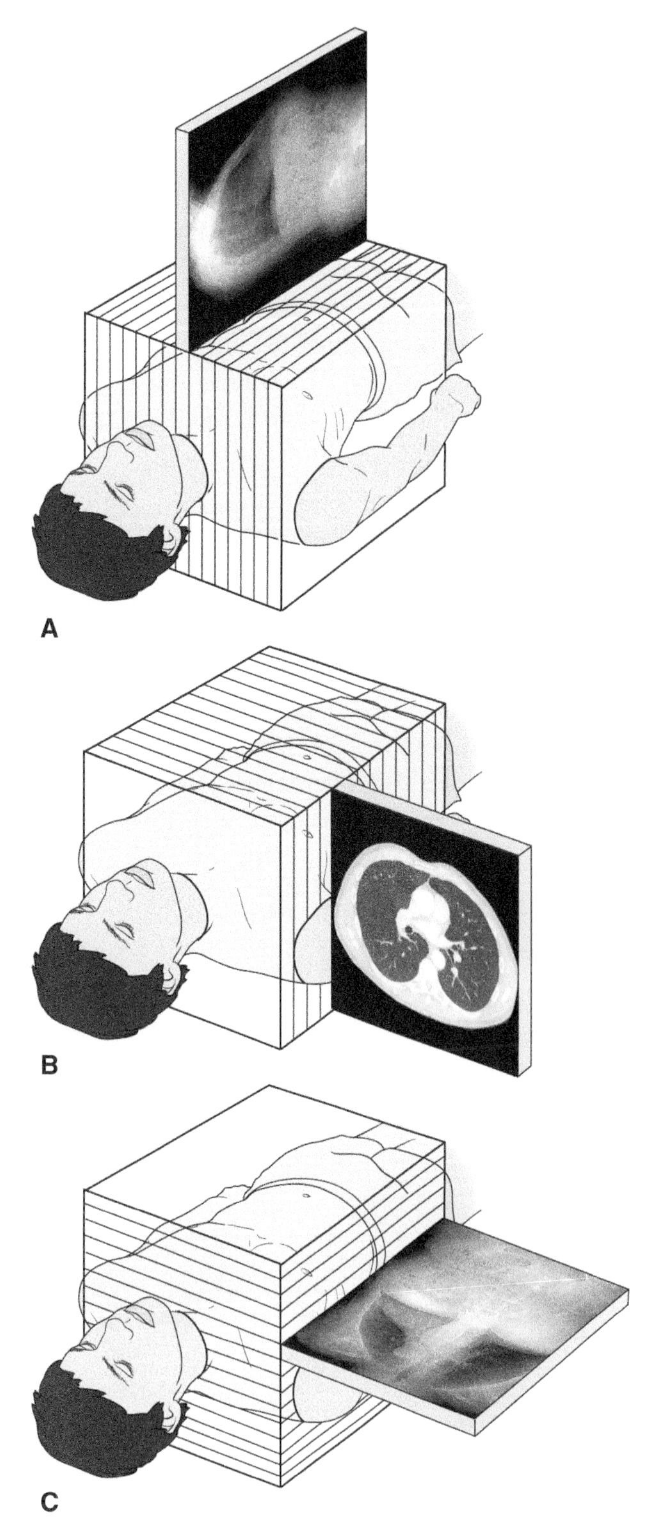

Figure 30.1. Scanning projections. (A) Sagittal. (B) Transverse. (C) Coronal.

The exact method a CT imaging system uses to produce a transverse image is extremely complex, understanding it requires knowledge of physics, engineering, and computer science. The basic principles can be understood if one has a firm understanding of a finely collimated x-ray beam and single detector. These components move synchronously. When the x-ray beam is turned on, it will pass through the patient, anatomic tissues, and structures that will attenuate the x-ray beam. The intensities in the remnant beam will be detected, and an intensity profile or projection is formed. This simple process occurs many times until the entire anatomical area is imaged, resulting in a large number of projections. The projections are stored in the computer in digital form. Computer processing of the projections involved reconstructing all the anatomic structures in relation to one another to form a "slice" or complete picture of that specific area. This simple explanation will be expanded upon throughout the following sections.

CT Scanner Generations

Since the original EMI scanner, there have been rapid advancements in CT scanners. As technology has progressed, the development of scanners has kept pace. Currently, there are seven generations of scanners with each generation providing faster scan times and improved image manipulation.

First Generation

The first-generation CT scanner was a single x-ray system designed to examine only the head. This scanner used one or two detectors and a single finely collimated x-ray beam so that two continuous slices could be imaged (Fig. 30.2).

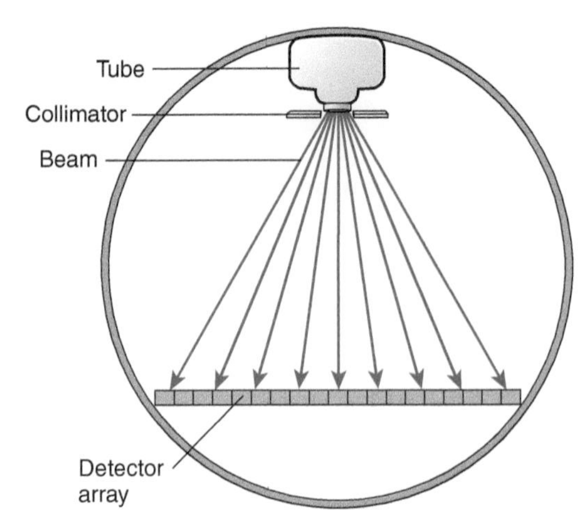

Figure 30.3. **Second-generation CT scanner.**

The x-ray beam was a pencil-thin field, which scanned 180 degrees around the patient's head. The first-generation scanner used a translate-rotate system. The x-ray tube and detectors were connected and moved synchronously from one side to the other while scanning the patient; this is called **translation**. The x-ray tube and detectors then rotate 1 degree into the next position and then translates or moves across the patient in the opposite direction. The x-ray beam was turned on while translating and off during rotation. This back-and-forth process was performed 180 times for each scan. The major drawback to the first-generation units was that it took nearly 5 minutes to complete one slice.

Second Generation

The second-generation CT scanner used a single-projection fan-shaped beam and a linear array with up to 30 detectors in the **detector array** (Fig. 30.3). The x-ray tube and detectors move in unison just like the first-generation scanner. The translate-rotate mechanism was used, and with the increased number of detectors, the translations

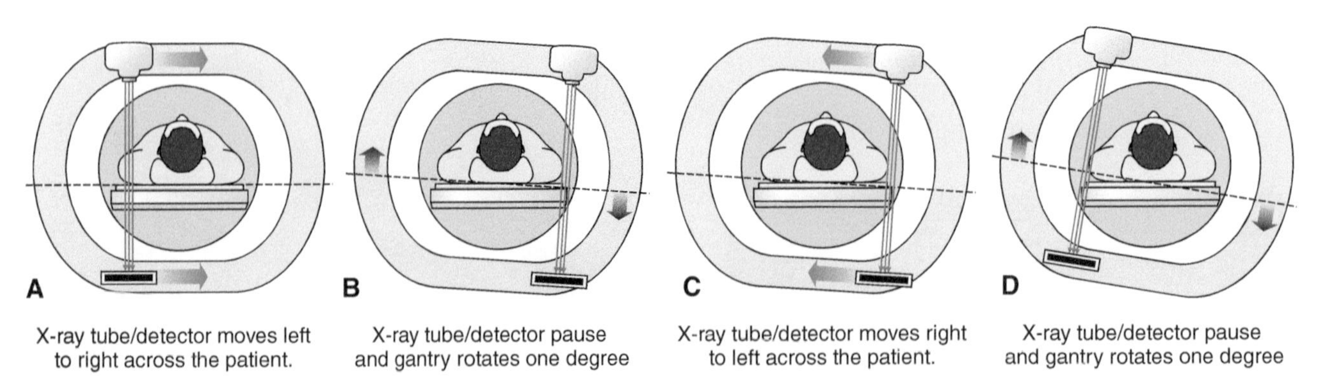

Figure 30.2. **Shows a schematic view of a first-generation CT scanner.**

were separated by rotation increments of 5 degrees or more. When a 10-degree increment rotation is used, only 18 translations would be needed for the 180-degree image acquisition. Scan time was reduced to ~30 seconds per slice; this allowed for the patient to hold his or her breath long enough for a complete scan. With these advancements, the rest of the body could be scanned.

Third Generation

A primary limitation with prior generations of scanners was the scanner's inability to rotate in a 360-degree arc around the patient. Third-generation scanners use a wider fan-shaped beam and a curvilinear detector array that forms an arc of 30 to 40 degrees or greater (Fig. 30.4). For the first time, the detectors and x-ray tube had the ability to continuously rotate. The translate-rotate mechanism was replaced with this rotate-rotate mechanism. The x-ray tube and detectors both rotate in a circle around the patient and the x-ray beam slices through the body to produce the image data. The support couch and the patient advance, and the tube again rotates around the patient to generate data for the next image. With this generation of scanner, the entire patient can be viewed with each scan. The scan time was reduced to 1 second per slice.

The curvilinear detector array produces a constant x-ray source to detector path length. This allows for better x-ray beam collimation and reduces the effect of scatter radiation.

Fourth Generation

Fourth-generation imaging systems use a single-projection fan-shaped beam with up to 4,000 detectors mounted to circular array, which forms a ring on the inside of the gantry. The system uses a rotate and stationary configuration where the ring of detectors remains stationary, while the x-ray tube rotates within the gantry (Fig. 30.5). As the tube moves within the circle, single x-rays strike a detector. The x-rays are produced sequentially during the circular travel. These scanners are capable of subsecond scan times, can accommodate multiple slice thickness through automatic prepatient collimation, and image manipulation capabilities. The image reconstruction algorithm is for fan beam geometry in which the apex of the fan is now at the detector.

Fifth Generation

The fifth-generation scanner was designed as a dedicated cardiac unit. These scanners are considered high-speed CT scanners because they acquire data in milliseconds. This type of scanner is also called the electron beam CT scanner (EBCT). The design of the EBCT scanner produces high-resolution images of moving organs such as the heart without motion artifact. The scanner can be used for imaging the heart and other organs in adults and children.

The x-ray tube has been replaced with an electron gun that generates a 130-kV electron beam. The beam

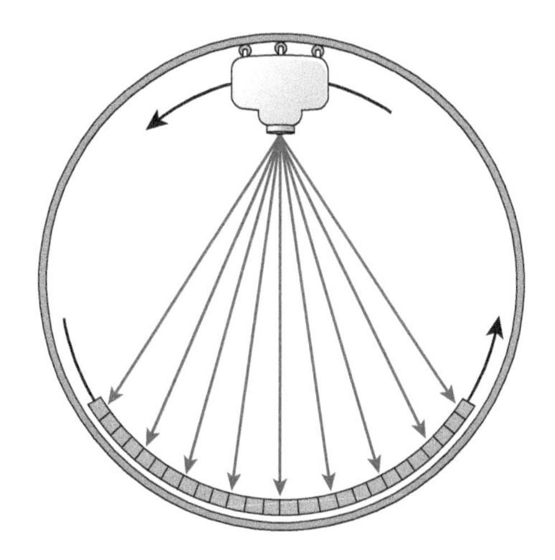

Figure 30.4. Third-generation CT scanner.

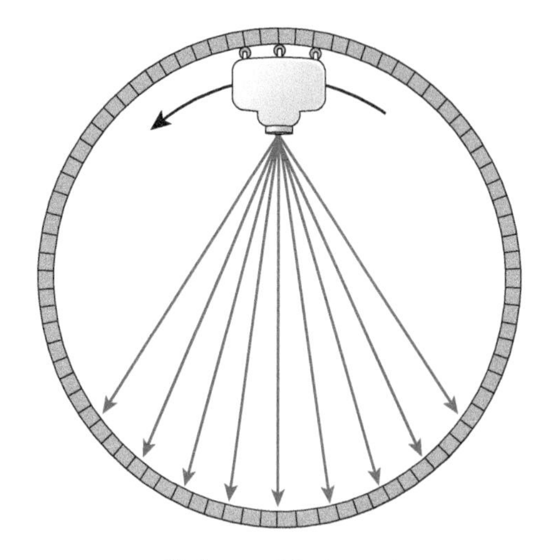

Figure 30.5. Fourth-generation CT scanner.

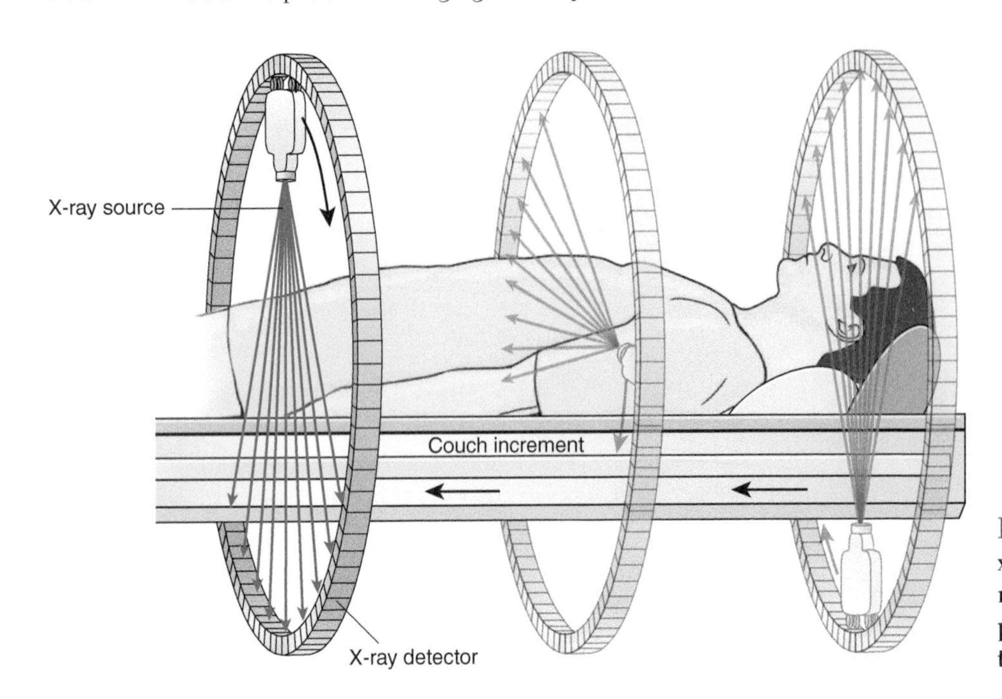

Figure 30.6. **Illustrates how the x-ray tube of a spiral CT scanner rotates around the patient, while the patient support table moves through the CT scan plane.**

is accelerated, focused, and deflected at a precise angle by electromagnetic coils to strike one of four adjacent tungsten target rings. These rings are stationary and span a 210-degree arc. The electron beam is steered along the rings, which are used individually or in any sequence.

When the electron beam strikes the tungsten ring, x-rays are produced. Collimators shape the x-rays into a fan beam that passes through the patient to strike a curved, stationary array of detectors across from the tungsten rings. The detector array of the two rings makes up a 216-degree arc of detectors. The first ring holds 864 detectors, while the second ring holds 432 detectors, which are twice as large as those in the first ring. The arrangement of the detector array allows for either two slices to be acquired with one target ring or eight slices when all four target rings are used in sequence. This scanner is 10 times faster than conventional CT scanners, which makes it fast enough to provide real-time dynamic sectional images of the beating heart.

Sixth Generation

Generations one through four utilized cables to provide the electricity necessary to move the components of the scanner while also providing kilovoltage for the x-ray exposure. The cables limited the scanners because the cables could only rotate a certain amount before they had to be "unwound." The sixth-generation scanner was designed to use slip-ring technology to replace the cables. The slip-ring technology allows continuous rotation of the x-ray tube and detectors around the patient.

As the x-ray tube circles around the patient, the patient table is continuously moved through the bore of the gantry. This allows for a continuous set of attenuation data to be obtained in a helical manner; therefore, this generation of scanner is referred to as a helical scanner (Fig. 30.6). Helical scanning differs from conventional CT scanning in that the support table is not stopped at the center of each slice location while the data are collected.

The primary advantage of the helical scanning is a dramatically shorter scan time; helical CT examinations can be completed in <1 minute. Other advantages include the ability to complete the entire exam with the patient holding his or her breath one time, lower amount of contrast media to produce a diagnostic image, and a decrease in motion artifacts.

The acquisition time is the time required to collect the CT data. The acquisition time for conventional axial CT scans is typically several seconds per slice. The acquisition time for helical scans is about 30 seconds. The examination time is the total time required to collect the CT data.

Multislice CT Scanners

The use of helical/spiral geometry is the most recent development in CT data acquisition. The terms spiral and helical are synonymously used to describe the data acquisition of continuous rotation scanners. Although the actual shapes of a spiral and helix are somewhat different, the terms have the same meaning when describing CT scanners with continuous rotation. Many authors and radiographers use both terms, but for this text, helical is the term of choice.

Multislice scanners or multisection scanners are able to expose multiple detectors simultaneously due to detector technology, which permits an array of thousands of parallel bands of detectors to operate at the same time (Fig. 30.7). This coupled with helical scanning that drastically reduces the total exam time for an entire chest or abdomen to 15 to 20 seconds. The **multislice CT** scanners (MSCT) is designed to be more efficient, reduces patient exposure to radiation, improves image resolution, and allows unprecedented postacquisition reconstruction of acquired data.

The need for faster scan times and sophisticated 3D and multiplanar reformation has encouraged the development of continuous rotation scanners where data are collected in volumes instead of single slices. CT scanning in helical geometry is based on slip-ring technology, which shortens the high-tension cables to the x-ray tube to allow continuous rotation of the x-ray tube. The overall goal of MSCT is to improve the volume while providing

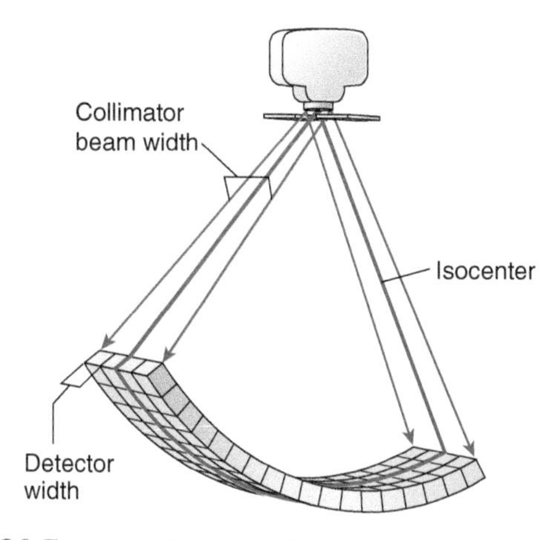

Figure 30.7. **Seventh-generation CT scanner.**

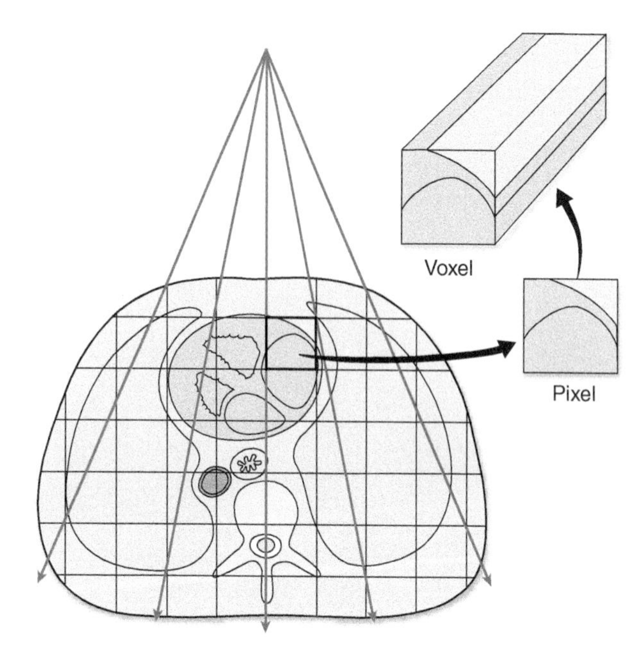

Figure 30.8. **Shows a fan-shaped beam from a CT scanner and the relationship between an individual pixel and voxel.**

improved spatial resolution compared to the older four slices per 360-degree rotation scanner. Current 64-slice volume scanners produce better spatial resolution of ~0.4-mm isotropic voxels and temporal resolution compared to 16-slice scanners. The thickness of the beam determines the slice thickness or amount of tissue irradiated and the volume of each pixel element (Fig. 30.8). The volume element is called a **voxel.**

Once the scan begins, the x-ray tube rotates continuously, and the couch continuously moves the patient through the plane of the rotating x-ray beam. The x-ray tube is on for the entire scan time, data are collected continuously, and an image can be reconstructed at any *z*-axis position along the length of the patient.

Interpolation Algorithms

During helical CT, image data are received, and data points are assigned at prescribed intervals as seen in Figure 30.9. When the image is reconstructed, the image plane does not contain sufficient data for reconstruction. To provide a complete set of information in the plane, the data must be estimated using **interpolation algorithms.**

Interpolation algorithm is a special computer program used to "fill in" missing data. The first interpolation algorithm used 360-degree linear interpolation. Referring to Figure 30.9, the dots represent known

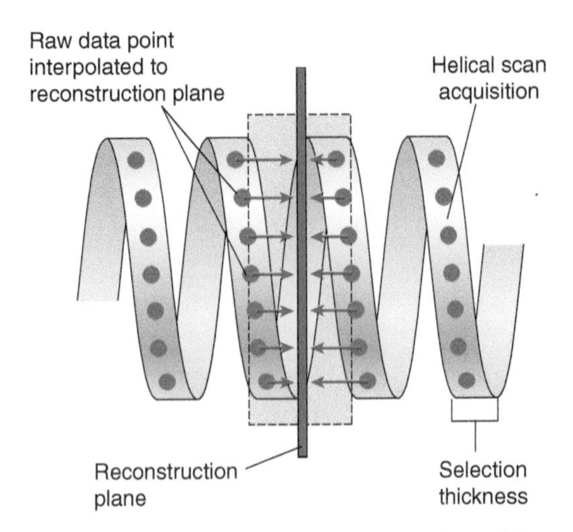

Figure 30.9. **Helical interpolation. The *dotted line* indicates the location where the raw data are projected. This section forms the image that is displayed.**

values of measured data. The interpolation algorithm will use these values to estimate the value between the two dots of known values. When you want to estimate a value between known values, that is called interpolation. The plane of the reconstructed image was interpolated from data acquired one revolution apart.

The transverse plane images will display with a high level of clarity. When sagittal or coronal views are formatted, there is a significant amount of blurring in the image. The solution to the blurring problem was to interpolate values separated by 180 degrees, half a revolution of the x-ray tube. This results in improved resolution for images from all scan planes.

Pitch

Helical pitch ratio, known simply as **pitch**, is the relationship between couch movement and the width of the x-ray beam in the time the x-ray tube makes one full 360-degree rotation. Pitch is expressed as such as 0.5:1, 1:1, 1.5:1, or 2:1. In a 1:1 ratio, the couch movement is equal to the section thickness. A pitch of 0.5:1 results in overlapping images and increased patient dose. A 2:1 pitch results in extended imaging and reduced patient dose. Increasing the pitch more than 1:1 increases the volume of tissue that can be imaged at a given time. This is an advantage of multislice helical CT: the ability to scan a larger volume of tissue during a single breath-hold. In clinical practice, the pitch for multislice helical CT is usually 1:1. Because multiple slices are obtained and reconstruction methods can be performed after imaging, overlapping images is not necessary.

Regardless of the generation of CT scanner, the latent image is acquired and archived in a similar manner. The exit radiation is detected and converted into a digital signal by the analog-to-digital converter or ADC. Data from many different entrance angles are processed in a computer to determine the transmission and attenuation characteristics of the tissues in the section under examination (Fig. 30.10). The data are stored in a matrix of pixels. The digital pixel data are processed in a digital-to-analog converter (DAC) before being displayed. The DAC converts the digital data into an analog signal for display.

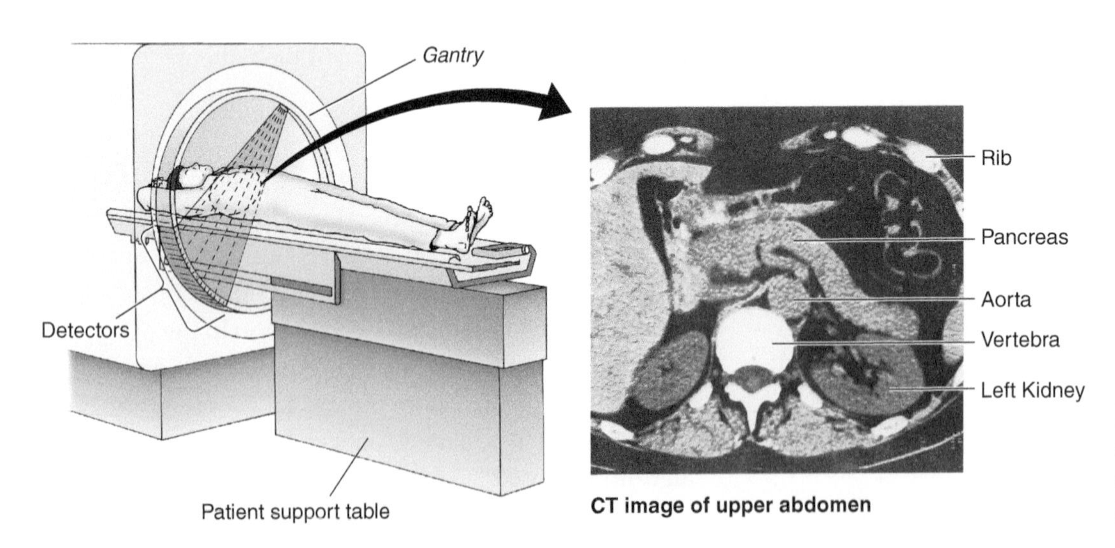

Figure 30.10. **Shows a schematic view of a CT scanner and the resultant image.**

Components of a CT Scanner

A CT imaging systems consists of four major components: a gantry, a patient support couch, a computer system, and an operating console (Fig. 30.11).

The Gantry

The gantry is a doughnut-shaped structure containing the x-ray tube, the detector array, the high-voltage generator, the patient support couch, and the mechanical supports for each. These subsystems receive electronic commands from the operating console then transmit data to the computer for image production and postprocessing.

The gantry frame maintains the proper alignment of the x-ray tube and detector array. The frame also contains the components necessary to perform scanning movements. The gantry has an aperture for the patient to pass through during the scan. Inside the gantry cover is a large ring that holds the detector array and the track for the x-ray tube while it rotates around the patient.

Most CT gantries can be angled to permit positioning the patient for coronal images and to align the slice plane to certain anatomy such as the base of the skull or lumbar spine curvature. The gantry can be angled toward or away from the patient couch and may permit coronal scanning of body areas, especially the head. There are also positioning lights mounted on the gantry. There are intense white lights and low-power red laser lights, which assist the positioning of the body. There can be three lights, which are used to accurately line the patient up for sagittal, coronal, and transverse centering.

X-Ray Tube

Multislice helical CT x-ray tubes are very large. Because of the size of the x-ray tube, multislice helical CT scanners place a considerable thermal demand on the x-ray tube. The x-ray tube can be energized up to 60 seconds continuously. The x-ray tube produces a continuous beam; it is a high-heat capacity tube that is capable of

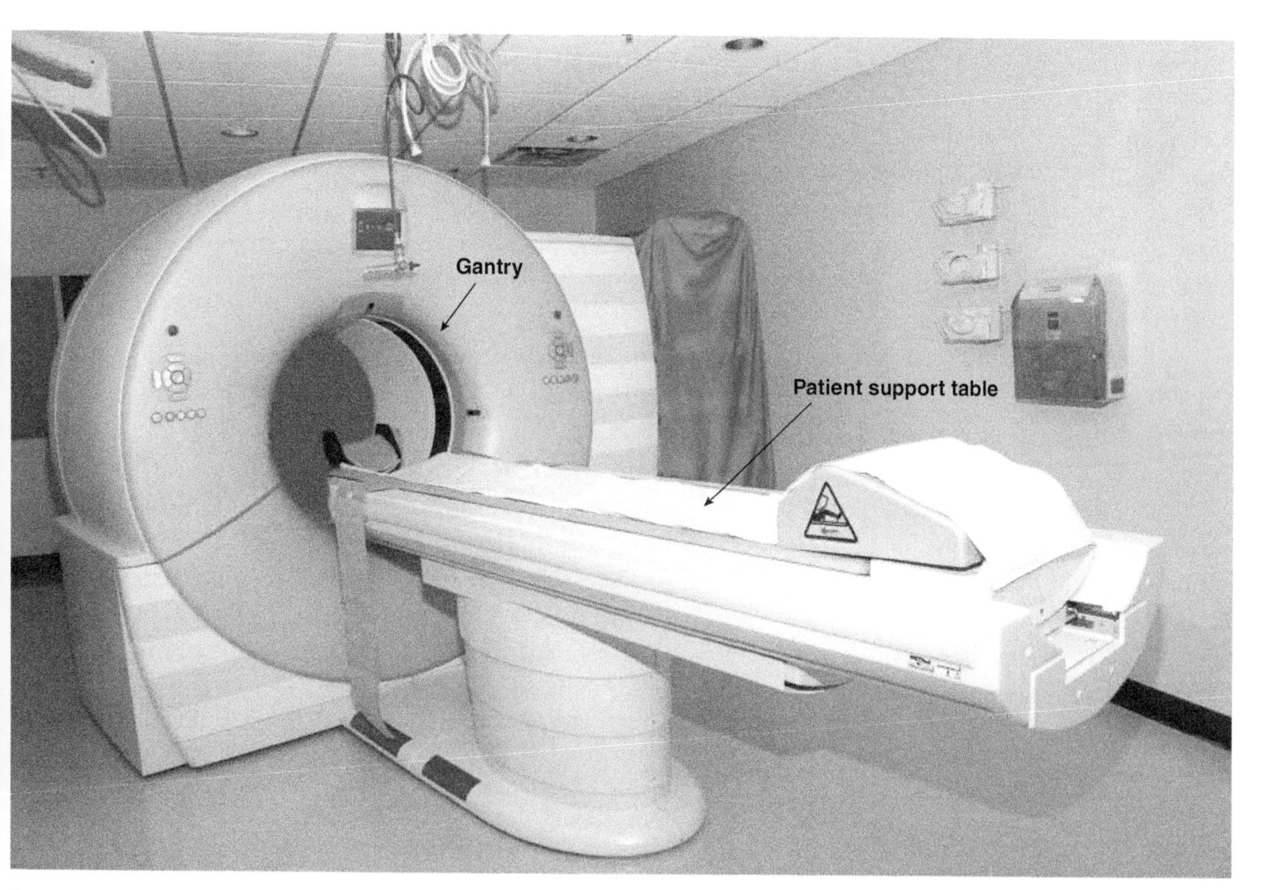

Figure 30.11. Shows the gantry and patient support table of a modern CT scanner.

operating up to 400 milliamperes (mA) and 120 to 150 peak kilovolts (kVp) for several seconds. High-speed rotors are commonly used because of their ability to dissipate heat. Tube failure is a main cause of CT imaging system malfunctioning and is a primary limitation for helical imaging.

The design of the focal-spot size is a consideration for CT imaging systems. In order to have high spatial resolution imaging, the x-ray tubes need to have a small focal spot.

Because the multislice CT x-ray tube is large, it has anode heat storage capacities up to 8 MHU or more. The anode disc has a large diameter and is thicker, which results in a greater mass. This design allows for anode cooling rates of ~1 MHU/min.

One notable company has developed a CT x-ray tube that uses liquid–metal technology to improve heat dissipation during helical procedures. The traditional x-ray tube has ball bearings, which allow the anode to spin rapidly; the high heat associated with helical scanning can cause the bearings to wear prematurely or to weld together. The liquid metal acts as a lubrication medium, which is a good conductor of heat. The tube is capable of cooling at a rate over 100 KHU/min.

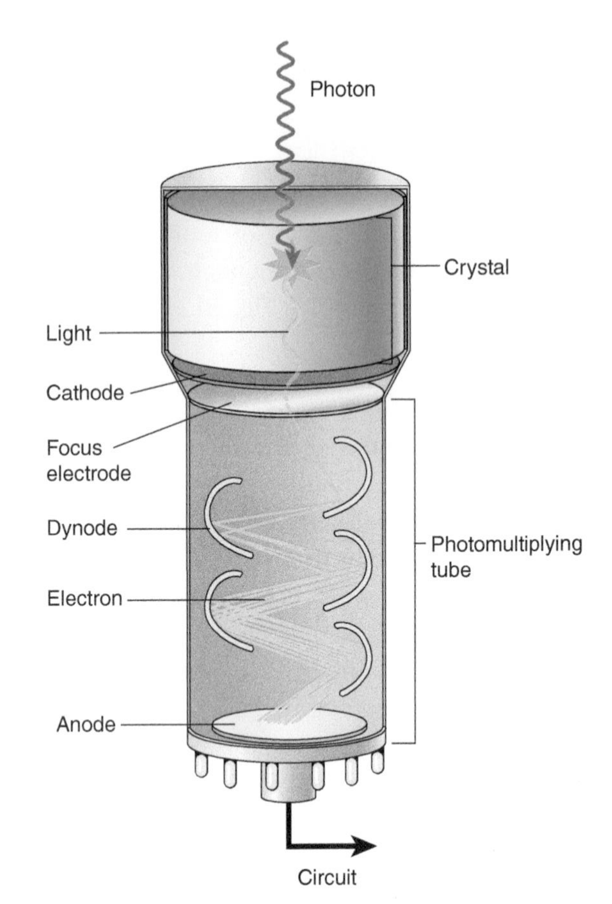

Figure 30.12. **Shows a typical scintillation detector.**

Detector Array

Multislice helical CT scanners have multiple detectors in an array that numbers into the thousands. Rotating detector systems use enough detectors to intercept the entire fan beam. The image quality, resolution, and efficiency of the stationary and rotating detector systems are effectively the same.

CT scanners employ scintillation crystals or **solid-state detectors**. The image quality and detection efficiency of the different types of detectors are approximately the same.

Scintillation detectors in early systems were comprised by sodium iodide (NaI) crystals. The radiation produces light in proportion to the intensity of the photon and at the site where the photon struck the crystal. The light from the scintillation crystal is detected by a photomultiplier (PM) tube (Fig. 30.12). The light photon strikes the cathode of the PM tube where it is converted into electrons. The electrons are then amplified by a chain of dynodes as they pass through the PM tube. The dynodes have progressively higher voltage, which causes an increase in the number of electrons as they move toward the anode. Once the electrons bombard the anode, they are converted into an amplified electrical signal, which is then processed by the computer. The scintillation crystals and PM tubes were used in early generations of scanners but are not conducive to the modern scanners because of the phosphorescent afterglow properties of the scintillation crystals.

The sodium iodide was replaced by bismuth germinate (BGO) and cesium iodide (CsI). The current crystals of choice are special ceramics and cadmium tungstate. The concentration of scintillation detectors is an important feature of a CT imaging system that affects the spatial resolution of the system. Scintillation detectors have high x-ray detection efficiency where ~ 90% of the x-rays that strike the detectors are absorbed; this contributes to the output signal. Improvements in design have made it possible to place the detectors next to each other with no space between them. This results in overall detection efficiency approaching 90%. There are several advantages to this type of design: reduced patient radiation dose, faster imaging time, and improved image quality because of increased signal-to-noise ratio. The detector design is especially crucial to multislice helical CT scanners.

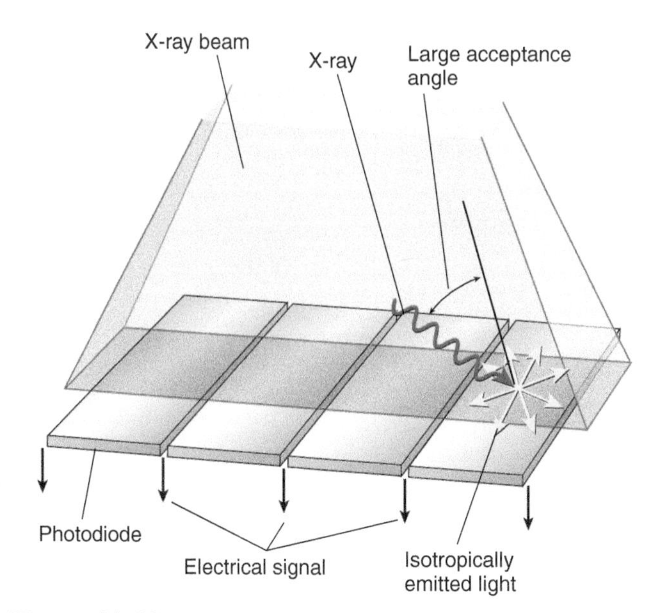

Figure 30.13. **Solid-state detector. The photodiode is coated with a scintillator. When the remnant x-ray photons activate the scintillator, light photons are emitted and detected by the photodiode. The photodiode then gives off an electrical signal.**

Solid-state detectors are used in helical and MSCT scanners. Solid-state detectors combine a calcium tungstate, yttrium, or gadolinium ceramic scintillator with a photodetector. As seen in Figure 30.13, when the x-ray photon interacts with the solid-state scintillator, light photons are emitted isotropically in proportion to the intensity of the light. The scintillator is able to accept incoming x-ray photons because it is sensitive to the divergence of the fan-shaped beam. This permits the entire array of detectors to operate simultaneously. The photodiode detects the light photons emitted by the scintillator and converts them into an electrical signal, which is used by the computer to form the digital image.

The arrangement and type of detectors used in a particular CT scanner are selected by the manufacturer for commercial reasons. The processing of the signal from any type of detector is essentially the same in all CT scanners. The image quality of all modern CT scanners is effectively the same.

Collimation

Collimation is required in CT scanning for exactly the same reasons as in radiography. Proper collimation reduces patient dose by restricting the amount of tissue that is irradiated. Collimation also enhances image contrast by limiting scatter radiation. Multislice helical CT units use two collimators. The **prepatient collimator** is mounted on the tube housing and limits the area of the patient that is exposed to the primary beam. This collimator determines the slice thickness and patient dose. The **predetector collimator** restricts the x-ray field viewed by the detector array, thereby reducing scatter radiation on the detector. When properly coupled with the prepatient collimator, the predetector collimator helps to determine the slice thickness. The predetector collimator reduces scatter radiation that reaches the detector array that improves image contrast.

Patient Support Couch

The patient support couch is constructed of low atomic number carbon graphite fiber so it does not interfere with transmission of the x-ray beam and patient imaging. It is motor driven to move smoothly and accurately to allow precise positioning of the patient. It must be able to support the entire weight of the patient when moved into the gantry aperture.

The positioning of the couch is called **indexing**. Couch indexing must be accurate and reproducible within 1 millimeter (mm). In conventional axial CT scanning, the tube rotates around the patient to collect data for one slice, the couch indexes into the gantry at a preset distance, and the tube rotates again to collect data for the next slice. The x-ray beam is on only during tube rotation. A typical axial CT examination involves collecting data from 10 or more sections and requires several minutes to complete. In spiral scanning, the support couch moves steadily through the gantry, while the tube continuously rotates around the patient.

Slip-Ring Technology

Slip-ring technology uses slip rings that are electromechanical devices that conduct electricity and electrical signals through rings and brushes from a rotating surface onto a fixed surface. One ring remains stationary, while an inner rotating ring has brushes that remain in electrical contact with the inside of the stationary ring. Brushes that transmit electricity to the gantry components glide in contact grooves on the stationary slip ring. Composite brushes made of silver graphite alloy (a conductive material) are used as the sliding contact. As a result, the inner ring is free to rotate continuously without interruption. In the slip-ring system, power and electrical signals are transmitted through the stationary rings, which eliminate the need for electrical cables. Recall that in early CT systems, the gantry would rotate one direction then it had to rotate the opposite direction to unwind the cables.

Computer System

The CT computer is a unique component of the CT system. The computer must have sufficient speed and memory to solve as many as 250,000 calculations simultaneously. The CT computer is designed to control data acquisition, processing, display, and storage. At the CT console, the radiographer has access to software programs that allow processing and display of the images. The computer system microprocessor calculates the attenuation of the individual voxels using the x-ray exit radiation data collected at many different tube positions around the patient. The computer programs used to perform these calculations are called algorithms. The calculations of the CT microprocessor must be very fast to produce images for immediate viewing. The time it takes from the end of scanning to the appearance of an image is called the **reconstruction time**. Because of the number of scans produced for one CT exam, the microprocessor may not be fast enough. Many CT systems now use an **array processor**, which is capable of performing many calculations simultaneously and is significantly faster than the microprocessor.

Operating Console

CT imaging systems can be designed to use two or three consoles. The CT radiographer will use one console to operate the imaging system. This console permits control of all scan parameters including selecting proper technical factors, movement of the gantry and patient couch, and computer commands that allow reconstruction and transfer of image data for storage in a data file. The CT console operates a menu of directory operations including preprogramming with the kVp and mA values for individual anatomic sites. The radiographer uses a keyboard and mouse to indicate the desired operation for the anatomy to be scanned.

A second console may be available for the radiographer to postprocess images to annotate information on the images. This console also allows the radiographer to view the images before transferring them to the PACS and radiologist.

The third console is part of the physician's work station and has a separate cathode ray tube or LCD flat panel display with controls. The console is a separate workstation that allows radiologists to retrieve previous images, display, and manipulate images to optimize diagnostic information. CT display consoles permit a wide range of features to enhance the digital image. These features include:

- Scanogram: A scout image of the area to be scanned. Dotted lines corresponding to the section intervals provide a convenient reference guide when viewing the images.
- Multiplanar reformations (MPRs): A computer process that stacks transverse images on top of each other to form a three-dimensional (3D) set of data.
- Reverse display: Allows the image to be reversed from right to left and to reverse density so that black appears white and white appears black.
- Magnification: Enhances visualization of small structures but can distort the image if used beyond three-times magnification.
- Suppression: Allows a problem area to be outlined and deleted from the reconstruction data.
- Region of interest (ROI): An area of an anatomic structure that is measured to display the average Hounsfield unit.
- Annotation: Text that is added to images for anatomical labeling or descriptive purposes.
- Maximum intensity projections (MIP): A type of 3D process, reconstructing an image by selecting the highest value pixels along a line through the data set and exhibiting only those pixels.
- Three-dimensional imaging: Specialized software and image processing units allow the manipulation of the image to visualize structures that are hidden. The image can be rotated, tumbled, or tilted, and densities can be made more translucent or divided.

Image Characteristics

Section Interval and Thickness

The section interval is the distance between scan sections, while the section thickness is the width of the volume of tissue being imaged (voxel). The section thickness is typically less than voxel width due to the divergence of the x-ray beam. The divergence of the x-ray beam causes a problem where either overlapping or excluding tissue between sections occurs. The radiographer must take this into consideration when setting up the section interval and thickness for a given scan. CT units have preset programs, which standardize scanning parameters for given procedures that take into account the correct amount of overlap needed; however, the parameters can be modified to accommodate special circumstances.

Exposure Factors

Most CT scanners operate at a preset kVp. Because of helical scanning, time is not a factor because it is controlled by the scanning program so that the sufficient exposure can be made to the detectors. The radiographer can change the mA setting to control the primary beam. It is critical that the correct amount of mA be used to keep the dose to the patient as low as possible while providing optimum images.

Algorithms

When setting up a scan, the radiographer must select the appropriate algorithm for the scan. The operator's console combines the correct algorithm with the scanning procedure. The use of the correct algorithm will make it possible for the CT unit to filter unwanted artifacts so they are not displayed in the final image.

Image Matrix

The CT image format consists of a matrix of pixels, which are assigned a number for the level of density in the pixel. The pixel is displayed as an optical density or brightness level on the monitor. Modern systems provide matrices of 512 × 512, which results in 262,144 pixels of information. Each pixel contains numerical information called a **Hounsfield unit** or CT number. The pixel is a two-dimensional representation of the tissue volume.

The field of view (FOV) or scan field size is set to accommodate the size of the body area being scanned. The matrix size is fixed, and when the FOV is increased, for example, from 12 to 20 cm, the size of each pixel will be increased proportionally. When the FOV is increased from 512 × 512 to 1,024 × 1,024, the size of each pixel is smaller. As previously discussed, the smaller the pixel size, the better the image resolution is.

CT Numbers

The CT number of each voxel is calculated from the transmission data collected as the beam passes through the patient at many different angles. Each pixel is displayed on the video monitor as a level of brightness, which corresponds to the level of optical density in the pixel. The relative attenuation characteristics of a voxel are reported as a CT number and referred to as Hounsfield units. The CT numbers range from −1,000 to +3,000 for each pixel. A CT number of −1,000 corresponds to air, while a CT number of +3,000 corresponds to dense bone. A CT number of zero indicates water. Table 30.1 shows the CT values of various tissues.

Changing the size of either the matrix or the slice thickness may change the CT number because different tissues will be included in the voxel. The CT number of a tissue is always calculated relative to the attenuation of water. The CT number of a tissue is given by:

$$\text{CT number} = \frac{k(\mu_t - \mu_w)}{\mu_w}$$

where μ_t is the attenuation coefficient of the voxel and μ_w is the attenuation coefficient of water, and k is a constant that determines the scale factor for the range of CT numbers. Because the CT number is based on the difference between the attenuation coefficient of each voxel and the attenuation coefficient of water, the CT number

TABLE 30.1 HOUNSFIELD UNITS OF VARIOUS TISSUES

Tissue	Hounsfield Unit or CT Number
Air	−1,000
Lung	−200
Fat	−100
Water	0
Tumors	+5 to 35
Blood	+20 to 40
Cerebrospinal fluid	+15
Gray matter	+40
White matter	+45
Muscle	+50
Liver	+40 to 70
Blood, clotted	+55 to 75
Dense bone	+700 to 3,000

of water is always equal to zero. Tissues with densities greater than water have positive CT numbers; tissues with densities less than water have negative CT numbers. Tissues with negative CT numbers are displayed as darker densities, while tissues with positive CT numbers appear as lighter densities. For the CT system to operate with precision, the detector response must be routinely calibrated so that water is always represented by zero. When *k* is 1,000, the CT numbers are called Hounsfield units and range from −1,000 to +1,000.

Image Quality

Image quality is controlled by the resolution of the image and the amount of noise in the image. There are five basic characteristics, which determine the overall quality of a CT image. These include spatial resolution, contrast resolution, noise, linearity, and uniformity.

Spatial Resolution

Spatial resolution is defined as the minimum separation of two objects that can be distinguished in the image as two separate objects. In CT imaging, an image of a geometric structure that has a sharp border, such as the vertebral spine, the image at the border will be somewhat blurred. The amount of blurring is a measure of the spatial resolution of the imaging system. The CT systems have certain limitations; the expected sharp edge of CT values is replaced with a smoothed range of CT values at the interface between the pixels at the border of the spine and the adjacent tissue. The ability of the CT imaging systems to reproduce with a high degree of accuracy and the high-contrast edge is expressed mathematically as the **edge response function (ERF)**. The measured ERF can be transformed into another mathematical expression called the **modulation transfer function (MTF)**. The MTF along with its graphic depiction are most often mentioned to express the spatial resolution of the CT imaging system.

Increasing the matrix size decreases the pixel size and improves spatial resolution. Spatial resolution in CT scanning depends on a combination of factors, including focal spot size, beam collimation, detector size, matrix size, pixel size, and subject contrast. Larger matrices with small pixels and high subject contrast have better spatial resolution. Utilizing small focal spots and narrow collimation provides better spatial resolution.

Spatial frequency is measured in line pairs per centimeter (lp/cm). A low spatial frequency represents large objects, and a high spatial frequency represents small objects. When comparing two objects, the low-frequency larger object will be represented more accurately than the high-frequency smaller object. The loss in accurate reproduction with increasing spatial frequency occurs because of limitations in the imaging system. Limitations that contribute to the degradation of the image include collimation, detector size and concentration, mechanical and electrical gantry control, and the reconstruction algorithm.

Contrast Resolution

One of the major advantages of CT scanning is its ability to image tissues with similar attenuation characteristics. **Contrast resolution** is the ability to distinguish two objects with similar attenuation values regardless of their size or shape. Multislice helical CT images have high-contrast resolution, which is the biggest advantage of CT imaging. For example, Figure 30.14 demonstrates how blood and liver are very close in attenuation characteristics but have different appearance on a CT scan of the abdomen.

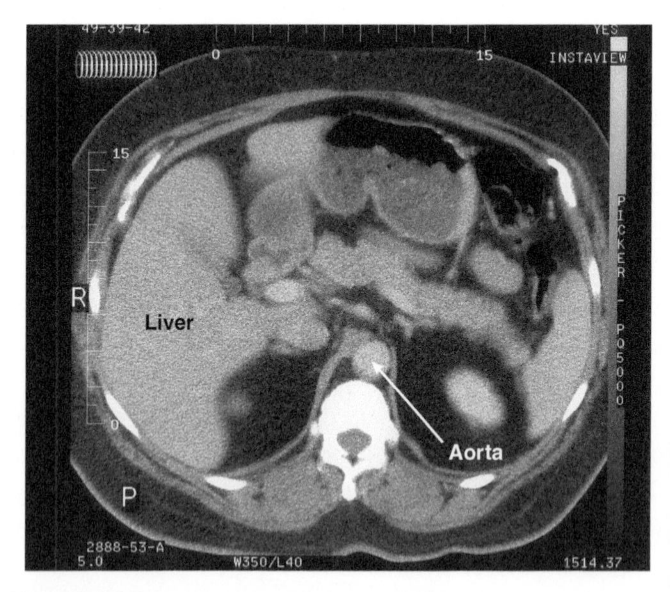

Figure 30.14. Demonstrates the difference in appearance between blood in the aorta and liver tissue in a CT examination of the abdomen.

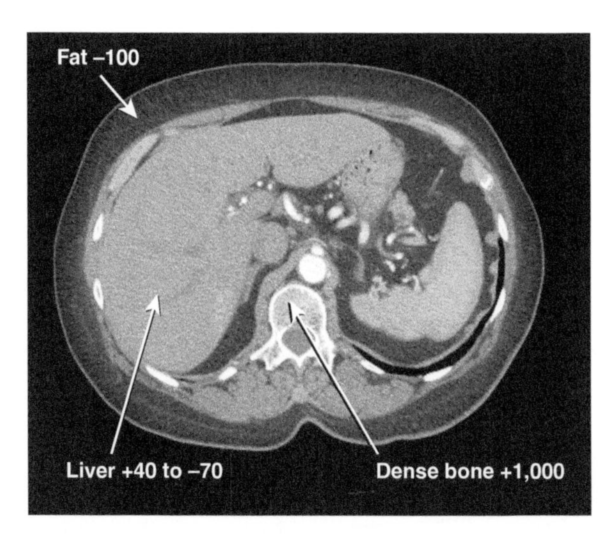

Figure 30.15. The soft tissues in the abdomen are very similar in density. The CT scanner is excellent in distinguishing between these small differences and allows a clear image of all the structures.

Contrast resolution is determined by the number of density differences stored in each matrix. A low-contrast image has many density differences in the entire image, while a high-contrast image has few density differences. The level of contrast in each pixel is determined by the absorption of x-ray photons in tissue, which is characterized by the linear attenuation coefficient. Tissue with a higher atomic number will attenuate more photons and will have a higher linear attenuation coefficient (Fig. 30.15).

The CT imaging system can amplify the differences in subject contrast so the image contrast is high. The range of the CT numbers seen in Figure 30.15 are 100, 50, and 1,000. The amplified contrast scale allows CT to better resolve adjacent structures that are similar in composition. CT is superior to conventional radiography in the realm of contrast resolution because of the scatter radiation rejection of the prepatient and predetector collimators. The ability of CT to image low-contrast objects is limited by the size and uniformity of the object as well as the noise of the system.

Noise

When a homogenous object such as water is imaged, each pixel value should be zero. This will never happen because the contrast resolution in the system is not perfect. This means that the CT numbers may average zero; however, a range of values greater than and less than zero exist. This variation in CT numbers above and below the average is the noise in the system. All digital images have problems with system noise.

Noise in the CT image is directly related to a number of factors:

- kVp and filtration
- pixel size
- slice thickness
- detector efficiency
- patient dose

The noise is seen as graininess on the image. Low-noise images appear very smooth to the eye, while high-noise images appear blotchy. System noise should be evaluated daily by scanning a 20-cm diameter water phantom. The CT imaging system has the ability to measure a ROI on the image. The system will compute the mean and standard deviation of the CT numbers in the ROI. To accurately measure noise, the ROI must include at least 100 pixels. The noise measurements should include five control areas: four on the periphery and one in the middle.

Linearity

The CT scanner must be calibrated so that water is consistently represented as zero HU, and other tissues are represented by their appropriate CT value. A calibration check that can be performed daily uses a five-pin phantom of the American Association of Physicists in Medicine (AAPM). Each pin is made of a different plastic material that has known physical and x-ray attenuation properties. The phantom is scanned, and the CT number for each pin is recorded. When plotted on a graph, the CT number versus the linear attenuation coefficient should travel in a straight line going through zero. Any deviation from linearity is an indication of a malfunction or misalignment in the scanner.

Uniformity

When a uniform object is imaged, each pixel should have the same value because each pixel represents exactly the same object. If the CT system is properly calibrated, the value should be zero. As previously discussed, a CT imaging system is an extremely complex electronic mechanical device, and it is not possible to have such consistent precision. The CT value for water may drift from day to day or even hourly.

When the water bath is imaged and the pixel values are constant in all areas of the reconstructed image, it is considered to have **spatial uniformity**. Spatial uniformity is easily tested by using a software package to plot the CT numbers along any axis of the image as a line graph. If all values along the line graph are within two standard deviations of the mean value, the system is considered to exhibit acceptable spatial uniformity.

Image Reconstruction

As the patient is being scanned, the detectors transmit information proportional to the attenuation coefficient of the voxel of tissue. The projections acquired by each detector are stored in computer memory. The image is then reconstructed by the computer using complicated mathematical algorithms called Fourier transform. The Fourier transform is primarily used in MRI to reconstruct images, while a modern CT scanner uses filtered back projection or convolution. Helical CT scanners are also capable of producing 3D images using multiplanar reformation.

Filtered Back Projection

Filtered back projection is the process of modifying pixel values by using a mathematical formula; an actual filter is not used. We will first describe back projection to explain the foundation of this technique. Figure 30.16 View 1 demonstrates simple back projection where all the pixels have the same value along the x-ray path. The peak on

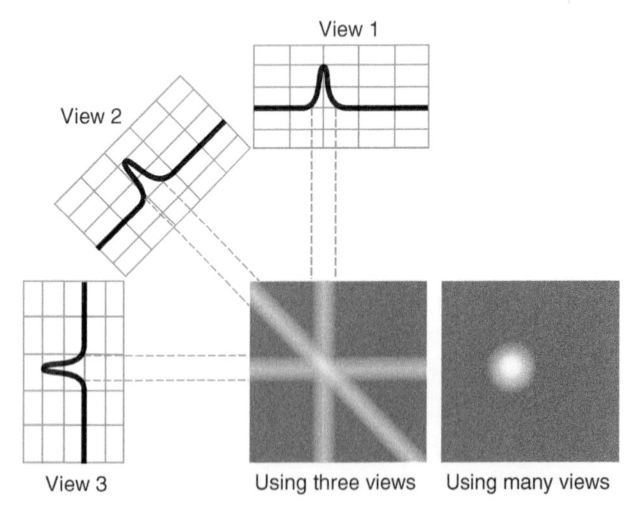

Figure 30.16. Back projection. Notice how the object has a blurry appearance after many views are used.

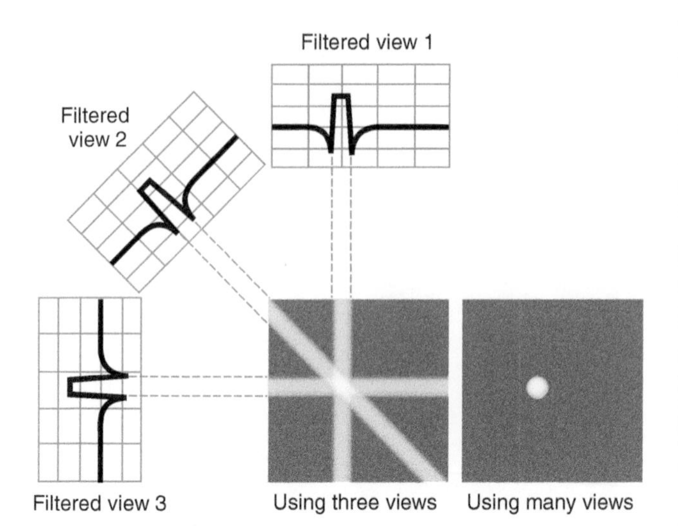

Figure 30.17. Filtered back projection. Modifying the projection results in sharp borders in the object.

the graph represents pixels of a certain value as the x-ray beam traveled through the object. The arrow represents that the view is "smeared" backward through the image in the direction it was originally acquired. This back projection occurs for each of the three views in Figure 30.16. Using many views to construct the entire image, a single point in the image is reconstructed as a circular area that has increased intensity in the middle and decreased intensity at the periphery. This is because the back projected image is blurry.

Filtered back projection is a technique to correct the blurring of the image in back projection. As demonstrated in Figure 30.17, each view is filtered before the back projection to counteract the blurring. Each of the one-dimensional views is convolved with a one-dimensional filter kernel to create a set of filtered views. The kernel overlies each pixel and changes the value of the pixel. Notice how the view graphs have been changed by the filter. The top of each pulse is flattened, resulting in the final back projection creating a level uniform signal within the circle; negative spikes have been added at the sides of each pulse. When the spikes are projected backward, these negative regions counteract the blur. This removes the blurring seen in simple back projection and results in a mathematically exact reconstruction of the image. The image will now appear crisp and sharp.

The filtered back projection proved effective, but a more robust reconstruction algorithm has been developed—iterative reconstruction. This type of reconstruction technique uses small steps to calculate the final image. There are several variations of this method with the difference between them being how the successive corrections are made. Iterative reconstruction requires more computer capacity, but it can result in improved contrast resolution with lower radiation dose to the patient.

Reformatting

Reformatting uses data from a series of sectional images to produce an image in a new scan plane without actually rescanning the patient. Reconstruction algorithms can take the scanned transverse sections and extract coronal or sagittal images to provide additional views of the patient's anatomy (Fig. 30.18). Multidetector CT coupled with reconstruction software excels in producing three-dimensional **multiplanar reformation (MPR)** images. Transverse images are stacked to form a three-dimensional data set; this new data set can be used to construct an image in a variety of ways. There are three 3D MPR algorithms that are used the most commonly: **maximum intensity projection (MIP)**, **shaded surface display (SSD)**, and **shaded volume display (SVD)**.

MIP selects the highest value pixels along a line through the data set to reconstruct an image; only those pixels will be displayed. MIP is excellent for CTA examinations because the images can be reconstructed quickly. Only a small portion of the 3D data points are used to make an image. This results in a very high-contrast 3D image of contrast-filled vessels. The software on the computer allows the image to be rotated to demonstrate 3D features.

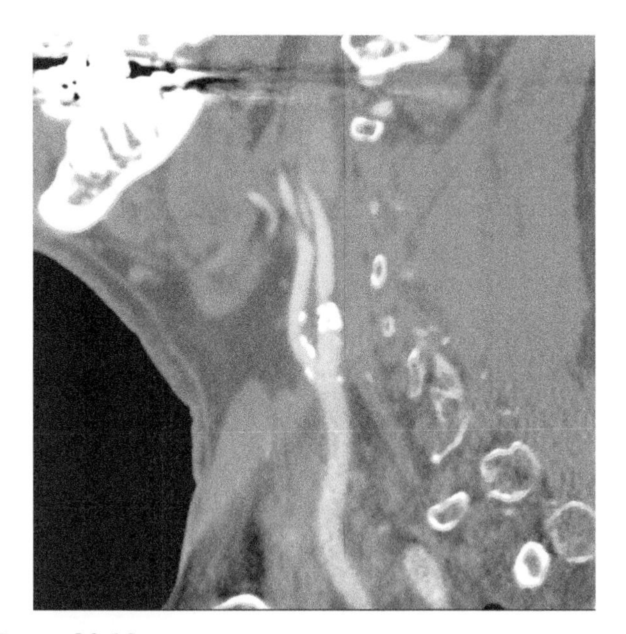

Figure 30.18. Sagittal image. Image produced from transverse plane with postacquisition algorithms.

SSD is a computer-aided technique, which was initially used for bone imaging but is now used more regularly for virtual colonoscopy imaging. The operator selects the SSD identified range of values, and when the range is displayed, it appears as the surface of the organ or structure such as the colon. Regardless of the algorithm used, MPR allows improved visualization of the normal anatomy and anatomic variants. It also provides greater diagnostic accuracy in the evaluation of organs and blood vessels.

Artifacts

As with conventional radiographic imaging, CT images can be produced with various types of artifacts.

Motion

Motion artifact on a CT image appears as a streak through the image. This type of artifact occurs when an error in the algorithm does not detect the changes in attenuation that occur at the edges of the moving part. The CT image will have blank pixels, which appear as a streak in the areas of algorithm error.

Metal or Star

Metallic materials in the patient can cause streak artifacts but may also cause a star artifact (Fig. 30.19). The artifact

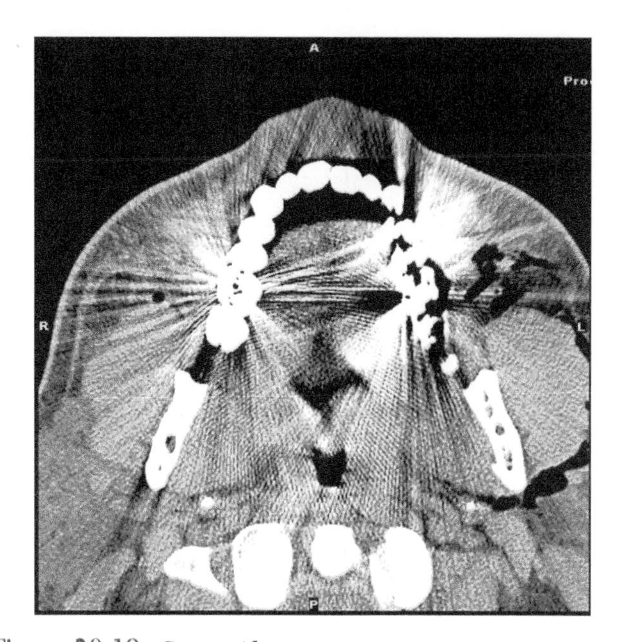

Figure 30.19. Star artifact.

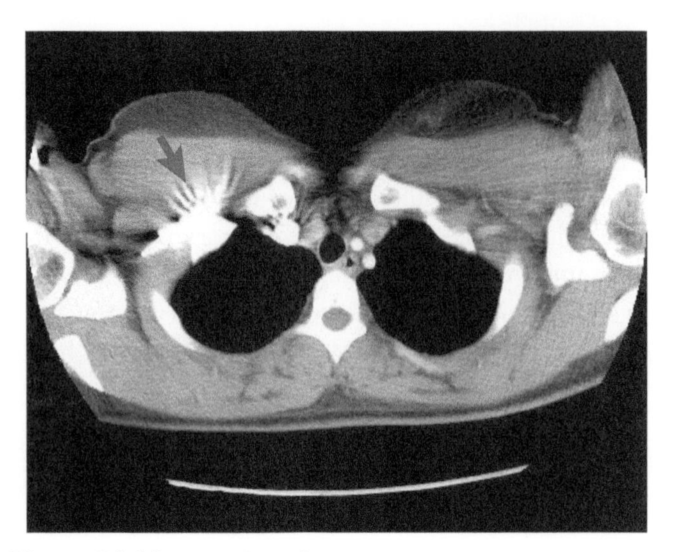

Figure 30.20. **Metal artifact.**

is caused when the metal object attenuates 100% of the primary beam, thereby producing an incomplete projection. If the algorithm is not able to create a full set of surrounding projections to smooth the edges of the object, the star artifact will be visible.

Figure 30.20 demonstrates a metallic artifact. In this image, the arrow is pointing to the area where there may be a metallic object such as a Port-A-Cath implanted at the chest wall. Because the metal is attenuating a large amount of radiation in this area, there is not sufficient information for the computer algorithm to adequately produce an image.

Beam Hardening

Beam hardening artifacts occur as the beam is attenuated when it passes through the patient. This type of artifact results from the beam being significantly attenuated as it passes through the patient. These artifacts appear as broad dark bands or streaks in the image.

Partial Volume Effect

Partial volume effect occurs when tissue that is smaller than the section thickness or voxel width is hidden from the view on the image. This artifact is produced because the data from the whole section thickness are averaged together to form the image. This type of artifact can also occur if a tiny portion of a large structure is located in the section thickness; the tiny portion is simply averaged in with the rest of the information.

Ring Artifacts

Ring artifacts occur when a single detector goes out of calibration and does not properly record attenuated data. The detector error has a unique annular or ring appearance in the image (Fig. 30.21).

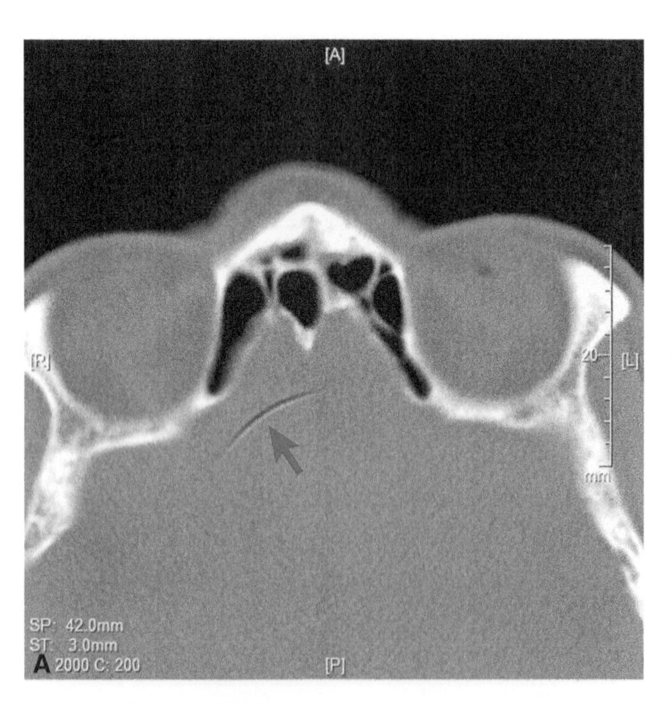

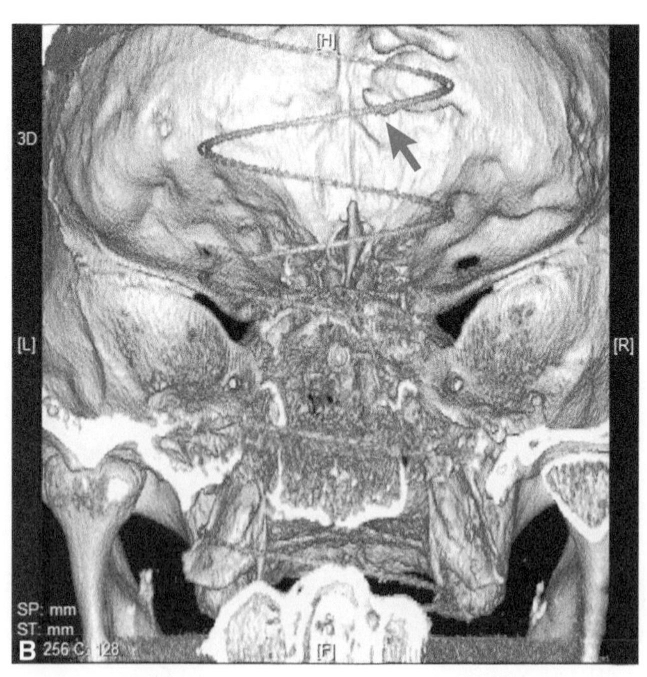

Figure 30.21. **(A) Ring artifact. (B) Ring artifact in volume rendered 3D reconstructed image.**

Computed Tomography Quality Control

Computed tomography has many moving parts, which could experience instability, misalignment, miscalibration, and malfunction. These parts include the gantry, detectors, console, computer, and patient couch. Computed tomographic QC includes annual tests of system noise and uniformity, linearity, spatial resolution, contrast resolution, slice thickness, patient exposure, laser localizer, and support table increment accuracy. An effective QC program will encompass daily, weekly, monthly, and annual measurements and visual inspection that coincides with a preventive maintenance program. The measurements should also be performed when the equipment has had a repair of a major component or when new equipment has been installed. Table 30.2 provides a quick reference of the QC tests, frequency of testing, and limits.

Noise and Uniformity

The test for noise and uniformity is performed weekly. A 20-cm water bath is scanned, and the average value of water should be within ±10 Hounsfield units (HU) of zero. The uniformity should be such that there is variation of not more than ±10 HU across the image.

Linearity

CT linearity is measured using the AAPM five-pin phantom with plastic rods of different calibrated densities and HU. The coefficient correlation for the relationship between the electron density and HU should equal or exceed 0.96% or two standard deviations. The unit is initially calibrated so that water has a HU of 0, and air has a HU of −1,000. The assessment is performed semiannually. Systems that are used to perform quantitative CT must precisely determine the value of tissue in HU.

TABLE 30.2 **CT SCANNER QC TESTS**

Factor	Frequency	Limits
Noise	Weekly	±10 HU
Uniformity	Weekly	±0.04%
Spatial resolution	Semiannual	±20%
Contrast resolution	Semiannual	±0.5%
Slice thicknesses <5 mm	Semiannual	0.5 mm
Slice thicknesses >5 mm	Semiannual	1 mm
Support table indexing	Monthly	±2 mm

Spatial Resolution

Monitoring spatial resolution is the most critical component of the CT program. It is crucial to ensure the spatial resolution is at a maximum. This ensures that the detector array and reconstruction electronics are performing properly and that the mechanical components of the CT unit are also performing as expected.

The QC tests for spatial resolution include imaging a wire or an edge to obtain the ERF. These functions are then mathematically converted to obtain the MTF. The specific test used is the preference of the medical physicist. The spatial resolution should be assessed semiannually to be certain the unit stays within the manufacturer's specifications.

Contrast Resolution

The contrast resolution of the CT scanner is of superior quality. The specifications vary from one manufacturer to another and even between the different models. The current standard for all scanners is the ability to resolve 5-mm objects at 0.5% contrast. Contrast resolution testing should be performed semiannually and can be performed with low-contrast phantoms, which have built-in analytical schemes.

Couch Increment Accuracy

The patient couch moves with precision through the gantry while the patient is scanned. It is imperative that the patient couch be evaluated monthly to make sure it is working correctly. The test is performed when a patient is on the couch. During the scan, make note of the position of the couch at the beginning and ending of the examination by using a tape measure and a straightedge on the table rails. Compare the measurement with the expected couch movement; it should be within ±2 mm.

Slice Thickness

A specially designed phantom that has a ramp, spiral, or a step wedge is used to measure slice thickness. The slice thickness should be ±1 mm of an expected 5 mm or greater slice thickness. A slice thickness <5 mm has an acceptable tolerance of 0.5 mm. The assessment should be performed on a semiannual basis.

Laser Localizer

Most CT scanners utilize internal and external laser lights for patient positioning. There are several specially designed phantoms for determining the accuracy of the laser localizers. The accuracy should be tested semiannually and can be performed at the same time as the evaluation of the couch incrementation.

Patient Dose

Due to the broad range of examinations in CT, there are no recommended limits specified for the permissible dose to the patient. The dose will vary according to the scan parameters with high-resolution scanning requiring increased dose. There are some examinations that utilize a fixed technique from one patient to the next. Patient radiation dose is specified as CT dose index or dose-length product and can be monitored with specially designed pencil ionization chambers or thermoluminescent dosimeters.

Chapter Summary

1. CT scanners provide cross-sectional images, also called transaxial images, of the body by measuring the x-ray transmission through the body.
2. The x-ray tube is mounted on a circular frame inside the gantry together with the radiation detectors. The detectors are mounted either on a stationary ring or on a support frame that rotates opposite the x-ray tube.
3. The x-ray tube has collimators to set the size of the x-ray beam and a high heat capacity rotating anode.
4. The patient support couch moves the patient through the gantry at preset increments in conventional CT scanning.
5. In helical CT scanning, the tube and detectors rotate continuously, while the support couch and patient are moved through the gantry.
6. Helical CT scans produce a complete examination in a shorter time because the tube rotates continuously around the patient instead of starting and stopping for each slice.
7. The spatial resolution of CT scans depends on the focal spot size, pixel size, and matrix size. Smaller pixel sizes give better spatial resolution.
8. The CT number of a tissue describes the difference in density between the tissue and water. The CT number of water is always 0.
9. Contrast resolution describes how close in density two tissues can be and still be recognized as separate tissues.
10. High mA CT scans with large pixels have superior contrast resolution because they have more x-ray counts in each pixel.
11. Helical CT units have the computer software abilities to reconstruct or reformat data to display various images. This permits additional images for the radiologist while sparing the patient additional radiation exposure.
12. There are several artifacts that are unique to computed tomography. The more common artifacts include motion, star, beam hardening, partial volume effect, and ring artifacts.
13. Each CT unit must have quality control testing performed on a regular basis to ensure the unit is operating at an optimal level.

Case Study

CT scanners utilize radiation detectors to gather remnant radiation that contains the latent image. Various generations of scanners have used scintillation detectors, gas-filled ionization detectors, or solid-state detectors.

Critical Thinking Questions

1. Which type of detector is used in a helical scanner?
2. What materials are used in the detector?
3. How is the digital image formed?

Review Questions

Multiple Choice

1. CT scanning provides a(n) __________ view of the body.

a. axial
b. linear
c. longitudinal
d. transaxial

2. The gantry of a spiral CT scanner contains:

a. the tube
b. the detectors
c. high-voltage circuit
d. all of the above

3. The x-ray beam in a second-generation CT scanner is shaped into a __________ beam.

a. pencil
b. circular
c. fan
d. hypocycloidal

4. In helical CT scanning, pitch is the ratio of:

a. the rotation speed to the patient motion per revolution
b. the amount of couch movement per revolution to the section thickness
c. the section thickness to the revolutions per second
d. the section thickness to the revolutions per patient motion

5. The CT number of water is:

a. −1,000
b. −50
c. 0
d. +1,000

6. When the field of view increases and the matrix size remains unchanged, the contrast resolution will be:

a. improved
b. degraded
c. unchanged

7. The number of pixels required to image one line pair is:

a. 1
b. 2
c. 4
d. 8

8. The Hounsfield unit for blood is:

a. +60
b. −40
c. −300
d. +40

9. **Slip-ring technology uses a stationary ring and a rotating ring with ________ that make contact with the stationary ring.**

   a. needles
   b. brushes
   c. metallic pads
   d. metallic shoes

10. **Where is the predetector collimator located?**

    a. Between the x-ray tube and the patient.
    b. CT units do not use predetector collimators.
    c. It is located between the patient and the detector array.

Short Answer

1. **Who is the person credited with the invention of computed tomography?**

2. **The patient support table is made up of which material?**

3. **Using Table 17.1, the CT number of −100 relates to which type of tissue?**

4. **Explain why the CT computer must be high speed and have a large capacity?**

5. **Why is collimation important in CT scanning?**

6. **What are the components of the gantry?**

7. **Which device controls the slice thickness of a CT scan?**

8. **The numerical information contained in each pixel is a(n) ________ or ________?**

9. **Define linearity and contrast resolution.**

10. **Define the terms transaxial, translation, and reformatting.**

PART VI

Radiation Biology and Protection

31

Radiation Biology: Cellular Effects

Objectives

Upon completion of this chapter, the student will be able to:

1. Describe the reproductive cycle of the human cell.
2. Identify the relative radiation sensitivity of human cells, tissues, and organs.
3. Discuss target theory of radiobiology.
4. Relate the Law of Bergonie and Tribondeau.

Key Terms

- anabolism
- catabolism
- chromosomes
- codon
- cytoplasm
- deoxyribonucleic acid (DNA)
- endoplasmic reticulum
- fractionation
- genetic cells
- homeostasis
- interphase
- linear energy transfer (LET)
- lysosome
- meiosis
- metabolism
- mitochondria
- mitosis
- nucleus
- oxygen enhancement ratio (OER)
- precursor cells
- protraction
- relative biological effectiveness (RBE)
- ribonucleic acid (RNA)
- ribosomes
- somatic cells
- stem cells
- undifferentiated cells

Introduction

Radiation biology is the study of the effects of ionizing radiation on biological tissue. Radiobiology research is striving to accurately describe the effects of radiation on humans so that safe levels of exposure to radiation can be determined. The advent of using radiation to image the human body has provided unparalleled information for radiologists to diagnose and image pathologies. Radiation must be used with respect for the potentially damaging effect it can have on tissue. It is the responsibility of the radiographer, radiologist, and medical physicist to produce high-quality images while using the least amount of radiation possible.

With this approach, there will be a lower risk of radiation exposure to patients and radiation workers. This chapter examines the concepts of human biology and the body's response to radiation.

Human Biology

The human body is composed of ~80% water. Water plays a very important role in delivering energy to target molecules, which contributes to radiation effects. These effects will be discussed later in the chapter. The remainder of the molecular composition in the body consists of about 15% proteins, 2% lipids, 1% carbohydrates, 1% nucleic acid, and 1% of other materials. These molecules are organized into the living cells of the body including epithelial (skin) cells, osteocytes (bone cells), nerve cells, and blood cells. The cells of a specific type combine to form tissues, and tissues combine to form organs. The functions of cells can differ greatly, but all cells in the body have many common features. They absorb nutrients, produce energy, and synthesize molecular compounds. These activities are called metabolism. There are two types of cells in the body: genetic and somatic. Genetic cells are cells of the reproductive organs, which carry the task of preserving the species through reproduction. Somatic cells are all the other cells in the human body (skin, nerve, muscle, etc.) that specialize in a particular organ function for survival and thriving of the organism.

Cell Theory

At the very basic level, the human body is composed of atoms. When the atoms are exposed to ionizing radiation, damage may occur at the atomic level. The atomic composition of the body as well as the molecular and tissue composition all define the type of response to radiation.

When radiation strikes a cell, the interaction at the atomic level will result in molecular change; this can produce a cell, which is deficient in normal growth and metabolism. If the radiation dose is high enough, it could mean cell death.

Molecular Structure

There are five primary types of molecules in the body. Four of these are considered to be macromolecules: proteins, lipids, carbohydrates, and nucleic acids. Each of these molecules contains carbon and supports the life of the organism. Nucleic acid molecules are the rarest molecule and are considered to be the most critical and radiosensitive target molecule. The two types of nucleic acid molecules will be discussed in the next section.

Water is the most abundant molecule in the body yet it is the most simple. The water molecules are very important in delivering energy to target molecules and also contribute to the radiation effects of the cell. Recall that the water molecule consists of two atoms of hydrogen and one atom of oxygen. Water molecules assist the body in maintaining the proper balance of the internal environment, which is called **homeostasis**. When the body is out of balance, for example, when electrolytes are depleted, the body is no longer in homeostasis. The body will go through biochemical reactions in an attempt to restore homeostasis so that the systems in the body can properly perform their functions.

During a normal cycle, the cell will break down large molecules into smaller molecules; this is called **catabolism**, which results in the waste products of water and carbon dioxide being exuded by the cell. **Anabolism** is the production of large molecules from small molecules. The term **metabolism** is the sum of catabolism and anabolism, which happen in a cell.

Proteins comprise ~15% of the molecular configuration in the body. Proteins are macromolecules that are a linear arrangement of amino acids connected by peptide bonds. Twenty-two amino acids are used in protein synthesis, the production of proteins. The linear arrangement of the amino acids determines the exact function of the protein molecule. Proteins are used in many areas of the body. They provide structure and support to tissue. Muscles are tissues that are very high in protein content. Proteins can also function as enzymes, hormones, and antibodies.

Enzymes are molecules that allow a biochemical reaction to continue in the cell. Enzymes are used in small quantities and are not part of the reaction, but they are critical in the continuation of the biochemical reaction.

Hormones are molecules that exert regulatory control over select body functions such as growth. Endocrine glands (pituitary, adrenal, thyroid, parathyroid, pancreas, and gonads) produce and secrete hormones for specific body functions.

Antibodies are the body's primary defense mechanisms against infection and disease. The configuration of the antibody is designed for attacking a particular type of antigen, which is an invasive pathogen or infectious agent.

Lipids (fats) are macromolecules made up of carbon, hydrogen, and oxygen. Lipids are made of two smaller molecules: glycerol and fatty acid. Each lipid molecule is made up of one glycerol and three fatty acid molecules. Lipids are the structural components of cell membranes and therefore are found in all body tissues. Lipids concentrate just under the top layer of skin and act as a thermal insulator from environmental temperatures. Lipids also act as fuel for the body because they are energy stores; however, it is very difficult to convert lipids into energy.

Carbohydrates are also made of carbon, hydrogen, and oxygen; however, their structure is different from lipids. Carbohydrate atoms have a 2:1 ratio of two hydrogen atoms for each oxygen atom; the majority of the atom is made up of hydrogen and oxygen. Carbohydrates are also called saccharides. Monosaccharides and disaccharides are sugars. Glucose is a simple sugar that is contained in a small molecule. In the human body, polysaccharide is stored in the tissues of the body and used as fuel when there is an insufficient amount of glucose.

Glucose is the primary molecule that provides fuel to the body. Lipids can be catabolized into glucose for energy, but this is a very difficult process. Polysaccharides are much easier to transform into glucose. When a quick burst of energy is needed, eating a food high in glucose (candy or chocolate) will do the trick!

Cell Structure

Figure 31.1 is the common model for the basic cell structure. The cell has two main components: the cytoplasm and nucleus. Most of the cell is composed of **cytoplasm**, a watery medium in which the organelles are suspended. The cytoplasm contains organelles that produce energy, synthesize proteins, and eliminate waste and toxins.

The organelles include the **mitochondria**, which digest macromolecules to produce energy for the cell. This makes the mitochondria the power source for the cell.

The small round orbs are the **ribosomes** whose main function is to produce proteins, which are essential for cell function.

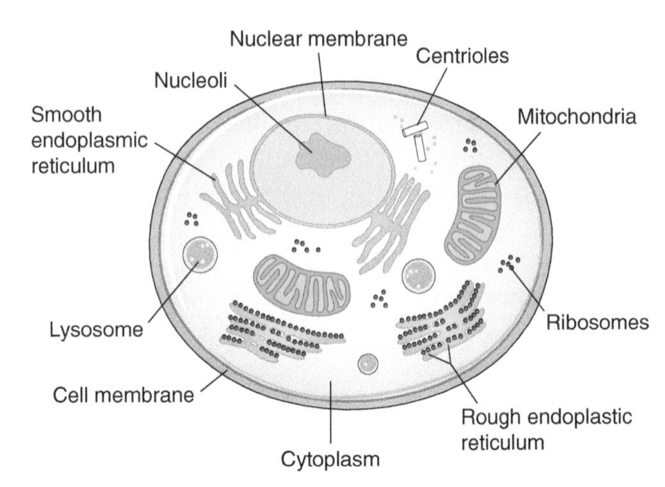

Figure 31.1. **The structure of a human cell.**

The **lysosomes** are small pea-like structures, which contain enzymes that digest cell fragments and are responsible for the removal of waste products.

The **endoplasmic reticulum** is a membrane-enclosed channel or series of channels that serve as a transport system between the nucleus and cytoplasm. There are two types of endoplasmic reticulum: *smooth* that is the channel and *rough* that is a channel bordered by numerous ribosomes.

All of these structures are surrounded by membranes. The membranes are comprised mostly of lipid–protein complexes that selectively allow water and small molecules to diffuse from one side to the other. The cell membranes also provide structure and form for the cell and its internal components.

Cell Function

The central **nucleus** of a human cell is the other main component of the cell and contains the genetic code, which is held in large macromolecules of **deoxyribonucleic acid (DNA)**. The nucleus also contains some **ribonucleic acid (RNA)**, protein, and water. RNA molecules are similar to DNA molecules, but they have only a single strand of nucleic acid, whereas the DNA molecules have two strands.

There are two types of RNA cells: messenger RNA (mRNA) and transfer RNA (tRNA). These molecules are distinguished according to their biochemical functions. They are involved in the growth and development of the cell by way of protein synthesis and other biochemical pathways.

The nucleolus is a rounded structure that contains the majority of RNA in the nucleus; often there are multiple nucleoli in the nucleus. The nucleoli are attached to the nuclear membrane, a double-walled structure that is connected to the endoplasmic reticulum. This connection controls the passage of RNA molecules from the nucleus to the cytoplasm. The nucleoli assist in the formation of the ribosomes; the RNA and ribosomes both play crucial roles in the production of proteins. It is the specific types of proteins produced by the cell that determine its function as part of an organ in the body.

The synthesis of proteins from small to large molecules is known as anabolism. Protein synthesis requires the transfer of information from the nucleus (the plans) out to the cytoplasm (the factory). This transfer occurs primarily along the endoplasmic reticulum.

The DNA contains all the hereditary information representing the cell. Germ cells contain all the hereditary information for the whole individual. The cell's genetic information is transferred by **chromosomes**. Within the cell nucleus, there are 23 pairs of chromosomes for a total of 46. Two of these are the "sex" chromosomes, which determine the gender of the individual; the other 44 are referred to as autosomes and determine the traits and characteristics of the organism.

The genetic information about a cell's form and function is contained in the DNA molecule. This molecule is shaped in the form of a double helix. The double helix is made of chains of sugar–phosphate molecules and is connected by nitrogenous base pairs attached to the side chains like the rungs of a ladder (Fig. 31.2). The rungs are made up of four different nitrogenous base pairs: adenine, guanine, thymine, and cytosine, abbreviated as A, G, T, and C, respectively. Adenine and guanine are purines. Thymine and cytosine are pyrimidines. The sequence of these bases and how they are connected to the side chains encode the information in the DNA molecule. The adenine (A) is chemically bonded to thymine (T), and the cytosine (C) is chemically bonded to the guanine (G). In this sequence of bases, four bonding combinations are possible: TA, AT, GC, and CG.

There are thousands of base molecules along a strand of DNA. A series of three base pairs, called a **codon**, identifies one of the 22 amino acids available for protein synthesis. The physiologic functions of every organ and the cells that make up the organ are controlled by the synthesis of protein molecules. The synthesis of protein molecules within a cell is very complex but can be simplified as follows: when a molecule of DNA splits down the middle of the rungs, each pair of nitrogenous bases separate, leaving an exposed side. Other molecules that are capable of chemical bonds with the four bases will begin to attach to them to form a shorter chain molecule called messenger RNA (mRNA) (Fig. 31.3).

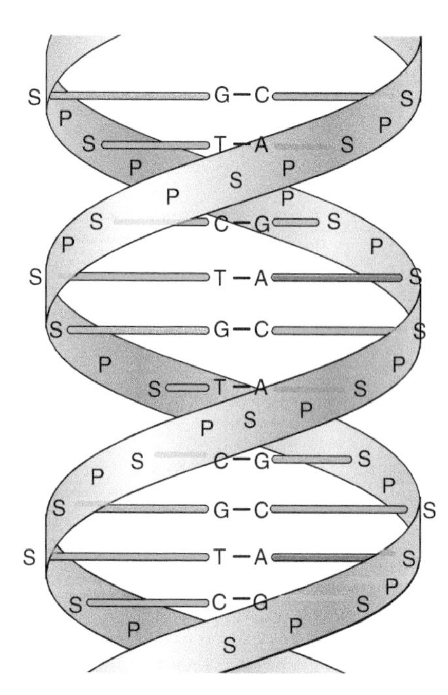

Figure 31.2. A schematic diagram of a DNA molecule.

The mRNA then travels out of the nucleus into the cytoplasm through the rough endoplasmic reticulum and makes its way to a ribosome. Close to the ribosome are molecules of transfer RNA (tRNA). Each tRNA molecule has only a short segment of genetic code on it, and it has a chemical structure that tends to bond with a specific amino acid. When the tRNA comes into contact with the specific amino acid, the two will connect. The mRNA is considered the messenger that physically brings the code from the nucleus to the ribosome. The tRNA is considered to be the translator in this process.

In the biochemical reactions that occur, the ribosome acts as a protein-building unit. The ribosome travels along the mRNA strand, effectively "translating" the code and matching the short code segments of nearby tRNA molecules to the mRNA (Fig. 31.4). As the process continues, the tRNA molecules are brought into contact with the mRNA. This process lines up the amino acids attached to the tRNA molecules in a sequence. The amino acids will bond to each other to form a chain; a complete protein molecule is formed.

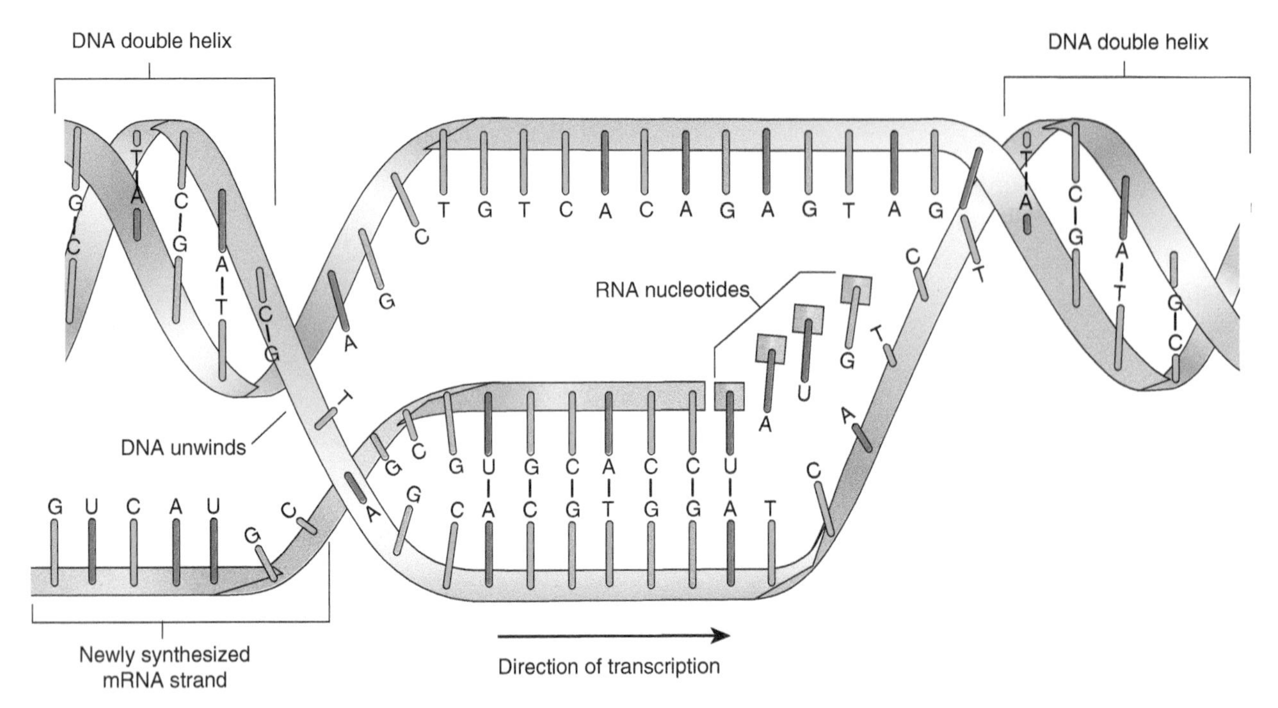

Figure 31.3. **Formation of mRNA alongside the broken DNA molecule in the nucleus.**

Notice that the tRNA code segments mirror the code of the mRNA, which in turn is a mirror image of the original DNA code. By undergoing the process, the original code sequence of DNA can be replicated. The result is a protein whose sequence of amino acids has ultimately been dictated by the original DNA in the nucleus.

Once the complete chain of amino acids has formed the correct protein, the amino acids separate from the tRNA molecules, and the resulting protein moves away to become part of an organelle and to perform its biochemical function upon the cell (Fig. 31.5). The tRNA molecules detach from the mRNA strand. The tRNA molecules will then be recycled and go in search of another loose amino acid in the vicinity; the tRNA is then reused by a ribosome in the production of another protein.

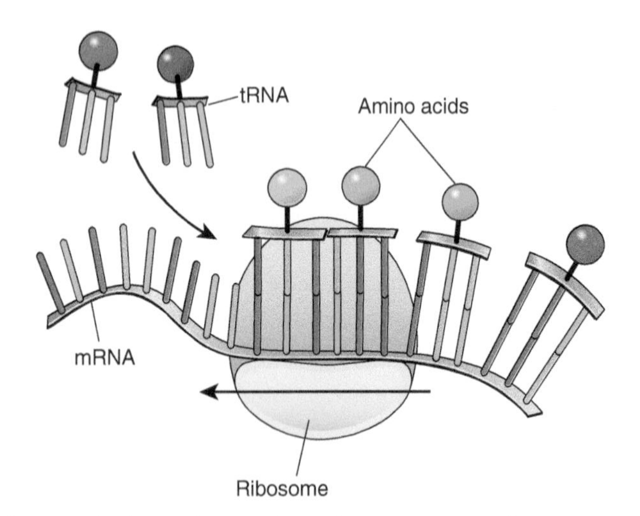

Figure 31.4. **In the rough endoplasmic reticulum, ribosomes move along the mRNA molecule and ensure the correct tRNA molecules attach in sequence. Each tRNA is attached to a specific amino acid resulting in the amino acids lining up in sequence to form a protein molecule.**

Cell Proliferation

Cell proliferation is the act of a single cell or group of cells reproducing and multiplying in number. Cells go through a cycle during proliferation or division. The end result of the cycle is the division of a single cell into

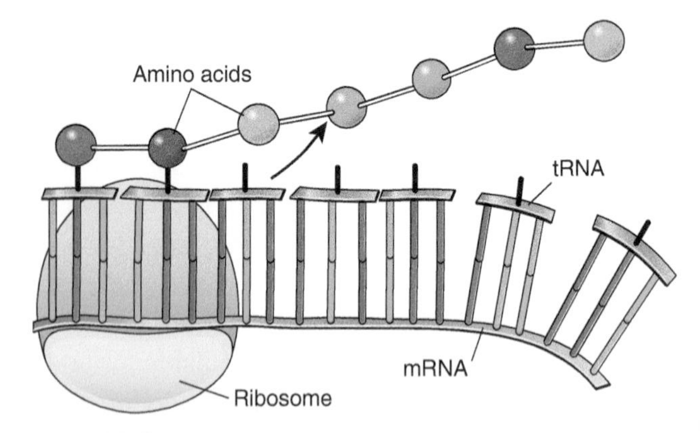

Figure 31.5. **Once the entire protein molecule is properly formed, it will break off from the tRNA molecules.**

two cells. Two types of cells exist in the human body: **somatic cells** and **genetic cells**. The genetic cells are the oogonium of the female and the spermatogonium of the male; the rest of the cells are somatic cells. The proliferation or division of somatic cells is called **mitosis**, and the proliferation or division of genetic cells is called **meiosis**.

Life Cycle of the Cell

The lifetimes of cells vary greatly; a typical cell has a life cycle of 24 hours. In order for the organism to grow normally and to repair tissues, somatic cells must go through reproductive phases called mitosis. These phases of active reproduction are separated by periods called **interphase** (Fig. 31.6).

During interphase, the cell is not dividing; the 46 chromosomes appear in the nucleus as a diffuse, granular mass called chromatin. The chromosomes consist of very loosely coiled strands of chromatin fiber. The chromatin fiber is made from twisting strands of chromatin together.

Mitosis and interphase can both be broken down into subphases. Interphase consists of three stages: G_1 (Gap-1), DNA synthesis phase (S), and G_2 (Gap-2) as seen in Figure 31.6.

During G_1, the cell is metabolically active; the organelles are duplicating, but the DNA is not. In the nucleus, the chromatin fibers holding the DNA are organized into a pair of chromatids, which are held together at a

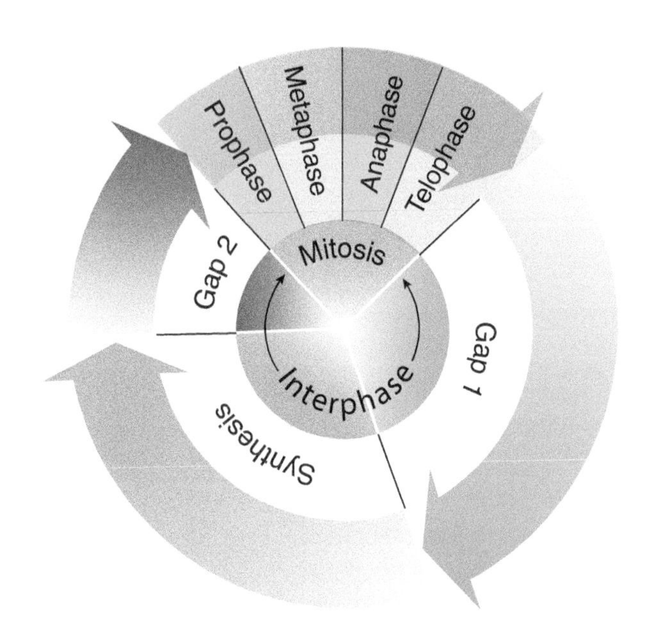

Figure 31.6. **Phases of mitosis and interphase with the subphases of the cell's life cycle.**

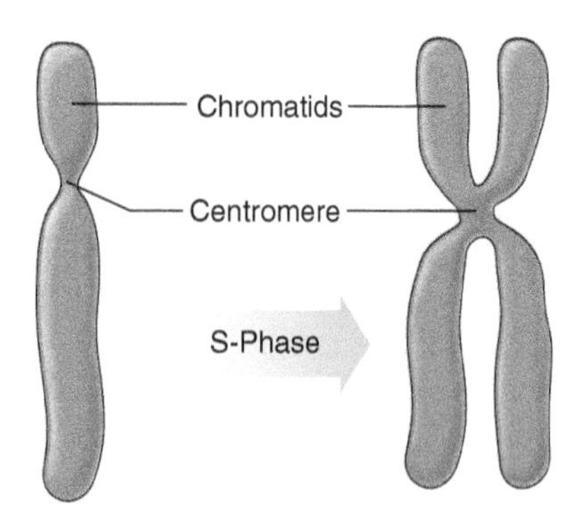

Figure 31.7. **During the synthesis portion of interphase, the chromosomes replicate from a two-chromatid to a four-chromatid structure.**

constricted point by the centromere (Fig. 31.7). The G_1 phase typically lasts 8 to 10 hours. This phase is followed by the DNA synthesis phase, S.

During the S phase, each DNA molecule is duplicated to form two identical daughter DNA molecules. These two DNA molecules will combine to form duplicate chromosomes whose structure has four chromatids attached to a centromere. The S phase typically lasts 6 to 8 hours.

After synthesis is completed, the cell enters into the post-DNA synthesis, or G_2 phase, during which the cell continues to grow, and enzymes and proteins are formed in preparation for cell division. G_2 normally lasts 4 to 6 hours. Although the chromosome structure has been doubled, the chromatin fibers are still loosely coiled together, which makes them impossible to observe with a microscope. The cell is now ready to divide through the process of mitosis.

The sensitivity of the cell to radiation exposure will vary with the stage of its life cycle. At the very beginning of the S phase is the most sensitive time during the cell's entire life cycle. If radiation strikes the cell and ionizes genetic molecules, various genetic mutations can be induced or biochemical changes can cause the next cycle of cell division to result in nonviable daughter cells.

Mitosis

Mitosis is the cellular reproduction process used for the normal growth and repair of somatic cells. Mitosis is also called replication division because it results in a full set of genetic material in each daughter cell. In other words, each daughter cell is an exact replica of the parent cell. There are four subphases of mitosis: prophase, metaphase, anaphase, and telophase. The part of the cell

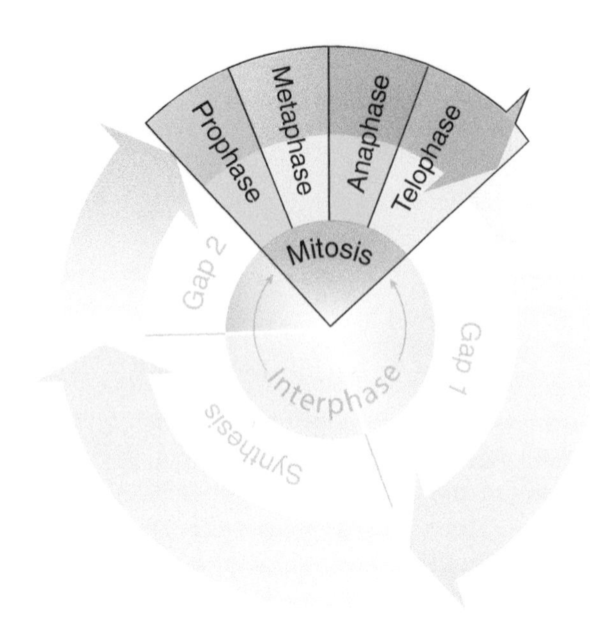

Figure 31.8. **Subphases of mitosis: prophase, metaphase, anaphase, and telophase.**

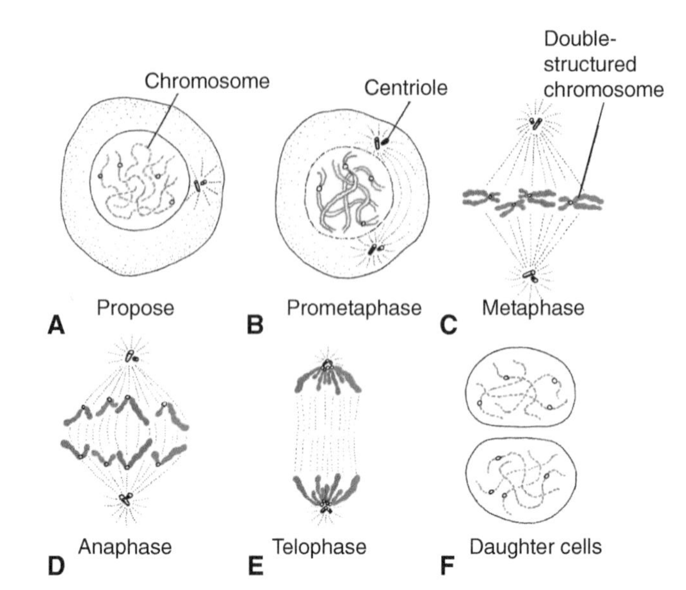

Figure 31.9. **Mitosis is the phase of the cell cycle where the chromosomes become visible, divide, and migrate to daughter cells. (A) Prophase. (B) Prometaphase. (C) Metaphase. (D) Anaphase. (E) Telophase. (F) Daughter cells. (Reprinted from Sadler T. *Langman's Medical Embryology*. 9th Ed. Baltimore, MD: Lippincott Williams & Wilkins, 2003, with permission.)**

cycle between the subphases is called interphase, which is characterized by a period of growth of the cell between each division (Fig. 31.8).

- Prophase: The nucleus begins to swell and become more prominent; it begins to take form.
- Metaphase: The loosely coiled chromatin tightens and condenses making the chromosomes visible under a microscope. The nucleus elongates; the chromosomes align themselves on fibers along the center of the nucleus.
- Anaphase: The chromosomes divide at the centromere so that two chromatids and a centromere are connected by a fiber to the poles of the nucleus. The poles are called spindles, and the fibers are spindle fibers. This division leaves each new cell with 23 pairs of chromosomes, which slowly migrate toward the spindle. Two identical sets of chromosomes have been formed.
- Telophase: The two sets of chromosomes lose their structure to become two masses of DNA. The nuclear membrane temporarily dissolves in the middle, while a new cell membrane forms through the middle of the cell, effectively completing the division of the cell. Each new cell has one-half the cytoplasm of the original cell and the new mass of DNA, thereby forming the two daughter cells. Each daughter cell nucleus contains 23 pairs of chromosomes and contains exactly the same genetic material as the parent cell (Fig. 31.9). The newly formed daughter cells are immature or young somatic cells and are called **stem cells**. They remain stem cells until they grow, develop, and mature.

Metaphase is the most radiosensitive phase during mitosis and the second most radiosensitive phase of the entire life cycle of the cell. The tightly packed and condensed chromosomes are extremely vulnerable to damage from ionizing radiation. Any damage or mutations of the chromosomes can be observed under a microscope.

Meiosis

Meiosis is the term that describes the reproduction of gametes or genetic cells. Reduction division is the division of a cell in which the number of chromosomes is reduced to one-half of the normal 46 chromosomes from the parent cell so that each daughter cell contains only 23 chromosomes.

The genetic cell begins meiosis with 46 chromosomes that appear the same as a somatic cell at the end of the G_2 phase (Fig. 31.10). The reproduction cycle is identical to that for mitosis, forming two daughter cells. At this point, the process changes. During interphase before the next cell

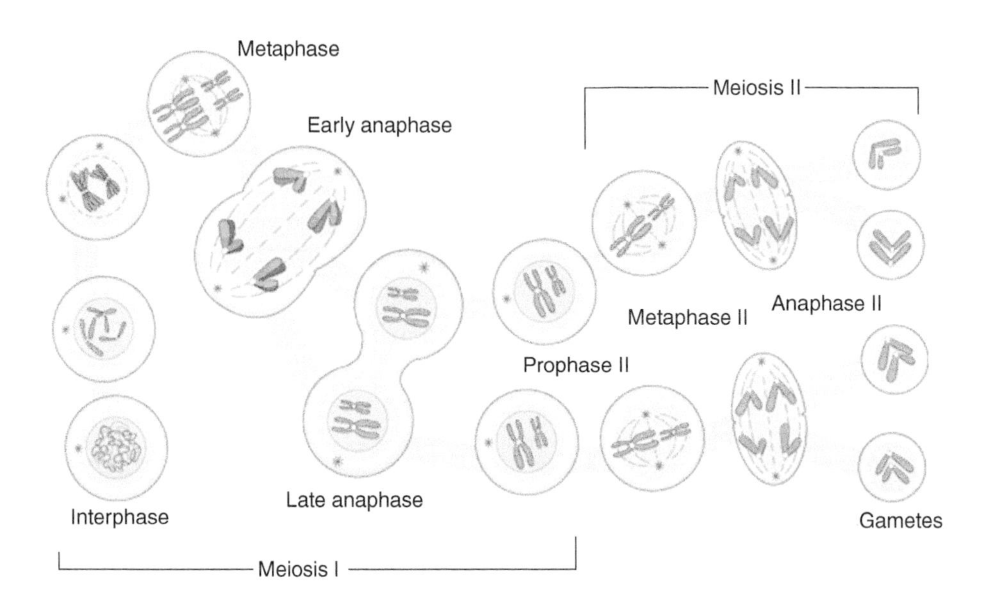

Figure 31.10. **Cell meiosis. Meiosis is the process of reduction and division of germ cells. (Image from *LifeART Super Anatomy Collection 2, CD-ROM*. Baltimore, MD: Lippincott Williams & Wilkins.)**

division takes place, the S phase is skipped (Fig. 31.11); therefore, the DNA is not replicated and the chromosomes are not duplicated. Each parent cell has undergone two division processes, which resulted in the four daughter cells that each contains only 23 chromosomes. Following conception, each of the two germ cells contributes half of the chromosomes when they combine to form a daughter cell containing the standard number of 46 chromosomes.

Radiation Effects

Cells in the body with similar structure and function combine to form specific tissues. These tissues combine in a precise manner to form organs. Organ systems perform specific functions. Different types of tissues and organs have cells with different structures and functions.

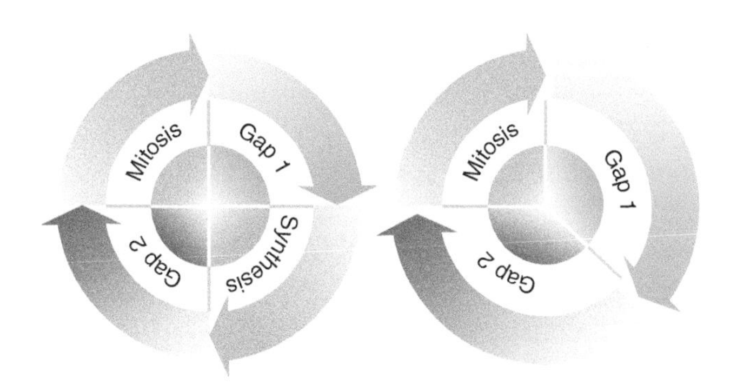

Figure 31.11. **Meiosis cycle diagram demonstrating the S phase is skipped in the second cellular division.**

Examples of major organ systems include the nervous, respiratory, digestive, endocrine, circulatory, and reproductive systems. The effects of radiation exposure that appear at the whole body level begin with damage at the cellular level and progress to the organ systems.

The cells of a tissue system are characterized by their rate of proliferation and their stage of development. Immature cells are called **undifferentiated cells**, **precursor cells**, or stem cells. When the cell grows and matures, it goes through various stages of differentiation into a complete functional cell.

The state of maturity and its functional role in the organ system influence the cells' sensitivity to radiation. Typically, immature cells are more sensitive to radiation than mature cells. Table 31.1 lists various types of cells according to their degree of sensitivity to radiation.

Law of Bergonie and Tribondeau

Two French scientists, Bergonie and Tribondeau, studied the effect of radiation on cells, tissues, and organs. Their observations relate to the sensitivity of cells, tissues, and organs, which were being exposed to ionizing radiation. Important points of the Bergonie and Tribondeau law are as follows:

1. Younger or immature cells are more radiosensitive.
2. Rapidly dividing cells are more radiosensitive.
3. Mature cells are radioresistant.
4. As the growth rate of cells increases, so does their radiosensitivity.

TABLE 31.1 RADIATION SENSITIVITY OF SOME CELLS, TISSUES, AND ORGANS

Most sensitive	Lymphocytes
	Spermatogonia
	Oogonia
	Hemopoietic tissues/erythroblasts
	Intestine/intestinal crypt cells
Intermediate	Bone/osteoblasts
	Skin/epithelial cells
	Lens of eye/cornea
	Thyroid
	Spermatids
	Fibroblasts
Least sensitive	Muscle cells
	Nerve cells
	Spinal cells
	Brain cells

These points are more important in diagnostic radiology because the fetus, which contains younger or immature cells, and cells that are rapidly dividing, are more sensitive to radiation than adult cells. Cells are most sensitive to radiation exposure during the M phase of the cell cycle when the proliferation and division are occurring.

Medical physicists use the laws of Bergonie and Tribondeau as their basis for treating cancer. Cancer cells are cells that grow and divide more rapidly than many of the normal cells around them. The rapid division of the cancer cells places them in a radiosensitive phase. Radiation works by making small breaks in the DNA inside cells. These breaks prevent the cancer cells from growing and dividing, which often cause them to die.

Germ and stem cells are more radiosensitive than mature cells of the same type. Stem cells of a particular type are identified with the suffix "-blast." For example, immature red blood cells are known as erythroblasts, and bone stem cells are known as osteoblasts. Blastic cells are more radiosensitive than mature cells of the same type.

Cells that are less sensitive to radiation are called radioresistant. Radioresistant cells show fewer biologic effects of radiation than do radiosensitive cells. In keeping with the law of Bergonie and Tribondeau, nerve cells of the brain and spinal cord are most radioresistant because once they are developed, these nerve cells do not undergo further cell division. Lymphocytes and gonadal cells are the most radiosensitive because they undergo rapid cell division and are constantly developing.

Factors Affecting Radiosensitivity

When irradiating tissue, the response to the radiation is determined by the amount of energy deposited per unit mass: the dose in Gray (rad). During experiments to test the response of tissue to equal doses of radiation to an equal number of tissue specimens, the results will vary depending upon physical factors that affect the degree of response to the radiation dose.

Linear Energy Transfer

thePoint® *An animation for this topic can be viewed at http://thepoint.lww.com/Orth2e*

The characteristics of particulate and electromagnetic radiation can affect the amount of biologic damage. The radiation characteristic that is most important in determining cell damage is the rate at which the radiation deposits its energy.

The term **linear energy transfer (LET)** describes how the ionizing radiation energy is deposited along a tract or path in tissue. LET has units of kiloelectron volts per micrometer (keV/mm). As the radiation passes through tissue, it deposits energy and produces ionization of the cells in the tissue.

Different types of ionizing radiation have different LET values. As high LET radiation passes through tissue, it deposits large amounts of energy, which increases the likelihood of interaction with the target molecule. Accordingly, high LET radiation has a greater biologic effect but very little penetrating ability because it loses all its energy in a short distance. LET is always inverse to penetration—more penetrating radiations have a lower LET.

Low LET radiation is more penetrating because it spreads its energy over large distances. There is little chance that a low LET radiation will deposit more than one ionization in any one cell. Current theories suggest that two or three ionizations in a cell nucleus are required to produce biologic effects (Fig. 31.12). Because the ionizations from low LET radiation are spread over many cells, this radiation does not usually cause significant damage in any one cell.

Alpha and beta particles and protons are types of high LET radiation, with alpha particles having the highest LET. High LET radiation has values from 10 to 200 keV/mm, which can travel a few millimeters in tissue. X- and gamma

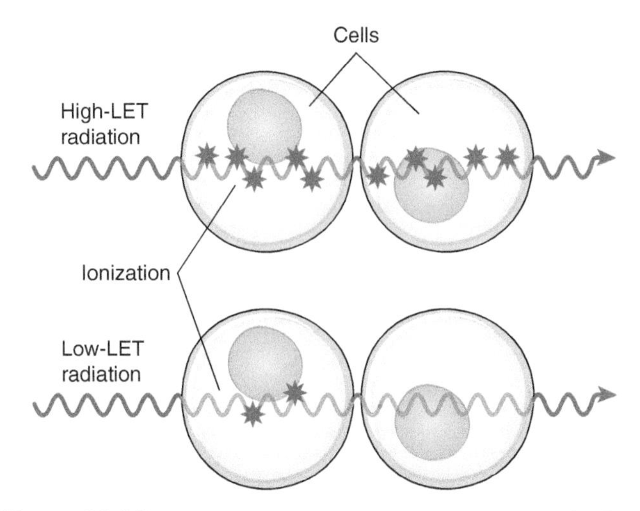

Figure 31.12. **The ionization along the tracks of a high and a low LET radiation.**

rays are types of low LET radiation, with values from 0.2 to 3 keV/mm radiation that will travel many centimeters in tissue.

Relative Biological Effectiveness

The quantity or amount of radiation is expressed in terms of absorbed dose, a physical quantity with the unit of Gray (Gy). Absorbed dose is a measure of the energy absorbed per unit mass of tissue. Equal doses of different types of radiation do not produce the same biologic effect. As an example, 1 Gy of alpha particles produce a greater biologic effect than 1 Gy of x-rays.

When comparing different types of radiation, it is expected to use x-rays as the standard. The National Bureau of Statistics in 1954 defined **relative biological effectiveness (RBE)**: the RBE of test radiation compared with x-rays is defined by the ratio of D_{250}/D_r, where D_{250} is the dose of x-rays and D_r is the test radiation required for equal biologic effect. The formula can be set up as:

$$\text{RBE} = \frac{D_{250}\ (\text{Dose of 250 kVp x-rays required})}{D_r\ (\text{Dose of test radiation})}$$

Let us consider the formula in regard to an experiment. Two Petri dishes have the same number of epithelial cells. When one dish is irradiated with 250 kVp, it takes 6 Gy to kill one-half of the cells. When the other dish is irradiated with alpha radiation only, 2 Gy are needed to kill one-half of the cells. What is the RBE for the alpha radiation?

$$\text{RBE} = \frac{6\ \text{Gy}}{2\ \text{Gy}} = 3$$

This means that alpha radiation is three times more effective at killing one-half of the epithelial cells compared to x-rays.

When radiation is absorbed in biological material, the energy is deposited along the tracks of charged particles in a pattern that is characteristic of the type of radiation involved. After exposure to x-rays or gamma rays, the ionization density would be quite low. After exposure to neutrons, protons, or alpha particles, the ionization along the tracks would occur much more frequently, thereby producing a much denser pattern of ionizations. These differences in density of ionizations are a major reason that neutrons, protons, and alpha particles produce more biological effects per unit of absorbed dose than do more sparsely ionizing radiations such as x-rays, gamma rays, or electrons (Table 31.2).

Protraction and Fractionation

Protraction is defined as extending the time over which a set dose of radiation is delivered. It will have the opposite effect to dose rates because the dose is delivered in smaller increments per minute, thereby keeping the overall dose amount the same. In other words, protraction reduces dose rates, which in turn reduces the effectiveness of the dose.

Fractionation is defined as breaking the total delivered dose into several equal portions or fractions. Fractionation is the basis for radiation therapy treatments. The doses to the patient are spread out over several treatments; this provides time periods between doses so that cells can undergo repair and recovery.

TABLE 31.2 **RADIATION WEIGHTING FACTORS**

Type and Energy Range	Radiation Weighting Factor
X-rays and gamma rays	1
Electrons	1
Protons	5
Fast neutrons	10
Alpha particles	20

Direct and Indirect Effects

thePoint® *An animation for this topic can be viewed at http://thepoint.lww.com/Orth2e*

The amount of cell damage depends on both the quality of radiation and how the radiation is deposited in the cell. If the radiation directly damages the cell nucleus, the damage is called a direct effect. If the radiation deposits its energy outside the nucleus, the damage is called an indirect effect.

Direct effects result from ionizing radiation depositing its energy within the cell nucleus and breaking the DNA molecular bonds. The target for direct effects is the DNA molecule. High LET radiation primarily produces direct effects. High LET ionizations are deposited inside the cell nucleus and damage so many DNA molecules that the cell is unable to repair all the damage. High LET radiation usually results in cell death.

Indirect effects result from ionizing radiation depositing its energy within the cytoplasm outside of the cell nucleus. Low LET radiation primarily produces indirect effects. Free radicals have excess energy, and when they migrate to a target molecule, they transfer their energy, which results in damage to the target molecule.

Types of Cell Damage

Several things can happen when ionization occurs within a cell. The cell can die and form scar tissue. The cell can repair itself from the damage. Repaired cells can continue to function normally after repair. Alternatively, the cell can be transformed into an abnormal cell. Transformed cells may begin the process of becoming cancer cells.

If a large number of ionizations occur in a cell over a short period of time, the cell's repair mechanisms may be overwhelmed, and it may not be able to repair the damage. Biologic effects of low dose rate exposures are less than those from high dose rate exposures. Long-term exposures over months or years show about half the effect as those caused by short-term exposures involving the same dose.

Radiosensitivity Factors

In addition to the physical factors, which affect radiosensitivity, there are a number of biologic conditions, which alter the tissue's response to radiation. These factors have to do with the state of the host such as age and metabolic rate.

Age

The age of the individual directly affects his or her sensitivity to radiation. As seen in Figure 31.13, humans are most radiosensitive in utero because of their rapid growth and development rate, in accordance with the law of Bergonie and Tribondeau. In the first 6 weeks of pregnancy, the human embryo is ~10 times more sensitive to radiation than an adult. The late term fetus and newborn infant are approximately twice as sensitive as an adult. As the infant approaches childhood, their radiosensitivity continues to lower. The sensitivity is the lowest in adulthood when humans are the most radioresistant to radiation-induced effects.

During the elder years, humans become somewhat more radiosensitive but not to the same level as the fetus. Elderly humans are more sensitive to radiation and all other risk factors because their degenerative state weakens the entire organism and its defenses. These factors explain the necessity to use proper radiation protection for patients during imaging procedures where they will be exposed to ionizing radiation.

Oxygen Effect

Another factor to consider is the amount of oxygen present in tissue. Tissue is more sensitive to radiation when it is irradiated under aerobic or oxygenated conditions.

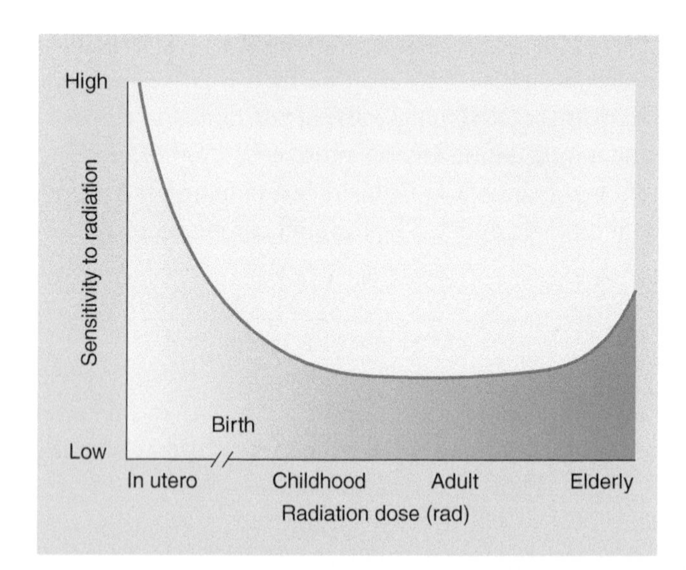

Figure 31.13. Radiosensitivity varies with the age of the person. Research shows that the very young and the elderly are the most sensitive to the effects of radiation.

Tissue that is anoxic or hypoxic is less sensitive to the effects of radiation. This characteristic of biologic tissue is called the oxygen effect.

Low LET radiation can damage the cell by producing an intermediate, toxic product in the cytoplasm, which then interacts with the DNA in the nucleus. The human body is comprised of 80% water molecules, and when irradiated, the water molecules will dissociate (break apart) into a toxic product. The most common toxic product is produced by the radiolysis of water. In radiolysis of water, the water molecule is broken into two ionized particles: HOH^+ and an electron.

At this point, various reactions can occur (Fig. 31.14). First, the ion pair may rejoin into a stable water molecule in which case no damage occurs. Second, the ions do not rejoin, and the negative ion (the electron) attaches to another water molecule and produces yet another ion HOH^-. The HOH^+ and HOH^- ions are unstable and can dissociate into still smaller molecules as follows:

$$HOH^+ \rightarrow H^+ = OH^*$$

$$HOH^- \rightarrow OH^- + H^*$$

Finally, radiolysis of water results in the formation of an ion pair, H^+ and OH^-, and two free radicals, H^* and OH^*. The ions can recombine, and there would be no biologic damage. Although free radicals are uncharged, they have an unpaired electron in the valence or outer shell and are very chemically reactive. Free radicals, which are produced primarily in the cytoplasm, have a short life, but they exist long enough to reach the nucleus and damage the DNA molecules by easily breaking the DNA bonds. Free radicals produced from the radiolysis of water can also combine to form hydrogen peroxide, H_2O_2, which is toxic to cells. Most damage from low LET radiation is caused by indirect effects because the low LET ionizations are separated by distances much larger than a cell.

Free radicals are produced more readily when there is an abundance of oxygen present. The cytoplasm, which consists primarily of H_2O, is an abundant reservoir of oxygen. The effect of oxygen is measured by the **oxygen enhancement ratio (OER)**, which is the ratio of the radiation doses necessary to produce the same effect with and without oxygen present. OER values for high LET radiations are close to 1 because the high LET radiations are so effective in producing damage that the presence or absence of oxygen does not matter. Low LET radiations typically have OER values of 2 to 3, meaning that oxygen enhances the effects of radiation.

More indirect effects occur if there is more oxygen present because free radicals are readily produced by ionizations in the presence of oxygen. Oxygen is a radiosensitizer because cells in the presence of oxygen are more sensitive to radiation. Cells in tissues with a poor blood supply are more resistant to radiation damage because they have a diminished oxygen supply. Many tumors are radioresistant because they are avascular, that is, they lack an adequate blood supply.

Target Theory

Each cell in the body has an overabundance of cellular components. When the cell is irradiated, one or more of these components may be damaged. If the damaged component cannot continue to support the function of the cell, other similar molecules would be available to take its place. Other molecules are vital to the function of the cell, and in many cells, there may only be one such molecule. Radiation damage to such a molecule could have a severe effect on the cell, and there would be no similar molecules to take its place. The concept of a key sensitive molecule is the foundation for target theory. Target theory suggests that for a cell to die after radiation exposure, its target molecule must be inactivated or damaged beyond repair.

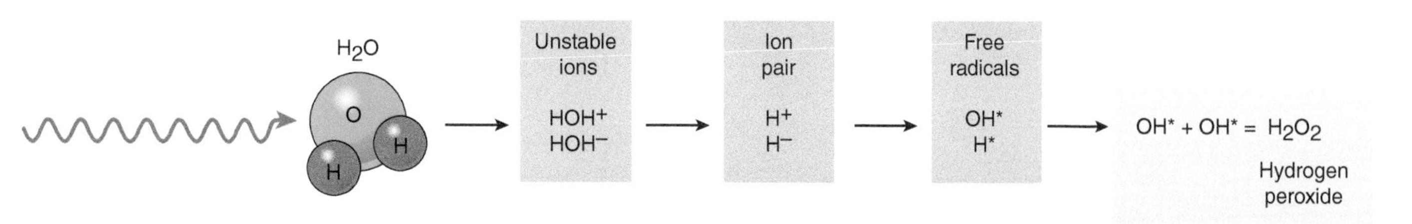

Figure 31.14. **The formation of a free radical pair by radiolysis of water.**

In target theory, the target is considered to be an area of a cell occupied by the target molecule, usually the DNA. The act of irradiating the target molecule is completely random, and its sensitivity to radiation is simply because of its vital function in the cell. The interaction between the radiation and target molecule can either be direct or indirect as it is impossible to know for sure. Regardless of the type of interaction, the target molecule is hit by the radiation, which inactivates the target molecule and ultimately leads to cell death.

Chapter Summary

1. Cell division consists of four phases: M, G_1, S, and G_2. The M phase consists of mitosis or meiosis. Somatic cell division is called mitosis, and the division of genetic cells is called meiosis.
2. Cells are most sensitive to radiation exposure during the M phase and most radioresistant in the late S phase.
3. Immature somatic cells are called stem cells, and immature genetic cells are called germ cells. Germ and stem cells are more radiosensitive than mature cells.
4. The Law of Bergonie and Tribondeau states that younger, immature, and rapidly dividing cells are more radiosensitive.
5. Direct effects result from ionization and breaking of DNA molecule bonds in the cell nucleus. Indirect effects are produced when radiation interacts with the cytoplasm to produce free radicals that damage the cell.
6. The effect of oxygen on tissue radiosensitivity is measured by the OER.
7. LET describes how energy is deposited along the radiation path in tissue. High LET radiation produces direct biologic effects; low LET radiation produces biologic effects through indirect effects.
8. The effects of radiations with different LET values can be evaluated by comparing their RBE values. X-rays and gamma radiations are forms of low LET radiations. Alpha and beta particles are high LET radiations.

Case Study

Laura is a 2nd year radiologic technology student. During her course in radiation biology, she was assigned to describe the process of meiosis to her classmates. In her assignment, she is to answer the following questions.

Critical Thinking Questions

1. Which type of cells undergo the meiosis process?
2. How is the reproduction cycle different from mitosis?
3. What is the significance of the daughter cells having 23 chromosomes?

Review Questions

Multiple Choice

1. The most radiosensitive tissues and organs are:

1. muscle
2. nerve
3. gonads
4. intestine

a. 1 and 3
b. 1 and 2
c. 1 and 4
d. 3 and 4

2. A direct effect of radiation exposure to the cell involves the:

a. DNA bond
b. cell membrane
c. cytoplasm
d. organelles

3. The fetus is most sensitive to radiation during the __________ trimester of pregnancy.

a. first
b. second
c. third
d. fourth

4. Alpha particles have which of the following properties?

1. Emitted from uranium and radium
2. Large particles
3. Deep penetrating power

a. 1 only
b. 1 and 2
c. 2 and 3
d. 1, 2, and 3

5. Which of the following will have the highest LET?

a. Alpha particles
b. X-rays
c. Beta particles
d. Fast neutrons

6. If the quality factor of ionizing radiation is higher, the RBE:

a. is also higher
b. is lower
c. remains the same
d. changes with LET

7. Biologic material is MOST sensitive to irradiation under which of the following conditions?

a. Anoxic
b. Hypoxic
c. Oxygenated
d. Deoxygenated

8. What unit of measure expresses the amount of energy to which tissue has been subjected?

a. roentgen (C/kg)
b. rad (Gy)
c. rem (Sv)
d. RBE

9. During radiolysis of water, which type of toxic chemical can be produced when free radicals combine?

a. Water
b. Sulfahydryls
c. Oxygen
d. Hydrogen peroxide

10. __________ refers to damage in a DNA nucleotide sequence as a result of radiation exposure.

a. Target theory
b. Radiolysis
c. Compton interaction
d. Mitosis

Short Answer

1. Who were the French scientists who theorized about the radiosensitivity of human tissue? Explain the law that bears their names.

2. How does age of the host affect the radiosensitivity of the tissue?

3. What is target theory in radiology?

4. What are the stages of cell division in a somatic cell?

5. Give a definition of RBE.

6. If the initial ionizing event occurs on a molecule, the effect is said to be ______.

32

Organism Response to Radiation

Objectives

Upon completion of this chapter, the student will be able to:

1. Describe dose–response models.
2. Identify stages of acute radiation syndrome.
3. Discuss the biologic factors that affect the degree of tissue damage in relation to radiation exposure.
4. Describe the three acute radiation syndromes.
5. Define lethal dose, $LD_{50/60}$.
6. Discuss local tissue damage after high-dose irradiation.
7. Review the three features of a deterministic radiation effect.

Key Terms

- acute radiation syndrome (ARS)
- carcinogen
- central nervous system syndrome
- desquamation
- deterministic effects
- doubling dose
- epilation
- erythema
- gastrointestinal (GI) syndrome
- genetically significant dose (GSD)
- hematopoietic syndrome
- latent period
- $LD_{50/60}$
- lethal dose
- linear, nonthreshold
- linear, threshold
- manifest illness stage
- mutagenic effects
- nonlinear, nonthreshold
- nonlinear, threshold
- nonstochastic effects
- organogenesis
- prodromal stage
- skin erythema dose (SED)
- somatic cells
- stochastic effects
- teratogenic effects
- threshold dose

Introduction

After the discovery of x-rays, some scientists conducted experiments on animals to observe the effects of radiation. Their efforts were not scientifically sound and were not applied. In the 1940s, the atomic bomb and resulting radiation exposure enormously increased interest in radiobiology. The purpose of radiobiological research has been to establish radiation dose–response relationships.

Radiation studies have demonstrated two applications in radiology. First, the dose–response relationships are used to design therapeutic radiation treatments for patients with cancer. Second, the relationships have led to information on the effects of low-dose irradiation. These studies and the dose–response relationships along with the response of the cell will be discussed in this chapter.

Cell Survival Curve

The number of cells that survive after being exposed to radiation depends on the radiation dose. A cell survival curve is a plot of the fraction of cells surviving as a function of radiation dose. It is obtained through a series of experiments in which groups of cells are exposed to different doses of radiation.

The cell survival curve can be divided into two parts: the S or shoulder region and the L or linear region, which is the straight-line portion. The shoulder of the curve in the S region indicates the amount of cell repair or recovery (Fig. 32.1). At very low doses, almost 100% of the cells survive. As the dose is increased, some of the cells are killed, but most recover from the radiation damage and survive. The dose at which an extrapolation of the straight-line portion of the survival curve intersects the 100% survival line is known as D_Q the threshold dose. D_Q is a measure of the width of the shoulder portion and is related to the amount of cellular repair or sublethal damage. Cells with greater repair or recovery capability have a larger shoulder region and a larger D_Q value. High Linear Energy Transfer (LET) radiations produce cell survival curves with almost no shoulder region and very small D_Q values. This is due to the high LET radiations' ability to overwhelm the cell's repair mechanism.

The linear region occurs at higher doses where the survival curve becomes a straight line when cell survival is plotted on a logarithmic scale. In the L region, cell survival is inversely proportional to dose. An increase in dose produces a decrease in cell survival. The dose required to reduce the population of surviving cells to 37% of the original value is D_O, the mean lethal dose.

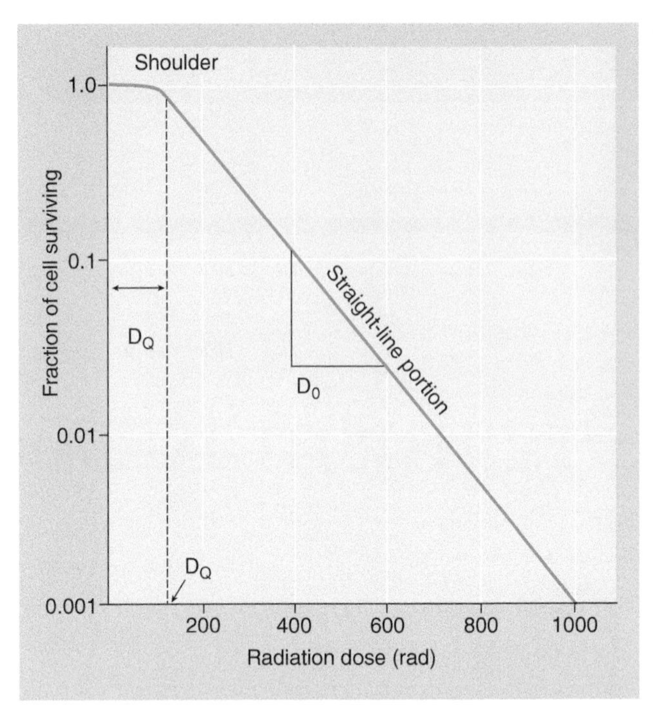

Figure 32.1. The fraction of surviving cells plotted against the radiation dose.

Different cell and tissue types have different D_O and D_Q values. Radioresistant cells have high D_O values because they require a high radiation dose to reduce the number of surviving cells to 37% of the original population. Radiosensitive cells have low D_O values because they require a lower radiation dose to reduce the number of surviving cells to this degree.

Stochastic Effects

Stochastic effects are defined as the increase in probability with increasing dose. Stochastic effects also occur randomly in irradiated tissue. Stochastic effects are those effects that occur by chance; they occur among unexposed as well as exposed individuals.

When a stochastic effect does occur, it is an "all-or-none" response. In the context of radiation exposure, stochastic effects mean cancer and genetic effects. The result of exposure to radiation increases the probability of occurrence of the effect, with the increase in response being proportional to the size of the dose. A larger exposure to radiation equates into a larger potential for cell damage or biological response. The incidence of the biological response in relation to the disease process will increase proportionally with the radiation dose, but there is no dose threshold. This means that no amount of radiation exposure is safe and that there is always a chance for tissue damage to occur.

Deterministic Effects

Deterministic effects of radiation are also called **nonstochastic effects** and are the biological responses that will cause an effect because of a threshold. In other words, a minimum dose of radiation will not cause any biological damage or any amount of radiation below the threshold is considered safe. The amount of biological damage will increase with an increase in radiation dose after the threshold. Deterministic effects are characterized by three qualities:

1. A certain minimum dose must be exceeded before the particular effect is observed.
2. The magnitude of the effect increases with the size of the dose.
3. There is a causal relationship between exposure to radiation and an observed effect.

The stochastic and deterministic effects are plotted on the linear and nonlinear dose–response models.

Dose–Response Models

Radiation dose–response relationships have important applications in radiology. First, these relationships are used to design radiation therapy protocols for cancer patients. Second, studies have been designed to determine the effects of low-dose radiation. The data gathered from these studies are the foundation for radiation control programs whose main goal is the reduction of radiation exposure in diagnostic imaging.

A dose–response curve shows the relationship between the radiation dose and the resulting biologic effects. Biologic data on humans are available only at doses greater than ~1 Gy (100 rad). No biologic effects have been observed at doses of a few milligray. These are the dose levels usually encountered in diagnostic radiology.

The dose–response models demonstrate the natural incidence of cancer in humans as well as the body's response to overexposure. There is a certain point on the dose–response models where there is no distinguishable difference between people who have not been irradiated and those who have received an overexposure. It should be emphasized that although overexposure to radiation increases the likelihood of cancer, it is impossible to definitely identify any particular cancer with any given exposure.

Data obtained at higher doses can be extrapolated to lower doses to estimate biologic effects at the lower dose levels. These extrapolations are done using dose–response models. There are two types of dose–response models: the linear and nonlinear models. Either model can exhibit a **threshold dose**, which is defined as the minimum dose at which biologic effects become evident.

Linear Dose–Response Model

The linear dose–response model demonstrates that any dose of radiation will produce an effect. This model also demonstrates that there is a natural incidence in the population of cancer, genetic diseases, and leukemia, which must be accounted for. A linear model predicts a doubling of the biologic effect if the radiation dose is doubled. A linear model can have either a **linear, threshold** or a **linear, nonthreshold** response with a stochastic effect. A linear response that begins at zero demonstrates a nonthreshold response. The nonthreshold response demonstrates that any dose, regardless of its size, is expected to produce a response. A linear response that rises at some dose greater than zero is a threshold response, meaning that for any dose below the threshold, no response will be demonstrated. The type of response that the patient experiences is stochastic. Figure 32.2 demonstrates a simple linear dose–response relationship.

The linear model extrapolates by using a straight line to connect the data for high doses to the 0 point of radiation dose from the graph. The linear model predicts that biologic effects are directly proportional to the radiation dose. The magnitude of the effects gradually increases with increasing radiation dose until the two models predict the same biologic effects at high doses, where human data are available. The linear, nonthreshold dose–response model is used to estimate radiation effects in the diagnostic energy range. Diagnostic x-rays are assumed to follow a linear, nonthreshold dose response.

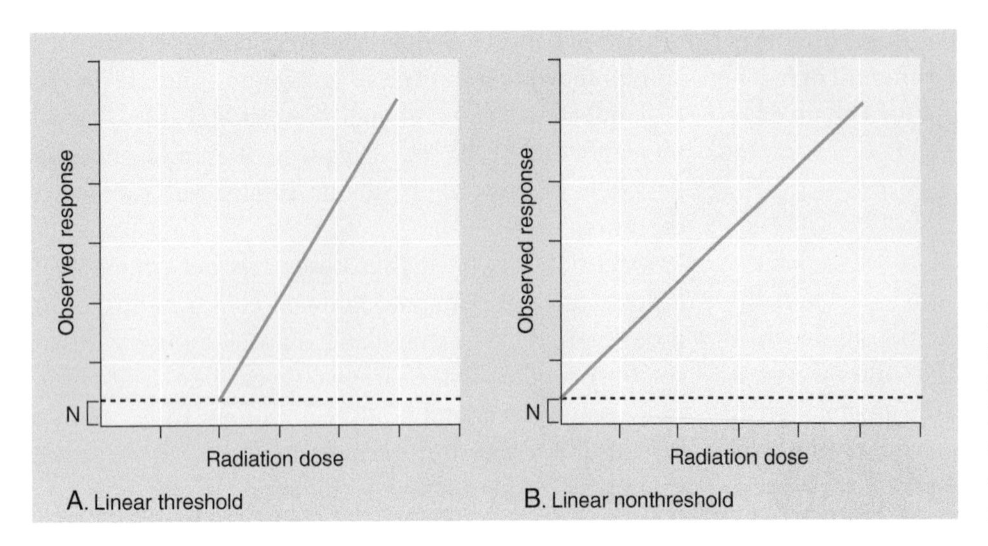

Figure 32.2. The linear dose–response model with and without a threshold, (A) and (B), respectively. Notice the natural incidence of radiation effects on the bottom of the chart and how the linear response begins on this line.

Nonlinear Dose–Response Model

A nonlinear model predicts a different type of relation between the dose and its effect; however, the effect will be stochastic or random in manifestation. A nonlinear model can have either a **nonlinear, threshold** or a **nonlinear, nonthreshold** response. The nonlinear, nonthreshold response curve represents that in a low-dose range, there will be very little biological response. At high doses, the same amount of dose will produce a much larger response. When the nonlinear model has a threshold, the curve is moved to the right on the graph to represent that a safe dose of radiation can occur at the low range (Fig. 32.3). As the dose is increased to above D_T, it becomes increasingly effective in creating a biologic response. This type of dose–response relationship is characteristic of a deterministic response.

Linear, Quadratic Dose–Response Model

In 1980, the Committee on Biological Effects of Ionizing Radiations (BEIR) of the National Academy of Sciences completed a thorough review of scientific information from several different studies including:

- The continuing studies of Japanese survivors of nuclear bombings during World War II
- Radiation accidents
- Patients who were exposed to radiation during medical treatment

This report dealt with the somatic effects and genetic effects of exposure to low doses of low-LET radiation. The findings of the study are directly applicable to diagnostic imaging. At this time, the committee concluded that effects followed a linear, quadratic dose–response

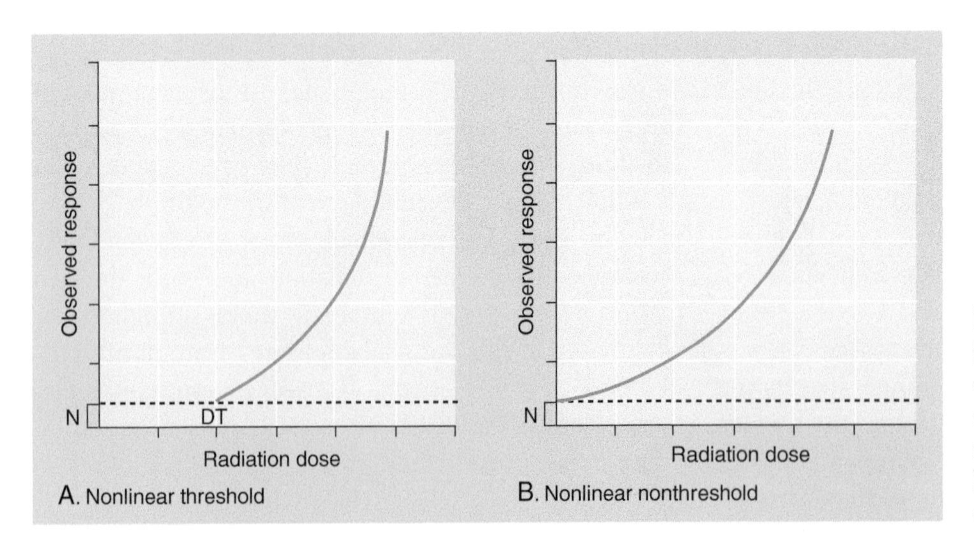

Figure 32.3. The curves obtained from the nonlinear model with and without a threshold, (A) and (B), respectively. In practice, almost all nonlinear curves have a threshold below in which there are no observable biologic effects.

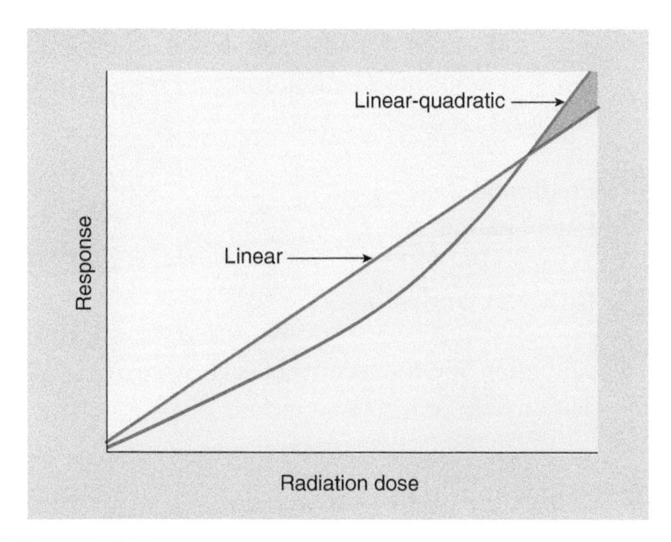

Figure 32.4. **Linear, quadratic dose–response relationship. Applies to low-dose low-LET radiation effects.**

relationship (Fig. 32.4). The linear quadratic model predicted small effects at low doses. Subsequent data that determined this type of dose–response relationship overestimated the risk associated with diagnostic radiation. In 1990, the BEIR committee revised its radiation risk estimates, leading to the use of the linear, nonthreshold model as the most appropriate model to use for establishing radiation protection guidelines that reflect a safe approach.

Lethal Doses

Estimating **lethal dose** levels for radiation exposure is very difficult to establish because it is based on complete annihilation of a population. The method using lethal dose 50 (LD_{50}) was developed as a more reliable approach. Acute radiation lethality is the radiation dose to the whole body that will produce death in 50% of the exposed population within a given time frame. The exact length of time used varies among authors, either 30 or 60 days. Humans develop sign of damage and recover from it at a slower rate than other mammals. The peak incidence of human death from hematologic damage occurs at ~30 days after exposure, but deaths continue for up to 60 days. **$LD_{50/60}$** is a more accurate way to assess lethal dose to humans than $LD_{50/30}$ because survival over a 60-day period would be a more relevant indicator of patient outcome. Table 32.1 lists the $LD_{50/30}$ for other species.

The $LD_{50/60}$ will be used to express the lethal dose of radiation to humans. $LD_{50/60}$ is a threshold response and

TABLE 32.1 **$LD_{50/30}$ FOR WHOLE-BODY RADIATION EXPOSURE**

Species	$LD_{50/30}$ (Rad)
Pig	250
Dog	275
Human	300
Guinea pig	425
Monkey	475
Opossum	510
Mouse	620
Hamster	700
Rat	710
Rabbit	725

nonlinear, meaning any amount of radiation will elicit a biological response. At lower dose of ~1 Gy (100 rad), no exposed individual is expected to die. When the dose is above ~6 Gy (600 rad), all individuals irradiated would be expected to die unless immediate, vigorous medical support is available. Irradiation doses above 10 Gy (1,000 rad) will result in death regardless of medical treatment. If death does occur, it will likely happen within 60 days of the exposure.

Gonadal Effects

The gonads have particular importance as target organs. They are particularly sensitive to radiation with responses at doses of 10 rad being reported. Data have been gathered from radiation therapy patients, radiation accident victims, and volunteer convicts to complete a description of the response of gonads to radiation.

Male Gonads

Data collected from patients who have undergone radiation therapy treatments for testicular cancer and volunteer convicts determined that after high doses of radiation, the testes will begin to atrophy. After irradiation of the testes, the maturing cells (spermatocytes) and spermatids are relatively radioresistant and will continue to mature. The spermatogonial stem cells are the most sensitive phase in development. There is no significant reduction in the number of spermatozoa until several weeks after exposure. Radiation doses as low as 100 mGy (10 rad) can result in the reduction in the number of spermatozoa. The reduction will continue to take place over a long period of time. Doses of up to 2 Gy (200 rad) will produce temporary infertility, which will begin at full 2 months after irradiation and will last ~12 months. If the dose is 5 Gy (500 rad), permanent sterility will occur.

Female Gonads

When the ovaries are exposed to radiation early in life, the ovaries will be reduced in size or will atrophy. After puberty, irradiation can suppress and delay the menstrual cycle. The oocyte in the mature follicle is the most radiosensitive cell in female reproduction. Doses as low as 100 mGy (10 rad) may cause suppression or delay in menstruation in the mature female. Temporary sterility will occur with a dose of ~2 Gy (200 rad) with permanent sterility occurring at ~5 Gy (500 rad).

Acute Radiation Syndrome

The early effects of high doses of radiation have been studied in animals in the laboratory, and there is limited information about human exposure. To date, no human has died from exposure to radiation following a diagnostic imaging procedure. The early pioneers in radiology were exposed to extremely high total radiation dose, which led to early deaths for some individuals. In modern diagnostic radiology departments, the exposures that are made are not sufficiently intense enough to cause death.

Historically, there have been accidental exposures of persons to extremely high doses of radiation. In April 1986, an accident with a nuclear reactor at Chernobyl caused 134 people to be exposed to high levels of radiation, which resulted in acute radiation syndrome; of these, 30 people died within 3 months of the accident. Individuals exposed to the radioactive fallout from Chernobyl will be followed for years to come to gather data on the effects of the radiation exposure. Humans exposed to high amounts of whole-body radiation up to 100 rad may experience nausea, vomiting, and diarrhea known as N–V–D syndrome. These symptoms would be accompanied by a feeling of general weakness or malaise. The symptoms will last for a few days and will then go away; the person will have no further somatic effects.

Acute radiation effects result from high radiation doses above 100 rads delivered to the whole body in a few hours or less. This is called **acute radiation syndrome (ARS)** and leads to death within days or weeks. The clinical signs and symptoms of radiation exposure present themselves in four stages:

1. Prodromal stage
2. Latent period
3. Manifest stage
4. Recovery or death

The duration and the severity of each stage depend on the radiation dose or whole-body dose.

Prodromal Stage

The first stage of radiation response following an exposure is the **prodromal stage** or N–V–D stage. The prodromal stage shows the clinical signs and symptoms resulting from radiation exposure to the whole body within hours of the exposure and can last up to a day or two. Individuals who are exposed to radiation levels >1 Gy (100 rad) usually show prodromal symptoms, which include nausea, vomiting, and diarrhea that may be accompanied with fever and/or faintness. The prodromal stage can begin within a few minutes to hours following exposure and last for a few hours to a few days. The time between the exposure and the onset of prodromal symptoms is an indication of the magnitude of the exposure. Higher exposure levels result in shorter times to the onset of the prodromal symptoms. The severity of the symptoms is dose related, and at doses exceeding 10 Gy (1,000 rad), the symptoms can be quite violent. The onset of prodromal symptoms shortly after exposure indicates a major radiation exposure to the whole body.

Latent Period

The second stage of high-dose effects is the **latent period.** During the latent period, the exposed individual has no clinical symptoms or illness from the radiation exposure and appears to have recovered with no ill effects. However, even though there are no visible symptoms, there may be ongoing cell damage. The latent period can extend from a few hours to several days, depending on the dose. Higher doses result in shorter latent periods.

Manifest Illness Stage

During the **manifest illness stage** of radiation response, the full clinical effects are evident. The prodromal symptoms will return, and additional life-threatening

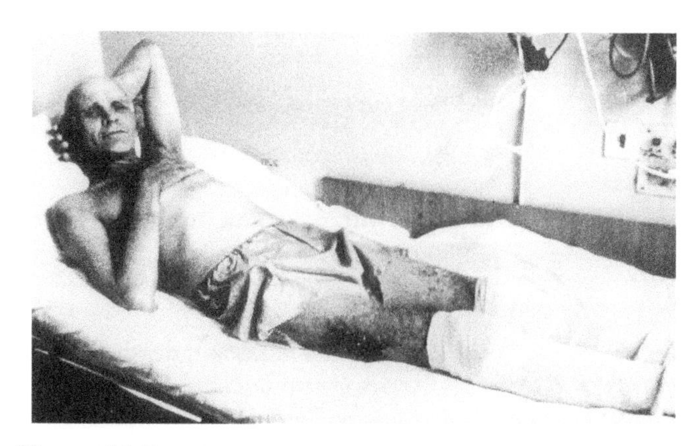

Figure 32.5. **Chernobyl victim suffering from acute radiation syndrome a few weeks after the accident. Note the hair loss, indicating a radiation dose of several hundred rem. Also, note injury to the skin of the lower extremities as a result of high (a few thousand rem) doses of beta (nonpenetrating) radiation.**

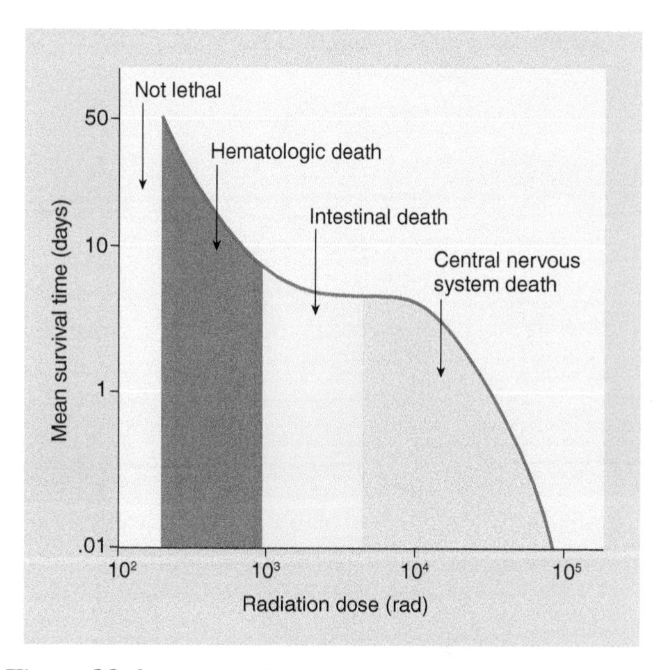

Figure 32.6. **Acute radiation syndrome (ARS). Hematopoietic, gastrointestinal, and central nervous system syndromes and relative dose associated with each syndrome.**

symptoms appear that are characteristic of the subsyndromes. The manifest illness stage can last several hours to ~2 months at which time the person either recovers or succumbs to the illness.

As seen in Figure 32.5, this victim of the Chernobyl nuclear power plant accident has experienced hair loss and radiation burns from the exposure to a few thousand rem.

ARS can be divided into three subsyndromes that are the hematopoietic (hematologic) syndrome, the gastrointestinal (GI) syndrome, and the central nervous system (CNS) syndrome.

The whole-body dose determines the effects that an individual will display during each stage. At higher dose levels, the effects observed may include more than one syndrome. The three syndromes resulting from high-dose whole-body exposures are dose related (Fig. 32.6). The first syndrome to appear is the hematologic syndrome; then, if the whole-body dose is high, the GI syndrome will appear. At very high doses, the CNS syndrome becomes evident. Thus, an individual exposed to 10 Gy (1,000 rad) will display the symptoms of all three syndromes (Table 32.2).

The threshold dose necessary to produce a given syndrome and related effects is often seen in a given range for each syndrome. It is expected that patients will experience each phase of the syndrome; however, the sequence of events in each syndrome is not always seen (Fig. 32.7). Exposure to very high radiation doses will often result in the latent period disappearing, while very low doses may have no prodromal stage and consequently no associated latent period.

Hematopoietic Syndrome

Hematopoietic or bone marrow syndrome will usually occur with a dose in the range of 0.7 to 10 Gy (70 to 1,000 rads) though mild symptoms may occur with a dose as low as 0.3 Gy (30 rads). The hematologic or hematopoietic syndrome is characterized by damage to the bone marrow and the physiological consequences of this damage. The major hematologic effect of radiation exposure is a decrease in leukocytes, erythrocytes, thrombocytes, and lymphocytes. This means that the body's defenses against infection are reduced or eliminated.

TABLE 32.2 DOSE LEVELS AT WHICH BIOLOGIC EFFECTS APPEAR

Dose Level (Gy)	Biologic Effect	Latent Period
<1	No observable effect	
>0.7	Hematopoietic	1–6 wk
>10	GI	3–5 d
>50	CNS	A few hours

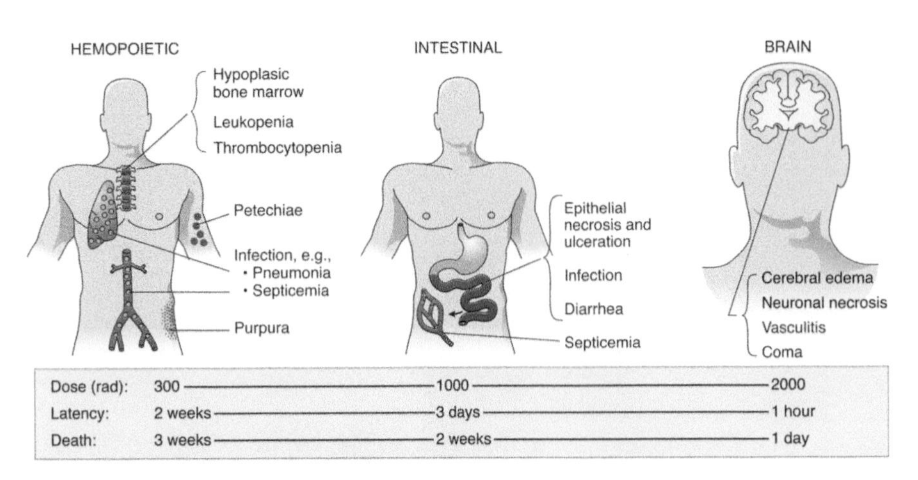

Figure 32.7. Whole-body radiation syndromes. At a dose of ~300 rad of whole-body radiation, a syndrome characterized by hematologic failure develops within 2 weeks. In the vicinity of 1,000 rad, a GI syndrome with a latency of only 3 days is seen. With doses of 2,000 rad or greater, disease of the CNS appears within 1 hour, and death ensues rapidly. (Image from Rubin E, Farber JL. *Pathology*. 3rd Ed. Philadelphia, PA: Lippincott Williams & Wilkins, 1999.)

Individuals experience nausea and vomiting during the prodromal stage, onset occurs within 1 hour to 2 days after exposure. Hematopoietic effects follow a latent period of 1 to 6 weeks. During the latent period, there are no apparent symptoms characterized by a general feeling of well-being, but blood cell damage is still being expressed.

During the manifest illness stage, symptoms include anorexia, fever, and malaise. The blood cell counts drop for several weeks. If the dose is not lethal, the body's defense mechanisms begin to recover 2 to 4 weeks after exposure, and a full recovery may take as long as 6 months. When these defense mechanisms against infection are fully active, complete recovery can be expected. Individuals exposed to doses as high as 6 Gy (600 rad) can recover if they are given vigorous medical care to prevent infection.

Survival rates of patients with this syndrome decreases with higher doses. The primary cause of death is the destruction of bone marrow, which results in infection and hemorrhage. Death at these exposure levels is due to infection, electrolyte imbalance, and dehydration. Depending on the dose, the $LD_{50/60}$ is about 2.5 to 5 Gy (250 to 500 rad).

Gastrointestinal Syndrome

Gastrointestinal syndrome symptoms appear at whole-body doses of 10 Gy (1,000 rad) or higher. Whole-body doses kill most of the stem cells in the bone marrow and GI tract. The patient will experience all the hematologic effects, with severe nausea, vomiting, and diarrhea that will begin very soon after exposure. The prodromal stage occurs within hours of the exposure and may last as long as 2 days. Following the prodromal stage, there is a latent period of about 3 to 5 days during which the patient experiences no symptoms. During the manifest illness stage, the individual experiences malaise, anorexia, nausea, vomiting, severe diarrhea, fever, dehydration, and electrolyte imbalance. This stage lasts <1 week. Massive infection occurs as the intestines break down, allowing a loss of body fluids and an invasion of bacteria. This occurs just as the body's defenses are beginning to fail because of the hematologic effects. Death usually occurs about 2 weeks after exposure.

Death occurs primarily because of the severe damage to the cells lining the intestines. These cells are normally in a rapid state of proliferation and are continually being replaced by new cells. The normal process of cell proliferation is ~3 to 5 days. These cells are very sensitive to the effects of radiation, and the high dose of radiation will kill the most sensitive cells, the stem cells, and this determines the length of time until death. When the intestinal lining is completely denuded of cells, the result is uncontrollable passage of fluids across the intestinal membrane, severe electrolyte imbalance, and dehydration. Bacteria are absorbed into the blood stream via the small bowel wall. The patient will experience a severe septic infection and intensified dehydration. Even with aggressive, immediate medical care, death is likely in 2 weeks due to the failure of the hematologic system. The LD is 100% with doses >10 Gy.

Central Nervous System Syndrome

The full **central nervous system syndrome** will typically occur with a dose >50 Gy (5,000 rad) although some symptoms may occur with a dose as low as 20 Gy (200 rad). The radiation damages the nerve cells, and the body's regulatory mechanisms begin to fail within minutes of the exposure and complete failure occurs within 3 days.

During the prodromal stage, there is onset of extreme nervousness and confusion, severe nausea, vomiting and watery diarrhea, loss of consciousness, and burning sensations of the skin. Symptoms will occur in minutes and may last a few hours. The latent period may be as short as a few hours with very high doses, while higher doses result in shorter latent periods. During the manifest illness stage, the symptoms include the return of watery diarrhea, convulsion, and coma. Onset of symptoms occurs in 5 to 6 hours after exposure with death occurring within 3 days. Exposures at these dose levels always result in death because the hematopoietic and GI systems have also been destroyed.

Final Stage

The survival of an individual depends on many complex factors, including the amount and distribution of the radiation, the individual's general health, individual's sensitivity to radiation, and the medical treatment obtained. Human data on exposures at these levels are limited, but it appears that survival from doses of 6 to 7 Gy (600 to 700 rad) is possible with vigorous medical treatment that includes large doses of antibiotics and maintenance of body fluids and electrolyte balance. The mean survival time is the average time of survival and is dose related; higher doses have shorter mean survival times. Although there are no absolute values, the mean survival time for the hematopoietic syndrome is 45 days, for GI syndrome is 8 days, and that for the CNS syndrome is 3 days.

Effects of Partial Body Irradiations

Radiation exposures to limited portions of the body require a higher dose to produce a response. Exposure of localized portions of the body to radiation produces different effects compared to exposure of the whole body. Tissues and organs in the exposed area can atrophy (shrink in size), which is caused by cell death. This can lead to a complete lack of function for the tissue or organ, or it can be followed by recovery. Localized exposures show striking, but nonlethal effects to tissues and organs. The type of response of the tissue will depend on the radiosensitivity as well as the phase of proliferation and maturation of the cell. Local tissues that show an immediate effect are the skin, gonads, and bone marrow.

All deterministic radiation responses follow a threshold-type dose–response relationship. This means that a minimum dose is necessary to produce a deterministic response. When the threshold has been exceeded, the severity of the response will increase as the radiation dose increases.

Effects on the Skin

Localized exposure to the skin will produce **erythema**, or sunburn-like reddening, at dose levels near 5 Gy (500 rad). Roentgen and many other early x-ray pioneers suffered erythema "burns." Fractions of the **skin erythema dose (SED)** were used to measure radiation exposure until the unit Roentgen was defined. For patients having radiation therapy treatments, the radiation caused local damage to the skin stem cells, producing reddening of the skin within a couple of days. The latent period for skin erythema is a few days. Higher doses of radiation to the skin can lead to damage at the cellular level; a second round of erythema is followed by **desquamation** (ulceration and denudation) of the skin.

Small doses of radiation will not cause erythema, while extremely high doses of radiation cause erythema in all people who received that dose. In regard to intermediate doses, the response of the tissue is dependent upon the radiosensitivity of the tissue, the dose rate, and the size of the area of irradiated skin. Using data of people who were treated therapeutically with superficial x-rays has shown that the SED necessary to affect 50% of the population (SED_{50}) is near 5 Gy (500 rad).

With the advent of cardiovascular and interventional procedures, the risk of serious skin injury has increased because of the lengthy amounts of fluoroscopy time used for the procedures. As seen in Figure 32.8, this localized skin lesion appeared to show some healing with a small, central area of necrosis at 16 to 21 weeks

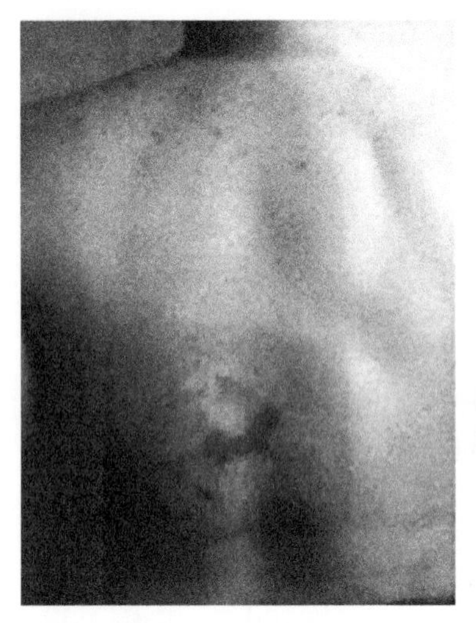
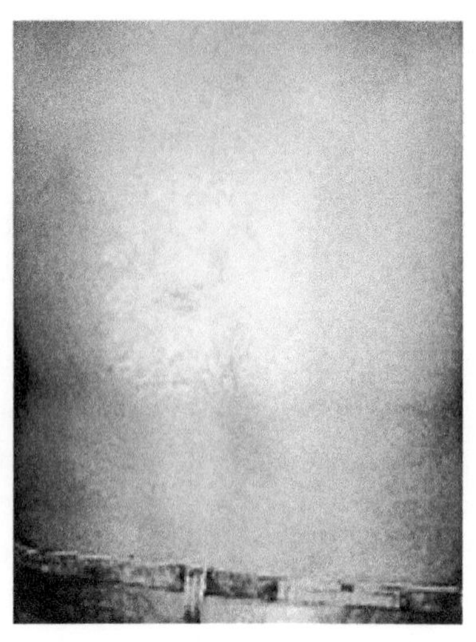
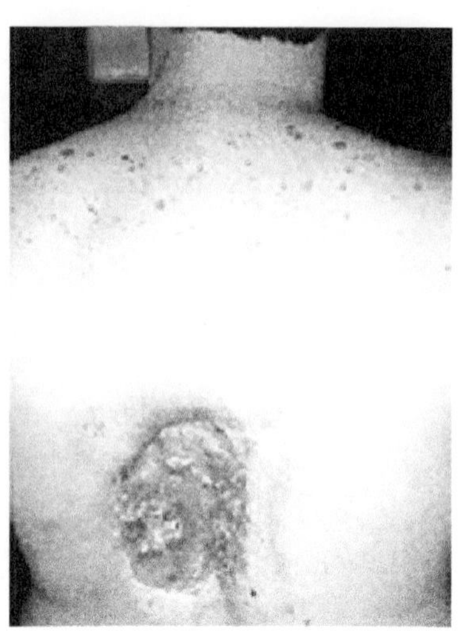

Figure 32.8. **Time line of a major radiation injury. Image at left is 6 to 8 weeks after exposure and shows prolonged erythema with mauve central area, which is suggestive of ischemia. The center image is at 16 to 21 weeks following exposure; depigmented skin with central area of necrosis is seen. Image on the right is at 18 to 21 months and shows deep necrosis with atrophic borders. (This sequence is available on the FDA Web site [NRCP 168, 2010].)**

postinjury. Over the course of 18 to 21 months, the skin has broken down and demonstrates deep necrosis with atrophic borders.

Another response of the skin to radiation exposure is **epilation**, or temporary hair loss. This occurs at doses above a threshold of 3 Gy (300 rad) with a latent period of a few weeks. Regrowth of the hair begins in about 2 months and is complete in about 6 months.

Late Somatic Effects

Somatic cells, which are exposed to radiation, often demonstrate an effect many months or years after the irradiation occurred. Late somatic effects can occur to the cells' response to either whole-body or partial-body exposure to high radiation doses, to individual low doses, or to chronic low doses sustained over several years. The cells respond to the radiation by mutating into cancerous cells, which leads to various types of cancer.

Leukemia

We have discussed that the bone marrow is one of the most radiosensitive tissues in the body. The exposure of the bone marrow to high doses of radiation suppresses the formation of normal red blood-cell precursors and lymphocytes. Leukocytes continue to accumulate unchecked until they overwhelm the system, resulting in a life-threatening disorder called leukemia.

Scientists have performed research on laboratory animals to study radiation-induced leukemia. Their research shows that the response is real, and the incidence rates increase with increasing radiation dose. The dose–response relationship is linear and nonthreshold. Scientists have studied the groups of human populations, which were exposed to high levels of radiation—atomic bomb survivors, radiotherapy patients, radiologists, and children irradiated in utero, among other groups. Their results concluded that these human groups have exhibited an elevated incidence of leukemia as a direct result of their radiation exposure.

Leukemia, caused by permanently damaged bone marrow, can appear after a latent period of 4 to 7 years. Individual risk is much longer, up to 20 years. Atomic bomb survivors had a 3:1 relative risk for leukemia. In the early decades of radiology, through the 1940s, it was common for radiologists to accumulate radiation exposures 10 to 20 times more than modern radiologists. The rates of leukemia were significantly higher for radiologists compared to other physicians. Out of the expanding knowledge of the dangers of radiation came the realization that personnel must protect themselves, and today, it is the standard of practice. Currently, radiologists do not exhibit an elevated incidence of leukemia compared to other physicians. A link between occupational exposure and leukemia for radiographers has not been shown.

Cancer

In general, the risk of acquiring some type of cancer is very high at ~33%. It has been estimated that for each exposure of 10 rad of total body exposure, risk will increase by another 1%. Currently, occupational exposure levels for radiation personnel are so low that excess risk for cancer is undetectable. Even at the maximum dose limits, the increased risk of death from cancer is not likely to exceed 1%, which is similar to other nonradiation industries.

Ionizing radiation can cause cancer; it is a known **carcinogen**. There are many other carcinogens, including smoking, diet, and environmental factors. It is difficult to determine the exact cause of any particular cancer because cancers induced by radiation have latent periods of 10 to 25 years.

Carcinogenesis has an increased frequency in the exposed population with long latent periods of 20 to 30 years for solid tumors to appear. As with other population exposed to radiation, there is a stochastic or random effect, so it is difficult to predict with absolute certainty which person will develop cancer. Various forms of cancer, which have been identified, include the following:

- Breast cancer: Several studies followed women who had multiple exposures to their chests during tuberculosis testing and/or fluoroscopy to identify their rates of breast cancer compared to women who did not receive the same amount or type of radiation. Relative risk for radiation-induced breast cancer was as high as 10%.
- Skin cancer: Early radiation workers were exposed to large amounts of radiation to their hands. Chronic, severe doses of radiation resulted in skin lesions. Presently near-epidemic proportions of skin cancer are because of cosmetic use of radiation and outdoor activities. The latent period can range from 5 to 10 years.
- Bone cancer: Identified in radium watch dial painters. The paint was laced with radium, which is a bone-seeking element. Patients developed osteogenic sarcoma as a direct result of ingesting the paint when they moistened the brush with their lips. The overall risk for bone cancer was estimated at 122:1!
- Liver cancer: Thorotrast was used in medical imaging as a contrast agent. Thorotrast contained thorium, which contained radioactive isotopes. After injection, the thorium particles concentrated in the liver and spleen. These patients demonstrated an increase in liver cancer due to the thorium-releasing alpha particles as the thorium decayed.
- Lung cancer: Uranium miners inhaled radioactive dust, which lead to their increased rates of lung and bronchial epithelium cancer. There was also an increased incidence of lung cancer in atomic bomb survivors and early radiologists. Presently, there is no occurrence of lung cancer for technologists or radiologists.

Radiation and Pregnancy

From early medical applications of radiation, there has been concern in regard to the effect radiation will have on the embryo and developing fetus. The **teratogenic effects** of radiation in utero are dose related and time related. Teratogenic effects should not be confused with **mutagenic effects**, which occur from radiation exposure to the gametes (sperm or egg) prior to conception. The teratogenic effects are caused by radiation exposure after conception and include preimplantation death, neonatal death, congenital abnormalities, malignancy induction, and general impairment of growth, genetic effects, and mental retardation. Figure 32.9 has been drawn from studies that observed the effects of a 2 Gy (200 rad) dose delivered at various stages in utero in mice. The data were extrapolated to indicate approximate comparable time in human gestation.

The embryo is very sensitive to radiation because it is made up of rapidly dividing cells. The fetus is most sensitive to radiation during the first trimester of pregnancy. The effects on the fetus depend on the stage of fetal development at which the radiation exposure occurs, and the fetus will experience an all-or-nothing effect, either the fetus will develop an abnormal defect or will be born without any sign of defect.

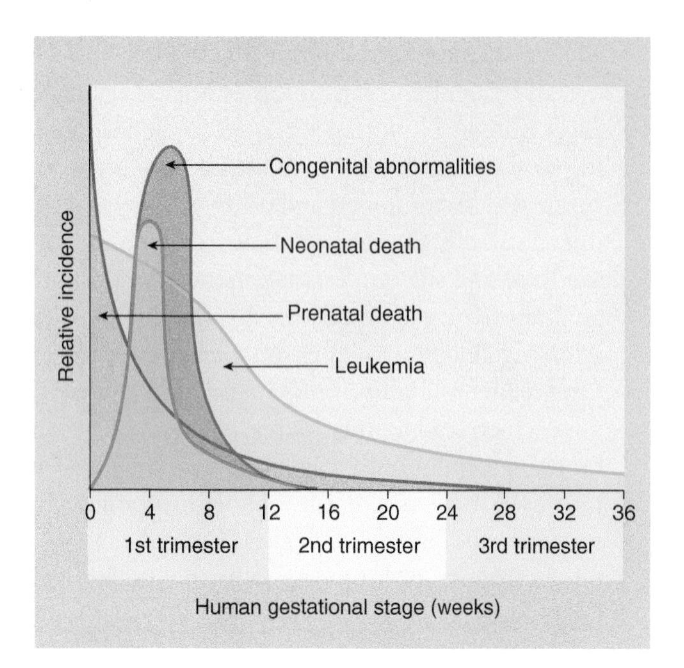

Figure 32.9. $LD_{50/60}$ of mice in relation to the age at time of irradiation. Human age extrapolated from mice experiment.

0 to 2 Weeks' Gestation

High-dose radiation exposure during the preimplantation stage of the first 2 weeks will result in spontaneous death or the embryo will be viable with no effects—it is an all-or-none effect. Observations of radiation therapy patients have confirmed this effect but only after very high doses. When considering animal experimentation, it appears that this response is very rare. The best estimate is that a 100 mGy (10 rad) dose during the first 2 weeks will possibly induce a 0.1% rate of spontaneous abortion. This is in addition to the 25% normal incidence of spontaneous abortions.

2 to 8 Weeks' Gestation

During the phase of major **organogenesis** from weeks 2 to 8, the embryo is experiencing rapid cell growth. Early in this phase, the tissues are differentiating, and identifiable organs begin to be formed. The main radiation risk during this time is for various congenital abnormalities to be induced. The natural incidence of congenital deformities is ~6%. Large doses of radiation appear to increase this ratio by about 1% to 7%.

The congenital deformities that occur during major organogenesis fall into two categories:

- Early 2 to 5 weeks: During this time, there are skeletal defects such as stunted limb, missing or extra finger, or other structural malformations. Organ abnormalities can also be induced.
- Later 6 to 8 weeks: Neurological deformities are common during this phase. The deformations may include anophthalmia where an eye fails to form properly or failure of the cranium to form properly resulting in anencephaly or exencephaly. Abnormalities to the CNS cannot be detected until after birth.

8 to 12 Weeks' Gestation

During this phase, the risk of morphological changes is gone for the developing fetus. The concern is the fetus is susceptible to radiation-induced mental retardation. The natural frequency of intellectual disability or mental retardation in nonexposed population is ~6%; with large doses of radiation, the incidence increases to ~6.5%.

When considering the first trimester in pregnancy, it becomes clear that this is the most radiosensitive stage of the pregnancy for the developing fetus. Studies have reported that while there is minimal evidence of injury to the fetus with doses <1 rad, there are detectable abnormalities to the CNS and congenital malformations and increased evidence of tumors when the dose is 5 rad. At doses of 50 rads, the fetus may have a decrease in the size of skeletal structures and a fivefold increase in intellectual disabilities. During the first 8 weeks, the embryo is ~10 times more sensitive to radiation than an adult; recall this is because of the rapid rate of cell differentiation during this critical time.

Beyond 12 Weeks' Gestation

During the remainder of gestation, the developing fetus continues to be susceptible to one radiation risk: latent carcinogenic effects. Various types of cancer may occur later in life due to the radiation exposure during gestation. These cancers can also be caused by other factors, such as genetic factors, so it is difficult to establish the specific factor that actually caused a particular type of cancer to proliferate. Of particular concern is adolescent leukemia, leukemia that develops during the teen years. Acquiring leukemia at this phase of life is more likely from radiation

TABLE 32.3 EFFECTS AFTER 100 mGy EXPOSURE IN UTERO

Phase at Exposure	Type of Response	Natural Occurrence	Radiation Response
0–2 wk	Spontaneous abortion	25%	0.1%
2–8 wk	Congenital deformities	6%	1%
8–12 wk	Mental retardation	6%	0.5%
0–9 mo	Malignant disease	8/10,000	12/12,000
0–9 mo	Impaired growth/development	1%	Zero
0–9 mo	Genetic mutation	10%	Zero

exposure in utero compared to other potential carcinogens. Table 32.3 summarizes effects to the embryo/fetus after 100 mGy of radiation is delivered.

It is critical to stress that most diagnostic radiography procedures pose little or no measurable risk to the fetus. The majority of radiography procedures do not place the fetus in the direct beam of x-rays. An abdomen procedure, such as a single abdomen exposure, may be determined to be worth the risk to the fetus when an emergency to the mother warrants medical procedures. The diagnostic imaging procedures that are of concern are those that are known to use higher doses such as any fluoroscopy procedure over the abdomen and computed tomography abdomen scans. All institutions should have a policy regarding x-ray examinations of potentially pregnant patients to ensure that all patients are treated the same way. Medically necessary examinations should never be delayed because of pregnancy as an examination that can be postponed until the birth of the baby is not a necessary examination.

Mutagenic Effects

The mutagenic effects of radiation exposure are those effects upon the chromosomes of human gametes, prior to fertilization, which may contribute to congenital defects, disease present at birth, or latent disease. Many experiments have been conducted on mice to evaluate the effect of radiation damage on future generations. Germ cells are radiosensitive because they are immature genetic cells. The mutagenic effects follow a linear, nonthreshold response curve. These are stochastic effects: as radiation exposure increases to the gametes, the frequency of mutations increases but not the severity. Although the frequency is proportional to dose, the frequency is estimated to be quite low, possible one mutation per 1,000 rad delivered to the population not to the individual.

Doubling Dose

The **doubling dose** is defined as that amount of radiation dose that produces twice the spontaneous genetic mutation rate in a population. For humans, the doubling dose is estimated to be between 0.5 and 25 Gy (50 and 250 rad). The term congenital defects refers to any defect present at birth and may be either mutagenic effects or teratogenic effects.

Genetically Significant Dose

The **genetically significant dose (GSD)** measures the effect on the genetic pool of radiation exposure to the gonads. The GSD is defined as that dose which, if delivered to every member of the population, would produce the same genetic effect as is produced by the actual dose to the individual members of the population. The GSD is an averaged quantity that indicates how much genetic harm is being caused to the entire human population due to the use of medical radiation. The GSD takes into account that some of the population is infertile and that not all exposed individuals will receive measurable gonadal dose.

The current GSD estimates to be about 200 mGy (20 mrad) per year. In other words, it is the rate of genetic mutations, and other genetic effects throughout the entire population would be expected if every person received 20 mrad of medical radiation every year. The GSD has been steadily increasing over time, possibly because of the use of computed tomography and fluoroscopy. The GSD should be monitored closely to determine trends that identify the medical imaging procedures which deliver the higher dose levels to patients. With this knowledge, technologists, medical physicists, and physicians can work together to produce medically needed procedures with the minimal radiation dose possible to the patient.

Chapter Summary

1. Radiation risks may be estimated by experimentation with laboratory animals and extrapolation of the data for humans.
2. Stochastic effects of radiation exposure increase in occurrence with increasing dose, but the level of severity is independent of the dose.
3. Deterministic effects increase in severity with increasing dose; they are certain to occur above threshold dose levels.
4. Early effects of radiation are those effects demonstrated in less than several weeks. Most early effects are somatic or random, cells can recover, and effects follow a nonlinear, threshold response curve.
5. Late effects occur after a delay measured in months or years from the time of radiation exposure. These effects include most genetic and carcinogenic effect.
6. The threshold dose for human deaths is ~100 rad to the whole body.
7. N–V–D syndrome is expected to occur when 50 to 100 rad of whole-body dose is experienced. At a threshold dose of 100 rad, some exposed people will begin to suffer the hematopoietic form of ARS and may die from infections.
8. At 600 rad, people will experience the GI syndrome with death resulting primarily from dehydration and malnutrition.
9. CNS syndrome occurs with doses of 5,000 rad, and death results from intracranial pressure.
10. The threshold dose for skin erythema is ~200 rad, for epilation 300 rad.
11. Temporary infertility in both genders can occur following a dose of 200 rad.
12. Teratogenic effects of radiation to the developing human embryo or fetus are dependent upon the stage of gestation when the exposure occurs. The first trimester is marked by the highest levels of radiosensitivity.
13. Mutagenic effects from radiation exposure are still under investigation; however, the effects are stochastic in nature.
14. The risk of acquiring cancer in a person's lifetime increases by about 1% for every 10 rads of radiation.
15. There is some concern for patients exposed to multiple high-dose level radiographic procedures; of particular concern is leukemia in adolescent patients.

Case Study

Laura is a 2nd year radiologic technology student. During her course in radiation biology, she was assigned to perform research on people who have received a whole-body exposure to 600 rad or 6 Gy of radiation. In her assignment, she is to answer the following questions.

Critical Thinking Questions

1. What does $LD_{50/60}$ represent?
2. How does the level of radiation exposure correlate to patient survival? Which symptoms will the patient likely experience?
3. Which late effect syndromes will be identified with this level of exposure?

Review Questions

Multiple Choice

1. The $LD_{50/60}$ represents a radiation dose that will kill:

a. 30 people in 50 days
b. 30% of the cells in 50 days
c. 50% of the people in 60 days
d. 50% of the cells in 30 days

2. The first stage of acute radiation response following an exposure is the __________ stage.

a. prodromal
b. latent
c. acute
d. final

3. The physical defects that are caused by radiation exposure to the developing embryo are referred to as __________ effects.

a. congenital
b. mutagenic
c. teratogenic
d. genetic

4. Hematologic syndrome is expected to occur at dose levels of:

a. 25 to 100 rad
b. 100 to 1,000 rad
c. 1,000 to 5,000 rad
d. more than 5,000 rad

5. Epilation is defined as the:

a. feeling of well-being
b. overproduction of skin cells
c. ulceration of the skin
d. loss of hair

6. Which of the following is NOT a symptom of the gastrointestinal syndrome?

a. Nausea
b. Vomiting
c. Seizures
d. Loss of appetite

7. Which factor has no influence on a human's response to radiation exposure?

a. Dose protraction
b. Age of organism
c. Gender of organism
d. Occupation

8. Congenital abnormalities of skeletal and neurological defects would have been most likely to be caused by radiation exposure during which stage of gestation?

   a. Conception to 2 weeks
   b. 2 to 8 weeks
   c. 3 to 8 months
   d. During the 9th month

9. When studying the hematological effects of radiation exposure, which of the following doses would be of the greatest importance?

   a. GSD
   b. Gonadal dose
   c. Skin dose
   d. Bone marrow dose

10. The minimum amount of radiation at which a particular biological response can be observed is called the:

    a. threshold dose
    b. GSD
    c. congenital dose
    d. tolerance dose

Short Answer

1. Define acute radiation syndrome. What was the outcome of the 33 people who were diagnosed with acute radiation syndrome after the Chernobyl nuclear power plant accident?

2. The clinical signs and symptoms of the manifest illness stage of acute radiation lethality can be classified into what groups?

3. Which stage of acute radiation syndrome simulates recovery?

4. Define early and late effects of radiation exposure.

5. With increasing radiation dose to a population, the deterministic or nonstochastic effects increase in their:

6. Which effects are caused by radiation exposure to the gametes prior to conception?

7. When a developing embryo is exposed to radiation during the 0 to 2 weeks of gestation, there is a small increase in the risk of __________.

8. Explain N–V–D syndrome.

9. Most deterministic effects of radiation follow which type of response curve?

10. During the first trimester, the embryo is __________ times more sensitive to radiation than an adult.

33

Radiation Protection: Principle Concepts and Equipment

Objectives

Upon completion of this chapter, the student will be able to:

1. Identify the units of exposure, dose, and effective dose.
2. State the requirements for personnel monitoring.
3. Identify devices used to detect and measure radiation.
4. Describe ALARA.
5. Name the dose limits for occupational and nonoccupational workers.
6. List the three types of natural radiation.
7. Discuss man-made radiation and its impact on radiation doses.

Key Terms

- absorbed dose
- ALARA
- Becquerel (Bq)
- cosmic radiation
- Curie (Ci)
- dose equivalent
- dose limits (DLs)
- effective dose
- exposure
- film badge dosimeters
- Geiger-Müller counters
- internal radiation
- ion chambers
- man-made radiation
- natural radiation
- occupational exposure
- occupationally exposed workers
- optically stimulated luminescence (OSL)
- rad
- radiosensitivity
- rem
- scintillation detectors
- Sievert (Sv)
- *Systeme International d'Unites* (SI)
- terrestrial radiation
- thermoluminescent dosimeter (TLD)

Introduction

In this chapter, we will begin by discussing the types of radiation humans are exposed during their everyday life. The amount of exposure to ionizing radiation that is received has been studied, and recommended dose limits have been determined. The tissues in the body have varying degrees of radiosensitivity to radiation and the different types of radiation will cause varied harmful effects in tissue or organs. We will discuss the weighting factors for each. Exposure to radiation is a particular concern for medical imaging personnel. Their dose to radiation must be closely monitored. During radiographic procedures, personnel monitoring devices are required to monitor the amount and type of radiation a radiographer is exposed to on a daily basis.

Sources of Radiation

There are many sources of radiation that are harmless. Ionizing radiation is harmful to humans. We can divide the sources into natural and man-made radiation.

Radiation is all around us in our natural environment. **Natural radiation** consists of three types: cosmic radiation, terrestrial radiation, and internal radiation (Fig. 33.1).

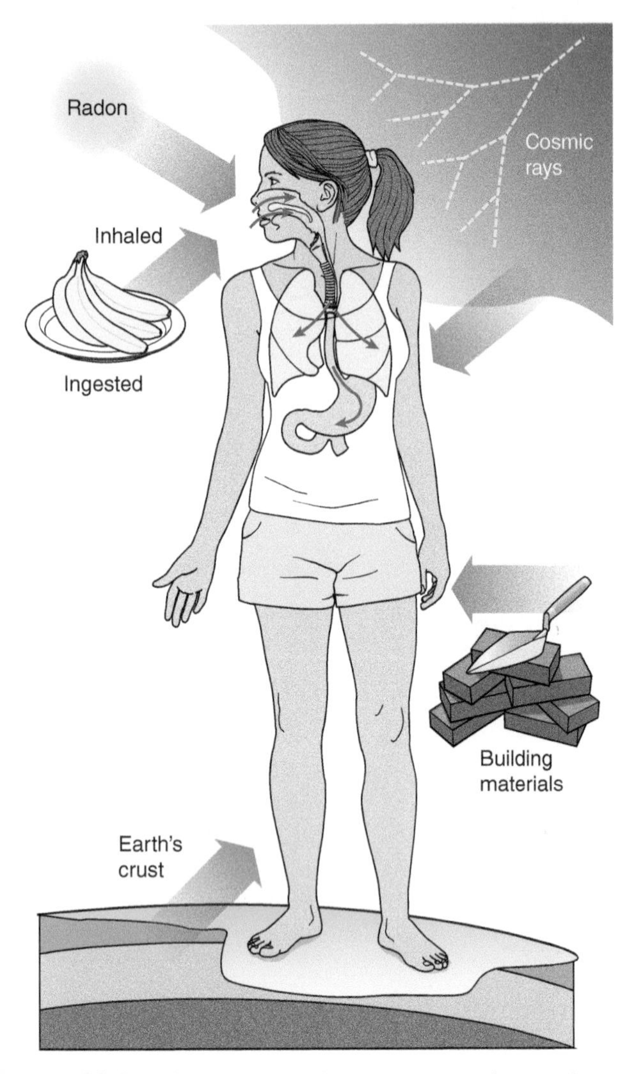

Figure 33.1. **Three principal components of natural background radiation; (1) cosmic rays from solar flares in the sun or from outer space; (2) ingested radioactivity, principally potassium 40 in food, and inhaled radioactivity, principally radon; and (3) radiation from the earth's crust, which in practice means radiation emanating from building materials, because most people spend much of their lives indoors. (Reprinted from Hall EJ, Giaccia AJ. *Radiobiology for the Radiologist*. 7th Ed. Philadelphia, PA: Lippincott Williams & Wilkins, 2012, with permission.)**

Cosmic Radiation

Cosmic radiation is emitted by the sun and stars. We are protected from most of the hazardous types of cosmic radiation by the earth's magnetic field, and the atmosphere provides additional shielding before the radiation can reach us. On earth, the intensity increases with altitude and latitude. People who live at higher elevations receive less protection from the thinner layers of atmosphere above them. The Rocky Mountains are beautiful but with their altitude comes a higher risk to people who live there. For instance, people living in the "mile-high" city of Denver receive about 70 mR per year more than people who live close to sea level.

Traveling on a transoceanic flight can bring you an additional 5 mR from the time spent at the high altitude. The high altitude is especially concerning for flight crew members who can accumulate 170 mR per year, because of this high level many airlines require radiation monitoring. The overall worldwide average exposure to cosmic radiation is ~30 mR per year.

Terrestrial Radiation

Terrestrial radiation comes from naturally occurring radioactive materials that are located throughout the earth's crust. Deposits of thorium, uranium, and other radionuclides are found in abundance. Many building materials use resources from the earth's crust, which means radiation is emanating from building materials. This is a consideration because most people spend the majority of their lives indoors.

In India, there are areas where the soil emits up to 4,000 mR of radiation per year. Commonly, the higher levels of radiation are found in mountainous terrain where the earth's crust has been thrust upward. Worldwide average exposure to terrestrial radiation, not including radon gas, is ~30 mR per year.

Internal Radiation

Lastly, **internal radiation** refers to the small amounts of radioactive minerals normally found in the body, ingested from the small amount present in food and inhaled as airborne particles. Radioactive thorium, radium, and lead can be detected in most people; however, the amounts are small and varied. These deposits account for <10 μSv per year. The most prominent radioactive isotope found

TABLE 33.1 ANNUAL NATURAL BACKGROUND RADIATION LEVELS

Type of Radiation	Radiation Level
Cosmic radiation	30 mR
Terrestrial radiation (nonradon)	30 mR
Internal radiation	40 mR
Radon gas	100–200 mR
Total	200–300 mR

in the human body is potassium 40, which attaches to the calcium in bones and radiates to nearby organs. The dose rate is ~0.2 mSv per year and must be considered when researching sources of mutations in humans. The total amount of radiation from internal sources, not including radon, averages 40 mR per year.

The largest source of natural background radiation is radon gas, which seeps into basements of homes from rocks underground. Radon gas is a natural by-product in the decay series for uranium. If the basement is not properly sealed with plastic, the radon gas will seep in through cracks or flaws in the concrete foundation. In the absence of proper ventilation, the radon gas can accumulate to dangerous levels over time. It is inhaled and attaches to the surface of the lungs and bronchi where it poses serious health risks, this is why it is being included in internal radiation.

When considering worldwide accumulation of radon gas, the average dose is estimated to be 100 to 200 mR per year, some areas have a high concentration of radon gas, while other areas have nonexistent levels. Table 33.1 summarizes the annual radiation levels for natural background radiation.

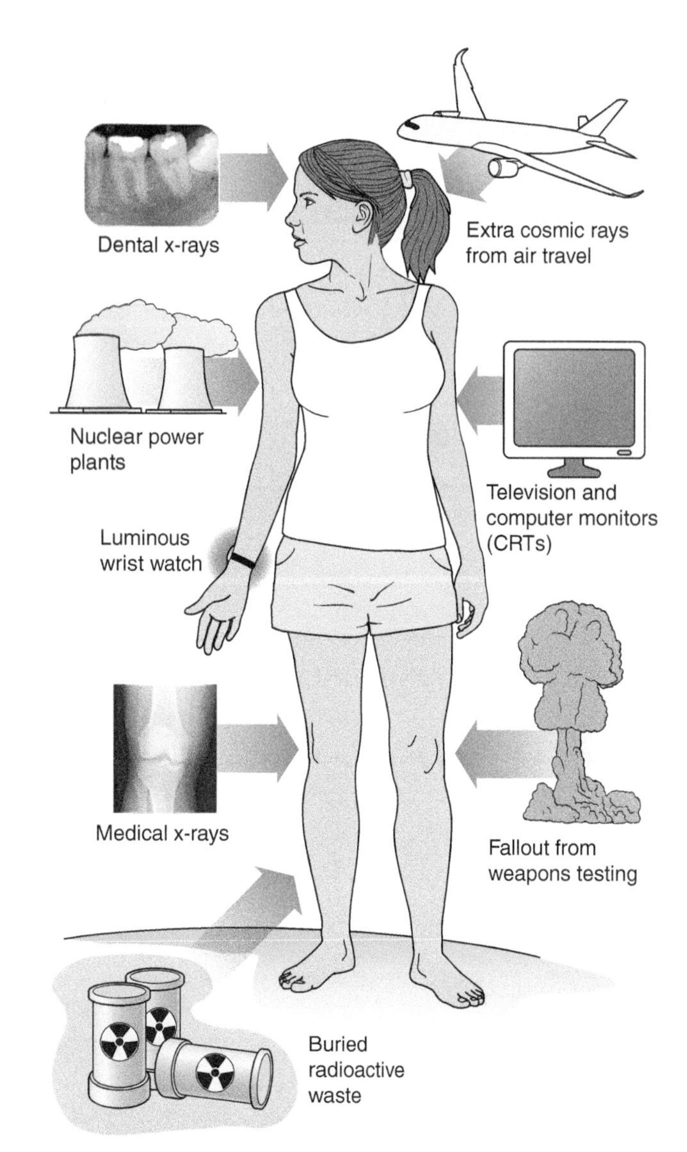

Figure 33.2. The various sources of radiation resulting from human activity to which the human population is exposed. In developed countries, the effective dose is dominated by medical radiation. (Reprinted from Hall EJ, Giaccia AJ. *Radiobiology for the Radiologist*. 7th Ed. Philadelphia, PA: Lippincott Williams & Wilkins, 2012, with permission.)

Man-Made Sources of Radiation

In addition to natural background and internal radiation, the human population is exposed to many other sources of radiation called **man-made radiation** (Fig. 33.2). Remember that humans have been exposed to all types of radiation throughout our existence. Figure 33.3 shows the contribution of a variety of sources of exposure; of these, diagnostic x-ray procedures make up the largest man-made source of ionizing radiation (3.2 mSv per year).

The National Council on Radiation Protection and Measurements (NCRP) estimated the radiation from man-made sources to be nearly 0.4 mSv per year in 1990. A follow-up report in 2006 stated the average effective dose per person in the US population was 6.2 mSv per year. This represents a large increase in dose, most of which is attributed to computed tomography, nuclear medicine, and interventional (fluoroscopy) medical procedures (Fig. 33.4).

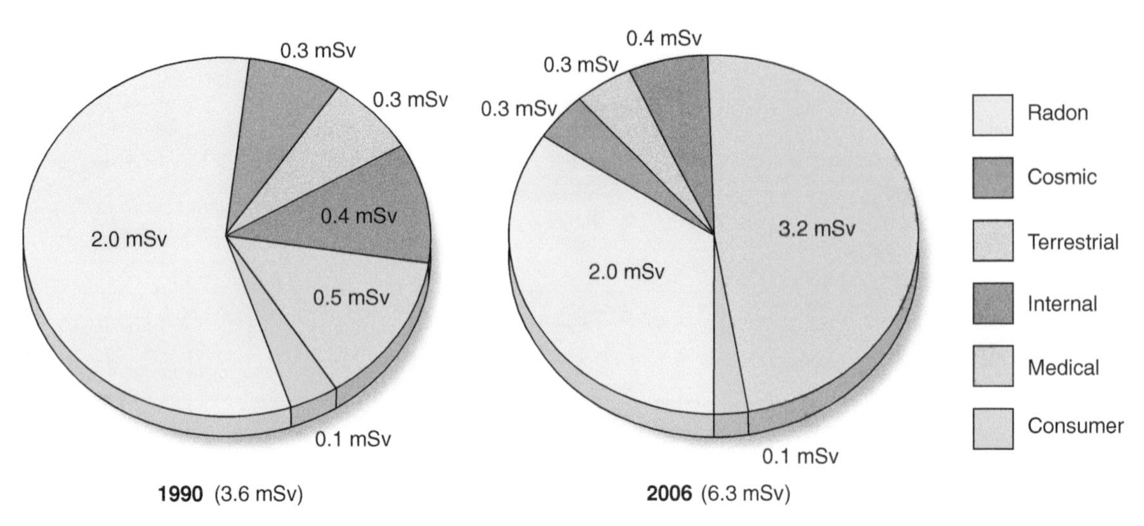

Figure 33.3. **The various sources of radiation resulting from human activity to which the human being is exposed.**

The benefits of diagnostic x-ray procedures cannot be disputed in the determination of the presence and treatment of disease. Computed tomography has seen the most growth in regard to the increased percent of man-made radiation a person is exposed to. The performance of these procedures or any procedure that uses ionizing radiation must be performed with caution so that the amount of ionizing radiation can be reduced. This will benefit patients and radiation personnel alike. The responsibility falls primarily to the radiographers because they control the operation of the equipment sued for the procedures. Consider this—75% of man-made radiation exposure is from medical procedures! This is a huge responsibility for the radiographer but we are up to the task!

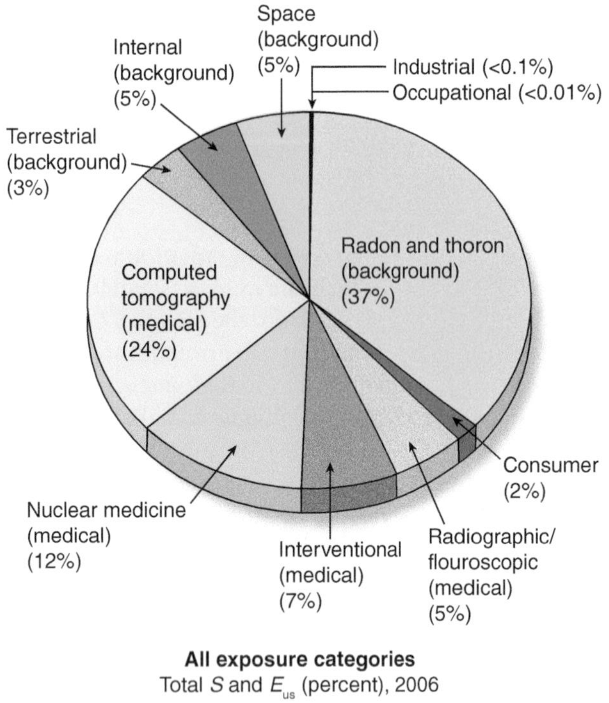

Figure 33.4. **Percentage contribution of the various sources of exposure. Medical radiation and natural background radiation make almost equal contribution. (Courtesy National Council on Radiation Protection and Measurements; NCRP Report 160.)**

Other sources of man-made radiation include nuclear power generators, consumer products, research applications, and industrial sources. Consumer products such as smoke detectors, camping lantern mantles, airport surveillance systems, color televisions, cigarettes, and enameled jewelry each contribute ~0.1 mSv per year to our annual dose.

Radiation Units

Historically, the quantities and units utilized to measure ionizing radiation included the roentgen (R), rad, rem, and curie. In 1948, an international system of units based on the metric system was developed. These units are called SI units or ***Systeme International d'Unites***. The SI units are the coulomb per kilogram (C/kg), gray (Gy), Sievert (Sv), and the Becquerel (Bq). Although the SI units were formally adopted, the older traditional units are still in use today. This may cause confusion in understanding which units to use and how they are related to each other. The following discussion reviews both systems of measurement.

Radiography utilizes the units of radiation to determine the amount of exposure that reached the patient, how much radiation was deposited in tissue, and how much damage occurred. The four fundamental units of radiation used in radiology are:

1. Exposure
2. Absorbed dose
3. Dose equivalent
4. Radioactivity

Exposure

Exposure is defined as the amount of ionization produced by radiation in a unit mass of air. We could count the number of x-rays, but it is easier to measure the amount of ionization produced by the x-rays. Exposure is measured in the SI system by coulombs per kilogram (C/kg) or in the conventional system using roentgen (R). The C/kg is a measure of the number of electrons liberated by ionization per kilogram of air. The roentgen or C/kg is generally used to express the output intensity of x-ray equipment or intensity in air. The relationship between the roentgen and coulomb per kilogram is $1\ R = 2.58 \times 10^{-4}$ C/kg. The roentgen is a fairly large unit so a smaller unit, the milliroentgen (mR), is more commonly used. One milliroentgen is 1,000 times smaller than one roentgen.

Absorbed Dose

The units of **absorbed dose** or absorbed energy are the gray (Gy) in the SI system and the **rad** (radiation-absorbed dose) in the conventional system. The rad is used to determine the damage or biologic effects of energy deposited by ionizing radiation in the patient tissues. The rad is an acronym for radiation-absorbed dose. One rad is defined as 100 ergs of energy absorbed per gram of tissue. An erg is a unit of energy where 1 erg equals 10^{-7} joules. When 1 rad is absorbed, each gram of exposed tissue will absorb 100 ergs of energy. Recall that some x-rays penetrate all the way through the body; therefore, we expect the absorbed dose to be slightly less than the exposure. 1 R of exposure generates ~0.96 rads of dose, or 96 ergs of energy is deposited as the radiation passes through the body. Because 0.96 rads is close to 1, we will round it up; this means that 1 R of x-ray exposure causes ~1 rad of absorbed dose.

$$1\ \text{R} \rightarrow 1\ \text{rad}$$

Absorbed dose is also stated as 1 gray is equivalent to 100 rads and 1 rad equals 10 mGy. Because the gray and rad are so large, the milligray (mGy) and the millirad (mrad) are more commonly used.

Dose Equivalent

The rem is used to quantify **dose equivalent** or **occupational exposure**. This unit is a true biologic unit because it addresses the different effects of different types of ionizing radiation to which a radiographer or any radiation worker may be exposed. The units of **Sievert (Sv)** in the SI system or **rem** (radiation equivalent man) in the conventional system are used. One Sievert is equal to 100 rem. Because the units are so large, the millisievert (mSv) and the millirem (mrem) are often used. The rem is a broad measurement that must be discussed in more detail to better develop an understanding of the effect of ionizing radiation on specific tissues.

Effective Dose

The **effective dose** relates the risk from irradiating a part of the body to the risk of total body irradiation. In other words, the tissues of the body are not equally affected by ionizing radiation. Some tissues are more sensitive to the effects of ionizing radiation. We know that a dose of 6 Sievert (Sv) to the entire body is fatal. However, a dose of 6 Sv to a patient's hand or foot is not fatal. The harm from a radiation dose depends on both the amount of radiation or dose and the part of the body irradiated. The combination of the dose and the body parts irradiated is measured by the effective dose.

At this point, you may be asking "How much biologic harm is there from radiation?" To answer this, we must use the rad and two weighting factors, symbolized as W_r and W_t. W_r refers to the relative harmfulness of the specific type of radiation. As seen in Table 33.2, the radiation weighting factor is dependent upon the type of LET associated with the different types of radiation. Radiation, which deposits more radiation in the tissue (high LET), has a higher weighting factor than radiation, which deposits a low amount of radiation. Alpha particles have a W_r of 20 because these are extremely low penetrating particles that deposit energy in a more concentrated area within the gram of tissue, which is more harmful.

TABLE 33.2 RADIATION WEIGHTING FACTOR FOR TYPES OF RADIATION

Type and Energy Range	Radiation Weighting Factor (W_r)
X- and gamma rays, electrons	1
Neutrons, energy <10 keV	5
10–100 keV	10
>100 keV–2 MeV	20
>2–20 MeV	10
>20 MeV	5
Protons	2
Alpha particles	20

The second weighting factor, W_t, refers to the sensitivity of different tissues in the body. Table 33.3 has the tissue weighting factor, which accounts for the relative **radiosensitivity** of various tissues and organs. In order to determine the effective dose, the following formula is used:

$$\text{Effective dose } (E) = \text{Radiation weighting factor } (W_r) \times \text{Tissue weighting factor} (W_t) \times \text{Absorbed dose}$$

When the absorbed dose in rads is multiplied by the two weighting factors, the dose equivalent or effective dose is obtained and expressed in rem. It is the most accurate unit to use to convey the effects of medical radiation exposure to patients and radiation personnel.

TABLE 33.3 WEIGHTING FACTORS USED IN CALCULATING EFFECTIVE DOSE

Tissue/Organ	Tissue Weighting Factor (W_t)
Gonads	0.20
Active bone marrow	0.12
Colon	0.12
Lungs	0.12
Stomach	0.12
Bladder	0.05
Breast	0.05
Esophagus	0.05
Liver	0.05
Thyroid	0.05
Bone surfaces	0.01
Skin	0.01

The effective dose from a posteroanterior (PA) chest examination is about 0.1 mSv (10 millirem [mrem]) although the entrance dose is about 0.70 mSv (70 mrem). The difference between the entrance dose and the effective dose occurs because many of the organs used to calculate the effective dose are not exposed to the primary beam during the examination.

For a specific tissue, we can base comparisons by only using the W_r factor; we can state that for x-rays, 1 R of exposure deposits 1 rad of absorbed dose into the body that causes 1 rem of harm or dose equivalent.

For a 50 keV neutron, a dose of 1 rad will generate 10 rems of dose equivalent. For alpha particles, 1 rad will cause 20 rem of biologic damage.

The units in the conventional system are arranged so that 1 R is equal to 1 rad, which is equal to 1 rem for x-rays.

Radioactivity

Radioactive atoms spontaneously decay by transforming or disintegrating into different atoms. The amount of radioactive atoms present is measured by their activity or the number of disintegrations per second, dps. The units of activity are the **Becquerel (Bq)** in the SI system and the **Curie (Ci)** in the conventional system. One Becquerel is equal to one disintegration per second. The Curie is based on the number of disintegrations per second from 1 g of radium. One Curie is equal to 3.7×10^{10} dps. Because the Curie is so large, the millicurie (mCi) is normally used. Table 33.4 summarizes the conventional and SI units.

Dose Limits

Over the years, there has been a continuous effort by health physicists to describe and identify occupational dose limits. The old term of maximum permissible dose (MPD) was used as the dose of radiation that would be expected to produce no significant radiation effects. At the MPD, the risk is not zero, but is small. The MPD is now considered obsolete and has been replaced by **dose limits (DLs)**.

TABLE 33.4 UNITS OF RADIATION

Quantity	SI Unit	Conventional Unit	Ratio of SI to Conventional
Exposure	Coulomb/kilogram (C/kg)	Roentgen (R)	2.58×10^{-4} C/kg = 1 R
Dose	Gray (Gy)	rad	1 Gy = 100 rad
Effective dose	Sievert (Sv)	rem	1 Sv = 100 rem
Activity	Becquerel (Bq)	Curie (Ci)	3.7×10^{10} Bq = 1 Ci

Whole-Body Dose Limits

The NCRP assessed risk based on data reported by the National Academy of Science (BEIR Committee) and the National Safety Council to establish dose limits. Current DLs are established for various organs and whole body across various industries. The NCRP recommendations ensure that all radiation workers have the same level of risk as workers in safe industries. The value 10^{-4} year^{-1} represents the approximate risk of death for workers in safe industries, or the risk of death would be <1 in 10,000. The DL is specified for **occupationally exposed workers** only, and particular care is taken to make sure that no radiation worker receives a radiation dose in excess of the DL.

The first DLs were recommended in 1902 and have been trending downward since that time. Current DL is 1 mSv per week (100 mrem per week). Currently, DLs are specified for whole-body and partial body exposure, organ exposure, and exposure of the general population. The DLs exclude medical exposures received as a patient and exposure from natural sources (Table 33.5). The DLs have been adopted by state and federal agencies and are law in the United States.

TABLE 33.5 DOSE LIMIT RECOMMENDED BY NCRP

	Dose Limit Values
Occupational Exposures	
Effective dose limits	
a. Annual	50 mSv (5 rem)
b. Cumulative	10 mSv × age (1 rem × age)
Equivalent annual dose limits for tissues and organs	
a. Lens of the eye	150 mSv (15 rem)
b. Skin, hands, feet, red bone marrow, and thyroid	500 mSv (50 rem)
Education and Training Exposures (Annual)	
Effective dose limit	1 mSv (0.1 rem)
Equivalent dose limits for tissues and organs	
a. Lens of the eye	15 mSv (1.5 rem)
b. Skin, hands, and feet	50 mSv (5 rem)
Embryo/Fetus Exposures	
a. Total equivalent dose limit	5 mSv (0.5 rem)
b. Monthly equivalent dose limit	0.5 mSv (0.05 rem)
Negligible Individual Dose (Annual)	0.01 mSv (1 mrem)
Public Exposure (Annual)	
Effective dose limit	
a. Exposure	5 mSv (0.5 rem)
Equivalent dose limits for tissues and organs	
a. Lens of the eye	15 mSv (1.5 rem)
b. Skin, hands, and feet	50 mSv (5 rem)

The limit on the whole-body dose for a radiation worker is 50 mSv (5 rem or 5,000 mrem) per year. The DL for the lens of the eye is 150 mSv per year, while the DL for other organs is 500 mSv per year. There is also a limit on the total dose that can be accumulated in a lifetime, which is called the cumulative limit. The cumulative effective dose limit (*E*) is the age in years (N) times 10 mSv.

CRITICAL THINKING BOX 33.1

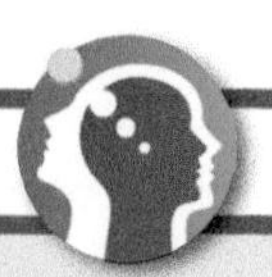

What is the cumulative limit for a 32-year-old radiographer?

Although most radiographers never receive even a small fraction of the annual dose limit, they are still issued personnel radiation monitors. The regulations require issuing a personnel dose monitor to any staff member who might be exposed to more than 10% of the limits listed in Table 33.5. Most radiology departments change the personnel monitors monthly, but the monitoring interval can be as long as 3 months. The personnel monitoring reports should be available for review by all monitored individuals.

The occupational exposure is described as dose equivalent and expressed in units of mS (mrem). DLs are specified as effective dose. The effective dose designation accounts for many types of radiation because of their varying relative biological effectiveness. Effective dose also takes into consideration the radiosensitivity of different tissues and organs.

Dose Limits for Tissues and Organs

The NCRP has recommended DLs for several specific tissues and organs. The DL for skin is 500 mSv per year, which is significantly higher than the whole-body DL. Radiographers who work in nuclear medicine are exposed to radioactive isotopes as they are drawing up doses for procedures. Even with this type of activity, it is highly unlikely for them to sustain exposure to the skin in excess of 10 mSv per year.

Radiologists and any physician who performs interventional procedures often have their hands near the primary fluoroscopy beam, which makes exposure of the extremities a concern. The DL for extremities is 500 mSv per year, although these levels are quite high, under normal working conditions, the levels should not be approached. Any occupational worker whose hands are routinely near radiation wears an extremity radiation monitor on their finger or wrist to track their level of exposure.

Radiation is known to cause cataracts. The DL for the lens of the eye is 150 mSv per year and should never be reached much less exceeded.

Alara

All radiation protection programs must operate under the principle of keeping the radiation exposure to staff, patients, and the public **as low as reasonably achievable (ALARA)**. This means that it is the responsibility of the radiographer that steps must be taken to reduce radiation exposure well below maximum regulatory limits. Technical factors such as kVp, mA, and length of exposure, distance, shielding, filtration, collimation, SID, beam area, and type of image receptor all influence the radiation levels to the staff and public.

Radiation Detectors

There are various dose-measuring devices that are used to measure or detect radiation exposure from x-rays. Dose-measuring devices are also known as dosimeters. These devices are classified as field survey instruments or personnel monitoring devices.

Gas-Filled Detectors

Ion chambers and **Geiger-Müller counters** are gas-filled detectors that collect the ions produced by ionizing radiation. The ions are collected, measured, and amplified to produce the output signal. Geiger-Müller counters are most efficient in detecting charged particles like beta particles but are inefficient in detecting x- and gamma-radiation. Geiger-Müller counters are sensitive to low levels of radiation. They are used in survey instruments to detect radioactive contamination in a nuclear medicine department, as detectors in CT scanners, and as calibration instruments for the calibration of x-ray tubes and nuclear medicine dose calibrators.

The ion chambers are primarily used to measure the primary and secondary radiation beam for the purposes of

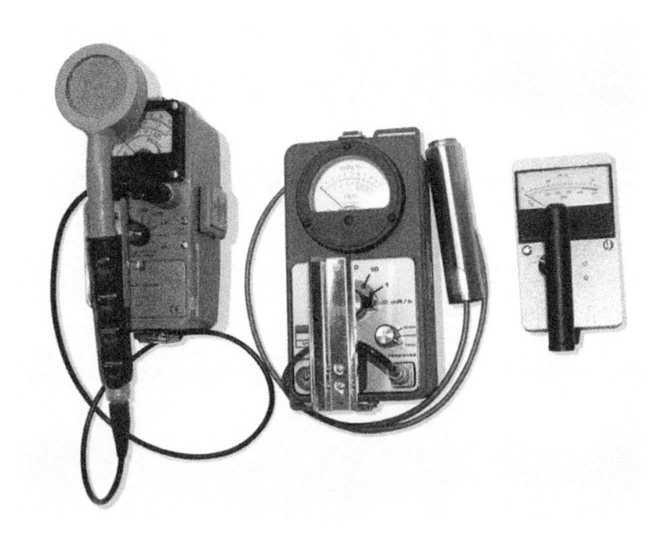

Figure 33.5. **Portable Geiger-Müller counters and ion chambers used for radiation surveys.**

evaluating equipment performance, assessment of scatter and leakage radiation, and to measure patient dose. The ionization chamber has a certain volume of air and an electrode. This chamber works on the principle that when radiation interacts with the electrons in the air, positive ions are produced. These positive ions then produce an electrical charge that can then be measured (Fig. 33.5).

Scintillation Detectors

Scintillation detectors use crystals that give off light when struck by radiation. The amount of light depends on the radiation energy deposited in the crystal. Higher radiation energy deposited results in greater light emission. The light emitted by the crystal is detected by a photomultiplier tube, which converts the light output into an electrical output signal, which is then measured. Scintillators are used as detectors in CT scanners and nuclear medicine gamma cameras.

Personnel Monitors

People who work in imaging departments and who are routinely exposed to ionizing radiation should be supplied with personnel monitoring devices that will estimate the amount of exposure they received. The personnel monitoring device measures the quantity of exposure it has received during the radiographers' occupational duties (Fig. 33.6). The radiographer is typically given one personnel monitoring device to wear; however, some facilities use two monitors for each radiographer. When one monitoring device is used, it should be worn on the anterior surface of the body between the chest and waist level. Some of these devices are meant to be worn at the level of the collar with the clip on the monitor closest to the body and with the face of the monitor directed outward away from the body.

The method commonly used for two monitoring devices is to wear one at the collar, outside the protective gear, while the other is worn at the waist and inside the protective gear. Pregnant radiographers must be issued a second badge to be worn at the abdominal level under the

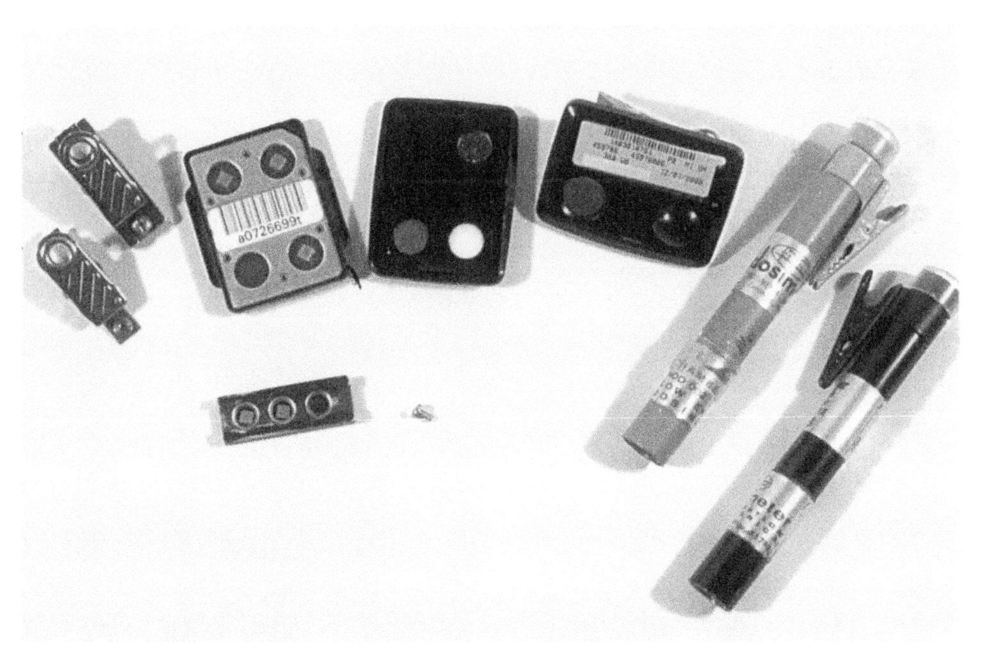

Figure 33.6. **A variety of personnel monitors.**

lead apron to estimate the dose to the fetus. Regardless of the location, the personnel monitoring devices must be worn each day while the radiographer is producing x-radiation, and the device should be worn at the same location every day.

The monitoring devices are not to be stored in any room where ionizing radiation procedures are performed or next to a radiation area. For each exposure performed, the monitoring device will be exposed to radiation; this will result in a falsely high reading when the monitoring device is processed. The monitoring device should be worn at all times by the radiographer during their work shift and then stored in an area away from radiation at the end of the shift. Preferably, it is kept in an office or other location far away from sources of radiation.

There are several types of personnel monitors: film badge dosimeters, thermoluminescent dosimeter (TLD), and optically stimulated luminescent (OSL) dosimeters.

Film Badge Dosimeters

Film badge dosimeters contain a small piece of film that will have a specific optical density after exposure to radiation and development. The silver halide in the film emulsion makes the film response very sensitive to x-ray energy. Radiation energies near the K-edge of silver are preferentially absorbed and produce correspondingly higher optical densities. The higher the exposure, the greater the optical density. Personnel monitors using film as a detector have copper, cadmium, and aluminum filters to estimate the energy of the incident radiation.

An energy correction, obtained from the optical densities under the filters, is applied to calculate the radiation dose from the unfiltered optical density. Readings lower than 10 mR are generally not detectable and may be reported as minimal on a film badge dosimetry report.

Film is sensitive to heat, light, and moisture as well as radiation. Personnel monitor dosimeters that use film must be kept dry and cool. Storing them in a hot car during the summer or passing them through a washing machine will render them useless.

Thermoluminescent Dosimeters

A **thermoluminescent dosimeter (TLD)** uses a lithium fluoride crystal as the radiation detector. When it is exposed to x-rays, the lithium fluoride crystal traps the radiation energy. This trapped energy can be released as light by heating the crystals to over 100°C. The light is detected by a photomultiplier tube and converted into an

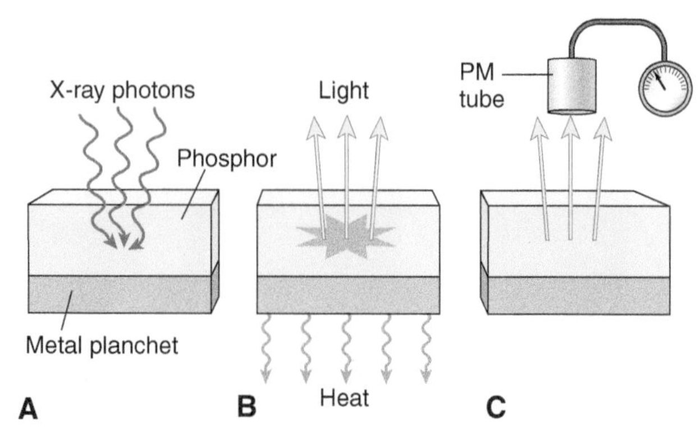

Figure 33.7. **The process of reporting the exposure absorbed by a TLD. (A) Crystal is exposed to ionizing radiation. (B) Crystal is heated and emits visible light. (C) Photomultiplier tube measures intensity of light.**

electrical output signal. These dosimeters are called TLDs because they give off light after heating. The amount of light is proportional to the radiation dose absorbed in the crystal (Fig. 33.7). Lithium fluoride has almost exactly the same energy response to radiation as human tissue.

TLDs are often used instead of the film badge dosimeter. Like a film badge dosimeter, it is worn for a period of time (typically 3 months or less) and then must be processed to determine the dose received, if any. TLDs can measure doses as low as 1 mrem, but under routine conditions, their low-dose capability is approximately the same as for film badge dosimeters. TLDs are very small and typically used in ring badges to monitor radiation exposure to the extremities (Fig. 33.8).

Optically Stimulated Luminescence

In the late 1990s, Landauer designed a radiation dosimeter especially for personnel monitoring. The dosimeter uses a process called **optically stimulated luminescence (OSL),**

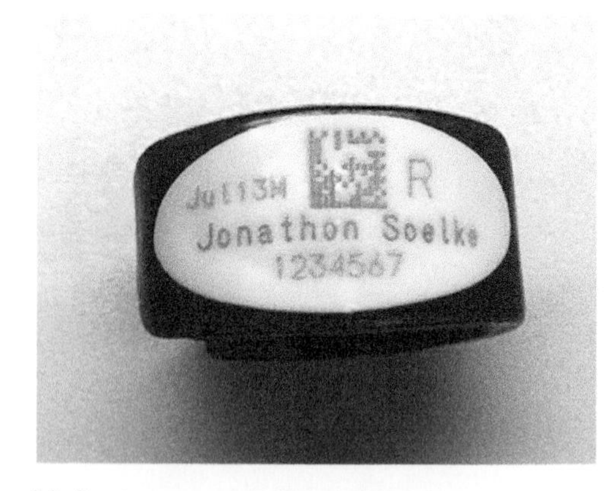

Figure 33.8. **Saturn ring dosimeter uses thermoluminescent technology to identify radiation exposure to extremities. (Courtesy Landauer, Inc.)**

which uses aluminum oxide (Al_2O_3) as the radiation detector. When the aluminum oxide is irradiated, some of the electrons are stimulated into an excited state. The OSL is processed using laser light, which causes the electrons to return to their normal state with the emission of visible light.

The intensity of the visible light emission is proportional to the amount of radiation exposure received by the aluminum oxide. The OSL reports doses as low as 10 µg, which makes them more sensitive than TLDs and more precise. The OSL has many features including further analysis for confirmation of dose, qualitative information about exposure conditions, wide dynamic range, and excellent long-term stability (Fig. 33.9).

Instadose Dosimeter

The Instadose dosimeter is a breakthrough in technology, which provides radiation workers with a precise measurement of radiation dose. The device is small and provides immediate dose readings by using an Internet-enabled computer. The dosimeter is a USB-compatible device that enables customers to view a reading on a computer that has specialized software installed to perform dose readings. The dosimeter is a direct ion storage device that is capable of detecting a dose as low as 1 mrem (0.01 mSv) with a useful dose range of 1 mrem to 500 rem (0.01 mSv to 5 Sv). The Instadose dosimeter can be read up to a cumulative dose of 12 rem. Dosimeter reports are stored on a secure server for long-term storage (Fig. 33.10).

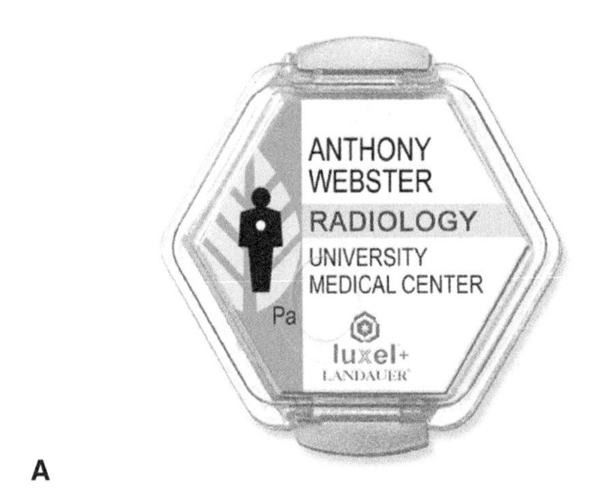

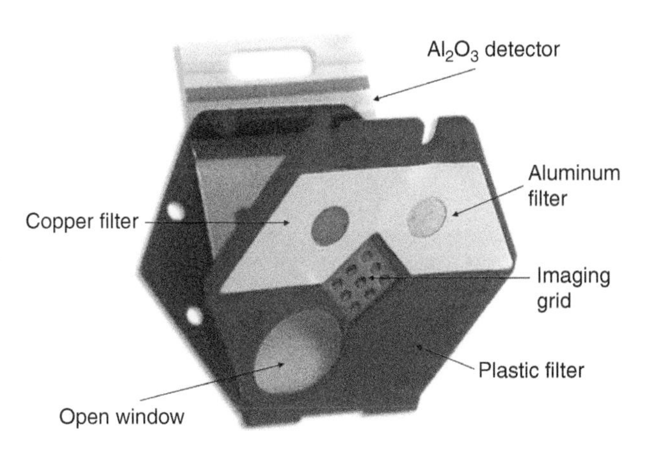

Figure 33.9. **Optically stimulated luminescence dosimeter. (A) Representative OSL dosimeter worn by imaging personnel. (B) Internal components include various filters to help identify the type of radiation and its energy. (Courtesy Landauer, Inc.)**

Monitoring Period and Report

The monitoring period for personnel dosimeters is usually 1 month; however, the wear date periods can range from annually, quarterly, monthly, or weekly. After the monitoring period is over, the control monitor and all film badge dosimeters or TLD monitors are returned to the supplier for reading. After processing, the response of the control monitor is subtracted from the response of

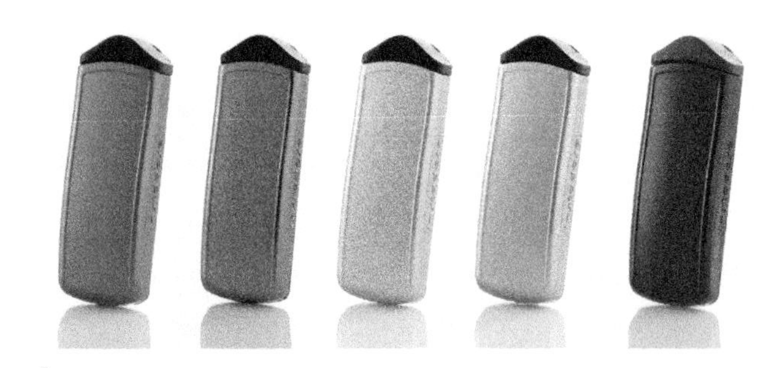

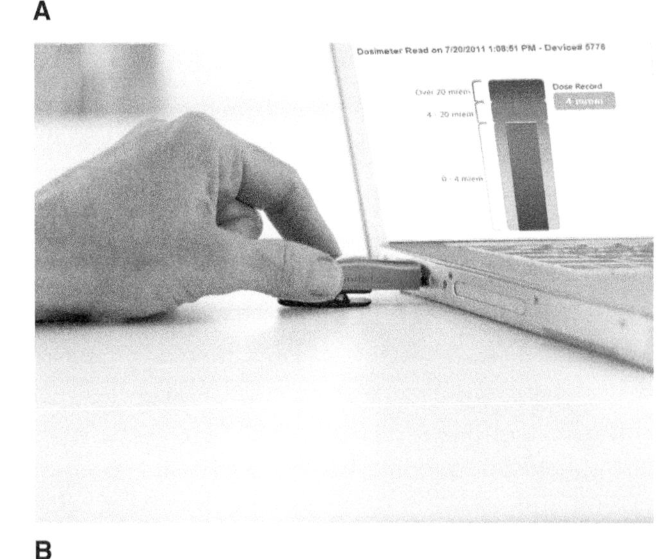

Figure 33.10. **(A and B) Instadose dosimeter provides an immediate read of radiation exposure. (Photo courtesy of Mirion Technologies Inc.)**

SAMPLE HOSPITAL
ATTN: RSO
4242 MAIN STREET
SMALLVILLE, MA 01432

Received Date / Reported Date	2014-05-30 / 2014-06-03
Page	1 of 4
Analytical Work Order / QC Release	1415095001 / NHE
Copy / Version	1 / 2 (1)

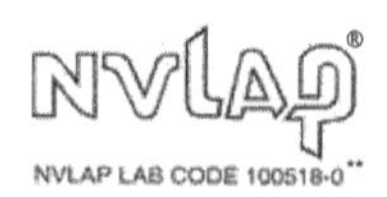

LANDAUER®
Landauer, Inc., 2 Science Road
Glenwood, Illinois 60425-1586
www.landauer.com
Telephone: (708) 755-7000
Facsimile: (708) 755-7016
Customer Service: (800) 323-8830
Technical: (800) 438-3241

Radiation Dosimetry Report

Account: 709008 Subaccount: 1431640 Series: CST

(2) Corrected

**No NVLAP accreditation is available from NVLAP for thermal neutron or X type dosimeters. When exposure results are reported for thermal neutrons or X type dosimeters, this report contains data that are not covered by the NVLAP accreditation.

Copy 1 : Original sent to SAMPLE HOSPITAL, ATTN: RSO, 4242 MAIN STREET SMALLVILLE, MA 01432

Participant Number	Name / ID Number	Birth Date	Dosimeter	Use	Rad. Type	Rad. Quality	Period Shown Below DDE	Period Shown Below LDE	Period Shown Below SDE	Quarter to Date DDE	Quarter to Date LDE	Quarter to Date SDE	Year to Date DDE	Year to Date LDE	Year to Date SDE	Lifetime to Date DDE	Lifetime to Date LDE	Lifetime to Date SDE	Inception Date	Serial Number
For Monitoring Period:							2014-05-01 to 2014-05-31			QUARTER 2			2014			LIFETIME				
(3) ***01067***	***Halpert, Jim***		*Pa*	*COLLAR*	*P*		***10***	***10***	***10***										2005/03	***6794392C***
	********2222***	***1979-10-20***		ASSIGNED			3	10	10	5	12	12	5	12	12	55	67	72		
				NOTE			Assigned dose based on EDE2 Calculation													
				NOTE			Participant active in other account(s) or subaccount(s)													
For Monitoring Period:							2014-06-01 to 2014-06-30			QUARTER 2			2014			LIFETIME				
00CST	CONTROL		Ja	CNTRL																7254728C
	CONTROL		Pa	CNTRL																7254729C
	CONTROL		Ta	CNTRL																7254730C
(4) 01068	Beesly, Pam		Pa	COLLAR			**M**	**M**	**M**										2005/03	7254731C
	********3333	1974-05-07		ASSIGNED			**M**	**M**	**M**	M	M	M	M	M	M	M	M	M		
				NOTE			Participant active in other account(s) or subaccount(s)													
01069	Reynolds, Malcolm		Pa	COLLAR	P		**18**	**18**	**18**										2014/06	7254733C
	*******4444 (5)	1971-03-27		ASSIGNED			**5**	**18**	**18**	8	30	34	8	30	34	8	30	34		
				NOTE			Assigned dose based on EDE2 Calculation													
				NOTE			Participant active in other account(s) or subaccount(s)													
01070	White, Walter		Pa	COLLAR	P		**1078**	**1078**	**1078**										2008/01	7254734C
	*******5555	1956-03-07		NOTE			Imaging indicates an irregular exposure. Dosimeter reprocessed, second read agrees with reported dose.													
				ASSIGNED			**1078**	**1078**	**1078**	2092	2123	2124	2092	2123	2124	2092	2123	2124		
				NOTE			Participant active in other account(s) or subaccount(s)													

Dose Equivalent (mrem) for Periods Shown Below. DDE-Deep Dose Equivalent LDE-Lens Dose Equivalent SDE-Shallow Dose Equivalent

Italicized and bolded participant line indicates corrected participant

This report must not be used to claim product certification, approval, or endorsement by NVLAP, NIST, or any agency of the federal government.

Figure 33.11. **Occupational radiation-monitoring report must include the items of information shown in this report. (Courtesy Landauer, Inc.)**

each individual monitor. This results in the report accurately stating the occupational radiation exposure for each individual monitor.

The supplier generates a report that is sent to the facility (Fig. 33.11). The report includes participant identification information, the type of dosimeter used, and the radiation exposures that were received. The radiation exposure is given as the dose equivalent in millirem for the wear period, a quarterly accumulated dose equivalent, a year-to-date dose equivalent, and a lifetime dose equivalent for each participant. The report also provides exposure rates for deep dose, lens of the eye, and shallow dose equivalents. The report should be reviewed by each participant for each wear date period.

Chapter Summary

1. Early in radiography history, there were many dangers to radiation workers. Today, radiography is classified among the safest of professions by following three foundational principles: time, distance, and shielding. All radiation exposure should follow the ALARA principle!
2. Sources of radiation include cosmic radiation, natural radiation, and internal radiation. Each of these contributes a small amount to the overall amount of radiation a human experiences each year.

3. Man-made sources of radiation include nuclear power generators, consumer products, industrial sources, and medical radiation. The average effective dose per person is ~6.2 mSv per year. Medical radiation accounts for 75% of this yearly exposure.
4. Routine medical x-rays contribute a very small amount to the medical radiation with computed tomography, nuclear medicine, and interventional procedures contributing the most.
5. There are two systems of radiation units, the SI and the conventional. The units of exposure are the roentgen (R) and the coulombs per kilogram (C/kg). The units of dose are the gray and the rad. The units of the effective dose are the Sievert and the rem.
6. The lower the penetration capability of a particular type of radioactivity, the more hazardous it is because the tissue damage is more concentrated.
7. DLs are determined by the NCRP for various organs, whole body, and different working conditions.
8. A cumulative whole-body DL of 10 mSv times age in years is the recommended dose.
9. Personnel who work in radiation departments are required to wear radiation-monitoring devices. The personnel monitor should be worn on the outside of the protective apparel near the collar.
10. Gas-filled detectors are used to calibrate x-ray units. TLDs are used in personnel monitors and must be heated to obtain a reading. Film badge dosimeters use a piece of film and specialized filters to absorb incident radiation.
11. The OSL uses an aluminum oxide crystal to absorb radiation, and when exposed to a laser, the crystal will emit light with an intensity proportional to the radiation exposure.

Case Study

Joanie is studying the various types of natural radiation the human population is exposed to. She is having a difficult time remembering the types and dose levels. As Joanie is eating a banana and thinking about her flight from Florida to Denver, she can't help but think about her annual dose levels.

Critical Thinking Questions

1. What are the average levels for cosmic, terrestrial, and internal radiation?
2. How does altitude affect cosmic radiation levels?
3. Why are people who live in mountainous regions exposed to higher levels of terrestrial radiation?
4. How does the food Joanie eats add to her internal radiation levels?

Review Questions

Multiple Choice

1. **The personnel monitor should be worn:**

   a. under the protective apparel near the waist
   b. outside the protective apparel near the collar
   c. under the protective apparel near the collar
   d. outside the protective apparel near the waist

2. **Methods to reduce radiation exposure to the staff include:**

   1. reduce time
   2. increase distance
   3. reduce shielding
   4. reduce field size
   a. 1, 2, 3, and 4
   b. 1, 2, and 4
   c. 2, 3, and 4
   d. 1 and 2

3. **ALARA is the acronym for:**

   a. as low as readily achievable
   b. achievable
   c. as low as reasonably achievable
   d. always low and readily accessible

4. **What is the conventional unit of absorbed dose?**

   a. Curie
   b. Roentgen
   c. rem
   d. rad

5. **People who live in Denver, Colorado, receive more cosmic radiation than those who live in Florida because:**

   a. there is less atmosphere to shield people in Denver
   b. the atmospheric pressure is higher at sea level
   c. the altitude is lower in Denver
   d. there is less mineral content in the ground in Denver

6. **When all the sources of natural background radiation, including radon gas, are combined what is the worldwide average exposure each year?**

   a. 20 mR
   b. 100 mR
   c. 300 mR
   d. 500 mR
   e. 1,200 mR

7. **Potassium 40 is an example of which source of radiation?**

   a. Internal
   b. Terrestrial
   c. Cosmic
   d. Man made

8. **Which type of radiation has the lowest average penetration capability through human tissue?**

   a. Alpha particles
   b. Beta particles
   c. X-rays
   d. Gamma rays

9. **Of the following man-made technologies, which is the largest source of human exposure to radiation?**

   a. Nuclear power generators
   b. Diagnostic x-rays
   c. Fallout from nuclear weapons
   d. Radioactive materials in consumer products

10. **In the broadest terms, background radiation can be divided into which two categories?**

    a. Internal and external
    b. Confluent and regressive
    c. Cosmic and terrestrial
    d. Natural and man made

Short Answer

1. How are film badge dosimeters to be worn and where are they placed on the body?

2. What exposure data are included in the personnel monitoring report?

3. What is the annual dose limit for diagnostic imaging personnel?

4. What does the value 10^{-4} year^{-1} mean with regard to the NCRP recommended dose limits?

5. What source of natural background radiation poses the greatest hazard in modern times?

6. What percentage of all man-made radiation exposure is due to medical practice?

7. List the exposure data that must be included in the personnel monitoring report.

8. How do nuclear medicine radiographers monitor their extremity doses?

9. A patient was exposed to 3 rads of proton radiation in their chest. What is the effective dose?

10. What is the cumulative occupational DL for a 33-year-old radiographer?

34

Minimizing Exposure to Ionizing Radiation

Objectives

Upon completion of this chapter, the student will be able to:

1. Explain the construction of protective barriers.
2. Identify factors that determine the thickness of lead in primary and secondary barriers.
3. Describe the methods of reducing radiation exposure.
4. Describe ALARA.
5. State the three methods of radiation reduction to staff.
6. Name the dose limits for occupational and nonoccupational workers.
7. Discuss the radiosensitivity of pregnancy.

Key Terms

- ALARA
- contact shields
- controlled area
- half-value layer (HVL)
- primary barrier
- protective apparel
- secondary barrier
- shadow shields
- 10-day rule
- tenth-value layer (TVL)
- time of occupancy factor
- uncontrolled area
- use factor
- workload

Introduction

The gold standard in medical imaging departments is to minimize exposure of patients and personnel to ionizing radiation. There are many items to consider from designing the x-ray room to the type of lead shields that will be used. The methods of performing an exam so that radiation dose is kept at a minimum are also important aspects to consider. Finally, the ethical responsibility to perform duties in the best interest of the patient as well as managing radiation exposure all fall on the shoulders of the radiographer. At the end of this chapter, the student will have the foundational knowledge needed to minimize dose to ionizing radiation.

Room Shielding

Whether designing a single x-ray room or an entire imaging department, great attention must be given to the location of the imaging exam room and the areas adjacent to the room. When radiation safety is discussed, the types of protective barriers and their placement must be thoroughly considered. There are a large number of factors to consider when a protective barrier is designed. This section only touches on the fundamentals and some basic definitions. Any time a facility is being renovated or a new one built, a medical physicist must be included on the design team to ensure proper radiation shielding is part of the design.

Room protective barriers are designed to prevent the transmission of radiation through the walls. Almost all diagnostic and fluoroscopic rooms have shielding in at least some of the walls. The radiation shielding required is specified in terms of thickness of lead or concrete. The thickness of the protective barrier depends on the distance from the radiation source, the workload, the use of the space on the other side of the wall, and the amount of time the beam is pointed at the wall. Room shielding must protect against both primary and secondary radiation.

Primary Barriers

In each radiographic imaging room, there are three types of radiation that must be considered when determining the protective barriers (Fig. 34.1): primary, scatter, and leakage. Primary radiation is the direct, collimated, useful x-ray beam. Any wall to which the primary beam can be directed is designated a **primary barrier**. The wall on which the vertical or chest Bucky is mounted is considered to be a primary barrier because of the intensity of radiation directed toward the wall.

Sheets of pure lead are bonded to typical panels of "Sheetrock" (drywall) and are the most commonly used primary barrier. The objective is to ensure that the radiation must scatter twice before reaching the radiographer. A primary barrier in diagnostic room walls must be 1/16th inch (1.58 mm) thickness of lead. This barrier needs to extend 7 ft upward from the floor leaving a foot or more of Sheetrock close to the ceiling; it is not necessary to

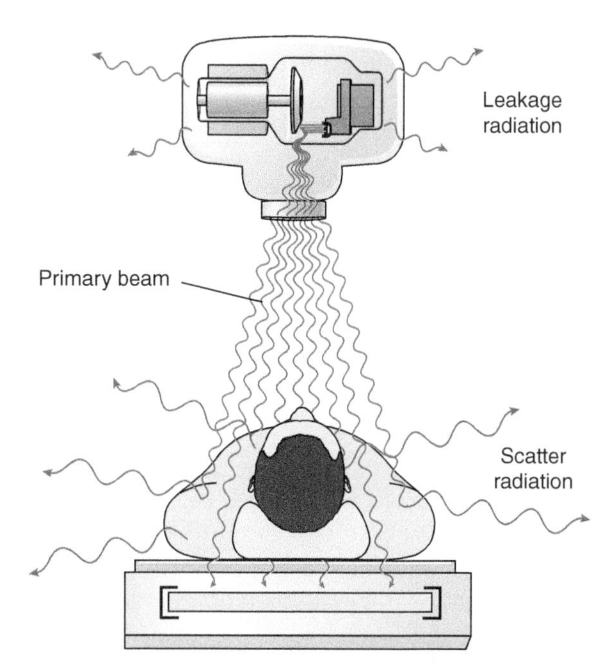

Figure 34.1. **The three types of radiation that are considered when designing protective barriers for imaging rooms.**

have the lead extend from the floor to the ceiling. In the corners of the room or anywhere there is a seam in the lead, strips of lead must be added so that all joints overlap at least 1 cm or double the lead thickness, whichever is greater.

Concrete, concrete block, and brick can be used instead of lead, 4 inches of masonry is equivalent to 1/16th inch (1.58 mm) of lead. The floors and ceilings of diagnostic x-ray rooms do not require additional shielding if they are made of concrete because the thickness of concrete supporting the floor also provides adequate shielding against scattered radiation. The primary beam is never directed at a secondary barrier.

Secondary Barriers

Secondary radiation is made up of scattered and leakage radiation. Scatter radiation results when the primary beam strikes any object, causing some x-rays to scatter. During radiography and fluoroscopy, the patient is the most important scattering object. Leakage radiation is that radiation that is emitted in all directions from the x-ray tube housing, the exception to this is that the leakage radiation does not emit toward the primary beam. Regulations require that leakage radiation be <100 mR/h at 1 m. Leakage radiation is not a problem with modern x-ray tubes because they are manufactured with adequate shielding in their housing.

Secondary barriers protect against secondary radiation. Secondary radiation has lower energy than the primary beam, and so less shielding thickness is required. The required thickness of lead is 1/32nd inch (0.79 mm). The control booth is a secondary barrier, and it has a window for viewing the patient during the exposure. This window can be made of leaded glass and must have a radiation absorption efficiency such that ¼ inch is equivalent to about 2 mm of pure sheet lead. A good method to follow in determining appropriate thickness for windows is to use four times the recommended sheet lead thickness. The control booth walls require 1/32 inch (0.79 mm) lead equivalent, four times this amount is 1/8 inch (3.175 mm), which would be sufficient for the control booth window.

Regulations for practice forbid ever pointing the x-ray tube toward the control booth; therefore, the control booth and its window are always a secondary barrier whose purpose is to protect personnel from secondary radiation. Figure 34.2 illustrates the design of a room with barrier thicknesses and locations.

Protective Barrier Thickness Considerations

Several factors must be considered when determining the thickness requirements for protective barriers. These factors include distance, occupancy, workload, and use factor.

Distance

The thickness of the barrier depends on the distance from the x-ray source to the barrier. If the design of the room allows the x-ray tube to be positioned by a wall, then this wall will require more shielding because of the hazard of leakage radiation. It may be best to position the x-ray unit in the middle of the room because then no one wall is subjected to especially intense radiation exposure.

Occupancy Factor

The use of an area that is being protected is of primary importance. An area that is rarely occupied, such as a closet, requires less shielding compared to an office that is occupied 40 hours per week. This description reflects the **time of occupancy factor**. Table 34.1 lists the occupancy levels for various areas as suggested by the NCRP.

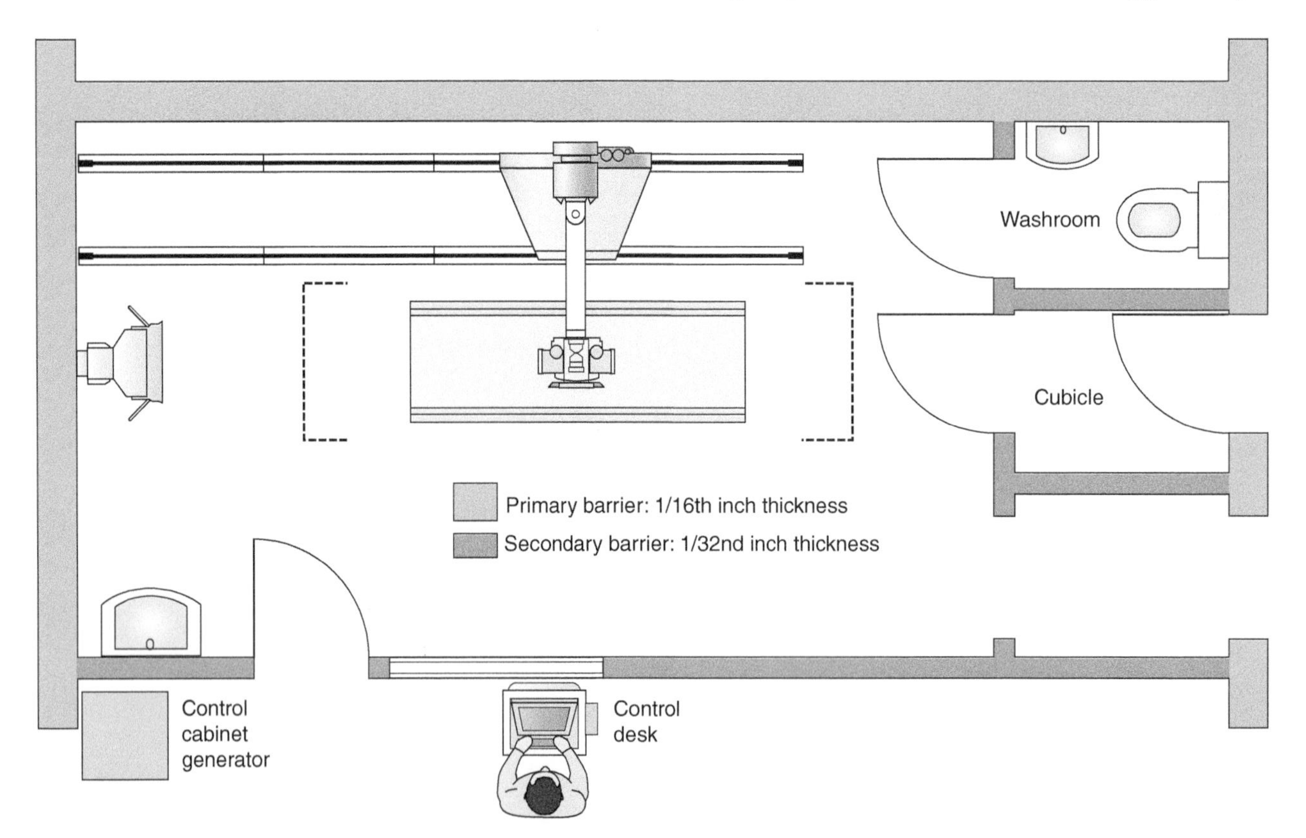

Figure 34.2. **Schematic representation of a general x-ray room with barriers and barrier thicknesses identified.**

TABLE 34.1 LEVELS OF OCCUPANCY OF AREAS AS SUGGESTED BY THE NCRP

Occupancy	Area in Hospital
Full	Work areas: offices, laboratories, nursing wards, nursing stations
Frequent	Hallways, restrooms, patient rooms
Occasional	Waiting rooms, stairways, closets, storerooms, elevators

The rooms in a hospital are considered to be either a controlled area or an uncontrolled area. The term **controlled area** includes areas occupied primarily by personnel and patients. Design limits for a controlled area are based on the annual recommended occupational dose limit of 50 mSv/y. The barrier is required to reduce the exposure rate to a worker to 1 mSv/wk (100 mrem/wk).

Uncontrolled areas are those areas where the general public can be found. This includes waiting rooms, stairways, hallways, the outside of the hospital, and restrooms with general hospital access. The maximum exposure rate allowed is based on the recommended dose limit for the public of 1 mSv/y (100 mrem/y). This is equivalent to 20 μSv/wk (2 mrem/wk), which is the design limit for uncontrolled areas. In addition, the protective barrier should ensure that no one person will receive more than 25 μSv (2.5 mrem) in any single hour.

Workload

The amount of shielding required for an x-ray room depends on the amount of procedures performed in the room. The higher the number of procedures performed each week the thicker the shielding must be. The **workload** is a combination of the number of patients and the technical exposure factors used. The workload is measured in milliampere-minutes per week (mAmin/wk). A busy, general purpose x-ray room might have a workload of 500 mAmin/wk.

CRITICAL THINKING BOX 34.1

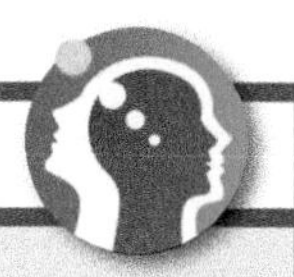

A hospital is adding on three x-ray exam rooms. The patient load for each room is estimated at 10 patients per day, each patient will average four images taken at 80 kVp, and 65 mAs. What is the projected workload for each room?

Workloads are typically meant to be an overestimation of the amount of procedures performed in a given room so that shielding will be more than adequate to ensure the protection of personnel and the public.

Use Factor

The **use factor** indicates the amount of time during which the x-ray beam will be energized and directed toward a particular barrier. The NCRP recommends that primary wall barriers be assigned a use factor of ¼ and the floor a use factor of 1. Secondary and leakage radiations are present 100% of the time the x-ray tube is energized. The ceiling is most often considered to be a secondary barrier for radiographic procedures.

Half-Value Layer

The **half-value layer (HVL)** is that amount of shielding required to reduce the radiation intensity to half the original value. The **tenth-value layer (TVL)** is the amount of shielding required to reduce the radiation to one-tenth its original value. The TVL is used in determining the amount of shielding required for primary and secondary barriers.

Reduction of Radiation Exposure to Staff

Basic Principles

When performing radiographic procedures, the radiographer must apply the three methods or cardinal rules for radiation protection. The three methods of reducing the radiation exposure of the staff are to:

1. Reduce *time* spent in the vicinity of radiation
2. Increase *distance* from the radiation source
3. Wear appropriate *shielding* to attenuate radiation

The radiation exposure of the radiographer and radiologist can be decreased by reducing the time the individual is exposed to radiation, increasing the individual's distance from the radiation source, and increasing the amount of shielding between the radiation source and the individual. The major source of radiation to the radiologist and radiographer is scatter radiation from the patient. The diagnostic x-ray beam should always be collimated to the smallest field size applicable for each examination. Smaller field sizes produce less scatter because less tissue is irradiated. The radiographer should never be in the direct beam or in the room during a diagnostic radiographic exposure. The radiographer should never hold a patient during the exposure. This being said, there are certain caveats that must be taken into consideration, and these will be covered later in the chapter.

Time

Routine radiographic procedures utilize extremely short exposure time to minimize motion artifact, and during these procedures, the radiographer should not be in the room with the patient. During fluoroscopy procedures, whether in the x-ray room or surgery, the radiographer is often required to be operating equipment while the beam is turned on. The length of time can be several minutes to as long as an hour or more. The dose to an individual is directly related to the length of time the beam is on. If the length of the exposure to radiation is doubled, then the exposure to the person will also be doubled.

Patient exposure during fluoroscopy is determined by the length of time the patient is in the x-ray beam. Shorter fluoroscopic exposure times result in lower doses to patients and staff. Regulations require that fluoroscopic units be equipped with a timer to indicate the total fluoroscopic beam on time. This timer must provide an audible reminder to indicate when 5 minutes of beam on time has elapsed; many mobile fluoroscopy units also use a light that turns on when the beam is on. Most fluoroscopic procedures require <5 minutes, although the timer can be reset when necessary.

During fluoroscopy, the patient's dose and therefore the dose to the radiographer can be reduced if pulsed fluoroscopy is used. This prevents the beam from being on continuously while still providing the physician with the image necessary for the exam. If the fluoroscopy unit does not have pulsing capability, the radiologist should alternate between beam on and beam off during the course of the procedure. This will decrease the dose to the patient and all persons in the room.

Distance

During fluoroscopy, the patient is the source of scattered radiation. The intensity of scattered radiation is less than that of the primary beam by a factor of 1,000. That is, the intensity of the scattered radiation 1 meter (m) from the patient is 1/1,000 of the primary beam intensity. During the procedure, the radiographer should stand as far away from the patient and fluoroscope as possible while still being able to render assistance to the patient when needed.

Increasing the distance from the patient decreases the scattered radiation reaching the staff. According to the inverse square law, doubling the distance from the source reduces the radiation intensity to one-fourth its original value (Fig. 34.3). Moving one step away from the edge of the fluoroscopic table reduces the radiation exposure significantly.

If the patient does not require assistance during the procedure, the radiographer must stand in the control

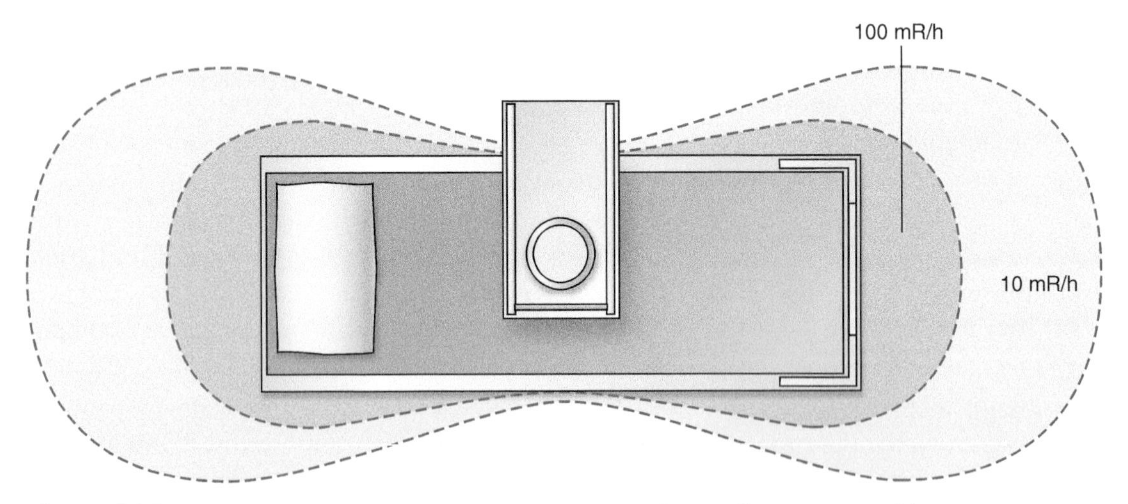

Figure 34.3. Typical exposure levels at various distances from a fluoroscopic table.

area and as far away from the scattered radiation as possible. The radiographer should be wearing appropriate protective apparel so that if he or she needs to assist the patient, there will not be a delay in providing that assistance.

The patient is also the source of scatter radiation during portable examinations. Increasing the distance from the patient during portable examinations decreases scattered radiation to the radiographer. The backscatter created during the exposure is more intense in line with the primary beam. To reduce exposure, the radiographer should stand at a diagonal angle to the primary beam. Portable units are equipped with an exposure switch on the end of a 180-centimeter (cm) (6-foot [ft]) cord to allow the radiographer to move away from the patient before making the exposure. The radiographer must use caution to place the portable unit in a manner that would prevent the x-ray tube from emitting primary radiation toward the portable unit or radiographer.

Shielding

Shielding is used when the radiographer must be in the room when the x-ray beam is turned on. Placing protective shielding between the radiation source and the radiographer will greatly reduce the level of exposure. Protective shielding in the radiography department typically consists of lead apparel, mobile shields, and building materials that are all designed to provide the maximum protection possible to shield the radiographer from radiation. The lead apparel and mobile shields must be used any time it is not possible to take advantage of the fixed structural barriers.

Protective Apparel

Radiographers are trained to wear **protective apparel** for examinations where they will be exposed to ionizing radiation. Protective aprons have equivalent lead thicknesses of 0.25, 0.5, or 1 millimeter (mm) lead. The protection is equivalent to that of pure lead of the thickness indicated. Drapes hanging from the image intensifier, protective aprons, gloves, Bucky slot covers, and moveable shields are designed to intercept the scattered radiation and reduce the radiation exposure of the staff. During fluoroscopy procedures, the Bucky tray should be moved to the foot of the table when possible to ensure that the Bucky slot cover is in place.

TABLE 34.2 PROTECTIVE APPAREL THICKNESS IN MILLIMETERS LEAD EQUIVALENT AND ATTENUATION VALUES

Apparel	Thickness (mm)	Attenuation (%)
Apron	0.50	99.9
Gloves	0.25	99
Thyroid	0.50	99
Glasses	0.35	99
Fluoroscopic drape	0.25	99

Lead glasses and thyroid shields can also be worn to protect the eyes and thyroid during fluoroscopy procedures in surgery and interventional procedures. Scatter radiation to the lens of the eyes can be substantially reduced by wearing protective eyeglasses with optically clear lenses that contain a minimum lead equivalent protection of 0.35 mm.

Table 34.2 presents the types of protective shielding, their equivalent lead thickness, and the approximate attenuation of scattered radiation.

Lead aprons are worn to protect vital organs. They are made of a vinyl-lead mixture covered with a smooth vinyl surface to aid in cleaning. The interior vinyl-lead composition is flexible but will crack if it is bent too far or bent repeatedly in the same location. Lead aprons must never be tossed in a heap or folded over for storage. They must be stored properly on reinforced hanging racks or laid flat on a table (Fig. 34.4). Because they are susceptible to cracking when stored improperly, lead aprons and other protective apparel should be inspected annually, both visually and under fluoroscopy or by taking radiographic images. This inspection must be documented. If a defect in a protective apron, glove, or shield is detected, the item must be immediately removed from service.

Because there is no protective barrier present, lead aprons must always be worn by radiographers during mobile radiographic procedures. A protective apron should be assigned to every C-arm and portable unit. If no lead apron is present on a portable unit, the radiographer must locate a lead apron to use for the procedure. Aprons vary in weight from a few pounds to ~ 25 pounds depending on the design and lead content. Figure 34.5 is an example of a thyroid shield and a lead apron that covers the front of the body, wraps completely around the

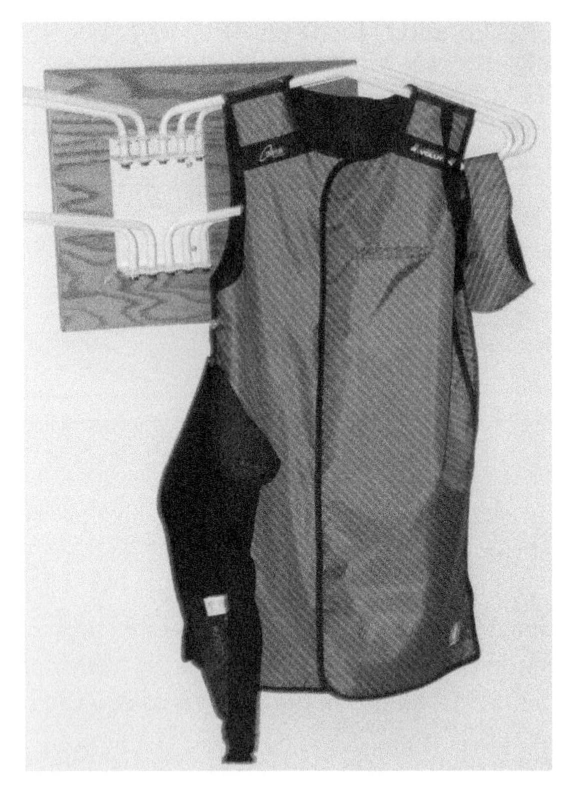

Figure 34.4. **A photograph of a hanging rack with protective aprons.**

person, and extends from the shoulders to the knees. Lead aprons with 1-mm lead equivalent will possess a significant weight and will cause fatigue for the radiographer if the apron is worn for extended periods of time. This type of apron is commonly used for fluoroscopic and mobile procedures but lacks protection for the persons back. The protective aprons must have a minimum of 0.5-mm lead equivalent when used for procedures where the x-ray beam peak energy will reach 100 kVp. Most departments will use aprons with 0.5-mm lead equivalent as a balance between weight and protection.

Protective lead aprons for interventional suites or cardiac catheterization labs should be of the wraparound type. The procedures that are performed in these settings require personnel to move around the room where their back may be exposed to scatter radiation from the patient. Radiographers who work in these areas must wear their lead aprons for a significant portion of each day, which can lead to fatigue in the shoulders and back. To provide complete protection and to minimize fatigue, a two-piece wraparound lead equivalent apron is preferred. The weight of the apron is divided between the shoulders and pelvis while providing complete wraparound protection.

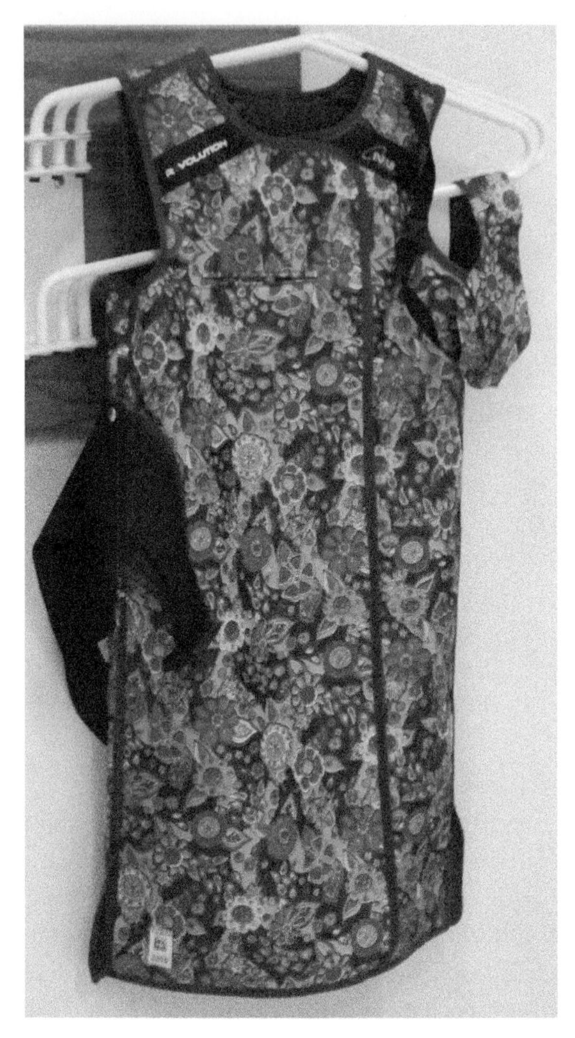

Figure 34.5. **Lead apron and thyroid shield.**

Holding the Patient

Radiographers should never stand in the primary or useful beam to immobilize or hold a patient during an exposure; however, there may be instances when the radiographer must hold a patient during an exposure. The radiographer should stand at right angles or 90 degrees to the scattering object, which is the patient; when the protection factors of distance and shielding have been accounted for, this is where the least amount of scattered radiation will be received. Nonoccupational persons who are wearing appropriate protective apparel or mechanical immobilization devices should be used to perform this function instead of a radiographer if such individuals are present.

Holding a patient may be necessary when an ill or injured person is not able to physically support himself or herself. For example, weak elderly patients may be unable to stand alone and raise their arms above their head for

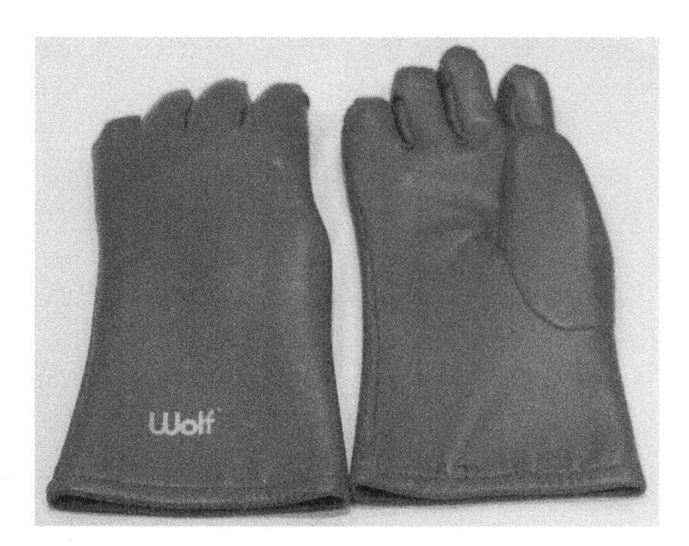

Figure 34.6. **Lead gloves for holding patients.**

a lateral chest x-ray. In this situation, a relative or friend may need to hold the patient in position during the exposure. A mechanical immobilization device may be used to hold an infant in the proper upright position for chest radiographs. Supine imaging of the chest will not result in the maximum quality necessary for diagnosing pneumonia or fluid in the lungs, only an upright position will demonstrate the air-fluid levels appropriately. If the infant is too small for the immobilizer or the device is not available, appropriate nonoccupational individuals would be needed to hold the infant upright during the exposure.

When nonoccupational individuals such as nurses, orderlies, relatives, or friends assist in holding the patient during an exposure, suitable protective apparel should be worn by each person participating in the examination. Suitable protective apparel includes lead apron, thyroid shield, and lead gloves (Fig. 34.6). The radiographer must be sure the person does not stand in the useful beam. Pregnant females should never be permitted to assist in holding a patient during an exposure as this could result in exposure to the embryo or fetus.

Reduction of Radiation Dose to the Patient

The radiation dose to the patient can be reduced by careful selection of exposure techniques and adherence to good radiographic procedures. Selection of higher-kVp, lower-mAs techniques reduces the patient dose.

Radiographic Techniques

Reducing the exposure time by using a higher mA station with a corresponding shorter time or by selecting a faster film/screen combination when one is available will reduce retakes due to patient motion. Increasing the kVp is always associated with decreased mAs to obtain an acceptable optical density that results in a reduced exposure to radiation. The relationship between mAs and patient dose is linear, as the mAs decreases so does the dose the patient receives. When selecting technical factors, the radiographer must use care to select the appropriate kVp. In digital imaging, the use of a higher kVp is much less a factor because of the digital imaging systems linear contrast response. Film screen is very different because using kVp, which is too high, will produce a poor quality image that will likely not provide the radiologist with the necessary quality to make a diagnosis.

Using good collimation practices is essential to good radiographic technique. The radiographer has the ability to reduce the field size for each radiographic image. By reducing field size, the patient receives a lower dose of radiation, and the image quality will also be improved due to the reduction of scatter radiation.

Repeat Exposures

The single most important factor in reducing the patient dose is limiting or eliminating repeat exposures. A repeat image doubles the patient dose to obtain information that should have been obtained with the initial exposure. Repeating an image can be reduced by careful patient positioning, selection of correct exposure techniques, and good communication so that the patient knows what is expected of her or him.

Prior to digital radiographic imaging, the majority of repeated x-ray exposures (~ 60%) were due to images that were too light or too dark. This resulted from improper technique, improper chemical processing, chemical fog, light leaks, multiple exposures on one image, artifacts, and patient motion. Digital imaging has significantly reduced the amount of repeats to <10%. The primary cause of repeat images with digital imaging is due to positioning errors on the part of the radiographer.

In digital imaging, when an image is repeated by the radiographer, the new image is stored as a replacement file for the nondiagnostic image. The system will permanently erase poor image. When the radiographer selects the "reject image" option, the PACS requires the radiographer to enter the reason for rejecting the image from a drop-down menu. The menu options are typically limited to a few very broad selections, such as "PACS problem, equipment problem, or positioning error."

As great as digital imaging is, one unfortunate aspect is that these rejected images are lost, and there is no way to follow up with a more targeted repeat analysis. When using conventional film screen imaging, the images that were repeated were kept for a more thorough analysis. The images were divided into categories for specific procedures such as chest, abdomen, skull, extremity, etc. The images were then reviewed to determine common reasons for repeating images, and this facilitated planning of continuing education for the radiographers and students. The in-service meetings were then customized to specific areas for improvement. This repeat analysis was performed monthly for the purposes of tracking improvement.

Digital imaging does not afford radiographers and students with the luxury of viewing repeated images to determine the actual causes for the repeat image. From the limited selections on the reject menu, many radiographers have formed a habit of entering "other" rather than "positioning" to cover up their mistakes.

Regardless of the imaging system used, careful attention to detail will result in the production of a quality radiographic image. Procedures with the highest repeat rates are the lumbar spine, thoracic spine, chest, and abdomen.

Shielding Devices

The nature of radiographic examinations results in a partial body exposure to radiation. To ensure the other areas of the body are spared exposure to radiation, the radiographer can use collimation and area shielding. The use of area shielding is indicated when an organ or tissue that is radiosensitive will be near or in the useful beam. The lens of the eye, the breasts, and the gonads are frequently shielded from primary radiation.

Gonadal shielding should be considered as a secondary measure against radiation exposure to the reproductive organs and not a substitute for a properly collimated beam. Proper collimation of the useful beam must always be the first step in gonadal protection.

The gonads (ovaries and testes) are frequently shielded from primary radiation to minimize the possibility of any genetic effect occurring with future children. Gonadal shielding is only necessary for use on pediatric patients and adults of childbearing age. Gonadal shields are made in two basic types: flat contact shields and shadow shields (Fig. 34.7).

Flat Contact Shields

Flat **contact shields** are flat, flexible shields made of lead strips or lead-impregnated materials. These shields are placed directly over the patient's reproductive organs. Flat contact shields are most effective when used for patients who are recumbent on the radiographic exam table whether in the anteroposterior (AP) or

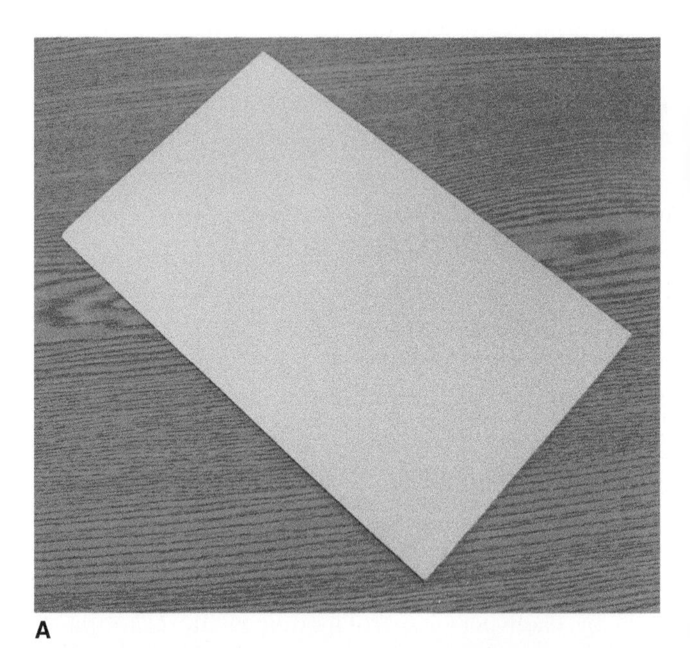

A

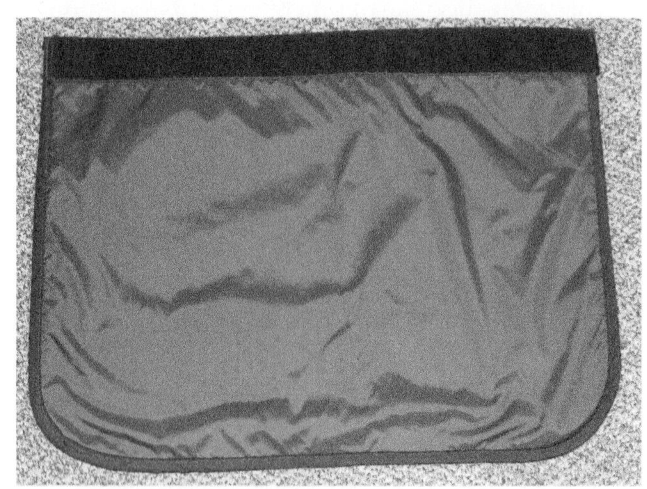

B

Figure 34.7. (A) Flat contact shield for recumbent imaging. (B) Lead apron for upright imaging.

posteroanterior (PA) position. Lead aprons with a wrap-around strap can be secured around a patient's waist and are suitable for use during upright imaging and fluoroscopy examinations.

Breasts shields are recommended for scoliosis exams, which often consists of an AP projection that subjects the juvenile breasts to primary beam. The PA projection works equally as well in producing a satisfactory image; there will be some magnification in the image but it is of little importance. The dose for the PA projection is a mere 1% of the AP projection dose.

Shadow Shields

Shadow shields are made of a radiopaque material. These shields are suspended above the collimator and are placed within the light field over the area of clinical interest to cast a shadow over the patient's reproductive organs. To ensure proper placement of the shadow shield, the light field must be properly positioned. In this manner, the shadow shield will not interfere with adjacent tissue. Improper positioning of the shadow shield can result in a repeat radiograph, which causes an increase in dose to the patient.

Radiation Dose

Each year, more and more individuals are undergoing diagnostic radiologic procedures, which equate into more irradiation of the general population. Because there is great concern about the risks associated with irradiation, it is imperative that risk to the patients be reduced whenever possible. In Chapter 33, the effects of whole-body irradiation were discussed and were mainly concerned with genetic effects or somatic effects. In addition to these considerations, we must consider the effect to the skin during a radiographic procedure where only a portion of the body is receiving radiation. It is obvious that the maximum exposure occurs at the skin entrance to the body and not at the area of interest. This is called the skin entrance dose or ESD.

Radiographic procedures of the lumbar spine, pelvis, and hip have the highest ESD due to the higher kVp and mAs that are required for quality images of the dense bone in these areas. When performing these examinations, the radiographer must carefully consider the purpose for the examination, correct positioning protocols, patient instructions, optimal technical factors based on body habitus, and shielding. Each of these factors plays a vital role in producing a quality image the first time the exposure is made.

Table 34.3 provides representative values of ESD, gonadal dose, and mean marrow dose for a variety of x-ray procedures. These are only approximate values and should not be used to estimate patient dose at any given facility; the actual doses delivered may be significantly different. There are many variables that are taken into consideration when determining actual dose.

Pediatric Considerations

When considering the potential for biological damage from exposure to ionizing radiation, children are more vulnerable to late somatic effects and genetic effects than adults. Imaging children requires special consideration to make sure the principles of **ALARA** are followed as well as shielding appropriately.

TABLE 34.3 **RADIATION QUANTITIES FOR VARIOUS IMAGING PROCEDURES**

Procedure	kVp/mAs	ESD (mGy)	Mean Marrow Dose (mGy)	Gonad Dose (mGy)
Abdomen	74/60	4.0	0.30	1.25
Cervical spine	70/40	1.5	0.10	<1
Chest	110/3	0.1	0.02	<1
Extremity	60/5	0.5	0.02	<1
Lumbar spine	72/60	3.0	0.60	2.25
Pelvis	70/50	1.5	0.20	1.50
Skull	76/50	2.0	0.10	<1
CT head	125/300	40.0	0.20	0.50
CT pelvis	125/400	20.0	0.50	20

To image a child, smaller doses of radiation are used to obtain diagnostic quality images than the doses used for adults. The entrance exposure below 5 mR will result from an AP projection of an infant's chest where the same projection of an adult's chest will yield an entrance exposure ranging from 12 to 26 mR.

Patient motion is the most common problem encountered in pediatric radiography. When working with children, the radiographer needs to be aware of the child's limited ability to understand the procedure, to cooperate, or to remain still for the exposure. To minimize this problem, the radiographer must use communication to explain what the child is to do and to elicit cooperation from the child. If the child is not able to hold completely still, the radiographer will need to utilize various immobilization devices. There are specially designed pediatric immobilization devices on the market to hold the patient securely and safely in the required position. The use of such devices along with the use of appropriate technical factors greatly reduces or eliminates the need for repeat images that increase patient dose. The techniques of gonadal shielding must also be applied to the pediatric patient any time the shield will not obscure anatomy. There are many different sizes of lead shields that can be used even on the smallest patient.

TABLE 34.4 REPRESENTATIVE ESD AND FETAL DOSE FOR RADIOGRAPHIC PROCEDURES USING A 400-SPEED IMAGE RECEPTOR

Procedure	ESD (mR)	Fetal Dose (mrad)
Abdomen (AP)	220	70
Chest (PA)	10	0
Cervical spine (AP)	110	0
Hip[a]	220	50
Intravenous urogram[a]	210	60
Lumbar spine (AP)[a]	250	80
Thoracic spine (AP)[a]	180	1
Wrist or foot	5	0

[a]Gonadal shields must be used when possible.

Reducing Exposure During Pregnancy

In medical imaging, there is heightened concern for the damaging effects of irradiation to the developing embryo or fetus. Special care is taken in medical radiography to prevent unnecessary exposure of the abdominal area of pregnant females. There is concern for the pregnant radiographer and for the pregnant patient. Table 34.4 lists the representative entrance exposures and fetal doses for radiographic procedures frequently performed using a 400-speed image receptor.

Pregnant Radiographer

The pregnant radiographer has the right to choose whether or not to declare her pregnancy. When the pregnant radiographer notifies her supervisor in writing of her pregnancy, the pregnancy becomes declared and the dose limit for the fetus becomes 0.5 mSv/mo. The equivalent dose limit for the fetus is 5 mSv for the entire pregnancy.

Most radiographers receive <1 mSv/y as determined with a personnel monitoring device, which is worn at the collar outside of protective lead aprons. The exposure at the waist under the protective apron will not normally exceed 10% of the dose registered at the collar.

Lead aprons with 0.5-mm lead equivalent provide ~90% attenuation of radiation at 75 kVp, which will sufficiently protect the pregnancy. Some aprons have a 1-mm lead equivalent; however, such thickness creates a heavier apron, which could cause back problems during pregnancy. A wraparound lead apron will provide maximum protection while distributing the weight to the shoulders resulting in fewer back problems. A facility should make a special effort to provide an apron of proper size for the pregnant radiographer to wear.

It is advisable for a pregnant radiographer to wear a second personnel monitoring device under lead aprons and at the waist level, this measures fetal dose. The report for both the collar and waist monitoring devices should be maintained on a separate record with the waist device being identified as exposure to the fetus. Historically, review of these additional monitors consistently reflects that exposures to the fetus are insignificant.

Fetal Dose

The NRC regulations state that the dose equivalent to the embryo or fetus during the entire pregnancy cannot exceed 5 mSv (0.5 rem). The NRCP recommends that the fetal exposure be restricted to an equivalent dose of 0.5 mSv (50 mrem) per month. These two limits complement each other since the normal gestation period is 10 months; therefore, 0.5 mSv/mo equates to 5 mSv for the entire pregnancy.

Pregnant Patient

Unfortunately, most women are not aware that they are pregnant during the earliest stage of pregnancy so there is concern over the exposure to the abdominal area in potentially pregnant women. To minimize the possible exposure to an embryo in the earliest days of a pregnancy, a guideline known as the **10-day rule** has been recommended by various advisory agencies. This guideline states that elective abdominal x-ray examinations for women of childbearing age must be postponed until the 10-day period following the onset of menstruation. It is considered unlikely that a woman would be pregnant during these 10 days. The risks of injury resulting from irradiation in utero are small. The physician ordering the radiologic examination will carefully weigh the risks of the irradiation to the fetus with the benefits of the exam.

It should be noted that only medically necessary examinations should be performed. The radiographer performing the examination must use precisely collimated field sizes and should carefully position protective shields where appropriate. High-kVp techniques are most appropriate in these situations so that the mAs, or dose to the patient, can be kept low.

A Final Word

The standard of practice for all personnel working around radiation is ALARA: As Low As Reasonably Achievable. This is a guiding principle for radiographers as they set technical factors based on body part thickness and pathology. It is their ethical responsibility to select the "best" technical factors. Sadly, with the advent of CR and DR, it has become a common practice for radiographers to use more mAs than is needed. As discussed previously in the text, the digital images will appear of diagnostic quality even if the patient has been overexposed.

Radiographers have the ethical responsibility to follow the ALARA principle because it is their way of demonstrating that all reasonable precautions were taken to keep the patient's and radiographer's exposure to radiation as low as achievable. The reason for this is that the effects of radiation are cumulative; therefore, the concern is the effects of exposure accumulated over long periods of time. This is especially true for people who work in a radiation industry like medical imaging.

Finally, every radiographer must be the champion of continuously educating themselves and others about radiation safety, whether the public or other health care workers. The medical imaging field is constantly changing with new equipment. Although it is fun to work with the new "toys" in the department, it is the radiographer who must become educated on each piece of equipment and its proper use. In this modern age, there are few occupations that require more constant updating of skills and knowledge than those of medical imaging.

Chapter Summary

1. This chapter has described the need for protecting the patient during radiographic procedures and the various tools and techniques used in radiography.
2. To reduce the dose to patients, the radiographer should use increased kVp, lower mAs, and faster film/screen combinations. Decreased exposure time will reduce patient motion artifacts.
3. Careful positioning and good communication with the patient will reduce retakes. The effective dose relates to the actual dose given to a portion of the body to the dose that would produce the same harm if delivered to the entire body.
4. The three methods for reducing radiation exposure to personnel are reduction of exposure time, increased distance, and increased

shielding. All radiation exposure should follow the ALARA principle.

5. The single most important factor for reducing the patient dose is to limit the amount of retakes for the image. Retakes double the patient dose. Careful positioning and good communication with the patient also helps reduce patient dose.
6. Primary barriers protect against primary radiation; secondary barriers protect against secondary radiation, which includes scatter and leakage radiation. Leakage radiation must be <100 mR/h at a distance of 1 m from the tube housing.
7. Scatter radiation is lower in intensity and energy than the primary beam.
8. The HVL is the amount of shielding required to reduce the intensity to one-half its original value. The TVL is the amount of shielding required to reduce the intensity to one-tenth its original value.
9. The primary barriers are those walls that have an upright Bucky or where the x-ray tube is stored.
10. The radiographer must wear protective apparel when remaining in the room while the x-ray beam is turned on and standing as far away from the radiation source as possible during exposures.
11. Nonoccupational individuals should hold patients when necessary for an exposure.
12. The use of immobilization devices should be incorporated into examinations where they will hold the patient still in order to prevent a potential repeat exposure.
13. The use of shielding devices is widely accepted in radiography departments. There are flat contact shields and shadow shields that are used to protect the gonads from exposure to primary radiation. These shielding devices are used on pediatric patients and those adults who are of childbearing age.
14. Care must be taken to reduce radiation exposure to any pregnant female, including pregnant or potentially pregnant patients and pregnant radiographers.
15. The recommendation for equivalent dose limit for the embryo or fetus is 0.5 mSv for any month after the pregnancy has been declared.

Case Study

Jessica is preparing to perform a fluoroscopic procedure on a 25-year-old patient. She has explained the examination to the patient and has answered the patient's questions. Jessica is certain the patient understands the expectations for the procedure. As Jessica is putting on her protective apparel, she is thinking of safe radiation practices she can take during the procedure.

Critical Thinking Questions

1. Name the primary practices Jessica is thinking of.
2. What is the purpose of putting on protective apparel?
3. Which apparel should she put on?
4. What is another method she can use to further decrease her exposure to scatter radiation?
5. If Jessica were to stand close to the patient, in which location would she receive the least exposure to scatter radiation?

Review Questions

Multiple Choice

1. **Lead aprons and other protective apparel should be inspected for hidden cracks at least:**
   a. daily
   b. weekly
   c. monthly
   d. annually

2. **The major source of scatter radiation exposure to radiology personnel is the:**
   a. primary beam
   b. Bucky
   c. image intensifier
   d. patient

3. **A protective apron should be assigned to __________ portable units.**
   a. all
   b. most
   c. many
   d. no

4. **Whenever scattered radiation decreases, the radiographer's exposure:**
   a. decreases
   b. increases slightly
   c. remains the same
   d. increases 100 times

5. **If the peak energy of the x-ray beam is 140 kVp, the primary protective barrier should consist of __________ and extend __________ upward from the floor of the x-ray room when the tube is 5 to 7 ft from the wall in question.**
   a. 1/32 in lead, 10 ft
   b. 1/32 in lead, 7 ft
   c. 1/16 in lead, 7 ft
   d. 1/16 in lead, 10 ft

6. **Primary barriers protect against __________ radiation.**
   a. direct
   b. leakage and scatter

7. **Secondary radiation is made up of __________ radiation.**
   a. scattered and direct
   b. leakage and scattered
   c. primary, leakage, and scattered
   d. leakage and scattered leakage and primary

8. **Which of the following is a primary barrier?**
   1. Wall with vertical Bucky cassette holder
   2. Wall of the control booth
   3. Floor

   a. 1
   b. 1 and 3
   c. 2 and 3
   d. 1, 2, 3, and 4

9. **HVL may be defined as the thickness of a designated absorber required to:**
   a. decrease the intensity of the primary beam by 50% of its initial value
   b. decrease the intensity of the primary beam by 25% of its initial value
   c. increase the intensity of the primary beam by 50% of its initial value
   d. increase the intensity of the primary beam by 25% of its initial value

10. **What is the amount of lead thickness for a thyroid shield?**
    a. 0.45 mm
    b. 0.25 mm
    c. 0.50 mm
    d. 0.35 mm

Short Answer

1. List the three cardinal rules of radiation protection. How are they applied to diagnostic imaging?

2. Explain the importance of gonadal dose.

3. Name the standard thickness of protective apparel.

4. Explain the procedure for holding patients during x-ray examinations.

5. List the four concepts of patient shielding during x-ray examinations.

6. What are the four factors that are taken into consideration when determining a barrier for a radiographic room?

7. Define controlled and uncontrolled areas in a hospital.

8. What are the three types of radiation exposure that are of concern when determining protective barriers?

9. During both fluoroscopy and radiography, the __________ is the single most important scattering object.

10. Leaded glass must normally be __________ times thicker than pure sheet lead to provide equivalent protection.

Glossary

15% rule changing the kVp by 15% has the same effect as doubling the mAs or reducing the mAs by 50%.

A

absorbed dose quantity of radiation in rad or gray (Gy).

absorption complete transfer of the x-ray photons' energy to an atom.

activator the chemical used in film developing to maintain the pH balance.

activity describes the quantity of radioactive material; expressed as the number of radioactive atoms that undergo decay per unit time.

active matrix array a large-area integrated circuit that consists of millions of identical semiconductor elements and acts as the flat-panel image receptor in digital radiographic and fluoroscopic systems.

active matrix liquid crystal display a type of flat-panel display that uses thin film transistors (TFTs) and capacitors.

actual focal spot the physical area on the focal track that is impacted.

acute radiation syndrome (ARS) an acute illness caused by irradiation of the entire body or most of the body by a high dose of penetrating radiation in a very short period of time.

additive disease processes a biologic process whereby tissue density is increased.

air core transformer a simple transformer made with two coils of wire placed close to each other to facilitate induction.

air gap technique a technique that uses increased OID to reduce scatter radiation reaching the image receptor.

ALARA a radiation safety principle that states that radiation exposure should be kept As Low As Reasonably Achievable.

aliasing loss of digital information because of a fluctuating signal.

alpha particle ionizing radiation having two protons and two neutrons emitted from the nucleus of a radioisotope.

alternating current (AC) current that flows in a positive direction for half of the cycle and then in a negative direction for the other half of the cycle.

ampere the unit of electric current; it is the number of electrons flowing in a conductor.

amplitude the maximum height of the peaks or valleys of a wave.

anabolism process of synthesizing smaller molecules into a larger macromolecule.

analog-to-digital converter (ADC) converts an analog signal to a digital signal for a computer to analyze.

anatomically programmed radiography (APR) a radiographic system that allows the radiographer to select a particular button on the control panel that represents an anatomic area; a preprogrammed set of exposure factors is displayed and selected for use.

angulation angle of the beam that creates a controlled or expected amount of shape distortion.

annihilation radiation gamma radiation produced when a particle and its antiparticle collide and annihilate. Most commonly, this refers to 511-keV gamma rays produced by a normal electron colliding with a positron.

annotation digital label or comment added to a digital image.

anode the positive electrode of an x-ray tube that contains the target that is struck by the projectile electrons.

anode angle the angle between the anode surface and the central ray of the x-ray beam.

anode heel effect phenomenon resulting from the angling of the anode target that causes the intensity of the x-ray beam to be less on the anode side because the "heel" of the target is in the path of the beam.

anti-halo layer a coating on the radiographic film that absorbs light that passes through the emulsion; prevents light from being reflected back through the emulsion.

aperture diaphragm a beam-restricting device constructed of a flat piece of lead that has a hole in it and is attached to the x-ray tube.

archive server consists of the physical storage device of the archive system; it commonly consists of two or three tiers of storage.

archives a collection of records that are no longer actively used that have been moved for long-term storage.

armature the rotating coil or coils of an electric motor.

array processor part of a computer that handles raw data and performs the mathematical calculations necessary to reconstruct a digital image.

artifact any unwanted optical density on a radiography or other film-type image receptor.

asthenic referring to the body habitus of a patient who is small or frail.

atomic mass number (A) the number of nucleons (neutrons plus protons) in the nucleus.

atomic number (Z) the number of protons in the nucleus.

attenuation the removal of incident x-ray photons from the beam by either absorption or scattering.

automatic brightness control (ABC) a circuit that maintains the fluoroscopic image at a constant brightness.

automatic collimator automatically limits the size and shape of the primary beam to the size and shape of the image receptor, also called a positive beam-limiting device.

automatic exposure control (AEC) a feature that uses an ionization chamber to detect the quantity of radiation exposing the patient and image receptor.

autotransformer a transformer with a single winding used to change the input voltage to a step-up or step-down transformer.

B

backscatter radiation x-rays that have interacted with an object and are deflected backward.

backup timer a timer that sets the maximum length of time the x-ray exposure will remain turned on when using an automatic exposure control system.

base the base material that the film or intensifying screen is made from; it is usually polyester, tough, rigid, stable, and uniformly radiolucent.

base plus fog (B + F) the density on the film at no exposure.

beam attenuation reduction in the energy or number of photons in the primary x-ray beam after it interacts with anatomic tissue.

beam quality the penetrating characteristics of the x-ray beam.

beam quantity the amount or intensity of the photons in the x-ray beam.

beam-restricting device alters the shape and size of the primary beam, located just below the x-ray tube housing.

Becquerel (Bq) special name for the SI units of radioactivity; one Becquerel is equal to disintegration per second.

beta particle ionizing radiation with characteristics of an electron; emitted from the nucleus of radioactive materials; it is very light and negatively charged.

bipolar every magnet has two poles; a north pole and a south pole.

bit depth number of bits that determines the precision with which the exit radiation is recorded; controls the pixel brightness or gray level that can be specified.

body habitus the general form or build of the body.

bone mineral densitometry measures the density of bone mineralization to assist the diagnosis of osteoporosis.

Bremsstrahlung interactions x-rays produced when projectile electrons are stopped or slowed in the anode.

brightness amount of luminance or light emission of a display monitor.

brightness gain ability of the image intensifier to increase the brightness level of the image.

Bucky the Potter-Bucky diaphragm located directly below the radiographic tabletop, which contains the grid and holds the image receptor.

Bucky factor the ratio of the mAs required with a grid to the mAs required without a grid to produce the same optical density. The amount of mAs increase required when a grid is added.

Bucky grids moving grids designed to blur out the grid lines and absorb scatter radiation.

C

calipers instrument that measures part thickness.

camera tube one of two devices used in a fluoroscopic system to convert the light image from the output phosphor to an electronic signal for display on a television monitor.

capacitors an electrical device used to temporarily store electrical charge.

carcinogen a substance capable of causing cancer in living tissue.

carriage the arm that supports the fluoroscopic equipment suspended over the table.

catabolism process that creates energy for a cell by breaking down molecular nutrients that are brought to and diffused through the cell membrane.

cathode the negative electrode of an x-ray tube, which contains the filament that emits electrons for x-ray production.

cathode ray tube television monitor used to display the fluoroscopic image.

central nervous system syndrome form of acute radiation syndrome caused by radiation doses of 50 Gy (5,000 rad) or more of ionizing radiation that results in failure of the central nervous system, followed by death within a few hours to several days.

characteristic cascade the process of electrons moving into the holes created during a characteristic interaction until there is only a hole in the outer shell.

characteristic curve a graph of optical density and relative exposure that is characteristic of a particular type of x-ray film.

characteristic interactions x-ray production that occurs when an orbital electron fills a vacancy in the shell of the atom.

charge-coupled device (CCD) solid-state device that converts visible light photons to electrons.

chromosomes a threadlike structure of nucleic acids and protein found in the nucleus of most living cells; carrying genetic information in the form of genes.

cine cine fluoroscopy is associated with rapid (30 frames per second or more) sequence filming.

clearing agent the primary agent, ammonium thiosulfate, in fixer that removes undeveloped silver bromine from the emulsion.

closed core transformer a transformer with two coils of wire each with an iron placed close to each other to facilitate induction.

codon series of three consecutive nucleotide bases in the DNA.

coherent scattering low-energy scattering involving no loss of photon energy, only a change in photon direction.

collimation restriction of the useful x-ray beam to reduce patient dose and improve image contrast.

collimator device used to restrict x-ray beam size and shape.

commutator rings a ring which is connected to an armature that rotates the armature through a magnetic field to convert alternating current to a direct current.

compression ratio the ratio between the computer storage required to save an original image and the storage required for the compressed data.

Compton scattering scattering of x-ray photons that results in ionization of an atom and loss of energy in the scattered photon.

computed radiography (CR) radiographic technique that uses a photostimulable phosphor plate as the image receptor that stores the x-ray energy in proportion to the intensity it receives.

computed tomography (CT) radiographic technique that creates cross-sectional tomographic sections of the body with a rotating fan beam, detector array, and computed reconstruction.

conductor a material in which electrons can move freely.
cone a metal cylinder that attaches to the x-ray tube housing to limit the beam size and shape.
contact shields shields that are flat and are placed directly on the patient's gonads.
contrast the difference between adjacent densities that makes detail visible.
contrast medium material added to the body to increase the subject contrast. Contrast media has densities and atomic numbers very different from body tissues.
contrast resolution used to describe the ability of the imaging system to distinguish between small objects that attenuate the x-ray beam similarly in digital imaging.
controlled area an area where imaging personnel occupancy and activity are subject to control and supervision for the purpose of radiation protection.
conversion efficiency a measure of a screen's efficiency in converting x-ray photon energy into light energy.
conversion factor a measure of the luminance intensity at the output phosphor to radiation intensity upon the input phosphor.
cosmic radiation particulate and electromagnetic radiation emitted by the sun and stars.
coulomb the standard unit of charge.
Coulomb's law the electrostatic force between two charges is directly proportional to the product of their quantities and inversely proportional to the square of the distance between them.
crossed grids two linear grids placed on top of one another so that the lead strips form a crisscross pattern.
crossover effect blurring of the image caused by light from one screen crossing into the light from another screen.
crossover network part of the automatic film processor system designed to bend and turn the film when it reaches the top of the transport rack and must be directed down into the next tank.
Curie (Ci) conventional system unit of radioactivity. Expressed as 1 Ci – 3.7×10^{10} disintegrations per second.
current the quantity or number of electrons flowing.
cylinder an aperture diaphragm that has an extended flange attached to it.
cytoplasm the material or protoplasm within a living cell, excluding the nucleus.

D

densitometer a device used to measure the amount of light transmitted through the film, giving the numerical value of its optical density.
density controls a component of the automatic exposure control device that allows the radiographer to adjust the amount of preset radiation detection values.
deoxyribonucleic acid (DNA) a self-replicating material present in nearly all living organisms as the main constituent of chromosomes. It is the carrier of genetic information.
desquamation denudation or ulceration of the skin.
destructive disease processes a biologic process whereby tissue density is decreased.
detail the degree of geometric sharpness or resolution of an object recorded as an image.
detective quantum efficiency (DQE) the radiation exposure level that is required to produce an optimal image.
detector array collection of detectors and the interspace material between them which absorbs the transmitted radiation and converts it to an electrical signal, which is displayed on a computer workstation.
detectors radiation measuring devices.
deterministic effects biologic response whose severity varies with radiation dose. A dose threshold usually exists.
developing the step in film processing where exposed silver halide crystals turn into metallic silver making the latent image visible.
dexel detector element; describes the elements in a detector that may be processed, combined, resampled, or manipulated to create an image.
diamagnetic materials magnetic materials that are weakly repelled by a magnet.
diaphragm device that restricts the x-ray beam to a fixed size.
dichroic stain two-colored stain that appears as a curtain effect on a radiograph.
differential absorption varying degrees of absorption in different tissues that results in radiographic contrast and visualization of anatomy.
diffuse reflectance the reflection of light from a surface such that an incident ray is reflected at many angles rather than at just one angle.
digital imaging and communications in medicine (DICOM) computer software standards that permit a wide range of digital imaging programs to understand each other.
digital radiography (DR) static images produced with an area x-ray beam that is intercepted by a photostimulable phosphor plate or a direct capture solid-state device.
digital-to-analog converter (DAC) converts a digital signal to an analog signal.
digital versatile disk (DVD) a type of compact disc able to store large amounts of data, especially high-resolution material.
direct current (DC) current that flows in only one direction.
direct square law maintains image density by changing mAs values to compensate for the change in distance.
display workstation special computer designed for technical applications.
distortion a misrepresentation of the size and shape of the anatomic structures being imaged.
D_{max} the maximum density the film is able to record.
dose-area product (DAP) the actual measurement of patient dose measured by a DAP meter embedded in the collimator. The DPA depends on the exposure factors and field size.
dose creep the slow rise of patient dose in digital x-ray studies which occurs over time.
dose equivalent radiation quantity that is used for radiation protection and that expresses dose on a common scale for all radiation. Expressed in rem or sievert (Sv).
dose limits (DLs) maximum permissible occupational radiation dose.

doubling dose the dose of radiation that is expected to double the number of genetic mutations in a generation.
drive system the mechanical system responsible for turning the rollers in the processor.
dynamic range the range of exposure intensities that an image receptor can respond to and acquire image data.

E

edge response function (EFR) mathematical expression of the ability of the computed tomographic scanner to reproduce a high-contrast edge with accuracy.
effective dose the dose to the whole body that would cause the same harm as the actual dose received from the examination; used to measure the radiation and organ system damage in man.
effective focal spot the area of the focal spot that is projected toward the object being imaged.
electric field the force field surrounding an object, resulting from the charges of the object.
electrification occurs when electrons are added to or subtracted from an object.
electrodynamics the study of moving electric charges.
electromagnet temporary magnet produced by moving electric current.
electromagnetic induction production of a current in a conductor by a changing magnetic field near the conductor.
electromagnetic spectrum describes the different forms of electromagnetic radiation.
electromagnetism deals with the relationship between electricity and magnetism.
electromotive force (EMF) electrical potential that is measured in volts (V) or kilovolts (kV).
electron binding energy the amount of energy needed to remove the electron from the atom.
electron volt measurement of the binding energy of an electron; the energy one electron will have when it is accelerated by an electrical potential of 1 V.
electronic medical record (EMR) a digital version of a paper chart that contains all of a patient's medical history; used by providers for diagnosis and treatment.
electrostatic focusing lenses negatively charged plates along the internal length of the image intensifier tube that repel the electron stream, focusing it on the small output phosphor.
electrostatics the study of stationary or resting electric charges.
elongation projection of a structure making it appear longer than it actually is.
emulsion layer a layer of gelatin containing the silver halide crystals; thin coating that acts as a neutral lucent suspension for the silver halide crystals.
endoplasmic reticulum channel or series of channels that allows the nucleus to communicate with the cytoplasm.
entrance skin dose (ESD) measure of radiation dose absorbed by the skin; expressed in milligray (mGy).
entrance skin exposure x-ray exposure to the skin; expressed in milliroentgen (mR).
epilation loss of hair.
erythema reddening of the skin which resembles a sunburn.
exit radiation the combination of transmitted and scattered radiation that passes through the patient.
exposure quantity of radiation intensity (R or C/kg).
exposure angle the total distance the tube travels while the exposure is being made.
exposure index method by which digital radiography estimates exposure on the image detector.
exposure latitude the range of exposure values to the receptor that will produce an acceptable range of densities for diagnostic purposes.
exposure linearity ability of a radiographic unit to produce a constant radiation output for various combinations of mA and exposure time.
exposure reproducibility the ability of a radiographic unit to duplicate the same exposure time after time.
exposure time the length of time required to end an exposure.

F

ferromagnetic materials materials that are easily magnetized.
filament the source of electrons in the cathode.
fill factor the percentage of the dexel devoted to the semiconductor detection area.
film badge dosimeters a device containing photographic film and filters that registers the radiation exposure to radiation workers.
film contrast the difference in optical density between a region of interest and its surroundings.
film speed a measure of film sensitivity; faster films require less exposure.
filtered back projection a reconstruction algorithm used in computed tomography, using a computer or electronic filter to reconstruct an image.
filtration the removal of low-energy x-ray photons from the primary beam with aluminum or other metal.
fixed kVp-variable mAs technique chart a type of technique exposure chart in which the optimal kilovoltage peak value for each anatomic part is indicated, and the milliampere/second value is varied as a function of anatomic part thickness.
fixing the process where the reducing action of the developer is stopped and the undeveloped silver halide crystals are removed; makes the image permanent.
flat-field correction technique used to remove artifacts from 2D images that are caused by variations in the pixel-to-pixel sensitivity of the detector and/or by distortions in the optical path.
flat panel detector plates used in direct digital imaging.
fluorescence the production of light in the intensifying screen phosphor by x-ray photons.
fluoroscopy dynamic x-ray technique for viewing moving structures.
flux gain a measurement of the increase in light photons due to the conversion efficiency of the output screen.
focal plane region of anatomy of interest in tomography; also object plane.
focal range the recommended range of source-to-image receptor distance measurements that can be used with a focused grid.
focal spot the area on the anode where the projectile electrons strike, the source of x-ray photons.

focal spot blur blurred region on the radiographic image over which the radiographer has little control.
focal track the area of the anode where the high-voltage electrons will strike.
focused grids grids whose radiopaque lead strips are tilted to align, at a predetermined SID, with the divergent x-ray beam.
focusing cup the shallow depression in the cathode that houses the filament or filaments.
fog unwanted exposure density on the radiographic image.
foreshortening projection of a structure making it to appear shorter than it actually is.
fractionation radiation dose delivered at the same dose in equal portions at regular intervals.
frequency the number of cycles per second that are in a wave.
fulcrum pivot point between the tube and image receptor.

G

gastrointestinal (GI) syndrome form of acute radiation syndrome that appears in humans at a threshold dose of approximately 10 Gy (1,000 rad). It is characterized by nausea, diarrhea, and damage to the cells lining the intestines.
gauss (G) the SI unit for magnetism.
Geiger-Muller counters radiation detection and radiation measuring instrument that detects individual ionizations.
generator a device that converts mechanical energy into electrical energy.
genetic cells oogonium or spermatogonium.
genetically significant dose (GSD) average gonadal dose given to members of the population who are of childbearing age.
geometric factors factors that affect radiographic quality; recorded detail and distortion.
gray scale the number of different shades of gray that can be stored and displayed by a computer system in digital imaging.
gradient processing in digital imaging, this is the manipulation of both the centering and the steepness of the curve.
grid scatter reduction device consisting of alternating strips of radiopaque and radiolucent material.
grid caps device that contains a permanently mounted grid; it is placed over the image receptor.
grid cassette an image receptor that contains a permanently mounted grid on the front of the receptor.
grid conversion factor (GCF) formula used when changing from one grid ratio to another.
grid cutoff the interception of transmitted x-ray photons by the radiopaque strips of a grid, resulting in lighter density at one or both edges of the field.
grid frequency the number of lead strips per cm or per inch.
grid ratio the ratio of the height of the lead strips to the distance between the lead strips in a grid.
guide-shoe mark appear as light lines or negative densities parallel to the direction the film traveled through the automatic processor.
Gurney-Mott theory a theory of how the silver halide crystals are exposed to form a latent image and developed to form a visible radiographic image.

H

half-life the time it takes for a radioisotope to decay to one half its activity.
half-value layer (HVL) the thickness of an absorbing material that will reduce the intensity of the primary beam by one half the original value.
half-wave rectification rectification resulting from one half of the incoming alternating current being converted to pulsating direct current.
hardener a chemical used to stiffen and shrink emulsion; prevents scratching and abrasions during processing.
health level 7 a set of international standards for transfer of clinical and administrative data between software applications used by various health care providers.
heel effect decreased intensity from the cathode side of the x-ray beam to the anode side. The lightest part of an image is at the anode side of the image.
helix an object having a 3D shape like that of a wire wound uniformly in a single layer, as in a corkscrew.
hematopoietic syndrome form of acute radiation syndrome that develops after whole body exposure to doses ranging from approximately 1 to 10 Gy (100 to 1,000 rad). It is characterized by reduction in white cells, red cells, and platelets in circulating blood.
high-frequency generator a generator capable of producing three-phase twelve-pulse wave forms.
high-kVp technique chart a type of technique exposure chart in which high kVp (greater than 100 kVp) is indicated, and the milliampere/second value is varied as a function of anatomic part thickness.
histogram a display of statistical information that uses rectangles to show the frequency of data items in successive numerical intervals.
histogram analysis a process in which a computer analyzes the histogram using processing algorithms and compares it with a preestablished histogram specific to the anatomic part being imaged.
histogram errors analysis errors that cause the image to be rescaled thereby affecting the curve of the histogram; displayed image will have excessive gray scale or excessive contrast.
homeostasis (1) state of equilibrium among tissues and organs. (2) Ability of the body to return to normal function despite infection and environmental changes.
hospital information systems (HIS) a comprehensive, integrated information system designed to manage all the aspects of a hospital's operation; medical, administrative, financial, legal issues, processing of services.
Hounsfield unit scale of computed tomographic numbers used to assess the nature of tissue.
hydroquinone a reducing agent in the developing solution that slowly changes the silver halide crystals into metallic silver.
hypersthenic referring to a body habitus of a patient who is large in frame and overweight.
hyposthenic referring to a body habitus of a patient who is thin but healthy in appearance.

I

image intensifier converts x-ray photons into a brighter visible image.

image manager a database that handles the workflow of the PAC system by moving images from storage to viewing or work stations and then back to the archive; interfaces with the RIS and HIS.

image storage stores or archives the data on a physical storage device such as magnetic tape, optical disk, or server.

imaging plate a device that receives the radiation leaving the patient.

incident electron the electrons from the thermionic cloud that bombard the anode target.

indexing positioning of the patient support couch in computed tomography.

inherent filtration filtration of useful x-ray beam provided by the internal components of an x-ray tube housing assembly and the glass window of the x-ray tube.

input phosphor a layer of the image intensifier tube made of cesium iodide and bonded to the curved surface of the tube.

insulator a material in which electrons are fixed and cannot move freely.

intensifying screens increases the efficiency of x-ray absorption and decreases the dose to the patient by converting x-ray photon energy into visible light energy.

intensity a measurement of the energy of x-rays.

internal radiation small amounts of radioactive minerals normally found in the body, ingested from the small amount present in food and inhaled as airborne particles.

interphase software and hardware that enable imaging systems to interconnect and to connect with printers.

interpolation algorithms a process that estimates of a value between two known values.

interspace material sections of radiolucent material that separates the strips of aluminum in a grid.

inverse square law the Electrostatic Law that states the force between two charges is directly proportional to the product of their quantities and inversely proportional to the square of the distance between them.

inversely proportional scales as one factor increases, the other must decrease to maintain the scale.

involuntary motion movement that is not in the control of the patient.

ion an atom that has gained or lost an electron.

ion pair two oppositely charged particles.

ionization the process of adding or removing an electron from an atom.

ionization chambers an air-filled cell that is connected to the timer circuit by an electrical wire.

isotopes atoms of the same element whose nuclei contain the same number of protons but a different number of neutrons.

K

keV kiloelectron volt. A measure of the energy of an x-ray photon or an electron.

kilovoltage peak (kVp) kilovoltage peak. A measure of the voltage applied to the x-ray tube.

L

latent image the unseen image stored in the exposed silver halide emulsion; the image is made manifest during processing.

latent period period after the prodromal stage of the acute radiation syndrome during which no sign of radiation sickness is apparent.

latitude range of exposures or densities over which a radiographic image is acceptable.

$LD_{50/60}$ dose of radiation expected to cause death within 60 days to 50% of the exposed population.

leakage radiation radiation outside the primary x-ray beam emitted through the tube housing.

lethal dose *see* $LD_{50/60}$

line focus principle used to reduce the effective area of the focal spot.

linear energy transfer (LET) measure of the rate at which energy is transferred from ionizing radiation to soft tissue. Expressed in kiloelectron volts (keV) per micrometer of soft tissue.

linear, nonthreshold any dose, regardless of its size, is expected to produce a response.

linear, threshold any dose below the threshold is not expected to produce a response.

linear tomography an imaging procedure using movement of the x-ray tube and image receptor in opposite directions to create images of structures in a focal plane by blurring the anatomy located above and below the plane of interest.

liquid crystal diode displays constructed of two thin flexible glass plates with the liquid crystal material sandwiched between the glass plates.

log relative exposure a measurement of the intensity of radiation exposure in increments by a factor of 2.

logarithmic scales a nonlinear scale used then there is a large range of quantities.

look-up table (LUT) matrix of data that manipulates the values of gray levels, converting an image input value to a different output value.

low-pass filtering a filter that passes signals with a frequency lower than a certain cutoff frequency and attenuates signals with frequencies higher than the cutoff frequency.

luminance emission of visible light.

luminescence the ability of a material to emit light in response to stimulation.

lysosome cell that contains enzymes capable of digesting cellular fragments.

M

magnetic dipole a group of atoms with their dipoles aligned in the same direction.

magnetic disk storage a flat rotating disk covered on one or both sides with magnetizable material.

magnetic domain a group of atoms with their dipoles aligned in the same direction.

magnetic field the force fields that are created when dipoles align in the same direction; also called lines of force or lines of flux.

magnetic induction temporary alignment of dipoles when acted upon by a strong magnetic field.

magnetism the ability of a magnetic material to attract iron, nickel, and cobalt.

magneto-optical disk (MOD) a plastic or glass disk coated with a compound with special optical, magnetic, and thermal properties. Disk is read with a low intensity laser.

magnification an increase in the image size of an object.
manifest illness stage stage of acute radiation syndrome during which signs and symptoms are apparent.
manifest image the observable image that is formed when the latent image undergoes proper chemical processing.
man-made radiation x-rays and artificially produced radionuclides used for nuclear medicine.
mAs/distance compensation formula a mathematical calculation for adjusting the mAs when changing the source-to-image receptor distance.
mAs readout immediate display of the amount of mAs used in the production of a radiographic image; used with automatic exposure control.
matrix a group of numbers arranged in rows and columns.
maximum intensity projection (MIP) reconstruction of an image through selection of the highest value pixels along any arbitrary line in the data set; only those pixels are exhibited.
meiosis process of germ cell division that reduces the chromosomes in each daughter cell to half the number of chromosomes in the parent cell.
metabolism anabolism and catabolism.
milliampere measure of x-ray tube current.
milliampere-second (mAs) product of exposure time and x-ray tube current; measure of total number of electrons.
minification gain resulting from the electrons that were produced at the input phosphor being compressed into the area of the smaller output phosphor.
minimum response time (MRT) the shortest exposure time that the automatic exposure control system can produce.
mitochondria structure that digests macromolecules to produce energy for the cell.
mitosis process of somatic cell division wherein a parent cell divides to form two daughter cells identical to the parent cell.
mobile the ability to be easily transportable.
modulation transfer function (MTF) a measure of the ability of the system to preserve signal contrast as a function of spatial resolution and describe the fraction of each component that will preserve the captured image.
Moiré artifact a zebra pattern artifact that can occur when a stationary grid is used during computed radiography imaging.
motor an electrical device used to convert electrical energy into mechanical energy.
multiplanar reformation (MPR) operation by the computer to display the image data in coronal, sagittal, or oblique planes.
multislice CT imaging modality that uses two detector arrays to produce two spiral slices at the same time.
mutagenic effects in genetics, a mutagen is a physical or chemical agent that changes the genetic material, usually DNA, of an organism and thus increases the frequency of mutations above the natural background level.
mutual induction the result of two coils being placed in close proximity with a varying current supplied to the first coil, which then induces a similar flow in the second coil.

N

natural radiation naturally occurring ionizing radiation, including cosmic rays, terrestrial radiation, and internally deposited radionuclides.
nonlinear, nonthreshold referring to varied responses that are produced from varied doses, with any dose expected to produce a response.
nonlinear, threshold referring to varied responses that are produced from varied doses, with a particular level below which there is no response.
nonmagnetic materials materials that do not react to magnetic fields. Examples: wood, glass, plastic.
nonstochastic effects biologic effects of ionizing radiation that demonstrate the existence of a threshold. Severity of biologic damage increases with increased dose.
normalization process of reorganizing data in a database so that it meets two basic requirements: (1) there is no redundancy of data (all data are stored in only one place), and (2) data dependencies are logical (all related data items are stored together).
nucleons nuclear particles; either neutrons or protons.
nucleus the central core of an atom made up fundamentally of protons and neutrons.

O

object plane region of anatomy of interest in tomography; also focal plane.
occupational exposure radiation exposure received by radiation workers.
occupationally exposed workers radiation workers who encounter radiation during the course of their work day.
off-centering placing the central ray either lateral or medial to the center of the anatomical part of interest.
off-focus radiation photons that were not produced at the focal spot.
ohm the unit of electrical resistance (Ω).
open core transformer two coils of wire each having an iron core placed close to each other to facilitate induction.
optical densitometer a device to measure the blackness or optical density of a film.
optical density a measure of the degree of blackness of the film expressed on a logarithmic scale. The primary controlling factor is mAs.
optically stimulated luminescence (OSL) a method for measuring doses of ionizing radiation.
optimal kVp the kVp value that is high enough to ensure penetration of the anatomical part but not too high to diminish radiographic contrast.
organogenesis the production and development of the organs of an animal or plant.
orthochromatic film sensitive to light from green light–emitting screens.
oscillating grid mechanism that moves the grid in a circular pattern above the image receptor.
output phosphor a layer in the image intensifier tube that absorbs the electron stream and emits light in response.
oxygen enhancement ratio (OER) ratio of the dose necessary to produce a given effect under anoxic conditions to the dose necessary to produce the same effect under aerobic conditions.

P

pair production an interaction between x-ray photons and the force field of the nucleus of an atom resulting in the x-ray photon energy being completely converted into a positive and negative electron.

panchromatic film sensitive to all wavelengths of visible light.
panoramic tomography (panorex) unit that is designed to image curved surfaces, typically the mandible and teeth.
parallel circuit circuit that contains elements that bridge conductors rather than lie in a line along a conductor.
parallel grids grids that have parallel lead strips.
paramagnetic materials materials that are weakly attracted to magnetic fields.
penetrometer aluminum step wedge with increasingly thick absorbers; uses x-ray beam to produce step wedge image for quality assurance.
period (of a wave) the time required for one complete cycle of a waveform.
permeability a quantity measuring the influence of a substance on the magnetic flux in the region it occupies.
phenidone a reducing agent in the developing solution that rapidly changes the silver halide crystals into metallic silver.
phosphor layer a layer of material used in intensifying screens that is capable of absorbing the energy from incident x-ray photon and emitting light photons.
phosphorescence the continuation of light emission from intensifying screens after the stimulation from the x-ray photons ceases (afterglow).
photocathode converts light photons into photoelectrons in the image intensifier.
photoconductor a device that absorbs x-rays and creates electric charges in proportion to the x-ray exposure received.
photodetector a device used to sense the light released from the photostimulable phosphor plate during scanning.
photodisintegration an interaction between an x-ray photon and the nucleus of an atom where the nucleus absorbs all the photons' energy and emits a nuclear fragment.
photoelectric effect complete absorption of the incident photon by the atom.
photoelectron an electron ejected from an atom following a photoelectric interaction.
photoemission electron emission after light stimulation.
photometer instrument that measures light intensity.
photomultiplier (PM) tube an electronic device that converts visible light energy into electrical energy.
photon small bundles of energy used to produce x-radiation; also called quantum.
photospot camera camera that exposes only one frame when active, receiving its image from the output phosphor of the image intensifier tube.
photostimulable luminescence the release of energy from trapped electrons by a laser during the scanning of the photostimulable phosphor plate.
photostimulable phosphor (PS) plate a plate made up of several layers that stores x-ray energy as a latent image for cassette-based digital systems.
phototimers automatic exposure control detectors that use a fluorescent screen and a device that converts the light to electricity.
pi mark occur at 3.1416-inch intervals because of dirt or a chemical stain on a roller.
picture archiving and communication system (PACS) an electronic network for communication between the image acquisition modalities, display stations, and storage.
pitch the relationship between slice thickness and the distance the table travels every time the tube rotates in spiral computed tomography.
pivot point a fixed point during the movement of the x-ray tube and image receptor that lies within the plane of the anatomic area of interest; also called the fulcrum.
pixel a picture element of a matrix that contains information on its location and intensity.
pixel density number of pixels per unit area.
pixel pitch the pixel spacing or distance measured from the center of a pixel to an adjacent pixel.
positive beam–limiting (PBL) device an automatic collimator that adjusts to the size of the cassette.
postprocessing manipulation and adjustments of the digital image after corrections have been made in the preprocessing stage.
potential difference the force or strength of electron flow; also known as electromotive force (EMF).
power the amount of energy used per second. Electric power is the current multiplied by the voltage and is measured in watts.
precursor cells an immature cell.
predetector collimator located just before the detector array in computed tomography imaging; controls how much of the detector is exposed.
prepatient collimator located just before the patient in computed tomography; a device that limits the beam size and therefore limits patient exposure and reduces the amount of scatter radiation produced in the patient.
prodromal stage first stage of the acute radiation syndrome; occurs within hours after radiation exposure.
proportional scales the relation of one part to another.
preprocessing takes place in the computer where the raw digital image data are corrected for flaws that are inherent in the x-ray beam, the elements and electrical circuitry of the particular imaging system or the physical elements and electrical circuitry of the processor; also be called image acquisition processing.
preservative a chemical additive that maintains chemical balance in the developer and fixer.
primary barrier any wall to which the useful beam can be directed.
protective apparel aprons and gloves lined with lead that are used to absorb radiation.
protective coat a material used in an intensifying screen that is applied to the top of the phosphor layer to protect it from abrasions and trauma.
protraction extending the time over which a set dose of radiation is delivered.

Q

quality assurance the activities that are performed to provide adequate confidence that high-quality images will be consistently produced.
quality control the measurement and evaluation of equipment to maintain superior standards.

quantization a process in which the continuous range of values of an analog signal is sampled and divided into non-overlapping (but not necessarily equal) subranges, and a discrete, unique value is assigned to each subrange.

quantum mottle the random speckled appearance of an image, similar to the "snow" seen with poor TV reception. Quantum mottle is greater when high-speed screens and low mAs techniques are used because there are fewer interactions.

quantum noise caused by too few photons reaching the image receptor to form the image; resulting in muted or grainy appearance.

R

rad special unit for absorbed dose and air kerma. 1 rad = 100 erg/g = 0.01 Gy.

radioactive decay the transformation of radioactive nuclei into a different element followed by the emission of particulate or electromagnetic radiation.

radiographic contrast a combination of film and subject contrast.

radiographic density the amount of overall blackness produced on the processed image.

radioisotopes an unstable isotope that spontaneously transforms into a more stable isotope with the emission of radiation.

radiology information system (RIS) the core system for the electronic management of imaging departments. The major functions of the RIS can include patient scheduling, resource management, examination performance tracking, examination interpretation, results distribution, and procedure billing.

radiolucent low attenuating material or tissue that appears dark on a radiographic image.

radiopaque highly attenuating material or tissue that appears bright on a radiographic image.

radiosensitivity relative susceptibility of cells, tissues, and organs to the harmful action of ionizing radiation.

rare earth screens rare earth phosphors employed in intensifying screens such as gadolinium, lanthanum, and yttrium.

raster pattern pattern produced on the screen of a television picture tube by the movement of an electron beam.

reciprocating grid a grid that moves while x-rays are being generated.

reciprocity law the same mAs, regardless of the values of mA and seconds, should give the same image density.

reconstruction time time needed for the computer to present a digital image after an examination has been completed.

recorded detail one of the geometric properties identified as the degree of sharpness in an image; also detail, sharpness, or spatial resolution.

rectifiers an electrical device that allows current to flow only in one direction to convert AC into DC.

redundant array of independent disks (RAID) system that consists of at least two disk drives within a single cabinet that collectively act as a single storage system.

reflective layer a layer of material used in an intensifying screen to reflect light back toward the film.

refresh time the amount of time it takes to reconstruct the next frame.

region of interest (ROI) area of an anatomical structure on a reconstructed digital image as defined by the operator using a cursor.

relative biological effectiveness (RBE) ratio of the dose of standard radiation necessary to produce a given effect to the dose of test radiation needed for the same effect.

rem special unit for dose equivalent and effective dose. Replaced by the sievery (Sv) in the SI system. 1 rem = 0.01 Sv.

remnant radiation x-rays that pass through the patient and interact with the image receptor.

resistance the opposition to current flow.

response time the amount of time the pixel requires to change its brightness.

restrainer a chemical added to the developer to restrict the reducing agent activity, acts as an antifogging agent.

retentivity the ability of a substance to retain or resist magnetization, frequently measured as the strength of the magnetic field that remains in a sample after removal of an inducing field.

ribonucleic acid (RNA) molecules that are involved in the growth and development of a cell through a number of small, spherical cytoplasmic organelles that attach to the endoplasmic reticulum.

ribosomes the site of protein synthesis.

ripple measures the amount of variation between maximum and minimum voltage.

rotating anode an anode that turns during an exposure.

rotor the central rotating component of an electric motor, used to rotate the anode.

S

sampling function of detecting and measuring radiation that occurs at the imaging plate or array of detectors.

scanning the process where the field of the image is divided up into an array of small cells.

scattering the photon interaction with an atom resulting in a change of direction and loss of energy.

scintillation detectors instrument used in the detector arrays of many computed tomographic scanners.

secondary barrier protective barrier designed to shield an area from secondary radiation.

section interval the distance between the fulcrum levels.

section level the variable location of structures of interest, controlled by the fulcrum.

section thickness the width of the focal or object plane, controlled by tomographic angle.

segmentation software which will cause the system to scan across the plate and determine the number and orientation of views on one image receptor; partitioned pattern recognition.

semiconductor a material that can act as a conductor or insulator, depending on how it is made and its environment.

sensitivity speck an impurity added to the silver halide crystals that attracts free silver ions during latent image formation.

sensitometer a device that uses light to produce a step wedge image for processor quality assurance.

sensitometric curve a graphic display of the relationship between the intensity of radiation exposure (x axis) and the resultant optical densities (*y* axis).

sensitometric strip a step-wedge density image produced after exposing the film in a sensitometer and then processing the film.
sensitometry the measure of the characteristic responses of film to exposure and processing.
series circuit a closed circuit in which the current follows one path, the current through each load is the same and the total voltage across the circuit is the sum of the voltages across each load.
shaded surface display (SSD) computer-aided technique that identifies a narrow range of values as belonging to the object to be imaged and displays that range.
shaded volume display (SVD) display which is sensitive to operator-selected pixel range that can make imaging of actual anatomical structures difficult.
shadow shields shield that is suspended over the region of interest; it casts a shadow over the patient's reproductive organs.
shell type transformer a central iron core with both the primary and secondary wires wrapping around the iron core to facilitate induction.
short-scale contrast a radiograph with few densities but great differences among them; described as high contrast.
shoulder region area of high exposure levels on a characteristic curve.
Sievert (Sv) special name for the SI unit of dose equivalent and effective dose. 1 Sv = 1 J/kg = 100 rem.
signal-to-noise ratio (SNR) white noise that interferes with the digital image.
single-phase circuits a circuit that allows the potential difference to build then drop to zero with each change in direction of current flow.
size distortion refers to an increase in the object's image size compared with its true or actual size.
skin erythema dose (SED) dose of radiation, usually about 200 rad or 2 Gy, that causes redness of the skin.
slip rings a ring in a dynamo or electric motor that is attached to and rotates with the shaft, passing an electric current to a circuit via a fixed brush pressing against it.
slip-ring technology technology that allows the shaft in an electric motor to rotate continuously without interruption.
solenoid helical winding of current carrying wire that produces a magnetic field along the axis of the helix.
solid-state detectors radiation detector in which a semiconductor material constitutes the detecting medium, called a semiconductor radiation detector.
solvent chemicals suspended in water that are used in developing film.
somatic cells all cells of the body except the oogonium and the spermatogonium.
source-to-image-receptor distance (SID) source to image receptor distance. The distance from the radiation source to the image receptor.
source to skin distance distance from the patient's skin to the fluoroscopic tube.
space charge effect with the buildup of electrons by the filament, the electrons' negative charges begin to oppose the emission of additional electrons.
spatial frequency measure of resolution; usually expressed in line pairs per millimeter (lp/mm).
spatial location processing that operates on individual pixels or groups of pixels.
spatial resolution the minimum separation at which two objects can be recognized as two separate objects.
spatial uniformity constancy of pixel values in all regions of the reconstructed image.
specular reflectance a reflection of light from a surface in which light from a single incoming x-ray is reflected into a single outgoing direction.
speed term used to loosely describe the sensitivity of film to x-rays.
spin magnetic moment the magnetic effect created by orbital electrons spinning on their axes around the nucleus of the atom.
SSD source to skin distance.
stator the fixed winding of an electric motor.
stem cells immature or precursor cell.
step-down transformer a transformer that has more turns in the primary winding than in the secondary winding, which decreases the voltage.
step-up transformer a transformer that has more turns in the secondary winding than in the primary winding, which increases the voltage.
sthenic referring to the body habitus of a patient who is strong and active; average body habitus.
stochastic effects effects that occur by chance and which may occur without a threshold level of radiation dose. Probability of effect is proportional to the dose and whose severity is independent of the dose.
storage phosphor also called a photostimulable phosphor plate (PSP).
straight-line portion the useful range of densities on the characteristic curve.
subject contrast the difference in x-ray photon transmission between different areas of the body. The primary controlling factor is kVp.
superconductor a material in which electrons can flow freely with no resistance when the material is cooled to an extremely low temperature.
***Systems International d'Unites* (SI)** modern form of the metric system; most widely used system of measurement. It comprises a coherent system of units of measurement built on seven base units.

T

target EI (EI_T) target exposure index value for each radiographic exam.
technical factors the kVp and mA as selected for a given radiographic examination.
10-day rule length of time used to determine possibility of pregnancy.
teratogenic effects radiation effects that affect the development of the embryo or fetus.
terrestrial radiation radiation emitted from deposits of uranium, thorium, and other radionuclides in the earth.
tesla (T) the SI unit for magnetism.
thermionic emission the emission of electrons by heating of the filament in the cathode.
thermoluminescent dosimeter (TLD) device that measures the emission of light by a thermally stimulated crystal.

thin-film transistor (TFT) a photosensitive array, made up of small pixels, converts the light into electrical charges.

three-phase circuit a full rectification circuit that produces a higher average voltage with less ripple.

threshold dose dose below which a person has a negligible chance of sustaining specific biologic damage or dose at which response to increasing x-ray intensity first occurs.

time of occupancy factor length of time that the area being protected is used.

tissue density matter per unit volume, or the compactness of the atomic particles composing the anatomic part.

toe region area of low exposure levels on a characteristic curve.

tomographic angle the total distance the tube moves during a tomographic exposure; also tomographic amplitude.

tomography a radiographic imaging technique that uses motion to demonstrate structures lying in a plane of tissue while structures above and below this plane appear blurred.

transformers electrical devices to change voltage from low to high or vice versa.

translation process of forming a protein molecule from messenger RNA.

transmission passage of an x-ray beam through an anatomical part with no interaction with atomic structures.

transport racks part of the automatic processing transport system consisting of three rollers located at the bottom of the processing tank that move the film through the tank.

transport system part of the automatic processor designed to move the film through developer, fixer, wash, and dryer sections.

U

ultra density optical (UDO) disk an optical disc format designed for high-density storage of high-definition video and data.

uncontrolled area area occupied by anyone; the maximum exposure rate allowed in this area is based on the recommended dose limit for the public.

undifferentiated cells immature or nonspecialized cell.

use factor proportional amount of time during which the x-ray beam is energized or directed toward a particular barrier.

V

values of interest (VOI) established values within histogram models that determine what part of the data set should be incorporated into the displayed image.

variable Vp-fixed mAs technique chart a type of exposure technique chart that changes the kVp for changes in part thickness.

vignetting the reduction of brightness at the periphery of an image.

voltage a measure of electrical force or pressure.

volts the unit of potential difference.

voluntary motion motion that can be controlled by the patient.

voxel volume element; determined by the size of the pixel and the thickness of the slice, the actual small amount of tissue that will be represented by one pixel.

W

wavelength the distance between adjacent peaks or adjacent valleys of a wave.

window level location on a digital image number scale at which the levels of grays are assigned; regulates the optical density of the displayed image and identifies the type of tissue to be imaged.

window width specific number of gray levels or digital image numbers assigned to an image; determines the gray scale rendition of the imaged tissue and the image contrast.

workload product of the maximum mA and the number of x-ray examinations performed per week. Expressed in milliamperes per minute per week (mA/min/wk).

X

x-ray beam quality a measurement of the penetrating ability of the x-ray beam.

x-ray beam quantity a measurement of the number of x-ray photons in the useful beam.

Index

Page numbers followed by *f* refers to figures and t refers to tables, respectively

Q

R

S